QUANTITATIVE CORONARY AND LEFT VENTRICULAR CINEANGIOGRAPHY

DEVELOPMENTS IN CARDIOVASCULAR MEDICINE

QUANTITATIVE CORONARY AND LEFT VENTRICULAR CINEANGIOGRAPHY

Methodology and Clinical Applications

by

J.H.C. REIBER, Ph.D.
P.W. SERRUYS, M.D.
C.J. SLAGER, M.Sc.

Department of Cardiology (Chief: P.G. Hugenholtz, M.D., F.A.C.C.)
Thoraxcenter, Erasmus University, and University Hospital Dijkzigt
Rotterdam, The Netherlands

1986 **MARTINUS NIJHOFF PUBLISHERS**
a member of the KLUWER ACADEMIC PUBLISHERS GROUP
BOSTON / DORDRECHT / LANCASTER

Distributors

for the United States and Canada: Kluwer Academic Publishers, 190 Old Derby Street, Hingham, MA 02043, USA
for the UK and Ireland: Kluwer Academic Publishers, MTP Press Limited, Falcon House, Queen Square, Lancaster LA1 1RN, UK
for all other countries: Kluwer Academic Publishers Group, Distribution Center, P.O. Box 322, 3300 AH Dordrecht, The Netherlands

Library of Congress Cataloging in Publication Data

```
Reiber, J. H. C. (Johan H. C.)
   Quantitative coronary and left ventricular
cineangiography.

   (Developments in cardiovascular medicine)
   Includes bibliographies and index.
   1. Cineangiography.  2. Coronary heart disease--
Diagnosis.  3. Heart--Diseases--Diagnosis.  I. Serruys,
P. W.  II. Slager, C. J.  III. Title.  IV. Series.
[DNLM: 1. Angiocardiography.  2. Cineangiography.
3. Heart Ventricle--radiography.  W1 DE997VME /
WG 141 R347g]
RC683.5.C54R45  1985      616.1'207572      85-21450
```

ISBN-13: 978-94-010-8382-9   e-ISBN_13: 978-94-010-8382-9
DOI: 10.1007/978-94-009-4239-4

Copyright

To Marjan Reiber

Danielle Serruys
and Michael, Gregory and Olivia

Jany Slager
and Janneke, Jos, Lenette, Koos and David

Table of contents

PART TWO – CLINICAL APPLICATIONS

Introduction

In recent years there has been an increasing interest in quantitative analysis of coronary cineangiograms and already for a longer time of left ventricular cineangiograms. The need for quantitation of coronary arterial dimensions has been stimulated by the introduction of new therapeutic procedures in the catheterization laboratory, such as the balloon dilatation technique (PTCA) and thrombolytic therapy, by the need to study the vasoactive responses of pharmaceutical agents, and also by the desire to study the progressive nature of coronary artery disease with the ultimate goal to find ways to bring a halt to the progression of coronary atherosclerosis or even achieve regression of the disease. Parallel with these clinical developments, rapid technical developments in computer architectures and semiconductor memories have made it possible to digitize and store cineframes or selected portions thereof in image processors and to analyze these pictorial data quantitatively at affordable prices.

More than 15 years of research have been directed by various groups towards the semi- or fully-automated delineation of the left ventricular boundaries on a frame-to-frame basis. Yet not a single system with fully-automated capability is commercially available. In the mean time many different left ventricular wall motion models have been developed, again with little consensus on which model is to be preferred as no golden standard exists.

Since the early nineteen seventies our department has been heavily involved in the development of image processing techniques for the semi- or fully-automated analysis of cineangiograms, to derive new, clinically relevant, parameters from these images; these techniques have been validated extensively and applied to clinical studies. This book describes our approaches and results in these areas. In addition, extensive overviews of the work of others have been included. Twelve chapters describe the various methodologies, followed by eleven chapters with clinical applications.

In the first chapter an extensive overview is presented of left ventricular and coronary angiographic procedures in terms of techniques, applications and their limitations. In the second chapter, the X-ray image forming process is described and technical information about the different components of the X-ray system is provided. In Chapter III the computer-based Cardiovascular Angiography Analysis System (CAAS) is described in detail, followed by a description of the left ventricular angioprocessing system, the Contouromat, in Chapter IV. The validations of these techniques are described in Chapter V. In the following chapters VI through IX, technical applications and new developments on the CAAS are presented, such as the definitions of selection criteria for coronary contrast catheters (Ch. VI), the densitometric analysis of coronary obstructions (Ch. VII), the three-dimensional reconstruction of coronary arterial segments from two projections (Ch. VIII) and the structural analysis of the entire coronary arterial tree (Ch. IX).

An extensive methodological review of existing quantification systems for coronary and left ventricular cineangiograms is presented in Chapter X. The basic principles of a new endocardial landmark motion model for left ventricular function are described in Ch. XI. Finally, in Chapter XII the cardiovascular database and coronary reporting system are described; all the database parameters that may be stored and retrieved are defined in the Appendix.

All clinical applications are presented in the second part of this book. In Chapter XIII the influence of the intracoronary administration of a calcium-antagonist (nifedipine) on left ventricular function, coronary vasomotility and myocardial oxygen consumption is described. The preliminary results of the Thoraxcenter randomized trial on intracoronary thrombolytic therapy and its influence on left ventricular function are presented in Chapter XIV. Various aspects of the percutaneous transluminal coronary angioplasty (PTCA) procedure are investigated and discussed, such as left ventricular chamber stiffness (Ch. XV), the question whether PTCA is mandatory after successful thrombolysis (Ch. XVI), diameter versus densitometric area measurements of coronary obstructions pre- and post-PTCA (Ch. XVII), and finally, left ventricular performance, regional blood flow, wall motion and lactate metabolism during PTCA (Ch. XVIII). Various aspects of coronary vasomotor tone are presented in chapters XIX (the role of vascular wall thickening) and XX (the effect of the cold pressor test on coronary dimensions). The functional significance of coronary obstructions in terms of transstenotic pressure gradients and defect sizes in exercise/redistribution thallium-201 scintigraphy is presented in Chapter XXI, while the changes in coronary arterial dimensions as related to lipid metabolism obtained in the Leiden Diet Intervention Trial are presented in Chapter XXII. Finally, the asynchrony in regional filling dynamics as a consequence of uncoordinated segmental contraction during transluminal coronary occlusion is described in Chapter XXIII.

Thus, this book should be of interest to all researchers and clinicians who are involved in cardiac catheterization procedures and/or the interpretation of the resulting images, either methodologically or clinically. Many of the techniques developed presently, will be applied routinely in the near future.

Many colleagues and friends have contributed in one way or the other to one or more chapters. We would like to mention (per group in alphabetical order): from the laboratory for clinical and experimental image processing: Frederik Booman, M.Sc., Ingrid P.M. Broeders, Pauli M. van Eldik-Helleman, Robert J.N. Kalberg, M.Sc., Cornelis J. Kooijman, M.Sc., Jan van Ommeren, M.Sc., Edwin J.B. van Ree, B.Sc., and Johan H.C. Schuurbiers, B.Sc.; from the catheterization laboratory: Ad den Boer, B.Sc., Marcel van den Brand, M.D., Pim J. de Feyter, M.D., Ton E.H. Hooghoudt, M.D., Juan Planellas, M.D., Vasco Ribeiro, M.D., Harry Suryapranata, M.D., and William Wijns, M.D.; from the information theory group of the Delft University of Technology: Jan J. Gerbrands, M.Sc., and the following colleagues, at that time students, who wrote their master of science theses on a particular part of the entire project: Bob H.D. van den Elskamp, M.Sc., Mark M. ter Kuile, M.Sc., M.BA; Gabe Langhout, M.Sc., Robert-Jan van Meenen, M.Sc., Ruud T. Rademaker, M.Sc., Bas Scholts, M.Sc., Cees Slump, Ph.D., Hong Sie Tan, M.Sc., and Gert-Jan Troost, M.Sc.; from the coronary care unit and nuclear cardiology laboratory: Maarten L. Simoons, M.D., Ph.D.; from the laboratory for clinical and experimental information processing: Ron van Domburg, M.Sc., Simon H. Meij, M.Sc., and Cees Zeelenberg, M.Sc.; from the laboratory of biomechanics: Ronald W. Brower, Ph.D. and Harold J. ten Katen, B.Sc.; from the Eye Hospital in Rotterdam: Guus V.M. Schulte, M.D. (Ch. IX); and our foreign friends Joerg Grimm, Ph.D., Otto M. Hess, M.D., and Hans P. Krayenbuehl, M.D., F.A.C.C. (Ch. XV) from the Cardiology Division, University Hospital in Zürich, Switzerland, and Michel E. Bertrand, M.D., and Jean Marc Lablanche (Ch. XIX) from the Cardiology Division, University of Lille, France.

We wish to thank Jaap Deckers, M.D., of the Thoraxcenter for his redaction of the special topic on the cold pressor test (Ch. XX), Jacques D. Barth, M.D., the Thoraxcenter, Hans Jansen, Ph.D., the Departments of Internal Medicine III and Biochemistry, Jan C. Birkenhäger, M.D., the Department of Internal Medicine III, all from the Erasmus University and University Hospital Dijkzigt, Rotterdam, and Alexander C. Arntzenius, M.D., the Department of Cardiology, University Hospital Leiden, the Netherlands, for their redaction and contributions to Chapter XXII: Quantitative coronary angiography in a lipid intervention study, and Federico Piscione, M.D. from the Clinica Medica I, 2nd Medical School, Napoli, Italy, who studied and described regional left ventricular filling dynamics during PTCA (Ch. XXIII) during his one year stay at the Thoraxcenter.

We also wish to acknowledge our photographer Jan Tuin, who has spent so many hours over the years in providing us with diapositives, films and prints. We are particularly grateful to our secretaries Ria Kanters-Stam and Saskia Spierdijk, who have typed and edited so many versions of the various chapters.

This work would not have been possible without the continuing support from Paul G. Hugenholtz, M.D., F.A.C.C., Chief of the Department of Cardiology, Geert T. Meester, M.D., Ph.D., Professor of Clinical Pathophysiology of the

Cardiovascular System and Nicolaas Bom, Ph. D., Head of the Bio-Engineering Group, Thoraxcenter. Finally, we are indebted to the Dutch Heart Foundation, which has supported the developments and clinical applications of the quantitative analysis of the coronary arteries from July 1978 until September 1984 under grants 77.084, 79.109 and 80.129.

Part One Methodology

I. Left ventricular and coronary cineangiography; overview of techniques, applications and limitations

Introduction

Left ventricular and coronary cineangiography are regarded as the definite procedures for the confirmation of cardiac disease. These invasive procedures produce high resolution, dynamic images of the left ventricle and the coronary arteries, respectively. The left ventricular angiograms may provide the clinician with detailed information about left ventricular anatomy, wall motion abnormalities and allow the computation of left ventricular volume and of global and regional ejection fraction. Likewise, the coronary cineangiograms allow the assessment of the presence and severity of coronary artery disease. In routine clinical practice, the angiographic data are still interpreted visually, which results in significant inter- and intraobserver variations. Moreover, the abnormalities as judged by the clinician can only be expressed in relative terms. It was recognized at an early stage, that quantitation of such images would be extremely desirable for a number of reasons: (1) availability of objective measurements; (2) communication between and comparison of results from different centers would be greatly facilitated; and (3) the state of disease of a given patient would be much better characterized. To obtain such objective measurements from the angiograms, many groups have been active over the last fifteen years in the development of methods for the quantitative analysis of the cineangiograms. These efforts have first been directed towards manual, semi- and fully-automated procedures for the outlining of the left ventricular boundaries and the subsequent analysis of these boundaries in terms of left ventricular volume, global and regional ejection fraction, as well as of regional wall motion. At a later point in time, methods for semi- or fully-automated boundary definition of the coronary arteries were being developed.

Use of such a system with semi- or fully-automated edge detection schemes have mainly been limited to research studies in the institutes where these were developed. Some of the reasons which have prevented widespread use of these techniques are: (1) quantitative measurements were hardly incorporated in the routine clinical management of the patients; (2) in general, relatively long processing times of the analysis procedures; (3) success rate of the quantitative procedures too low for routine use; (4) high cost of the computer equipment required; and (5) little interest from the manufacturers of X-ray systems and/or of computer systems for catheterization laboratories to invest money in these developments.

Since 1970 our group has been involved in the development of methodologies for quantitative analysis of left ventricular cineangiograms and since 1976 of coronary cineangiograms. It is the purpose of this book to describe such techniques developed and implemented in our institute and to present clinical applications. All the data will be based on the analysis of the standard 35 mm cinefilm, which has continued to be the medium of choice for registration of left ventricular and coronary angiograms for the following reasons: (1) its inherently high resolution, (2) relatively low cost of the medium; (3) readily accessible in a clinical environment; and (4) very practical to store and to send to other centers.

However, over the last few years we have seen very rapid changes in computer technology with micro- and miniprocessors now widely available at affordable and ever decreasing prices with simultaneously increases in computer power. Similar developments can be seen in the semiconductor memories with increasing memory sizes per single chip. Thanks to these developments digital cardiovascular imaging systems could be introduced a number of years ago which now enjoy a great interest from the clinical community. State-of-the-art systems allow on-line acquisition of left ventricular and coronary angiograms at matrix size of 512×512 pixels at a maximal rate of 30 frames per second. Further developments are towards 1024×1024 matrix size at 30 fr/s. At present, availability of application software packages on these systems is limited. Most of the basic principles of these analysis procedures are similar to those developed for cinefilm analysis.

For those studies requiring the highest spatial and time resolution, cinefilm remains the medium of choice. Thanks to these same hardware developments, special computer-based analysis systems are now becoming commercially available, an example of which is presented in Chapter III. Since these systems possess the computer power to allow quantitative analysis of angiograms, widespread use of these techniques may be anticipated.

In this introductory chapter a brief historic overview of the basic angiographic procedures will be given, to begin with for the left ventricular cineangiograms. The development of various clinically relevant left ventricular parameters, such as cardiac volume, regional wall motion and various wall motion models will be described. The second part of this chapter is devoted to the coronary cineangiography. Following a brief historic overview of the technique, the problems of inter- and intraobserver variations in the visual interpretation will be discussed, as well as the number of projections required and further limitations in the assessment of the severity of a coronary lesion. Although it is now possible to determine with high accuracy the dimensions of coronary arterial segments, it is still very difficult to determine the physiologic significance of a coronary obstruction. An extensive overview on the physiologic significance of a coronary obstruction, the hemodynamic aspects as well as the discrepancies between relative obstruction measures and its functional significance will be presented. Finally, indirect approaches towards the assessment of the functional significance of a coronary obstruction will be described.

Left ventricular cineangiography

Forssman showed in 1929 that a catheter could be introduced in the human heart without any harm [1]. Cournand developed heart catheterization to a clinical useful technique, which was used to determine intracardiac pressures, shunts and valve gradients in congenital and acquired heart disease [2–4]. In 1937 Castellanos visualized the cardiac chambers of children by rapid injection of a radiopaque substance in a peripheral vein [5]. Robb and Steinberg applied the method to adults, but dilution of the contrast medium during its long travel from the antecubital vein to the heart made the quality of these angiocardiograms in most cases very poor [6]. In 1947 Chavez solved this problem by putting 'the opaque substance in the place where it is needed' [7]. He introduced a 12–14 F rubber catheter through the external jugular vein into the right atrium or ventricle and injected 50–90 ml of a 70 percent solution of diodrast in 0.75–1.0 second. Injection of contrast in the cardiovascular system was shown to be relatively safe and to offer invaluable information about cardiac function. A detailed analysis of volume change and motion pattern of the cardiac chambers was made possible by the introduction of cinefluorography by Rushmer [8–10]. After injection of 25 ml of diodrast into the superior caval or right jugular vein of dogs, the circulation of the opacified blood was documented on 16 or 35 mm cinefilm. Examination of the motion picture films led to some interesting conclusions:
– the ventricles fill more rapidly than they empty,
– ventricular emptying is not complete; at end systole about one-third of the diastolic volume remains in the ventricle,
– the left ventricular volume is reduced during systole by reduction in diameter rather than by long axis shortening,
– wall thickness of both ventricles increases during systole.
Initially angiocardiography was applied on a small scale to patients with congenital and acquired valvular heart disease. However, after the introduction of selective coronary arteriography [11–13] and of coronary bypass surgery [14], an explosive growth of the number of performed studies took place. As there appeared to be a close relation between left ventricular function and the results of medical and surgical therapy in patients with heart disease [15–17], the need for quantification of left ventricular volume and wall motion was evident. Besides that, it was clearly demonstrated that the visual interpretation of left ventricular

wall motion is hampered by considerable inter- and intraobserver variations [18–20]. Quantitative angiocardiography has offered significant contributions to the assessment of ventricular size and function in patients with both coronary and valvular heart disease [21–27]. Various manual, semi- and fully-automated procedures for the definition of the left ventricular boundaries from the angiograms have been developed; an overview of these systems is given in Chapter X.

Cardiac volume

The complex configuration of the left ventricle in man precludes an accurate computation of ventricular volume or dimensions from X-ray ventriculograms without simplifying assumptions. Fortunately, stroke volume calculated from the measurement of end-diastolic and end-systolic volumes was shown to correlate well with stroke volume determined with the classic cardiac output techniques [28, 29].

Many methods have been proposed for the measurement of left ventricular volume from single or biplane views [30–32], but only few acquired general acceptance. Biplane methods have been demonstrated to be more accurate than single plane techniques from studies of models and man [33, 34]. Single plane X-ray techniques, however, have been used most frequently for human studies due to high cost and complexity of biplane equipment and the tedium associated with calculations from the resulting films, although computer-assisted methods have facilitated many of these latter difficulties. Single plane cine techniques also reduce the overall X-ray exposure to the patient and personnel.

For biplane films, the measurements can be made, either assuming that the left ventricle is ellipsoid [35–37], or that its cross-sectional outline is elliptical or circular [38]. Chapman's method divides the ventricle into thin slices [38]. The volume of each slice is computed following the formula:
$V = \pi \cdot h \cdot (A \cdot B) / 4$, where V is the volume of the slice in cm^3, h is the height of the slice, A is the axis in one view and B the axis in the perpendicular view at the same level (all in cm). Left ventricular volume is found by summing up the volumes of all segments. This method gives a relatively accurate approximation of actual volume, but comprises a great amount of calculations requiring computer facilities [39].

The basic assumption with single-plane methods is that the nonvisualized minor axis approximates the measured minor axis, so that the left ventricle is considered, in essence, a solid of revolution. Three methods have been proposed by Dodge and Sandler [33, 36, 40], Green et al. [41] and Snow et al. [42]. The first was initially applied to the AP-projection, the latter two to the RAO-projection. Dodge's area-length method [35], based on the assumption that the left ventricular cavity can be represented by an ellipsoid, is widely used. Though initially developed for biplane angiocardiograms, the method appeared also to be applicable to single plane films [40], in the antero-posterior and with higher accuracy in the right anterior oblique projection [43].

Due to the divergence of the X-ray beam, correction factors must be introduced in the applied formula's to correct for the X-ray magnification. Despite these corrections, the angiographic technique still tends to overestimate actual volume of the left ventricle, since papillary muscles and trabeculae displace contrast material within the cavity. Most laboratories, therefore, have derived regression equations from postmortem hearts injected with known amounts of contrast material and comparing the known volume with the calculated angiographic volume [30, 35, 41, 43–48]. Chatelain et al. described a method for in vivo determination of left and right ventricular volume correction factors, provided cardiac output can be measured without bias (e.g. from the cardiogreen cardiac output and heart rate) and first estimates of ventricular volumes are available [49]. In general, one single correction factor has been used for all cardiac phases and spatial positions of the heart. Lange et al. have clearly demonstrated that such correction factor is heavily dependent on the phase in the cardiac cycle and the spatial orientation [34]. They conclude, that on the basis of a given routine clinical angiocardiogram left ventricular volume can be estimated most exactly if the spatial position of the ventricle and the cardiac phase are determined, so that the appropriate correction factor can be applied. Moreover, a biplane method is preferable to a single plane one. The multiple slices and the area-length methods give equally good results, biplane as well as single plane.

The mechanical alterations of left ventricular function in heart disease are clearly visualized by a loop describing the relation between instantaneous left ventricular volume and pressure [44, 50]. The pressure-volume diagram reflects the phases of the cardiac cycle beginning at end-diastole and followed by iso-volumic contraction, systolic emptying, isovolumic relaxation and diastolic filling. Total mechanical work performed by the ventricle during a cardiac cycle, which is equal to the product of stroke volume and mean systolic pressure, is determined by planimetry of the area within and below this pressure-volume loop. To construct such a loop, frame-by-frame analysis of one or more cardiac cycles is essential, a time consuming and tedious activity, if performed manually. Such a procedure can be facilitated with automated left ventricular endocardial contour detection techniques.

Regional wall motion

The interest in regional wall motion and its hemodynamic significance was greatly stimulated by the work of Herman et al. [51, 52], who defined four types of local wall motion disturbance or 'asynergy':
– akinesis, or total lack of motion of a part of the left ventricular wall,
– asyneresis, or diminished motion of a part of the wall,

– dyskinesis, or systolic paradoxical motion,
– asynchrony, or a disturbed temporal pattern of contraction.
A rather close relationship between electrocardiographic findings, the angiographic site of coronary stenosis and regional wall motion abnormalities was
shown [53], although adequate collateral circulation may preserve a normal or
nearly normal contraction pattern in areas perfused by a severely narrowed
coronary artery [54], which explains why ventricular asynergy is not invariably
present at rest in patients with coronary artery disease. In some cases a stress such
as rapid atrial pacing [55, 56] may disrupt the balance between oxygen delivery
and metabolic demand, and consequently induce asynergy. Akinesis and dyskinesis are generally recognized by gross inspection of the ventriculogram, but
asyneresis and especially temporal disturbances of contraction require a detailed
and quantitative analysis. Evaluation of left ventricular wall motion is commonly
assessed from single or biplane angiograms in the RAO, LAO or in hemi-axial
projections. Bonzel et al. have demonstrated that the RAO-view is the most
sensitive view for the detection of hypokinetic walls [57].

With digital radiographic systems now increasingly becoming available,
Fourier techniques have been applied for the assessment of regional wall motion
from intravenously administered contrast administrations [58]. The phase image
reflects the synchronization of ventricular contraction and relaxation, whereas
the amplitude image reflects the extent of contraction. These techniques have
been adopted from the gated blood pool analysis procedures in nuclear cardiology [59].

Wall motion models

To perform an accurate description of wall motion, ideally, specific points along
the endocardial surface should be tracked. The only way to reach this goal is
implantation of endocardial metal markers, as was performed in animals [60–64],
but is impractical in humans. Epicardial clips [65–67] and midwall markers [68–
70] have contributed considerably to the understanding of myocardial dynamics,
but provide only remote information on actual endocardial motion.

Many wall motion models have been proposed to proximate actual endocardial
motion from the endocardial outlines [51, 71–76]. The various geometric models,
which were developed with the purpose to judge whether regional endocardial
motion is normal or abnormal, may be discussed on the basis of two items: the
reference system and the coordinate system.

Left ventricular reference systems
Several reference methods have been proposed in an attempt to separate regional
left ventricular wall motion from motion of the heart as a whole, caused by twist,
translation and rotation. Basically, two methods can be distinguished: (1) internal

reference system, or (2) external reference system. With the internal reference system, various methods have been proposed for the realignment of the end-diastolic and subsequent contours based on specific anatomical points of recognition of the heart such as (Fig. I.1):

(a) In the ED frame an indexing line is defined from the apex bisecting the ventricular area. In each subsequent frame the long axis was defined by the intersection of this indexing line with the aortic valve plane and the apex position. Subsequently, this new long axis is rotated such that it aligns with the ED indexing line [71]

(b) the contours are translated such that the midaortic points coincide [74]

(c) the contours are superimposed on the basis of the following fixed points:

(1) the center of gravity; and (2) the center of the aortic root [77].

With the external reference systems, the end-diastolic and end-systolic contours are allowed to move independently, that is no alignments take place [51, 72, 78–80]. However, modifications to the external reference system method have been proposed by a number of investigators.

Chaitman et al. have presented a method which utilizes two external markers (lead impregnated letters taped to the image intensifier) and the diaphragm as an

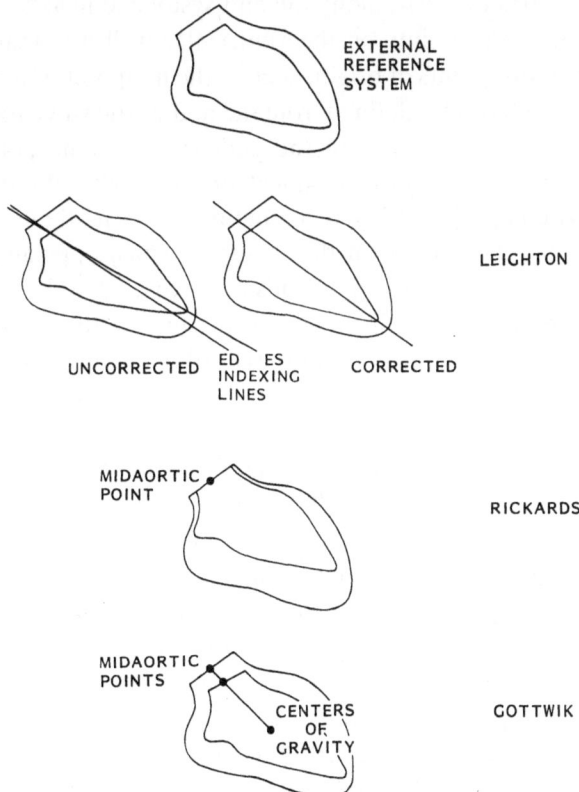

Fig. I.1. Overview of the various left ventricular reference systems.

internal marker [73]. If the diaphragm has moved over a cardiac cycle, for example due to patient and/or respiratory movement, this method cannot be used. Sasayama et al. superimpose sequential ventricular silhouettes on the end-diastolic frame by using two external reference markers [81]. A similar approach has been described by Lorente et al., who use two fixed external X-ray beam markers [82].

Left ventricular coordinate systems
After a particular reference system has been chosen, a coordinate system must be defined to assess left ventricular wall motion. Basically, one of three different coordinate systems are used most frequently:
- Rectangular coordinates: points on the wall are assumed to move in a direction perpendicular to a ventricular long axis along lines termed hemiaxes. The methods described by Herman et al., using hemiaxes perpendicular to a long axis defined from midaortic valve to apex at 25% intervals along the long axis [51] and Leighton et al. [71] are examples of such a method. Following Leighton's method, the origin of the rectangular coordinate system was defined for each frame at the intersection of the ED indexing line with the aortic valve plane of that particular frame. Shortening is measured along perpendiculars to the long axis at 20% intervals along the end-systolic long axis.
- Polar coordinates: the points on the ventricular wall are assumed to move towards one or more points of origin, such as the midpoint of the left ventricular long axis on each frame, defined from the mid-aortic valve to the apex [72], the geometric center of gravity of the end-systolic frame [74, 77], a point defined on the end-systolic aortic to apical long axis, 69% of the distance from the lateral aortic edge [78, 83, 84], or defined by a mathematical function, describing the x-y coordinates of the points to which opposing anterior and posterior endocardial boundary positions move [64, 79, 85].
- Centerline method: a centerline was constructed by the computer midway between the ED and ES contours and 100 chords were drawn perpendicular to this centerline, extending from the ED to the ES contour [80, 86].

Brower and Meester have studied the correlation between neighboring segments in regional wall motion studies using both a rectangular and a polar coordinate system to determine the required spatial resolution between segments [87]. They concluded that a total of 18 myocardial segments are required. A spatial resolution of 7.7 deg at the apex and 22 deg in the anterior and diaphragmatic regions was recommended. In addition to methods which are based on the motion of specific points along the endocardial left ventricular boundary, area-based methods have been developed. For example, Lorente et al. divide the end-diastolic and end-systolic outlines into e.g. 20 equal length segments [82]. An equal number of area segments are defined, with the areas bounded by the ED and ES contours and the straight lines connecting corresponding ED and ES contour points. For each segment, the segmental area ejection fraction index may be computed.

Validation studies various left ventricular wall motion models

Brower [88] compared six methods [51, 71–74, 89] to determine regional shortening from cine ventriculograms and concluded that no method proves to be ideal, as the majority of the methods shows a poor correlation with visual observation of regional wall motion. Chaitman's method [73] was considered unsatisfactory because of nonphysiological values for segmental wall motion in normals, while the other five methods were liable to false positive and false negative findings in severe akinesis. On the other hand, Chaitman's method yielded a 100% score for the detection of asynergy. Overall, the least errors occurred in the methods proposed by Leighton et al. [71] and Hernandex et al. [89], which align the major axes.

Daughters et al. [90] compared the following five techniques for left ventricular wall motion assessment: *external reference systems*: (1) polar coordinates with respect to 69% point on end-systolic long axis [78]; (2) rectangular coordinates perpendicular to ED and ES long axes [51]; (3) polar coordinates with respect to midpoint of long axes in each frame [72]; *realigned systems*: (4) contours superimposed around midaortic point, polar coordinates with respect to ES center of area [74]; (5) ED indexing line bisecting LV area and ES long axis rotated to align with ED indexing line and rectangular coordinates [71]. Based on a maximum number of correctly classified ventriculograms, they concluded that the first method [78] proved best in the clinical setting.

To filter out high-frequency noise components of wall motion, shortening fractions should not be computed from single points on the end-diastolic and end-systolic contours, but rather area shrinkage fractions of pie-shaped slices should be used [91]. Daughters et al. demonstrated that no improvement in the ability to detect wall motion abnormalities can be achieved by analyzing more than about 5 segments of the ventricular wall: two each on the anterior and inferior walls, and one apical segment [91].

Although most methods are based on the analysis of only two frames over a cardiac cycle, the end-diastolic and end-systolic frames, it has been shown that important information on regional left ventricular wall motion may be lost by such approach [92]. This has increasingly led to approaches for analysis of successive frames over a cardiac cycle, which can be facilitated by automated border detection techniques.

It has been demonstrated by Sheehan et al., that the beat-to-beat, intraobserver, and interobserver variabilities in the quantitative assessment of regional wall motion from manually traced LV boundaries, average 14%, 14% and 17%, respectively [93]. Study-to-study variability was significantly higher, averaging

30% of mean normal motion. Realignment to correct for cardiac rotation significantly increased variability. Gottwik et al. also concluded that a radial method in
combination with external coordinates is the most sensitive procedure to localize
regional dysfunction on the ventriculogram [77].

Clayton et al. also found significant patient-to-patient, region-to-region, beat-
to-beat, and study-to-study variability in the assessment of left ventricular wall
motion using an external reference system with polar coordinates [94]. This
variability appeared to be more substantial in diseased than normal ventricles. In
addition to the variabilities of the ventricle itself, interobserver error is also a
substantial factor in regional measurements [95].

Sheehan et al. concluded from their study that rectangular and centerline
methods are comparable, and identify abnormal wall motion better than the
radial method, all using external reference systems [86]. The centerline method
can measure motion near the apex and aortic valve, regions not accessible by the
rectangular method, and it does not use the apex as a landmark. On the other
hand, comparison of motion measured by the centerline method and normalized
by the length of the ED perimeter with motion measured by rectangular and
radial methods yields similar results.

From the above it will be clear that the assessment of left ventricular wall
motion has not been standardized. There are many wall motion models available,
either based on internal or external reference systems, with rectangular or polar
coordinate systems or modifications thereof, and each method has its own
advantages and disadvantages. There does not appear to be a consensus on a
particular model. Besides that, the reproducibility of the analysis has been
hampered by inter- and intraobserver variabilities in the manual tracing of these
left ventricular outlines. Such variabilities could be reduced if automated contour
detection techniques for the left ventricular outline were available.

Since the early 1970's our group has been involved in the development of a
system for semi- or fully automated analysis of left ventricular cineframes, that
would fulfill the following goals: (1) user-interactive, automated contour detection of the left ventricular outline with a clinically accepted speed of processing;
(2) a high success score of the contour detection such that it would be acceptable
on a routine basis; (3) development of a wall motion model based on physiological principles. The implementation of this system is described in detail in Chapter
IV, its validation in Chapter V and the derived model for LV wall motion in
Chapter XI.

Coronary cineangiography

Todate, selective coronary cineangiography has remained the only technique
available for the visualization of the coronary arterial system with such image
contrast and resolution that the presence and severity of coronary atherosclerosis

can be determined with sufficient accuracy. The basic technique was introduced in 1959 by Sones et al., who approached the right and left coronary arteries from the right brachial artery with a catheter designed by himself [96, 97]. A few years later, in 1962, Ricketts et al. introduced the percutaneous transfemoral technique with specially preshaped catheters [12]. Since then various authors have described the feasibility of these procedures for routine clinical studies, with further developments particularly directed towards the design of preshaped catheters [13, 98–103].

The femoral artery approach with preshaped catheters has many proponents for a number of reasons, such as: (1) the great simplicity of the procedure and the rapidity of execution; (2) the improvement in the quality of the angiographic documents through highly selective coronary artery injections [104]; and (3) the possibility of repeat investigations, since no arterial cutdown is necessary. However, experience with both techniques is useful, since peripheral arterial anatomy occasionally prevents the use of one technique or the other.

Adams et al. performed in 1970 and 1971 a US nationwide survey including 173 hospitals and a total of 46,904 coronary arteriograms on the complications of coronary arteriography [105]. They arrived at three conclusions. First, in the United States at that time, on the average, the risk of death, myocardial infarction, and cerebral embolus during or following coronary arteriography was greater with the transfemoral than with the transbrachial technique. Second, the risk of thrombosis at the site of catheter entry and contrast agent reaction during or following coronary arteriography was greater with the brachial technique. And third, the risk of death or serious nonlethal complications (myocardial infarction and cerebral embolus) was significantly enhanced in institutions performing a relatively small number of examinations whether the femoral or the brachial technique was employed. The mortality related to the technique should be maintained well below 0.1 percent. It has been stated that in institutions where the mortality exceeds 0.1 percent, the entire coronary arteriography program should be reevaluated and that in those where the rate exceeds 0.3 percent these studies should be discontinued.

From a study involving 5250 patients who underwent coronary arteriography by the percutaneous femoral technique, Bourassa et al. concluded in 1976 that in patients with normal coronary arteries, no fatal or serious nonfatal complications occurred [104]. However, major risk was proportional to the severity of disease in the left coronary system.

Gensini reported from a study involving 4000 patients, who were catheterized by the percutaneous femoral technique, an incidence of 1 death ($= 0.025\%$; presence of 99% obstruction of main left coronary artery confirmed at autopsy), 1 patient with myocardial infarction, 30 patients ($= 0.75\%$) with ventricular fibrillation and 40 patients ($= 0.1\%$) with cardiac arrest [106].

Inter- and intraobserver variations in visual interpretation

Conventional visual evaluation of the severity of coronary obstructions from the 35 mm cinefilm has been hampered by considerably large inter- and intraobserver variations [19, 107–114]. Interobserver variability was assessed by DeRouen et al. by requesting 11 experienced cardiac angiographers to estimate the percentage diameter narrowing of the worst lesions in 10 different standard arterial segments in each of 10 angiograms [108]. Observed standard deviations for the total of 100 coronary segments ranged from 0% to 51.32%; the largest deviation was found for the distal right coronary artery (RCA). Per vessel segment the average standard deviation (taken over all 10 cases) ranged from 8.0% for the proximal RCA to 28.5% for the diagonal branch. By averaging over all 10 cases and 10 segments an overall average standard deviation of 18% was found, being a crude estimate of general variability. If two standard deviations are used to indicate the possible error in reading an obstruction, this would indicate a possible error of 36%. Similar findings for the interobserver variability have been reported by Zir et al. [19]. From these studies it became evident that in addition to the problem of visually interpreting the severity of an obstruction, in particular the lack of uniformity in the designation of the location of lesions was one particular cause for the large interobserver variations.

These variations can be reduced by means of a consensus opinion based on several observers reading the coronary angiograms at the same time [114]. Sanmarco et al. studied the reproducibility of a consensus panel in the interpretation of coronary cineangiograms and found an overall standard deviation of the difference in panel reading of 14% [109].

Shub et al. have demonstrated that the intra- and interobserver variability varies with the severity of the stenosis [110] (Fig. I.2). For stenosis of less than 20% or more than 80% D-stenosis, the inter- and intraobserver differences were relatively small (mean differences less than 5%). For stenoses between 20 and 80%, the differences were slightly greater (mean differences 8 to 14%). The pattern of intra- and interobserver variability was similar.

The interobserver variability in the interpretation of coronary arteriograms by readers at two different clinics was determined in 870 arteriograms as part of the Coronary Artery Surgery Study (CASS) [111]. Of the seven segments studied, among the most difficult to read was the left main coronary artery, while among the easiest to read was the proximal right coronary artery. When one angiographer reads a stenosis of 50% or more in the left main, it was estimated that a second reader will report no lesion 18.6% of the time. In 94.7% of the films, the number of significantly ($\geq 70\%$ stenosis) diseased vessels was the same for both readers (72.1%) or differed by one vessel (22.6%). The reproducibility of interpretation of films of good or acceptable quality or completeness was better than the reproducibility of readings of arteriograms judged to be of poor quality or incomplete studies.

REPRODUCIBILITY OF ANGIOGRAPHIC INTERPRETATION

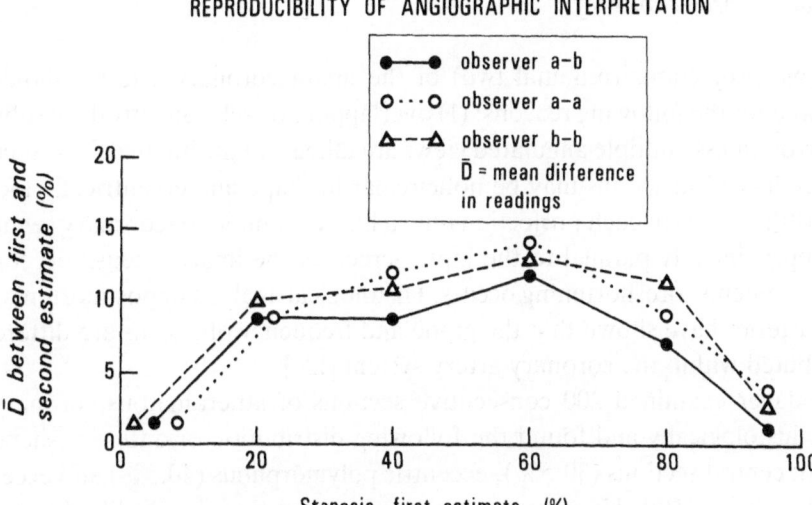

Fig. I.2. Reproducibility of angiographic interpretation. Twenty-five angiograms were randomly selected, read initially, and then reread 3 months later. Values for each stenosis were compared to assess intra-observer (a-a, b-b) and inter-observer (a-b) variability. D = mean difference in readings between first and second estimates. Lesions were grouped into following ranges of degree of stenosis (%): 0–9, 10–29, 30–49, 50–69, 70–89, 90–100, as shown on abscissa. Reproduced with permission from Shub et al. [110].

Meier et al. assessed the inter- and intraobserver variabilities in a PTCA-study, when using a calibrated magnifying glass for stenoses manually traced from a cineprojector [112]. The interobserver coefficients of variation (= standard deviation of differences between the measurements by the observers, divided by the mean value) were 7% for the one projection showing the most severe stenosis and 6.4% for the mean of three projections. The intraobserver coefficient of variation was significantly reduced from 16.0 to 10.5% by using the mean of three projections. They also made a visual assessment of the projection demonstrating the most severe stenosis and compared that to the severity of the stenosis obtained by tracing the lesions. In only 7/30 (23%) of the angiograms there was complete agreement among the three readers as to the projection demonstrating the most severe coronary stenosis before angioplasty.

Visual interpretation of left main coronary artery stenosis by three groups of experienced angiographers on a group consensus basis, demonstrated a 41% to 59% agreement on the severity of the lesion, with 80% agreement on whether the lesion was greater or less than 50% [113]. The severity of the lesion, its location, or presence of ectasia or calcium did not effect the discrepancy rate, whereas segments that were unusually short, diffusely diseased, or obscured by overlapping vessels were especially difficult to interpret.

Number of projections

Multiple projections (minimal two) of the major coronary arteries should be acquired for the following reasons: (1) overlapping vessels can introduce substantial error unless multiple angulated views are taken; (2) the luminal cross sections of coronary obstructions may be noncircular in shape and eccentrically located [115–119]; and (3) in each projection only a limited number of coronary segments are approximately parallel to the input screen of the image intensifier; for the other segments foreshortening occurs. Histological analysis of postmortem coronary arteries have shown that the grade and frequency of lesions are differently distributed within the coronary artery system [120].

Vlodaver examined 200 consecutive sections of atheromatous coronary arteries histologically and found the following distribution of different shapes of lumen: central sections (30.5%), eccentric polymorphous (40.5%) and eccentric slit-like (29%) [116]. However, it has been argued that the slit-like lumen is a product of postmortem arterial fixation with sectioning in the unpressurized state [121, 122]. On the other hand, if the slit-like lumen is a true phenomenon, in about one-quarter (29%) of the atheromas studied, severe obstruction might yield in certain angiographic views a luminal width suggesting an unobstructive segment. Similarly, angiographic evaluation post-angioplasty might be hampered by the eccentric nature of the mechanical disruption of the intima [123–125].

Because of the complex spatial orientation of the left coronary arterial system, usually four or five projections of this system are acquired. This allows the filming of an obstruction in at least one projection en face. For the right coronary system with a much simpler configuration two, preferably orthogonal, projections suffice.

Further limitations assessment lesion severity

Aside from the problems mentioned above, there are other factors which interfere with an accurate determination of the severity of coronary obstructions. Collateral flow to an obstructed segment may influence the estimation of distal vessel size [126]. If the severity of an obstruction is expressed in terms of percentage diameter reduction with respect to a so-called normal proximal or distal segment, diffuse atherosclerosis will produce an underestimation of the obstruction (Fig. I.3). Pathological studies have shown that coronary disease is often a diffuse process, which involves the entire length of a coronary artery [121, 127, 128]. Therefore, percent stenosis is an inadequate approach to assessing the severity of coronary obstructive disease in patients with coronary atherosclerosis. Spontaneous or catheter-induced coronary spasm may exaggerate abnormalities by causing different reactions in vasomotility of normal and obstructed segments. Conversely, preferential dilatation of a nonobstructive segment with respect to

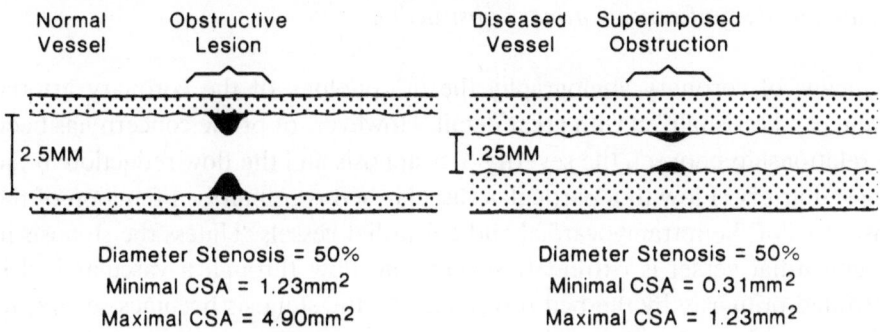

Fig. I.3. Both vessels would appear to contain 50% lesions at coronary angiography. The hemo-dynamic significance of the superimposed lesion on the right is greater than that of the lesion on the left. CSA = cross-sectional area. Reproduced with permission from Harrison et al. [175].

the obstructed segment may lead to a misleading interpretation of the otherwise beneficial effect of the vasodilator, since the absolute dimension of the obstructive lumen is actually increased. As a consequence of these problems associated with the relative measurements, the physiologic effects of the majority of coronary obstructions in terms of the reactive hyperemic response of coronary flow velocity studied with a Doppler technique at operation, could not be correlated accurately with the results from conventional angiography [129].

From the above, it is clear, that evaluation of the efficacy of modern therapeutic procedures in the catheterization laboratory, the effects of vasoactive drugs on the size of coronary arterial segments, the effects of short and long term intervention on the regression or progression of coronary artery disease as well as the examination of the correlation between severity of coronary narrowing and coronary blood flow, cardiac function and the electrocardiogram, an objective and reproducible technique for the assessment of coronary atherosclerosis is seriously needed. Such a technique should provide absolute measurements on the minimal diameter and extent of the obstructions, as well as on mean diameters of nonobstructed coronary segments, assessed from multiple projections. The increased accuracy and precision in the assessment of coronary obstructions as compared to the conventional visual interpretation, also may greatly reduce the number of subjects in intervention studies needed to obtain desired confidence levels. Ultimately, densitometric analysis will provide the most relevant information on luminal obstruction area, irrespective of the shape of the remaining cross section. Finally, developments should be directed towards the three-dimensional representation of coronary arterial segments.

Physiological significance coronary obstruction

By means of coronary angiography the morphology of the coronary arterial system can be visualized with great detail. However, of prime concern has been the relationship between the severity of a stenosis and the flow reduction in the stenosed artery. Flow to a particular vascular bed is primarily a function of the resistances of the intramyocardial and epicardial vessels. Unless the stenosis in the epicardial vessel is extremely severe, the flow through a vascular bed is controlled primarily by the bed resistance. As the stenosis becomes severe, its resistance to flow as evidenced by the pressure drop across the stenosis becomes highly significant and, in fact, can ultimately limit the flow to the peripheral bed, despite its maximal vasodilatation [130] (Fig. I.4.).

Haemodynamics coronary obstruction

In a narrowed segment, blood velocity (kinetic energy) increases and pressure (static energy) decreases in accordance with the Bernouilli principle. The reduction in luminal size at a coronary obstruction results in a pressure-drop or gradient over that obstruction influenced by four factors: entrance effects, viscous friction,

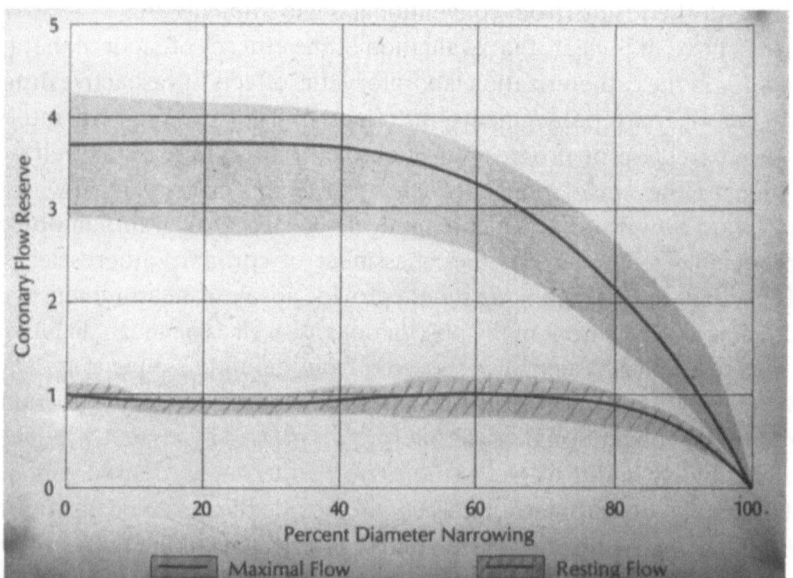

Fig. I.4. Coronary blood flow reserve in a stenotic artery is inversely proportional to the severity of stenosis. Resting coronary flow remains normal up to approximately 85% diameter narrowing, whereas maximal flow begins to fall at about 50% narrowing. With a stronger vasodilatory stimulus and a normal increase in flow of five times resting levels, even 30% to 40% narrowing may be detectable. Reproduced with permission from Kirkeeide et al. [166].

exit separation or vortex formation in the diverging portion of the stenosis and the inertia of the fluid [131–142] (Fig. I.5). Abrupt changes in entrance and exit angles are associated with substantial energy losses. These are usually the greatest at the exit, where turbulence may occur; these separation losses are a function of the blood flow velocity squared. Since myocardial oxygen delivery is proportional to coronary arterial blood flow, a high degree stenosis in a major coronary artery can cause significant ischemia under periods of increased oxygen demand (exercise etc.) by severely limiting flow, leading to either angina or myocardial infarction. Relations between this pressure loss $\triangle P$ and coronary velocity V or coronary flow Q have been derived from fluid mechanic equations for steady flow of an incompressible fluid in rigid tubes; these have been shown to apply in principle to the in vivo coronary circulation as well. An excellent study on the fluid mechanics of human coronary artery stenoses performed on 19 postmortem casts has been described by Logan [134]. The equations describing the relation between pressure loss $\triangle P$ across a stenosis and coronary flow velocity V is highly dependent on relative stenosis, as well as on absolute stenosis diameter. On the other hand, the relation between the pressure loss $\triangle P$ and coronary flow Q and thus coronary resistance defined as dP/dQ is dependent primarily on the absolute diameter of the stenotic segment, not on relative percent stenosis or diameter of the normal adjacent artery, although the latter has some minimal influence.

The problems associated with the assessment of the stenosis severity in terms of the $\triangle P$–V or the $\triangle P$–Q relation have been addressed in detail by Gould [143–145]. He concluded that the velocity equation and $\triangle P$–V relation, and therefore relative percent stenosis measurements are most appropriate to use for assessing or comparing stenosis severity in different-sized vessels normally carrying very different volume flow. The flow equation and the $\triangle P$–Q relation, and therefore absolute stenosis measurements are most appropriate to use for assessing or comparing the physiological effects of an intervention on volume flow or for

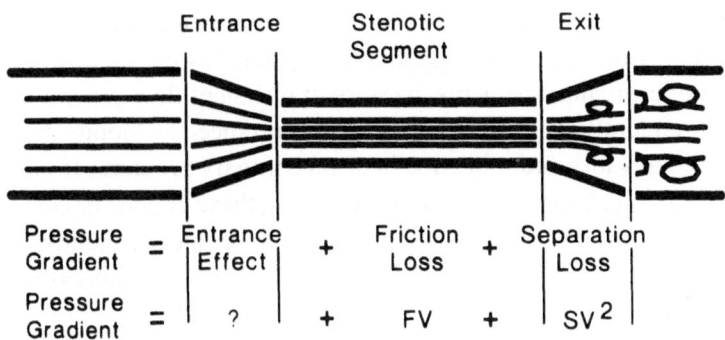

Fig. I.5. Sources of energy loss across a stenosis. The three segments of the stenosis which contribute to the pressure gradient across the lesion are entrance effects, friction losses in the stenotic segment, and separation losses at the exit of the stenosis. Reproduced with permission from Marcus et al. [141].

comparing the geometric severity before an intervention to the same stenosis in the same artery after the intervention.

Inherent in comparisons before and after an intervention is the underlying physiological question of whether coronary volume flow and pressure to the distal coronary bed are affected by that intervention. As long as the end point of the intervention is a physiological change of coronary blood flow and pressure to the distal coronary bed, the $\triangle$P–Q relation or absolute stenosis dimensions are the most useful measures of stenosis severity.

Although image processing techniques are now available to assess with high accuracy the anatomic severity to coronary obstructions, the determination whether an obstruction is hemodynamically significant remains a severe problem. In general, poor correlations have been found between percent diameter stenosis and the physiological significance of a given obstruction in patients [146]. The functional significance of a lesion depends not only on the degree of coronary narrowing, but also on its extent [147–150], the degree of asymmetry of the lesion [131, 132], the effect of multiple occlusions in series [149, 151], the shapes of the entrance and exits from the narrowed segment [152], blood viscosity and density [142], residual vasomotor tone, collateral perfusion to the given myocardial region [153], coronary bed resistance and blood flow velocity. Moreover, both active and passive increases in the severity of compliant coronary stenoses may occur [154–159]. Active changes in coronary stenosis diameter may result from either localized vasomotion superimposed on an atherosclerotic plaque or generalized changes in coronary diameter which include the stenotic segment. Passive narrowing of a compliant coronary stenosis may occur in response to a fall in coronary pressure or to any intervention which dilates the coronary arterial bed and lowers distending pressure distal to and within the stenotic segment.

It has been clearly demonstrated that the minimum cross-sectional area of an obstruction, and not percent diameter stenosis, is a major determinant of the obstruction resistance [137]. The length of a stenosis has a disproportionally small effect [134, 137, 147]; on the other hand, multiple stenoses in series have a greater effect on coronary flow than does a single stenosis of equal diameter and length [149, 160] (Fig. I.6). Kinetic energy loss across stenoses occurs primarily at the exits of stenotic vascular segments, because of turbulent flow generated at these points. Consequently, the greater number of entrance-exit points present, the greater the energy loss and reduction in distal coronary pressure. If stenoses are closely spaced, interaction may occur potentiating these effects, or conversely, if wide spacing is present, the various stenoses may act independently [161, 162]. Warltier et al. found that the effect of both upper and lower stenoses on coronary hemodynamics is essentially additive, when a fixed interstenotic segment of 10 mm was interposed, but this phenomenon may be dependent on the precise degree of vascular obstruction. For example, with two mild (30% occlusion) or very severe (95% occlusion) stenoses, additive effects may not be observed [163]. Gould and Lipscomb concluded that the concept that the more severe lesion

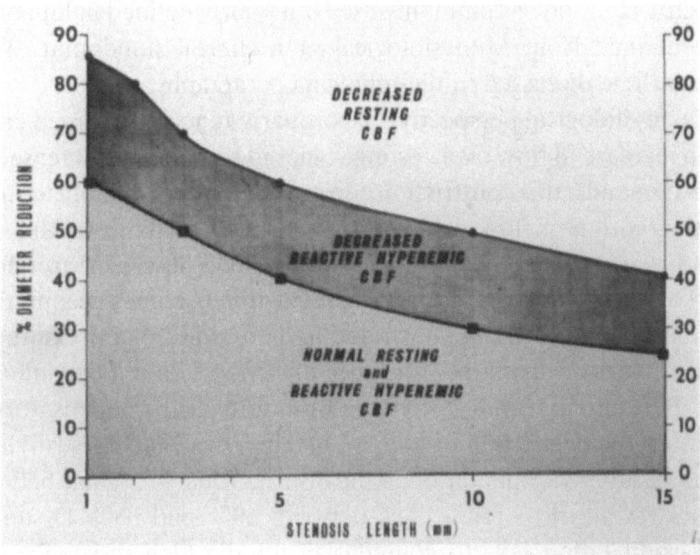

Fig. I.6. The effect of percent diameter reduction (vertical axis) and the length of diameter reduction (horizontal axis), on coronary blood flow. For example, 85 percent stenosis >1 mm. long decrease resting and reactive hyperemic flows; 50 percent stenosis >5 mm. long decrease reactive hyperemic flow but not resting flow. However, if the length of a 50 percent stenosis is increased to ≥10 mm., resting flow also decreases. A 20 percent stenosis fails to decrease resting or hyperemic coronary blood flow regardless of its length up to 15 mm. Reproduced with permission from Feldman et al. [160].

determines the hemodynamic effects of multiple stenoses is accurate only under restricted circumstances related to the severity of lesions and the extent to which hyperemic response or coronary flow reserve is elevated over basal resting levels [164].

The three most important determinants of the pressure gradient over a single stenosis, in descending order of importance, are the cross-sectional area of the stenosis, the flow through it and the length of the stenosis [137]. Particularly the length of an obstruction is often given little consideration when interpreting coronary cineangiograms. This is due to the fact that the length is difficult to estimate visually and the knowledge that the effect of length is relatively small. The possible presence of diffuse disease in the proximal and distal segments and unpredictable lesion geometry contribute greatly to the poor correlation between percent diameter stenosis and the physiological significance of a given obstruction in patients [146].

'Critical lesion'

The term 'critical lesion' is commonly used but poorly defined in human disease. It may be defined from a physiological or a clinical standpoint. These two approaches will be discussed in the following paragraphs.

From the physiological perspective, a coronary stenosis is defined critical, if it prevents an increase in flow over resting values in response to increased myocardial oxygen demands; this constriction corresponds approximately to the point at which resting coronary flow values start to decrease [165]. At this point the autoregulatory capacity of the coronary arterial bed has been stretched to the upper limit and the epicardial coronary obstruction becomes the limiting factor [134, 140, 166]. Gould et al. demonstrated in dog studies that pressure gradient-flow characteristics or hydraulic resistance of stenoses do not become abnormal enough to alter normal resting coronary flow nor to elicit compensatory changes for stenoses up to constriction of approximately 60% D-stenosis [167]. Furthermore, compensatory vasodilatation of the distal coronary vascular bed maintains near normal resting flow for lesions between 60% and 85% D-stenosis, but adaptive vasodilatation fails to compensate for the high resistance of lesions greater than 85% D-stenosis. Finally, there is vasodilator reserve still present when total coronary flow has been reduced below normal by a stenosis. In animal experiments hyperemic responses have been obtained either by intracoronary administration of a contrast medium or by a temporary complete occlusion of a coronary artery. The intracoronary injection of a contrast medium with high osmolality stimulates transient maximal vasodilatation and coronary flow, probably because of the high osmolality rather than its specific pharmacologic properties [165, 168].

In the animal laboratory, a coronary obstruction can be characterized precisely by simultaneous measurements of flow and pressure gradient throughout the cardiac cycle and a quantitative angiographic evaluation of stenosis geometry. Gould et al. found in dog studies that hyperemia after intracoronary injection of contrast material decreased when there was 30 to 45 percent D-stenosis and disappeared when there was 88 to 93 percent D-stenosis [165]. Results from model studies by Mates et al. predicted that an approximately 80–90% area stenosis (55–68% D-stenosis) is required to reduce resting flow; similar values have been published by Fiddian et al. [136, 147]. However, these threshold values cannot be projected to the clinical situation, because of two major differences with these dog and model studies. First, in the majority of the cases the human lesions are not symmetrical and secondly, the vascular segments immediately proximal and distal of the stenotic segment are usually not normal.

Dog studies by Dietze et al. showed that a significant decrease of coronary blood flow and poststenotic coronary pressure was closely related to the level of mean aortic pressure [169]. With lower aortic pressure the decrease occurred earlier than with higher aortic pressure. Resting coronary flow at 60 mmHg decreased significantly with a 70% D-stenosis and at 140 mmHg at 90% D-stenosis. In this range of aortic pressure between 60 and 140 mmHg reactive hyperemia was significantly diminished at a 60% D-stenosis and completely abolished when coronary stenosis was 90%. These results are in accordance with the observation that the hydraulic resistance across a nonfixed stenosis varies with intraluminal pressure passively; it increases as intraluminal pressure falls [155–157].

From the clinical perspective, a critical stenosis may be defined as one resulting in ischemic symptoms at rest. Using a semi-automated coronary analysis system, whereby elliptical cross sections of manually drawn contours in two orthogonal projections were computed, McMahon et al. found an average value of 92% cross-sectional area reduction for the critical stenosis in patients with unstable angina and single-vessel disease without angiographically demonstrable collaterals [170]. Rafflenbeul et al. quantifying lesions from 35 mm cinefilms in multiple projections using a vernier caliper found different values for the critical stenosis for arteries carrying normally different quantities of flow [171]. Although flow rates are normally higher in the LAD than in the RCA-artery, a smaller percent area stenosis (63%) in the RCA was found to be more critical than in the LAD (77%).

Discrepancy relative obstruction measure and its functional significance

The discrepancy between the anatomic presence or absence of 'significant' coronary artery narrowing and its functional significance has been clearly demonstrated in recent studies by Marcus et al., in which a newly developed single-crystal, pulsed Doppler probe was used to measure coronary artery flow reserve in patients sent to the operating room for coronary artery bypass graft surgery [129, 141, 172, 173]. The ultrasonic crystal was placed in a small silastic cup which is coupled to the epicardial coronary vessel being studied. Reactive hyperemic responses were measured following a 20 s. coronary occlusion. A poor correlation ($r = 0.10$) was found between coronary vasodilator capacity and percent diameter narrowing measured with micrometers on the patient's arteriogram with coronary obstructions of intermediate severity (10–90 percent D-stenosis). In a series of 23 patients with lesions in the proximal left anterior descending coronary artery, Harrison et al. compared percent diameter stenosis and percent area stenosis as measured from manually traced outlines of the arteries from optically magnified angiograms in 2 orthogonal projections using an elliptical model and the coronary reactive hyperemia results obtained immediately prior to bypass grafting. With both percent diameter stenosis and percent area stenosis there was substantial overlap between vessels with normal and abnormal reactive hyperemic responses. In contrast, all vessels with normal hyperemic responses had lesion minimal cross-sectional areas of greater than 3.5 mm^2 and 13 of 14 vessels with abnormal reactive hyperemic responses had minimal cross-sectional areas of less than $3.5\,mm^2$ [174, 175]. The same group has also shown that videodensitometrically measured absolute videodensity levels as a measure for the cross-sectional areas of coronary obstructions correlate well ($r = 0.85$) with peak-to-resting velocity ratio [176]. These data suggest that the absolute minimal cross-sectional area of the lesion can predict the coronary vasodilator capacity of obstructions in patients; such measurements require a procedure for accurate quantitative analysis of coronary cineangiograms.

Indirect approaches towards the assessment of the functional significance of obstructions

Videodensitometry
Aside from measurements during open heart surgery, indirect approaches must be used to assess the severity of coronary obstructions in patients with coronary artery disease. It is well known that the injection of contrast medium into coronary arteries or bypass grafts leads to an alteration of blood flow [177, 178]. The following phases can be distinguished: (1) the augmentation of the perfusion pressure in the vessel induced by the injection of contrast material causes an increase of the flow rate within the first second after injection; (2) the different hydromechanical properties (viscosity) of the contrast medium compared with blood cause a decrease of the flow rate; (3) the pharmacologic effect of the contrast medium on the coronary vessels and the myocardium lead to a reactive hyperemia with an increase of flow; (4) the flow returns after an average of about 13 sec after injection to the previous baseline level [179]. Therefore, measuring hyperemic responses in man during a cardiac catheterization requires a method for following rapid changes in coronary flow and of assessing its regional distribution. Videodensitometry provides a particular promising approach for measuring flow velocities in human coronary arteries from densograms [180]. At first only mean flow velocities could be assessed by measurement of the transit time of a bolus of contrast medium [181–184]. Further developments in this field have led to the determination of phasic flow pattern from ECG-triggered contrast boli [185], initially only in bypass grafts [178, 186], later also in coronary arteries [179, 187]; high film speeds of about 100 frs/s are hereby required. New developments in rapid sequential computed-tomography may allow quantitation of myocardial blood flow and perfusion using dynamic densitometry [188–190].

Pulsed Doppler coronary catheter
A pulsed Doppler coronary artery catheter which allows measuring rapid changes in coronary artery flow velocity, has also been used to assess hyperemic response produced by contrast media [191]. Until recently, a major problem of this technique was the inability to measure coronary blood flow in branches of the left

coronary system due to the physical size of the catheter. However, the group of Marcus have now developed a small (3F) coronary Doppler catheter, which can measure instantaneous changes in coronary blood flow velocity in individual coronary vessels at the time of cardiac catheterization [192].

Thallium-201 myocardial imaging
Noninvasive myocardial imaging with Thallium-201 (Tl-201) during pharmacologic coronary vasodilatation (e.g. with intravenously administered dipyridamole) or during exercise has been shown to be useful for noninvasively assessing regional flow reserve and the physiologic significance of moderate coronary stenoses [192–196]. Thallium-201, given intravenously during induced myocardial hyperemia, accumulates preferentially in regions where coronary flow is greatest. Animal studies have shown that the early myocardial thallium-201 distribution after intravenous dipyridamole infusion provides a reasonable estimate of the functional significance of the stenosis in terms of diminished reserve capacity [197]. Dipyridamole (DP) thallium-201 imaging has some theoretical and practical advantages compared to exercise thallium-201 imaging [194, 195]. The increased myocardial-to-background count ratio obtained from the DP method may result in improved image quality [196]. There may also be a greater increase in coronary blood flow following DP compared with maximal exercise. This difference would be even more significant in patients unable to perform near-maximal exercise. Albro et al. found the sensitivity of exercise and DP thallium-201 imaging, to be identical (67%) in detecting patients with coronary stenoses of $\geq 50\%$ D-stenosis [196]. On the basis of comparative studies on 33 patients with single-, double- and triple-vessel disease with the degree of obstructions measured quantitatively, Josephson et al. concluded that the sensitivity and specificity for detecting a $\geq 50\%$ diameter stenosis were 85% and 64%, respectively, for DP and 84% and 68% for exercise thallium-201 imaging [198]. Although the overall sensitivity and specificity of the two methods were not significantly different, DP-myocardial perfusion imaging (MPI) appeared more sensitive than exercise-MPI (70% vs 52%) in detecting coronary stenoses in the 40% to 60% range. Unfortunately, the specificity of both methods still appears to be relatively low with these visual interpretations of the thallium-201 scintigrams.

Although planar thallium-201 scintigraphy is useful for detecting coronary disease, it is much less reliable for determining the severity or location of coronary lesions [199]. From visual segmental analysis or early- and late-postexercise planar scintigrams, Rigo et al. found the following sensitivities for identifying individual vessel disease (D-narrowings > 50%) : 63% for LAD, 50% for RCA and 21% for LCX disease [200]. Sensitivity increased with the severity of stenosis, but even for 100% occlusions it was only 89% for LAD, 58% for RCA and 38% for LCX. Sensitivity diminished as the number of vessels involved increased: with single-vessel disease, 80% of LAD, 54% of RCA and 33% of LCX lesions were detected, but in patients with triple-vessel disease, only 50% of LAD, 50% of

RCA and 16% of LCX lesions were detected. Thus, although segmental analysis of thallium-201 myocardial scintigraphic imaging can identify disease in the individual coronary arteries with high specificity, only moderate sensitivity is achieved, reflecting the tendency of thallium-201 planar imaging to identify only the most severely ischemic area among several that may be presented in a heart [200–205]. Stenosed vessels supplying noninfarcted myocardium are much less readily recognized than those supplying infarcted or partially infarcted myocardium [206]. Even with critical stenoses, extensive collateralization to the involved artery results in poor sensitivity of the test as long as the artery supplying the collaterals is not significantly diseased [207]. Wijns et al. have shown that thallium-201 scintigraphy is highly predictive (74%) in the recurrence of restenosis after a primary successful PTCA; restenosis was predicted in only 50% of patients by exercise ECG [208].

Software packages for quantitative analysis of early- and late-postintervention planar thallium-201 scintigrams have been developed in a attempt to improve the sensitivity and diagnostic accuracy of the scintigraphic procedures [209–212]. Comprehensive computerized quantitative approaches minimize many of the problems associated with subjectivity of visual analysis of thallium-201 scintigrams [213–215]. Although the coronary angiogram has been used as the gold standard for the determination of the severity and extent of coronary artery disease in a given patient in these comparative studies, the angiograms were usually interpreted visually; because of all the known problems with the visual assessment, this has been an important limitation in the interpretation of the results.

It has been shown by various investigators, that the quantitative thallium-201 technique is more accurate than visual image interpretation for detection of disease in individual coronary arteries, especially in patients with multiple vessel coronary artery disease and those with moderate coronary artery stenosis [213, 214, 216, 217]. Maddahi et al. found that the quantitative analysis significantly increased the sensitivity of Tl-201 imaging over visual interpretation in the LAD (from 56% to 80%), LCX (from 34% to 63%) and RCA (from 65% to 94%) without significant loss of specificity [214, 217]. Importantly, the quantitative technique significantly enhances the potential of stress-redistribution scintigraphy for correct identification of patients with triple vessel and/or left main coronary artery disease [213, 214, 217]. Some of these improvements have been due to additional analysis of regional myocardial washout rate for Tl-201, which is a spatially nonrelative index of myocardial hypoperfusion. Nonetheless, three-vessel disease is still identified in only 78% to 86% of patients, and circumflex lesions are detected in only 63% of patients [213, 214, 217].

With planar thallium-201 scintigraphy 2-dimensional projections of a 3-dimensional activity distribution are obtained. It is obvious that this superimposition of myocardial muscle is an important limitation of this technique. In order to obviate these problems, new developments have been directed towards thallium-201 tomography, first with seven-pinhole and rotating slanthole collimators, later with rotating gamma camera's. With this new technique one hopes to be able to better determine the actual changes in the radioisotope distribution, which may possibly lead to an improvement in the localization of disease and the assessment of the severity of the disease in individual vessels.

Ritchie et al. compared the results from quantitatively analyzed tomograms obtained with a rotating gamma camera with the results from quantitative coronary angiography [218]. They found that all 14/14 RCA stenoses of $> 35\%$ D-reduction produced myocardial perfusion defects, while one out of four obstructions with $\leqslant 35\%$ D-stenosis was abnormal. All 16/16 LAD stenoses of $> 35\%$ D-stenosis were abnormal and 1/4 with $\leqslant 35\%$ D-stenosis was abnormal. However, only 8/16 circumflex lesions ($> 35\%$ D-stenosis) were identified and 3/5 stenoses with $\leqslant 35\%$ stenosis were abnormal by imaging.

In another tomographic study with a rotating gamma camera, Tamaki et al. obtained the following values for the sensitivity (Sn) and specificity (Sp) in the diagnosis of disease in the individual coronary arteries: overall $Sn = 92\%$, $Sp = 92\%$, RCA: $Sn = 79\%$, $Sp = 87\%$; LAD: $Sn = 85\%$, $Sp = 94\%$; LCX: $Sn = 64\%$, $Sp = 100\%$ [219]. Accurate diagnosis was made in 71% of single vessel disease and 91% of double vessel disease, while only 38% of three vessel disease was correctly predicted. These results show that quantitative thallium-201 tomography shows promise for detecting and assessing the severity of disease in individual vessels; however, LCX stenoses and three vessel disease seem to remain problematic.

Recently, Garcia et al. described a new comprehensive method for quantification of the relative 3-dimensional distribution of Tl-201 in the myocardium [220]. This is an extension of their work on quantitative planar Tl-201 scintigraphy [211]. The method uses maximal-count circumferential profiles of well-defined long- and short-axis tomograms to determine the 3-dimensional distribution of Tl-201. Subsequently, this distribution is mapped onto a 2-dimensional polar representation (Bull's eye display). Similar maps are available for the presentation of the extent and severity of uptake and washout defects. Another software package for quantitative analysis of thallium-201 tomograms is being developed by Reijs et al. [221].

Improved results may also be expected with the use of one of the technetium-99 m labelled cationic complexes currently under investigation as perfusion agents [222, 223]. These agents may improve image quality on the basis of less soft tissue attenuation and higher photon fluxes within current dosimetry restrictions.

Positron-emission tomography
The positron-emitting Rubidium-82 (Rb-82) can also be used to measure serial changes in myocardial blood flow, since Rb-82 uptake is proportional to myocardial blood flow [224, 225]. Serial images may be obtained in patients undergoing supine bicycle exercise tests as well as other interventions such as hand grip, cold pressor test, nitrate, dipyridamole or other pharmacologic interventions. Re-

gional changes in Rb-82 uptake in response to these interventions may be appreciated qualitatively as well as quantitatively due to the capabilities of positron tomography. This agent is well suited for the extensive investigation into the pathophysiology of coronary artery disease [166]. However, these studies are limited to these centers having a positron camera.

Radionuclide washout techniques

Washout techniques with radio-active tracers such as Xenon-133 have also been used to study the reduction of regional myocardial blood flow due to coronary obstructions; regional myocardial blood flow rates are expressed per unit mass of myocardium [226, 227]. This method requires direct injection of the radioisotope into the coronary arteries. Advantages of this technique are that one is able to separate flow through the right and left coronary circulations and that flow values can be directly correlated to the anatomic findings obtained on coronary arteriography. Lesions with area obstructions greater than 75% [228] and 80% [229] have been found to cause reductions in coronary flow.

Digital radiography

New approaches are being developed to assess the functional significance of a given anatomic lesion; in one approach digital radiographic techniques are used to determine the coronary flow reserve during contrast medium-induced hyperemia [230, 231] and after dipyridamole infusion [232]. Legrand et al. compared in a group of 19 patients percent diameter stenosis measurements with contrast-induced coronary flow reserve and noninvasive functional testing and found, that: (1) lesions with < 25% stenosis are hemodynamically insignificant; (2) those with ≥ 75% stenosis are hemodynamically significant; (3) those with 25–49% stenosis are hemodynamically insignificant about 75% of the time; and (4) those with 50–74% stenosis are hemodynamically significant about 75% of the time [233].

Digital subtraction angiography (DSA) techniques and digitized functional angiography (DFA) are being developed to quantitatively assess: (1) ischemic regions by reduced angiographic contrast in left ventricular wall segments; (2) the delayed washout of contrast medium from poststenotic vascular segments; and (3) abnormal vascular and myocardial flow [234].

It has been clearly demonstrated that with the present generation of X-ray systems, the morphology of the coronary arterial system cannot be visualized with sufficient accuracy following an intravenous injection of contrast agent. This is due to the fact that the contrast agent mixes in the left ventricle before the coronary arteries are filled; as a result, the mm-sized arteries are superimposed on the much larger left ventricular cavity. The X-ray equipment is not sensitive enough to distinguish between the contrast filled ventricle and arteries.

References

1. Forssman W: Die Sondierung des rechten Herzens. Klin Wochenschr 8: 2085–2087, 1929.
2. Cournand A, Ranges HA: Catheterization of the right auricle in man. Proc Soc Exper Biol and Med 46: 462–466, 1941.
3. Bing RJ, Van Dam LP, Gray FD Jr: Physiological studies in congenital heart disease. I. Procedures. Bull Johns Hopkins Hosp 80: 107–120, 1947.
4. Gorlin R, Gorlin SG: Hydraulic formula for calculation of the area of the stenotic mitral valve, other cardiac valves and central circulatory shunts. Am Heart J 41: 1–29, 1951.
5. Castellanos A, Pereiras R, Garcia A: La angiocardiografia, un metodo nueva para diagnostico de las cardiopatias congenitas. Archiv Soc Estud Clin Habana, 1937.
6. Robb G, Steinberg MF: Visualization of the chambers of the heart, the pulmonary circulation and great blood vessels in man. A practical method. Am J Roentgenol 41: 1–17, 1939.
7. Chavez I, Dorbecker N, Celis A: Direct intracardiac angiocardiography. Its diagnostic value. Am Heart J 33: 560–593, 1947.
8. Rushmer RF, Bark RS, Hendron JA: Clinical cinefluorography. Radiology 55: 588–592, 1950.
9. Rushmer RF, Crystal DK: Changes in configuration of the ventricular chambers during the cardiac cycle. Circulation 4: 211–218, 1951.
10. Rushmer RF, Thal N: The mechanics of ventricular contraction. A cinefluorographic study. Circulation 4: 219–228, 1951.
11. Sones FM, Shirey EK, Proudfit ML, Westcott RN: Cine-Coronary Arteriography. Circulation 20: 773–774, 1959.
12. Ricketts HJ, Abrams HL: Percutaneous selective coronary cine arteriography. JAMA 181: 620–624, 1962.
13. Judkins MP: Selective coronary arteriography. I. A percutaneous transfemoral technic. Radiology 89: 815–824, 1967.
14. Favaloro RG: Saphenous vein autograft replacement of severe segmental coronary occlusion – operative technique. Ann Thorac Surg 5: 334–339, 1968.
15. Bruschke AVG, Proudfit WL, Sones FM: Progress study of 590 consecutive nonsurgical cases of coronary disease followed 5–9 years. II. Ventriculographic and other correlations. Circulation 47: 1154–1163, 1973.
16. Hammermeister KE, DeRouen TA, Dodge HT: Variables predictive of survival in patients with coronary disease. Circulation 59: 421–430, 1979.
17. Tyras DH, Barner HB, Kaiser GC, Codd JE, Laks H, Pennington DG, Willman VL: Long-term results of myocardial revascularization. Am J Cardiol 44: 1290–1296, 1979.
18. Chaitman BR, DeMots H, Bristow JD, Rösch J, Rahimtoola SH: Objective and subjective analysis of left ventricular angiograms. Circulation 52: 420–425, 1975.
19. Zir LM, Miller SW, Dinsmore RE, Gilbert JP, Harthorne JW: Interobserver variability in coronary angiography. Circulation 53: 627–632, 1976.
20. Rogers WJ, Smith LR, Hood WP, Mantle JA, Rackley CE, Russell RO: Effect of filming projection and interobserver variability on angiographic biplane left ventricular volume determination. Circulation 59: 96–104, 1979.
21. Rackley CE, Dear HD, Baxley WA, Jones WB, Dodge HT: Left ventricular chamber volume, mass and function in severe coronary artery disease. Circulation 41: 605–613, 1970.
22. Hamilton GW, Murray JA, Kennedy JW: Quantitative angiocardiography in ischemic heart disease. The spectrum of abnormal left ventricular function and the role of abnormally contracting segments. Circulation 45: 1065–1080, 1972.
23. Moraski RE, Russell RO Jr, Smith M, Rackley CE: Left ventricular function in patients with and without myocardial infarction and one, two or three vessel coronary artery disease. Am J Cardiol 35: 1–10, 1975.
24. Jones JW, Rackley CE, Bruce RA, Dodge HT, Cobb LA, Sandler H: Left ventricular volumes

in valvular heart disease. Circulation 29: 887–891, 1964.

25. Miller GAH, Kirklin JW, Swan HJC: Myocardial function and left ventricular volumes in acquired valvular insufficiency. Circulation 31: 374–384, 1965.

26. Dodge HT, Baxley WA: Hemodynamic aspects of heart failure. Am J Cardiol 22: 24–34, 1968.

27. Kennedy JW, Twiss RD, Blackmon JR, Dodge HT: Quantitative angiocardiography. III: Relationship of left ventricular pressure, volume and mass in aortic valve disease. Circulation 38: 838–845, 1968.

28. Gribbe P: Comparison of the angiographic and direct Fick methods in determining cardiac output. Cardiologia 36: 20–29, 1960.

29. Wagner HR, Gamble WJ, Albers WH, Hugenholtz PG: Fiberoptic-dye dilution method for measurement of cardiac output. Comparison with the direct Fick and the angiographic methods. Circulation 37: 694–708, 1968.

30. Yang SS, Bentivoglio LG, Maranhao V, Goldberg H: From Cardiac Catheterization data to hemodynamic parameters. F.A. David Company, Philadelphia, 1972.

31. Sandler H: Dimensional analysis of the heart – a review. Am J Med Sci 260: 56–70, 1970.

32. Sandler H, Meier GD, Alderman EL: Ballistic motion of the heart. In: Ventricular Wall Motion. U. Sigwart, P.H. Heintzen (Eds.). Georg Thieme Verlag, Stuttgart/New York: 1–13, 1984.

33. Sandler H, Dodge HT: The use of single plane angiocardiograms for the calculation of left ventricular volume in man. Am Heart J 75: 325–334, 1968.

34. Lange P, Onnasch D, Farr FL, Straume B, Heintzen PH: Factors affecting the accuracy of angiocardiographic volume determination: left ventricle. In Roentgen-Video-Techniques for Dynamic Studies of Structure and Function of the Heart and Circulation: P.H. Heintzen, J.H. Bürsch (Eds.). Georg Thieme Publishers Stuttgart: 184–190, 1978.

35. Dodge HT, Sandler H, Ballew DW, Lord JD Jr: The use of biplane angiocardiography for measurement of left ventricular volume in man. Am Heart J 60: 762–776, 1960.

36. Dodge HT, Sandler H, Baxley WA, Hawley RR: Usefulness and limitations of radiographic methods for determining left ventricular volume. Am J Cardiol 18: 10–24, 1966.

37. Arvidsson H: Angiocardiographic determination of left ventricular volume. Acta Radiol 56: 321–339, 1961.

38. Chapman CB, Baker O, Reynolds J, Bonte FJ: Use of biplane cinefluorography for measurement of ventricular volume. Circulation 18: 1105–1117, 1958.

39. Reiber JHC: Special-purpose computer for real-time calculation of left ventricular volumes. Thesis, Electronics Laboratory, Delft University of Technology, 1971.

40. Sandler H, Hawley RR, Dodge HT, Baxley WA: Calculation of left ventricular volume from single-plane (A–P) angiocardiograms. J Clin Invest 44: 1094–1095 (Abstract), 1965.

41. Greene DG, Carlisle R, Grant C, Bunnell IL: Estimation of left ventricular volume by one plane cineangiography. Circulation 35: 61–69, 1967.

42. Snow JA, Baker LD, Leshin SJ, Messer JV: Validation of the single plane cineangiographic determination of canine left ventricular volume. II. Left ventricular dilatation. Fed Proc 28: 517 (Abstract), 1969.

43. Kennedy JW, Trenholme SE, Kasser IS: Left ventricular volume and mass from single-plane cineangiocardiograms. A comparison of anteroposterior and right anterior oblique methods. Am Heart J 80: 343–352, 1970.

44. Rackley CE, Behar VS, Whalen RE, McIntosh HD: Biplane cineangiographic determination of left ventricular function: Pressure – volume relationships. Am Heart J 74: 766–779, 1967.

45. Rackley CE, Hood WP Jr, Cleveland L, Stacy RW: Derivation of cardiac mechanical parameters from serial biplane angiocardiograms. J Appl Physiol 24: 254–258, 1968.

46. Graham TP Jr, Jarmakani JM, Canent RV Jr, Morrow MN: Left heart volume estimations in infancy and childhood: reevaluation of methodology and normal values. Circ 43: 895–904, 1971.

47. Bentivoglio LG, Griffith LD, Cuesta AJ, Geczy M: Radiographic evaluation of formulas for left

ventricular volume using canine casts. J Appl Physiol 33: 365–374, 1972.
48. Santamore WP, DiMeo F, Lynch PR: A comparative study of various single-plane cineangiocardiographic methods to measure left-ventricular volume. IEEE Trans Biom Eng BME–20: 417–421, 1973.
49. Chatelain P, Fleisch M, Doriot P–A, Rasoamanambelo L, Rutishauer W: In vivo determination of enddiastolic and endsystolic correction factors for left and right ventricular volumes – A new statistical method. Comp in Cardiol: 165–168, 1983.
50. Rackley CE, Hood WP Jr: Measurements of ventricular volume, mass and ejection fraction. In: Cardiac Catheterization and Angiography, W. Grossman (Ed.). Lea and Febiger, Philadelphia: 176–187, 1976.
51. Herman MV, Heinle RA, Klein MD, Gorlin R: Localized disorders in myocardial contraction. Asynsergy and its role in congestive heart failure. New Engl J Med 277: 222–232, 1976.
52. Herman MV, Gorlin R: Implications of left ventricular asynergy. Am J Cardiol 23: 538–547, 1969.
53. Herman MV, Eliott WC, Gorlin R. An electrocardiographic, anatomic, and metabolic study of zonal myocardial ischemia in coronary heart disease. Circulation 35: 834–846, 1967.
54. Sesto M, Schwarz F: Regional myocardial function at rest and after rapid ventricular pacing in patients after myocardial revascularization by coronary bypass graft or by collateral vessels. Am J Cardiol 43: 920–928, 1979.
55. Pasternac A, Gorlin R, Sonnenblick EH, Haft JI, Kemp HG: Abnormalities of ventricular motion induced by atrial pacing in coronary artery disease. Circulation 45: 1195–1205, 1972.
56. Dwyer EM, Jr: Left ventricular pressure – volume alterations and regional disorders of contraction during myocardial ischemia induced by atrial pacing. Circulation 42: 1111–1122, 1970.
57. Bonzel T, Löllgen H, Wollschläger H, Just H, Sigel H, Lippert R: Left ventricular wall motion analysis by conventional and hemiaxial biplane left ventricular angiography: choice of views. In: Ventricular Wall Motion. U Sigwart, P.H. Heintzen (Eds.). Georg Thieme Verlag, Stuttgart/New York: 43–49, 1984.
58. Widmann TF, Tubau JF, Ashburn WL, Bhargava V, Higgins CB, Peterson KL: Evaluation of regional wall motion by phase and amplitude analysis of intravenous contrast ventricular fluorangiography: technical aspects and computation. In: Ventricular Wall Motion. U Sigwart, P.H. Heintzen (Eds.). Georg Thieme Verlag, Stuttgart/New York: 24–33, 1984.
59. Adam WE, Bitter F: Advances in heart images. In: Medical Radionuclide Imaging. IAEA-SM-247/211: 195–218, 1981.
60. Rushmer RE, Crystal DK, Wagner C: The functional anatomy of ventricular contraction. Circ Res 1: 162–170, 1953.
61. Carlsson E, Milne ENC: Permanent implantations of endocardial tantalum screws: a new technique for functional studies of the heart in the experimental animal. J Ass Canad Radiol 19: 304–309, 1967.
62. Carlsson E: Experimental studies of ventricular mechanics in dogs using the tantalum-labeled heart. Fed Proc 28: 1324–1329, 1969.
63. Heikkila J, Tabakin BS, Hugenholtz PG: Quantification of function in normal and infarcted regions of the left ventricle. Cardiovasc Res 6: 516–531, 1972.
64. Slager CJ, Hooghoudt TEH, Reiber JHC, Schuurbiers JCH, Verdouw PD, Hugenholtz PG: Left ventricular wall motion as derived from endocardially implanted radiopaque markers and from contrastangiograms. In: Ventricular Wall Motion. U. Sigwart, P.H. Heintzen (Eds.). Georg Thieme Verlag, Stuttgart/New York: 150–159, 1984.
65. Harrison DC, Goldblatt A, Braunwald E, Mason D: Studies on cardiac dimensions in intact unanesthetized man. Circ Res 13: 448–467, 1963.
66. McDonald IG: The shape and movements of the human left ventricle during systole. Am J Cardiol 26: 221–229, 1970.
67. Brower RW, Katen HJ ten, Meester GT: Direct method for determining regional myocardial

shortening after bypass surgery from radiopaque markers in man. Am J Cardiol 41: 1222–1229, 1978.

68. Ingels NB Jr, Daughters GT, Stinson EB, Alderman EL: Measurement of midwall myocardial dynamics in intact man by radiography of surgically implanted markers. Circulation 52: 859–867, 1975.

69. Ingels NB Jr, Daughters GT, Stinson EB, Alderman EL: Evaluation of methods for quantitating left ventricular segmental wall motion in man using myocardial markers as a standard. Circulation 61: 966–972, 1980.

70. Amende I, Simon R, Hood WP, Hetzer R, Lichtlen PR: Intracoronary nifedipine in human being: magnitude and time course of changes in left ventricular contraction/relaxation and coronary sinus blood flow. JACC 2: 1141–1145, 1983.

71. Leighton RF, Wilt SM, Lewis RP: Detection of hypokinesis by quantitative analysis of left ventricular cineangiograms. Circulation 50: 121–127, 1974.

72. Harris LD, Clayton PD, Marshall HW, Warner HR: A technique for the detection of asynergistic motion of the left ventricle. Comput Biomed Res 7: 380–394, 1974.

73. Chaitman BR, Bristow JD, Rahimtoola SH: Left ventricular wall motion assessed by using fixed external reference systems. Circulation 48: 1043–1054, 1973.

74. Rickards A, Seabra-Gomes R, Thurston P: The assessment of regional abnormalities of the left ventricle by angiography. Eur J Cardiol 5: 167–182, 1977.

75. Sapoznikov D, Halon DA, Lewis BS, Weiss AT, Gotsman MS: Frame by frame analysis of left ventricular function. Cardiology 70: 61–72, 1983.

76. Shepertycki TH, Morton BC: A computer graphic-based angiographic model for normal left ventricular contraction in man and its application to the detection of abnormalities in regional wall motion. Circulation 68: 1222–1230, 1983.

77. Gottwik M, Stämmler G, Müller K–D, Siebes M, Kindler M, Winkler B, Schlepper M: Introduction and clinical evaluation of a computer-assisted method for the determination of regional wall motion of the left ventricle. In: Ventricular Wall Motion. U. Sigwart, P.H. Heintzen (Eds.). Georg Thieme Verlag, Stuttgart/New York: 113–121, 1984.

78. Ingels NB, Mead CW, Daughters GT, Stinson EB, Alderman EL: A new method for assessment of left ventricular wall motion. Comp in Cardiol: 57–61, 1978.

79. Slager CJ, Hooghoudt TEH, Reiber JHC, Schuurbiers JCH, Booman F, Meester GT: Left ventricular contour segmentation from anatomical landmark trajectories and its application to wall motion analysis. Comp in Cardiol: 347–350, 1979.

80. Bolson EL, Kliman S, Sheehan F, Dodge HT: Left ventricular segmental wall motion – a new method using local direction information. Comp in Cardiol: 245–248, 1980.

81. Sasayama S, Fujita M, Nonogi H, Kawai C, Eiho S, Kuwahara M: Quantitative assessment of regional disorders of left ventricular wall motion in patients with coronary artery disease by cineventriculography. In: Ventricular Wall Motion. U. Sigwart, P.H. Heintzen (Eds.). Georg Thieme Verlag, Stuttgart/New York: 62–73, 1984.

82. Lorente P, Adda JL, Creplet J, Masquet C, Babalis D, Piekarski A, N'guyen A, Azancot I: A new computerized segmental area based method to evaluate regional wall motion from cineangiograms and two dimensional echograms. In: Ventricular Wall Motion. U. Sigwart, P.H. Heintzen (Eds.). Georg Thieme Verlag, Stuttgart/New York: 130–139, 1984.

83. Ingels NB, Daughters GT, Stinson EB, Alderman EL: Evaluation of methods for quantitating left ventricular segmental wall motion in man using myocardial markers as a standard. Circulation 61: 966–972, 1980.

84. Alderman EL, Schwarzkopf A, Ingels NB, Daughters GT, Stinson EB, Sanders WJ: Application of an externally referenced, polar coordinate system for left ventricular wall motion analysis. Comp in Cardiol: 207–210, 1979.

85. Hooghoudt TEH, Slager CJ, Reiber JHC, Serruys PW: A new method to quantify regional left ventricular wall motion, as well as pump- and contractile function. In: Ventricular Wall Motion,

U. Sigwart, P.H. Heintzen (Eds.). Georg Thieme Verlag, Stuttgart/New York: 229—244, 1984.

86. Sheehan FH, Bolson EL, Dodge HT, Mitten S: Centerline method – Comparison with other methods for measuring regional left ventricular motion. In: Ventricular Wall Motion. U. Sigwart, P.H. Heintzen (Eds.). Georg Thieme Verlag, Stuttgart/New York: 139–149, 1984.

87. Brower RW, Meester GT: Spatial resolution and correlation between segments in regional wall motion studies of the left ventricle. Comp in Cardiol: 69–75, 1978.

88. Brower RW, Meester GT: Computer based methods for quantifying regional left ventricular wall motion from cine ventriculograms. Comp in Cardiol: 55–62, 1976.

89. Hernandez-Lattuf PR, Quinones MA, Gaasch WH: Usefulness and limitations of circumferential fibre shortening velocity in evaluating segmental disorders of left ventricular contraction. Br Heart J 36: 1167–1174, 1974.

90. Daughters GT, Schwarzkopf A, Mead CW, Stinson EB, Alderman EL, Ingels Jr. NB: A clinical evaluation of five techniques for left ventricular wall motion assessment. Comp in Cardiol: 249–252, 1981.

91. Daughters GT, Alderman EL, Ingels Jr. NB: A rational approach to the clinical detection of wall motion abnormalities. In: Ventricular Wall Motion. U. Sigwart, P.H. Heintzen (Eds.). Georg Thieme Verlag, Stuttgart/New York: 74–82, 1984.

92. Marier DL, Gibson DG: Limitations of two frame method for displaying regional left ventricular wall motion in man. Br Heart J 44: 555–559, 1980.

93. Sheehan FH, Stewart DK, Dodge HT, Mitten S, Bolson EL, Brown BG: Variability in the measurement of regional left ventricular wall motion from contrast angiograms. Circulation 68: 550–559, 1983.

94. Clayton PD, Klausner SC, Blair TJ, Jeppson GM, Liddle HV: Sources and magnitude of variability in measurements of regional left ventricular function. In: Ventricular Wall Motion. U. Sigwart, P.H. Heintzen (Eds.). Georg Thieme Verlag, Stuttgart/New York: 90–99, 1984.

95. Cohn PF, Levine JA, Bergeron GA, Gorlin R: Reproducibility of the angiographic left ventricular ejection fraction in patients with coronary artery disease. Am Heart J 88: 713–720, 1974.

96. Sones FM, Shirey EK, Proudfit ML, Westcott RN: Cine-Coronary Arteriography. Circulation 20: 773–774, 1959.

97. Sones FM, Shirey EK: Cine-coronary arteriography. Modern Concepts of Cardiovasc Dis 31: 735–738, 1962.

98. Amplatz K, Formanek G, Stanger P, Wilson W: Mechanics of selective coronary artery catheterization via femoral approach. Radiology 89: 1040–1047, 1967.

99. Bourassa MG, Lespérance J, Campeau L: Selective coronary arteriography by the percutaneous femoral artery approach. Am J Roentgenol 107: 377–383, 1969.

100. Wells DE, Befeler B, Winkler JB, Myerburg RJ, Castellanos A, Castillo CA: A simplified method for left heart catheterization including coronary arteriography. Chest 63: 959–962, 1973.

101. Wilson WJ, Lee GB, Amplatz K: Biplane selective coronary arteriography via percutaneous transfemoral approach. Am J Roentgenol 100: 332–340, 1967.

102. Spellberg RD, Ungar I: The percutaneous femoral artery approach to selective coronary arteriography. Circulation 36: 730–733, 1967.

103. Gensini GG: Coronary arteriography. Futura Publishing Com, Mount Kisco, N.Y., 1975.

104. Bourassa MG, Noble J: Complication rate of coronary arteriography. A review of 5250 cases studied by a percutaneous femoral technique. Circulation 53: 106–114, 1976.

105. Adams DF, Fraser DB, Abrams HL: The complications of coronary arteriography. Circulation 48: 609–618, 1973.

106. Gensini GG: Coronary Arteriography. In: Heart Disease. E. Braunwald (Ed.). W.B. Saunders Company, Philadelphia/London/Toronto: 308–362, 1980.

107. Detre KM, Wright E, Murphy ML, Takaro T: Observer agreement in evaluating coronary angiograms. Circulation 52: 979–986, 1975.

108. DeRouen TA, Murray JA, Owen W: Variability in the analysis of coronary arteriograms.

Circulation 55: 324–328, 1977.

109. Sanmarco ME, Brooks SH, Blankenhorn DH: Reproducibility of a consensus panel in the interpretation of coronary angiograms. Am Heart J 96: 430–437, 1978.

110. Shub C, Vlietstra RE, Smith HC, Fulton RE, Elveback LR: The impredictable progression of symptomatic coronary artery disease. A serial clinical-angiographic analysis. Mayo Clin Proc 56: 155–160, 1981.

111. Fisher LD, Judkins MP, Lespérance J, Cameron A, Swaye P, Ryan T, Maynard C, Bourassa M, Kennedy JW, Gosselin A, Kemp H, Faxon D, Wexler L, Davis KB: Reproducibility of coronary arteriographic reading in the Coronary Artery Surgery Study (CASS). Cath Cardiovasc Diagn 8: 565–575, 1982.

112. Meier B, Gruentzig AR, Goebel N, Pyle R, von Gosslar W, Schlumpf M: Assessment of stenoses in coronary angioplasty. Inter- and intraobserver variability. Int J Cardiol 3: 159–169, 1983.

113. Cameron A, Kemp HG, Fisher LD, Gosselin A, Judkins MP, Kennedy JW, Lespérance J, Mudd JG, Ryan TJ, Silverman JF, Tristani F, Vlietstra RE, Wexler LF: Left main coronary artery stenosis: angiographic determination. Circulation 68: 484–489, 1983.

114. Zir LM: Observer variability in coronary angiography. Editorial Note. Int J Cardiol 3: 171–173, 1983.

115. Levin DC, Baltaxe HA, Lee JG, Sos TA: Potential sources of error in coronary arteriography. I. In performance of the study. Am J Roentgenol, Rad Therapy and Nuclear Med 124: 378–385, 1975.

116. Vlodaver Z, Edwards JE: Pathology of coronary atherosclerosis. Prog Cardiovasc Dis 14: 256–274, 1971.

117. Vlodaver Z, Neufeld HN, Edwards JE: Pathology of coronary disease. Sem in Roentgenol 7: 376–394, 1972.

118. Hort W: Anatomy and pathology of the human coronary circulation. In: The Pathophysiology of Myocardial Perfusion. W Schaper (Ed.). Elsevier/North-Holland Biomedical Press, Amsterdam/New York/Oxford: 247–282, 1979.

119. Freudenberg H, Lichtlen PR: The normal wall segment in coronary stenoses. A postmortal study. Z Kardiol 70: 863–869, 1981.

120. Schlesinger MJ, Zoll PM: Incidence and localization of coronary artery occlusions. Arch Path 32: 178–188, 1941.

121. Arnett EN, Isner JM, Redwood DR, Kent KM, Baker WP, Ackerstein H, Roberts WC: Coronary artery narrowing in coronary heart disease: comparison of cineangiographic and necropsy findings. Ann Internal Med 91: 350–356, 1979.

122. Brown BG, Bolson E, Frimer M, Dodge HT: Computer-assisted measurements of coronary artery stenosis. Circulation 60: 1196 (Letter), 1979.

123. Block PC, Myler RK, Stertzer S, Fallon JT: Morphology after transluminal angioplasty in human being. N Engl J Med 305: 382–385, 1981.

124. Holmes DR, Vlietstra RE, Mock MB, Reeder GS, Smith HC, Bove AA, Bresnakan JF, Pichler JM, Schaff HV, Orszulak TA: Angiographic changes produced by percutaneous transluminal coronary angioplasty. Am J Cardiol 51: 676–683, 1983.

125. Essed CE, Brand M van den, Becker AE: Transluminal coronary angioplasty and early restenosis. Fibrocellular occlusion after wall laceration. Br Heart J 49: 393–396, 1983.

126. Levin DC, Baltaxe HA, Sos TA: Potential sources of error in coronary arteriography. II. In interpretation of the study. Am J Roentgenol, Rad Therapy and Nuclear Med 124: 386–393, 1975.

127. Roberts WC, Buja LM: The frequency and significance of coronary arterial thrombi and other observations in fatal acute myocardial infarction. A study of 107 necropsy patients. Am J Med 52: 425–443, 1972.

128. Isner JM, Wu M, Virmani R, Jones AA, Roberts WC: Comparison of degrees of coronary

arterial luminal narrowing determined by visual inspection of histologic sections under magnification among three independent observers and comparison to that obtained by video planimetry. An analysis of 559 five-millimeter segments of 61 coronary arteries from eleven patients. Lab Invest 5: 566–570, 1980.

129. White CW, Wright CB, Doty DB, Hiratza LF, Eastham CL, Harrison DG, Marcus ML: Does visual interpretation of the coronary arteriogram predict the physiologic importance of a coronary stenosis? N Engl J Med 310: 819–824, 1984.

130. Shipley RE, Gregg DE: The effect of external constriction of a blood vessel on blood flow. Am J Physiol 141: 289–296, 1944.

131. Young DF, Tsai FY: Flow characteristics in models of arterial stenoses. I. Steady flow. J Biomechanics 6: 395–410, 1973.

132. Young DF, Tsai FY: Flow characteristics in models of arterial stenoses. II. Unsteady flow. J Biomechanics 6: 547–559, 1973.

133. Young DF, Cholvin NR, Roth AC: Pressure drop across artificially induced stenoses in the femoral arteries of dogs. Circ Res 36: 735–743, 1975.

134. Logan SE: On the fluid mechanics of human coronary artery stenosis. IEEE Trans on Biom Eng BME-22: 327–334, 1975.

135. Brown BG, Bolson E, Frimer M, Dodge HT: Quantitative coronary arteriography. Circulation 55: 329–337, 1977.

136. Mates RE, Gupta RL, Bell AC, Klocke FJ: Fluid dynamics of coronary artery stenosis. Circ Res 42: 152–162, 1978.

137. Lipscomb K, Hooten S: Effect of stenotic dimensions and blood flow on the hemodynamic significance of model coronary arterial stenoses. Am J Cardiol 42: 781–792, 1978.

138. Gould KL: Pressure-flow characteristics of coronary stenoses in unsedated dogs at rest and during coronary vasodilation. Circ Res 43: 245–253, 1978.

139. Yongchareon W, Young DF: Initiation of turbulence in models of arterial stenoses. J Biomechanics 12: 185–196, 1979.

140. Klocke FJ: Measurements of coronary blood flow and degree of stenosis; current clinical implications and continuing uncertainties. J Am Coll Cardiol 1: 31–41, 1983.

141. Marcus ML: The coronary circulation in health and disease. McGraw-Hill Book Company New York, 1983.

142. Gottwik MG, Siebes M, Kirkeeide R, Schaper W: Hämodynamik von Koronarstenosen. Z Kardiol 73: 47–54, 1984.

143. Gould KL: Dynamic coronary stenosis. Am J Cardiol 45: 286–292, 1980.

144. Gould KL, Kelley KO, Bolson EL: Experimental validation of quantitative coronary arteriography for determining pressure-flow characteristics of coronary stenosis. Circulation 66: 930–937, 1982.

145. Gould KL, Kelley KO: Physiological significance of coronary flow velocity and changing stenosis geometry during coronary vasodilation in awake dogs. Circ Res 50: 695–704, 1982.

146. Wright C, White C, Furda J, Doty D, Eastham C, Laughlin D, Marcus M: Can the coronary arteriogram predict the functional significance of a coronary stenosis? Circulation 62 (Supp. III): III-214 (Abstract), 1980.

147. Fiddian RV, Byar D, Edwards EA: Factors affecting flow through a stenosed vessel. Arch Surg 88: 83–90, 1964.

148. Feldman RL, Nichols WW, Pepine CJ, Conti CR: Hemodynamic significance of the length of a coronary arterial narrowing. Am J Cardiol 41: 865–871, 1978.

149. Sabbah HN, Stein PD: Hemodynamics of multiple versus single 50 percent coronary arterial stenoses. Am J Cardiol 50: 276–280, 1982.

150. Feldman RL, Pepine CJ: Evaluation of coronary artery stenoses. Int J of Cardiol 4: 185–187, 1983.

151. Feldman RL, Nichols WW, Pepine CJ, Conti CR: Hemodynamic effect of long and multiple

coronary arterial narrowings. Chest 74: 280–285, 1978.

152. Clark C: The propagation of turbulence produced by a stenosis. J Biomechanics 13: 591–604, 1980.

153. Feldman RL, Pepine CJ: Determination of residual regional flow during acute coronary occlusion in conscious man. J Am Coll Cardiol 1: 684 (Abstract), 1983.

154. Schwartz JS, Carlyle PF, Cohn JN: Effect of coronary arterial pressure on coronary stenosis resistance. Circulation 61: 70–76, 1980.

155. Schwartz JS: Fixed vs nonfixed coronary stenosis: the response to a fall in coronary pressure in a canine model. Cath Cardiovasc Diagn 8: 383–392, 1982.

156. Schwartz JS: Compliant coronary stenoses. (Editorial Note). Int J Cardiol 4: 315–317, 1983.

157. Bove AA, Santamore WP, Carey RA: Reduced myocardial blood flow resulting from dynamic changes in coronary artery stenosis. Int J Cardiol 4: 301–313, 1983.

158. Maseri A, Chierchia S, Davies GJ, Fox KM: Variable susceptibility to dynamic coronary obstruction: an elusive link between coronary atherosclerosis and angina pectoris. Am J Cardiol 52: 46A–51A, 1983.

159. Epstein SE, Cannon III RO, Watson RM, Leon MB, Bonow RO, Rosing DR: Dynamic coronary obstruction as a cause of angina pectoris: implications regarding therapy. Am J Cardiol 55: 61B–68B, 1985.

160. Feldman RL, Nichols WW, Pepine CJ, Conetta DA, Conti CR: The coronary hemodynamics of left main and branch coronary stenoses. The effects of reduction in stenosis diameter, stenosis length, and number of stenoses. J Thorac Cardiovasc Surg 77: 377–388, 1979.

161. Brice JG, Dowsett DJ, Lowe RD: Haemodynamic effect of carotid artery stenosis. Br Med J 2: 1363–1366, 1964.

162. Young DF: Fluid mechanics of arterial stenosis. J Biomech Eng 101: 157–175, 1979.

163. Warltier DC, Buck JD, Brooks HL, Gross GJ: Coronary hemodynamics and subendocardial perfusion distal to stenoses. Int J Cardiol 4: 173–183, 1983.

164. Gould KL, Lipscomb K: Effects of coronary stenoses on coronary flow reserve and resistance. Am J Cardiol 34: 48–55, 1974.

165. Gould KL, Lipscomb K, Hamilton GW: Physiologic basis for assessing critical coronary stenosis. Instantaneous flow response and regional distribution during coronary hyperemia as measures of coronary flow reserve. Am J Cardiol 33: 87–94, 1974.

166. Kirkeeide RL, Gould KL: Cardiovascular imaging: coronary artery stenosis. Hospital Practice: 160–175, 1984.

167. Gould KL, Lipscomb K, Calvert C: Compensatory changes of the distal coronary vascular bed during progressive coronary constriction. Circulation 51: 1085–1094, 1975.

168. Lehan PH, Harman MA, Oldewurtel HA: Myocardial water shifts induced by coronary arteriography. J Clin Invest 42: 950 (Abstract), 1963.

169. Dietze W, Mittmann U, Schmier J, Wirth RH: Effects of coronary stenosis and mean aortic pressure on coronary blood flow, poststenotic coronary pressure, and reactive hyperemia. Basic Res Cardiol 71: 309–318, 1976.

170. McMahon MM, Brown BG, Cukingnan R, Rolett EL, Bolson E, Frimer M, Dodge HT: Quantitative coronary angiography: Measurement of the 'critical' stenosis in patients with unstable angina and single-vessel disease without collaterals. Circulation 60: 106–113, 1979.

171. Rafflenbeul W, Urthaler F, Lichtlen P, James TN: Quantitative difference in 'critical' stenosis between right and left coronary artery in man. Circulation 62: 1188–1196, 1980.

172. Marcus M, Wright C, Doty D, Eastham C, Laughlin D, Krumm P, Fastenow C, Brody M: Measurements of coronary velocity and reactive hyperemia in the coronary circulation of humans. Circ Res 49: 877–891, 1981.

173. Wright CB, Doty DB, Eastham CL, Marcus ML: Measurements of coronary reactive hyperemia with a Doppler probe. Intraoperative guide to hemodynamically significant lesions. J Thorax Cardiovasc Surg 80: 888–897, 1980.

174. Harrison DG, White CW, Hiratzka LF, Wright CB, Doty CB, Miller MR, Eastham CL, Marcus ML: Can the significance of a coronary stenosis be predicted by quantitative coronary angiography? Circulation 64 (Supp IV): 160. (Abstract), 1981.

175. Harrison DG, White CW, Hiratzka LF, Doty DB, Barnes DH, Eastham CL, Marcus ML: The value of lesion cross-sectional area determined by quantitative coronary angiography in assessing the physiologic significance of proximal left anterior descending coronary arterial stenoses. Circulation 69: 1111–1119, 1984.

176. Collins SM, Skorton DJ, Harrison DG, White CW, Eastham CL, Hiratzka LF, Doty DB, Marcus ML: Quantitative computer-based videodensitometry and the physiological significance of a coronary stenosis. Comp in Cardiol: 219–222, 1982.

177. Bussman WD, Rutishauser W, Noseda G, Preter B, Meier W: Influence of a new contrast medium (Metrizoate) on coronary blood flow. In: Roentgen-, Cine- and Videodensitometry. Fundamentals and Applications for Blood Flow and Heart Volume Determination. PH Heintzen (Ed.). Georg Thieme Verlag, Stuttgart: 133–139, 1971.

178. Hackbarth W, Bircks W, Pölitz B, Körfer R, Schmiel FK, Spiller P: Vergleich videodensitometrischer und elektromagnetischer Flussmessungen in aortokoronaren Bypassgefässen. Fortschr Röntgenstr 132: 554–560, 1980.

179. Spiller P, Schmiel FK, Pölitz B, Block M, Fermer U, Hackbarth W, Jehle J, Körfer R, Pannek H: Measurement of systolic or diastolic flow rates in the coronary artery system by X-ray densitometry. Circulation 68: 337–347, 1983.

180. Bürsch J, Johs R, Kirbach H, Schnürer C, Heintzen P: Accuracy of videodensitometric flow measurement. In: Roentgen-, Cine- and Videodensitometry. Fundamentals and Applications for Blood Flow and Heart Volume Determination. PH Heintzen (Ed.). Georg Thieme Verlag, Stuttgart: 119–132, 1971.

181. Rutishauer W, Noseda G, Bussman W–D, Preter B: Blood flow measurement through single coronary arteries by roentgen densitometry. Part II. Right coronary artery flow in conscious man. Am J Roentgenol, Rad Therapy and Nuclear Med 109: 21–24, 1970.

182. Smith HC, Frye RL, Donald DE, Davis GD, Pluth JR, Sturm RE, Wood EH: Roentgen videodensitometric measure of coronary blood flow. Determination from simultaneous indicator-dilution curves at selected sites in the coronary circulation and in coronary artery-saphenous vein grafts. Mayo Clin Proc 46: 800–806, 1971.

183. Simon R, Amende I, Lichtlen PR: Roentgen Videodensitometry in the analysis of coronary angiograms. In: Coronary artery disease today. Diagnosis, surgery and prognosis. AVG Bruschke, G van Herpen, FEE Vermeulen (Eds.). Excerpta Medica, Amsterdam/Oxford/Princeton: 176–182, 1982.

184. Simon R, Amende I, Oelert H, Hetzer R, Borst HG, Lichtlen PR: Blood velocity, flow and dimensions of aortacoronary venous bypass grafts in the postoperative state. Circulation 66 (Supp. I): I–34 – I–39, 1982.

185. Fermor U, Huber H, Neuhaus KL, Schmiel KF, Spiller P: Measurement of flow velocity in the model circulation by videodensitometry. Methodological investigations. Basic Res Cardiol 73: 361–377, 1979.

186. Pannek H, Neuhaus KL, Schmiel FK, Spiller P: Röntgenvideodensitometrische Flussmessungen in aortokoronaren Bypass-Gefässen. Z Kardiol 67: 787–796, 1978.

187. Sauer G, Krause H, Burmeister A, Tebbe U, Kreuzer H, Neuhaus KL: Determination of coronary flow velocities in man by a computer-aided cine-videodensitometric system. Z Kardiol 72: 207–214, 1983.

188. Lipton MJ, Boyd DP: Contrast media in dynamic computed tomography of the heart and great vessels. In: Contrast Media in Computed Tomography. Exerpta Medica, Amsterdam: 204–213, 1981.

189. Lipton MJ, Higgins CB, Farmer DW, Gould RG, Napel S, Boyd DP: Real time cardiac CT scanning using a millisecond focused electron beam (cine/CT) scanner: initial results in patients

and animals. JACC 3: 539 (Abstract), 1984.

190. Lipton MJ, Higgins CB, Farmer D, Boyd DP: Cardiac imaging with a high-speed cine-CT scanner: preliminary results. Radiology 152: 579–582, 1984.

191. Cole JS, Hartley CJ: The pulsed Doppler coronary artery catheter. Preliminary report of a new technique for measuring rapid changes in coronary artery flow velocity in man. Circulation 56: 18–25, 1977.

192. Wilson RF, Hartley CJ, Laughlin DE, Marcus ML, White CW: Transluminal subselective measurement of coronary blood flow velocity and coronary vasodilator reserve in man. J Am Coll Cardiol 3: 529 (abstract), 1984.

193. Strauss HW, Pitt B: Noninvasive detection of subcritical coronary arterial narrowings with a coronary vasodilator and myocardial perfusion imaging. Am J Cardiol 39: 403–406, 1977.

194. Gould KL: Noninvasive assessment of coronary stenoses by myocardial perfusion imaging during pharmacologic coronary vasodilatation. I. Physiologic basis and experimental validation. Am J Cardiol 41: 267–278, 1978.

195. Gould KL, Westcott RJ, Albro PC, Hamilton GW: Noninvasive assessment of coronary stenoses by myocardial perfusion imaging during pharmacologic coronary vasodilatation. II. Clinical methodology and feasibility. Am J Cardiol 41: 279–287, 1978.

196. Albro PC, Gould KL, Westcott RJ, Hamilton GW, Ritchie JL, Williams DL: Noninvasive assessment of coronary stenoses by myocardial imaging during pharmacologic coronary vasodilatation. III. Clinical Trial. Am J Cardiol 42: 751–760, 1978.

197. Beller GA, Holtzgrefe HH, Watson DD: Effects of dipyridamole-induced vasodilation on myocardial uptake and clearance kinetics of thallium-201. Circulation 68: 1328–1338, 1983.

198. Josephson MA, Brown BG, Hecht HS, Hopkins J, Pierce CD, Petersen RB: Noninvasive detection and localization of coronary stenoses in patients: comparison of resting dipyridamole and exercise thallium-201 myocardial perfusion imaging. Am Heart J, 103: 1008–1018, 1982.

199. Smalling RW: The spectrum of thallium-201 imaging in coronary artery disease. Teaching Editorial. J Nucl Med 24: 854–858, 1983.

200. Rigo P, Bailey IK, Griffith LSC, Pitt B, Burow RD, Wagner Jr, HN, Becker LC: Value and limitations of segmental analysis of stress thallium myocardial imaging for localization of coronary artery disease. Circulation 61: 973–981, 1980.

201. Lenaers A, Block P, van Thiel E, Lebedelle M, Becquevort P, Erbsmann F, Ermans AM: Segmental analysis of Tl-201 stress myocardial scintigraphy. J Nucl Med 18: 509–516, 1977.

202. McKillop JH, Murray RG, Turner JG, Bessent RG, Lorimer AR, Greig WR: Can the extent of coronary artery disease be predicted from thallium-201 myocardial images. J Nucl Med 20: 715–719, 1979.

203. Massie BM, Botvinick EH, Brundage BH: Correlation of thallium-201 scintigrams with coronary anatomy: factors affecting region by region sensitivity. Am J Cardiol 44: 616–622, 1979.

204. Dash H, Massie BM, Botvinick EH, Brundage BH: The noninvasive identification of left main and three-vessel coronary artery disease by myocardial stress perfusion scintigraphy and treadmill exercise electrocardiography. Circulation 60: 276–284, 1979.

205. Hör G, Kanemoto N: Tl-201 myocardial scintigraphy: current status in coronary artery disease, results of sensitivity/specificity in 3092 patients and clinical recommendations. Nucl Med 20: 136–147, 1981.

206. Rigo P, Bailey IK, Griffith LSC, Pitt B, Wagner HN Jr, Becker LS: Stress thallium-201 myocardial scintigraphy for the detection of individual coronary arterial lesions in patients with and without previous myocardial infarction. Am J Cardiol 48: 209–216, 1981.

207. Rigo P, Becker LC, Griffith LSC, Alderson PO, Bailey IK, Pitt B, Burow RD, Wagner Jr HN: Influence of coronary collateral vessels on the results of thallium-201 myocardial stress imaging. Am J Cardiol 44: 452–458, 1979.

208. Wijns W, Serruys PW, Reiber JHC, Feijter PJ de, Brand M van den, Simoons ML, Hugenholtz PG: Early detection of restenosis after successful percutaneous transluminal coronary an-

gioplasty by exercise-redistribution thallium scintigraphy. Am J Cardiol 55: 357–361, 1985.

209. Burow RD, Pond M, Schafer AW, Becker L: 'Circumferential profiles': A new method for computer analysis of thallium-201 myocardial perfusion images. J Nucl Med 20: 771–777, 1979.

210. Meade RC, Bamrah VS, Horgan JD, Ruetz PP, Kronenwetter C, Yeh E: Quantitative methods in the evaluation of thallium-201 myocardial perfusion images. J Nucl Med 19: 1175–1178, 1978.

211. Garcia E, Maddahi J, Berman D, Waxman A: Space/time quantitation of thallium-201 myocardial scintigraphy. J Nucl Med 22: 309–317, 1981.

212. Reiber JHC, Lie SP, Simoons ML, Wijns W, Gerbrands JJ: Computer quantitation location, extent and type of thallium-201 myocardial perfusion abnormalities. Proc. 1st. Intern. Symp. Medical Imaging and Image Interpretation ISMIII, IEEE Cat No CH 1804–4/82: 123–128, 1982.

213. Berger BC, Watson DD, Taylor GJ, Craddock GB, Martin RP, Teates CD, Beller GA: Quantitative thallium-201 exercise scintigraphy for detection of coronary artery disease. J Nucl Med 22: 585–593, 1981.

214. Maddahi J, Garcia EV, Berman DS, Waxman A, Swan HJC, Forrester J: Improved noninvasive assessment of coronary artery disease by quantitative analysis of regional stress myocardial distribution and washout of thallium-201. Circulation 64: 924–935, 1981.

215. Faris JV, Burt RW, Graham MC, Knoebel SB: Thallium-201 myocardial scintigraphy: improved sensitivity, specificity and predictive accuracy by application of a statistical image analysis algorithm. Am J Cardiol 49: 733–742, 1982.

216. Gibson RS, Taylor GJ, Watson DD, Stebbins PT, Martin RP, Crampton RS, Beller GA: Predicting the extent and location of coronary artery disease during the early postinfarction period by quantitative thallium-201 scintigraphy. Am J Cardiol 47: 1010–1019, 1981.

217. Maddahi J, Garcia EV, Berman DS: Quantitative analysis of the distribution and washout of thallium-201 in the myocardium: description of the method and its clinical applications. In: Nuclear Imaging in Clinical Cardiology. ML Simoons, JHC Reiber (Eds.) Martinus Nijhoff Publishers, Boston: 103–124, 1984.

218. Ritchie JL, Brown BG, Caldwell JH, Harp GD, Williams DL: Tl-201 quantitative tomographic imaging: comparison to quantitative coronary angiography. Circulation 68 (Supp III): III–386 (Abstract), 1983.

219. Tamaki N, Yonekura Y, Mukai T, Minato K, Nohara R, Kadota K, Kambara H, Kawai C, Ishii Y, Torizuka K: Values and limitations of segmental analysis of stress and redistribution Tl ECT for location of coronary artery disease. J Nucl Med 24: P18 (Abstract), 1983.

220. Garcia EV, Van Train K, Maddahi J, Prigent F, Friedman J, Areeda J, Waxman A, Berman DS: Quantification of rotational thallium-201 myocardial tomography. J Nucl Med 26: 17–26, 1985.

221. Reijs AEM, Reiber JHC, Blokland K, Gerbrands JJ, Simoons ML, Kooij PPM: Developments towards quantitative analysis of thallium-201 tomograms. Abstractbook 1984 European Gamma-11 Users' Meeting, Amsterdam, May 17–19: II:7 (Abstract), 1984.

222. Sullivan PJ, Werre J, Okada RD, Kopiwoda S, Castronovo F, McKusick KA, Strauss HW: Comparison of Tc-99m DMPE to 201-Thallium biodistribution. Am J Cardiol 49: 980 (Abstract), 1982.

223. Bushong WC, Weintraub WS, Bodenheimer MM, Akazuki S, Banka VS, Agarwal JB, Helfant RH: Assessment of myocardial perfusion using a newly developed technetium complex: comparison to 201-thallium and radioactive microspheres. Am J Cardiol 49: 979 (Abstract), 1982.

224. Selwyn AP, Allan RM, L'Abatta A, Horlock P, Camici P, Clark J, O'Brien HA, Grant PM: Relation between regional myocardial uptake of rubidium-82 and perfusion: Absolute reduction of cation uptake in ischemia. Am J Cardiol 50: 112–121, 1982.

225. Wilson R, Shea M, Landsheere C. de, Deanfield J, Lammetsma A, Terton D, Selwyn A: Myocardial blood flow: clinical application and recent advances. In: Nuclear Imaging in Clinical Cardiology. ML Simoons, JHC Reiber (Eds). Martinus Nijhoff Publishers, Boston: 39–54, 1984.

226. Ross RS, Ueda K, Lichten PR, Rees JR: Measurement of myocardial blood flow in animals and

man by selective injection of radioactive inert gas into the coronary arteries. Circ Res 15: 28–41, 1964.

227. Cannon PJ, Weiss MB, Sciacca RR: Myocardial blood flow in coronary artery disease: studies at rest and during stress with inert gas washout techniques. Progr in Cardiov Dis XX: 95–120, 1977.

228. Engel HJ, Hundeshagen H, Lichtlen P: Auswirkungen von Koronarstenosen und ventrikulären Funktionsstörungen auf die regionale Myokarddurchblutung bei koronarer Herzkrankheit. Schweiz Med Wschr 107: 1920–1927, 1977.

229. Smith SC, Gorlin R, Herman MV, Taylor WJ, Collins JJ: Myocardial blood flow in man: effects of coronary collateral circulation and coronary artery bypass surgery. J Clin Invest 51: 2556–2565, 1972.

230. Vogel R, LeFree M, Bates E, O'Neill W, Foster R, Kirlin P, Smith D, Pitt B: Application of digital techniques to selective coronary arteriography: use of myocardial contrast appearance time to measure coronary flow reserve. Am Heart J 107: 153–164, 1984.

231. Hodgson JMcB, LeGrand V, Bates ER, Mancini GBJ, Aueron FM, O'Neill WW, Simon SB, Beauman GJ, LeFree MT, Vogel RA: Validation in dogs of a rapid digital angiographic technique to measure relative coronary blood flow during routine cardiac catheterization. Am J Cardiol 55: 188–193, 1985.

232. Chappuis F, Ratib O, Meier B, Righetti A, Rutishauser W: Assessment of coronary flow reserve by computer analysis of digitized coronary angiograms at rest and after dipyridamol infusion. J Am Coll Cardiol 5: 475 (Abstract), 1985.

233. Legrand V, Hodgson JMcB, Aueron FM, Mancini J, Bates ER, Smith JS, LeFree MT, Vogel RA: The correlation of percent diameter coronary stenosis with the functional significance of individual coronary artery stenoses. J Am Coll Cardiol 5: 475 (Abstract), 1985.

234. Bürsch JH, Hahne HJ, Beyer C, Seemann S, Meissner L, Brennecke R, Heintzen PH: Myocardial perfusion studies by digital angiography. Comp in Cardiol: 343–346, 1983.

II. Cineangiocardiography

Introduction

Angiocardiography is an invasive X-ray imaging technique to visualize blood filled vessels and chambers. Since the X-ray absorption coefficient of blood differs little from that of tissue, special precautions need to be taken to obtain an image with the desired structures. This is achieved by selectively injecting a contrast agent via a catheter into the chamber(s) of interest or the arteries to be studied. A brief overview of various contrast agents which are in common use, will be given following this introduction.

Modern X-ray gantries allow multidirectional movements of the X-ray source and image intensifier around the patient with the patient remaining in the isocenter [1]. Table tops of carbon fibre reinforced plastic offer less absorption than previously used materials. For a number of reasons the tendency today is towards the use of biplane multidirectional systems: overall less amount of contrast medium, catheter tip in critical location during a minimum of the time and the facility for three-dimensional calculations and corrections. The biplane systems are most valuable in interventional procedures, like angioplasty. The main drawback is the impairment in access to the patient when he is surrounded by double sets of X-ray tubes and image intensifiers. Present biplane systems therefore combine single-plane and biplane modes of operation in such a way that one plane can be swung or moved aside when not necessarily needed.

The X-ray system basically consists of an X-ray source with adjustable kV (quality), mA (quantity) and pulse width and an image intensifier to convert the X-ray photons impinging on its input screen into visible light, while at the same time intensifying the signal (Fig. II.1). The images at the output screen of the image intensifier are registered with a video camera and a 35 mm cinecamera. The video images are displayed on a video monitor for visual feedback to the arteriographer during the catheterization procedure and stored on a video disk or tape for instantaneous replay and for backup reasons. For routine cine-angiographic procedures standard video systems with 625 lines in Europe and 525

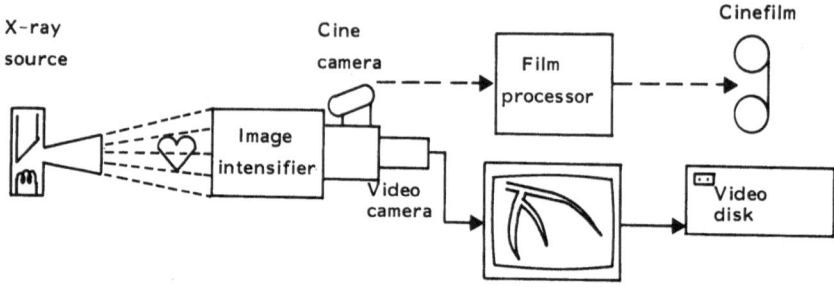

Fig. II.1. Diagrammatical scheme of X-ray system used in cardiac catheterization laboratories.

lines in the USA are utilized. Today, the l-inch plumbicon with a photo-sensitive layer of antimony trisulphide and lead oxide is used almost exclusively. This type of tube is characterized by a gamma of 1, good reproduction of movement and a high signal-to-noise ratio; however, its modulation transfer is poorer than that from vidicon tubes. Developments are towards tubes with better modulation transfer functions, solid state image sensors and high resolution X-ray television particularly to be used in digital vascular imaging [2–4]. The film speed for left ventriculography is usually taken at 60/50 frames/s, while 30/25 frames/s are used for coronary cineangiography. The 35 mm cinefilm is the medium on which all the angiographic image information is stored for later visual interpretation and quantitative analysis. Until to date it has remained the medium of choice because of its inherently high resolution and the relatively low cost associated with it. It is also a perfect medium for exchange of the pictorial information between cardiological departments.

It is the purpose of this chapter to describe the image forming process and to provide technical information about the different components of the X-ray system, i.e. the X-ray generator and tube, the image intensifier, the optics and the cinecamera. Furthermore, the process of cinefilm exposure and the cinefilm processing will be discussed. Finally, clinical factors in cineangiography will be presented, as well as a recommendation for different acquisition protocols for left ventricular and coronary cineangiographies. Guidelines for optimal resources for examination of the chest and cardiovascular system can be found in ref. 5; a related bibliography can also be found in this publication. An interesting paper describing causes of cine image quality deterioration has been published by Levin et al. [6]. A glossary of technical terms is also provided in this paper.

Contrast agents

Contrast medium must be of a high iodine concentration to cause a sufficient attenuation of the X-ray photons; typical concentrations are between 370 and 400 mg iodine/ml. Of equal importance to the high iodine concentration is a low toxicity to minimize cardiac changes and systemic discomfort that may result in motion and registration artefacts. Contrast materials cause numerous effects on the cardiovascular system [7–10]. The major direct actions on the heart are myocardial mechanical and electrophysiological alterations. The major direct action on the peripheral circulation is vasodilatation. The indirect effects, for the most part, are reflexly mediated and tend to offset the direct effects.

An excellent overview on contrast media toxicity in coronary arteriography has been published by Fischer and Thomson [11]. The flow of contrast material through the heart during coronary arteriography may result in a great number of effects on the physiology: heart rate and rhythm changes; changes observable in the electrocardiogram other than rate and rhythm alterations; changes in coronary blood flow; alterations in myocardial contractility; changes in systemic and cardiac chamber pressures; and alterations in biochemical processes. A survey of these changes is presented in the paper mentioned above.

Cardiodepressant effects caused by ionic contrast media include a reduction in left ventricular peak systolic pressure and both global and regional myocardial function, as well as adverse electrophysiologic changes [8]. Biphasic responses have been observed in conscious and anesthetized dogs; direct effects occurred within the first 10 seconds after injection, while secondary or indirect effects ensued near the end of the first 10 seconds or in the second 10-second period. These perturbations occur more frequently in the presence of coronary stenoses [12, 13]. The adverse effects of the conventional contrast media are related to the presence of single-valence cations, such as sodium and meglumine, to an imbalance in the ratio of sodium to calcium ions, to the high osmolality of the solutions and to their hyperviscosity. The hyperosmolality may exert its influence through the massive shifting of tissue water to the capillaries as the contrast medium flows through them, thus increasing the intravascular volume. Hyperosmolality is also one of the factors involved in the decrease of myocardial contractility, alterations of aortic pressure, and disturbances in the cardiac rhythm [13]. Ionic solutions cause more bradycardia and increase the PR-interval more than nonionic solutions [14]. Bentley and Henry, investigating the effect of the widely used ionic contrast agent Renografin-76 (diatrizoate) on animal arteries, demonstrated that the angiographic dye in concentrations not exceeding those during angiography exert potent dose- and time-dependent vasomotor effects [15]. Serrur et al. concluded from an experimental model that diatrizoate had an initial negative inotropic effect on isolated canine hearts, but contractile force returned to baseline within 1 minute during normal perfusion and within 2 minutes under ischemic conditions [16]. Griggs et al. found that following the administration of Hypaque-M (diatrizoate) coronary blood flow is increased to a degree equivalent to or greater than the peak hyperemic flow [17]. Table II.1 lists the most widely used ionic and nonionic contrast agents by their product and generic names.

To reduce these undesirable effects, much effort has been directed toward the

Table II.1. Product and generic names of widely used contrast media.

Generic name	Product name
1. *Ionic, high osmolality*	
Diatrizoate	Angiografin, Hypaque, Renografin, Urografin
Iotalamate	Conray, Vascoray
Ioxitalamat	Telebrix
Metrizoate	Isopaque Coronar
2. *Ionic, low osmolality*	
Ioxaglate	Hexabrix
3. *Nonionic, low osmolality*	
Iohexol	Omnipaque
Iopamidol	Niopam, Solutrast
Metrizamide	Amipaque

development of new water-soluble contrast media with reduced osmolality, which are either nonionic or contain physiologic concentrations of calcium ions [18, 19]. Collective studies offer experimental and clinical evidence for the advantages of the low osmolality agents in cardiac radiology [20]. These agents cause less subjective discomfort, less hemodynamic and biochemical effects, and less blood pressure and rhythm disturbance in coronary angiography. Amipaque (metrizamide) is such a nonionic water-soluble contrast medium, that has no sodium and approximately one third of the osmolality of conventional ionic water-soluble media [7, 21]. More recently, a new nonionic contrast medium Omnipaque (iohexol) has become available, which in addition to further improvements in pharmacological and clinical properties has the advantage over Amipaque of being supplied in solution, ready for use. It contains negligible amounts of sodium, and the osmolality is approximately half that of ionic contrast agents. Isopaque Coronar (meglumine metrizoate balanced with sodium and calcium) is an ionic contrast agent with added calcium ions resulting in a balanced concentration of sodium and calcium ions [7, 22].

Svenson compared the electrocardiographic and hemodynamic effects of Hexabrix (ioxaglate), an ionic low osmolality contrast agent with Renografin-76 in a crossover study of 41 patients [23]. He found no observable differences in opacification when used for left ventriculography and coronary arteriography. However, hemodynamic function was routinely affected less following the administration of Hexabrix as compared with Renografin-76 with statistically significant less change noted in the RR-interval following the LV and coronary arteriograms. Changes in aortic diastolic, systolic and mean pressures, as well as cardiac index changes and systemic resistance following left ventriculograms were all much less using Hexabrix.

These two contrast agents were also studied by Wolf in a randomized double-blind clinical trial of 50 patients undergoing cardiac angiography [24]. Cardiac output increased more significantly in the Renografin-76 group, and there was a significant difference in AV O$_2$ indicating less vasodilatation with Hexabrix; there was also dramatically less prolongation in the QT-interval for the Hexabrix group. In animal studies, he found that Renografin-76 significantly reduced the ventricular fibrillation threshold, whereas Hexabrix was much less toxic. Wolf concluded that Hexabrix is less hazardous in terms of total adverse effects and particularly indicated for certain risk groups.

It has been shown in anesthetized dogs that nonionic contrast media (Amipaque and Omnipaque) produced fewer alterations in coronary sinus blood chemistry and myocardial contractile state than ionic contrast media [12, 13]. Trägårdh et al. concluded that the nonionic contrast medium Amipaque produced a smaller coronary flow increase than the ionic medium Renografin-76 after injection into the main left coronary artery in dogs and also had a shorter transit time through the coronary vessels; in addition, the coronary veins were better filled with Amipaque [25]. In isolated canine hearts it has been demonstrated that Amipaque has a positive inotropic effect under normal perfusion as well as during ischemia. Calcium-enriched metrizoate (Isopaque) had only a positive inotropic effect under normal perfusion: during ischemia, however, the positive inotropic effect was followed by a decrease in contractile force to 93 ± 5% of baseline after 2 minutes [16].

Although much preliminary work has been done on the coronary circulation of experimental animals, trials in man are necessary since the responses of the experimental animal and of man may differ significantly [26]. It has been shown in man that Amipaque affected the aortic blood pressure and the ECG less than Isopaque [27]; it also resulted in reduced chest pain and heat sensation and longer coronary contrast transit time [22]. Mancini et al. found that Omnipaque produced fewer deleterious hemodynamic and electrocardiographic changes than Renografin-76 when studied in a typical adult population requiring diagnostic catheterization [28]. Bettmann et al. have demonstrated in a double-blind study in 51 patients that Omnipaque causes less alteration in cardiac function than Renografin-76 [29]. Wink and Heinrich demonstrated in a group of 80 patients that decreases in heart rate and aortic pressure during coronary angiography were significantly (p<0.05) stronger with the conventional ionic and high-osmolar ioxitalamat than with the ionic and nonionic low-osmolar ioxaglat or nonionic low-osmolar iopamidol [30]. Similarly, Brinker et al. found in a multicenter double-blind randomized trial of iopamidol, that diatrizoate has a more deleterious effect on ECG and hemodynamic parameters than iopamidol [31]. On the basis of similar findings, Gertz et al. concluded that iopamidol appears to enhance the safety of cardiac angiography [32].

The radiologic image

An important step in the angiographic image formation is the absorption of X-ray photons in the input phosphor of an image intensifier. An image with diagnostic quality must contain a minimum number of image forming events (X-ray quanta). For state-of-the-art image intensifiers with a 6–7″ field size 30–40 μR of radiation produces an acceptable cine-image; for a larger field of 9–10″ 15 μR per frame are required. The ability to obtain accurate diagnostic information from angiographic images depends upon three principle variables: contrast, noise and unsharpness.

Image contrast is influenced among others by the selected quality (kV) of the X-ray generator and by the receptor contrast. A lower level of the kV results in enhanced contrast (larger absorption differences between various anatomical structures), a higher level in decreased contrast (smaller absorption differences). The receptor contrast is determined by the response of the image forming components (image intensifier and cinefilm) to the radiation intensity pattern.

The total amount of noise in an image is determined by three sources: scatter radiation, quantum mottle and the receptor. Scatter radiation degrades image contrast; it can be reduced by a scatter grid at the expense of loss of sensitivity. The reliability of the grey level of a picture element in an image to represent the true amount of X-ray absorption in that particular projection depends to a great extent on the number of X-ray quanta received. Quantum mottle is the statistical fluctuation in the distribution of the image forming events, i.e. X-ray quanta. The quantum noise for a picture element is defined by the square root of the received number of photons for that element. In other words, elements within regions with a high absorption level, for example, elements belonging to contrast filled heart chambers or coronary vessels, are characterized by large amounts of quantum noise. On the other hand, pixels within regions with a relatively low amount of absorption, for example, regions representing tissue, are characterized by a very low quantum noise level. The image intensifier also introduces random fluctuations, while the noise component of the cinefilm is caused by the graininess of the film material. Usually, quantum mottle is the greatest component of noise in cineangiographic studies.

Sharp edges of distinct anatomical structures are blurred on the angiographic image due to a number of factors: patient and/or organ motion, geometric unsharpness, system unsharpness and absorption unsharpness. Patient or organ motion unsharpness can be reduced by using shorter cinepulse widths. Geometric unsharpness is affected by the finite size of the focal spot of the X-ray tube and is also related to target-to-object and object-to-receptor distances. This unsharpness can be reduced by using smaller focal spot size and a shorter object-to-receptor distance. System unsharpness is caused by the finite spatial frequency response of the image intensifier, while absorption unsharpness is due to the finite number of X-ray quanta forming the image.

The X-ray generator and tube

The X-ray generator and the radiographic tube are the power train for the production of the Roentgen ray. Three X-ray exposure factors determine the setting of the X-ray generator: kilovoltage (kV), tube current in milliamperes (mA) and pulse width in milliseconds (msec). Each X-ray tube has a maximum allowable kilowatt (kW) load, defined by $\frac{1}{1000} \times kV \times mA$ for modern X-ray generators. However, the anode in the X-ray tube has a certain heat capacity or thermal load, which limits the cinerun time. This maximal allowable time that the X-ray tube can be employed at a certain kW-level can be assessed from heating and cooling curves, that are available for each type of X-ray tube. The thermal load is dependent on the focal size used; a smaller focal spot results in a lower allowable load. Furthermore, there is an inverse relationship with the cinepulse width and the frame speed.

Two common modes of image recording are fluoroscopy and cinematography. During fluoroscopy the object is irradiated continuously at a low mA level (<4 mA). Although organ motion unsharpness is maximal in this mode, it is used advantageously at a low radiation level for patients and catheter positioning. The cinematographic mode is used for the definite documentation of the investigation. In this case X-ray photon flow from the radiographic tube to the image intensifier occurs for a predetermined number of milliseconds when the cine-camera shutter is open. This exposure time should be short enough to stop motion but long enough to allow a sufficient number of photons to expose the cinefilm. In those clinical circumstances where resolution of detail is essential, such as in coronary arteriography and congenital heart disease, a 20–40 μR exposure of each cineframe is required for a 7" image intensifier and 10–20 μR for a 9" image intensifier. Motion stopping exposures of 4–6 ms usually provide a good balance between quantum mottle and motion unsharpness, when a 40–60 kW or higher X-ray tube is used.

Optimal cine-imaging can be obtained if: (1) the X-ray quality (kV) is kept in the range of 70–90 kV for adult patients thus providing good radiation contrast; (2) exposure times of 4–6 ms are employed; (3) motion unsharpness is controlled; and (4) good filming geometry is maintained. Recommended is a cinepulse system with a working output of 40 kW or more. In modern cineangiographic generators, one or more of the X-ray exposure factors are adjusted by the unit automatically, which is accomplished by the automatic exposure control (AEC). To this end, a photomultiplier monitors the image brightness in a dominant region of interest in the center portion of the output screen of the image intensifier. The sensitivity of the photomultiplier tube is calibrated by a light- or radiation-sensing device to provide a selected radiation dose (μR/frame) at the input screen of the image intensifier. The following different procedures for the AEC have been implemented:

(a) The kV is regulated, while maintaining fixed pulse width and maximum allowable mA.

(b) A constant kilowatt output level is maintained with fixed pulse width and changing kV and mA. This procedure keeps the kV at an optimal low level and the mA as high as possible.

(c) Pulse width is adjusted, while mA is fixed at a maximum allowable level and the kV level is selected by the technologist.

Limitation of this dominant approach and a possible improvement is briefly discussed in this chapter in the section on clinical factors in cineangiocardiography.

The electrical efficiency of X-ray tubes is very low; less than 0.2% of the electrical energy is converted to X-ray photons. The remainder is converted into heat, most of which is generated in the anode of the X-ray tube. These tubes therefore must be cooled. Recent developments include replacement of the conventional glass tube with a metal envelope. Other developments are being directed toward improving focal spot geometry and providing nearly true Gaussian distribution of the X-rays, which should result in substantial improvements in image resolution; at present, the distribution of the X-rays is either homogeneous or square.

Modern tubes have 100 mm or larger black-coated rhenium-tungsten-molybdenum (RTM) or laminated anodes, or have rhenium-tungsten targets and graphite heat sinks capable of being rotated at high speed (10,000 rpm). The focal spot size, shape and intensity distribution are important to image quality. The focal spot of the radiographic tube should be as small as commensurate with the tube loadings necessary to produce a satisfactory balance between motion and geometric unsharpness within the angiographically acceptable X-ray quality (kV) range. Most standard X-ray tubes used for cineangiography contain both small (0.6 to 0.7 mm) and large (1.0 to 1.3 mm) focal spots (16° target angle). Allowable kW rating is substantially lower with the small focal spot. The principal advantage of tubes with small focal angles (6–9°) is their ability to maintain adequate X-ray quanta output during short exposures, while using focal spots of very small size, thus reducing geometric unsharpness. Their use is recommended in systems devoted to the study of ischemic heart disease, where angled views increase the demand for high tube loading. The disadvantages of tubes with smaller target angles are marked heel effect and limited useful field size.

For the investigation of ischemic heart disease by cinematography the radiographic facility should have a tube with a target angle of 6–9° and a diameter of 100–125 mm with a (nominal) 0.3–0.6 mm, 20–50 kW small focal spot and a 0.8–1.0 mm, 50–100 kW large focal spot coupled with a 6–7″ size image intensifier. The tube should be capable of rotation of 10,000–20,000 rpm.

X-ray absorption

In the ideal case with a monochromatic X-ray source emitting parallel beams of X-rays passing through a homogeneous absorbing medium without scattering, the absorption process is described by the Lambert-Beer Law:

$$I(E) = I_0(E) \cdot \exp(-\mu \cdot d) \tag{II.1}$$

where $I_0(E)$ is the number of photons of energy E incident on a small area of the medium, $I(E)$ the number of photons transmitted through the object, $\mu[cm^2/g]$ the mass attenuation coefficient of the medium and $d[g/cm^2]$ the irradiated mass per cm^2. The mass attenuation coefficient for different materials depends to a great extent on the energy of the impinging X-rays. In clinical practice with the commercially available X-ray systems the ideal case sketched above does not exist. The primary X-rays produced by conventional X-ray equipment are characterized by a wide continuous spectrum with a distribution depending on the kV of the X-ray source, the radiation beam is divergent and reduced in intensity by absorption and scattering. Due to the fact that μ is a function of the X-ray energy, beam hardening of the X-rays occurs when a particular medium is irradiated by polychromatic X-rays. This results in different attenuation coefficients for different medium thicknesses. This property can also be employed advantageously to homogenize the spectral distribution of the primary X-ray photons. By placing a copper and/or aluminum filter between the X-ray source and the object, the secondary spectrum will be more narrow and shifted towards the higher energy levels (smaller wavelength).

In addition to the fact that scattered radiation disturbs the exponential absorption law, it also produces a spatially nonuniform opacification of the film resulting in loss of contrast. The influence of the scatter can be limited by the use of a scatter grid positioned against the input screen of the image intensifier. This grid only allows penetration of X-ray photons from the direction of the X-ray focus. For angiocardiographic cinefilm imaging, a ratio 8:1 focussed 40 lines per centimer fiber-spaced grid is recommended.

Despite these imperfections in the X-ray absorption process it has been demonstrated by Bürsch and Heintzen that by the use of appropriate filters and scatter grids the Lambert-Beer Law is applicable for densitometric measurements in clinical studies with a sufficient degree of accuracy [33, 34]. Pochon and Rutishauser have shown that the Lambert-Beer Law is applicable for coronary arteries with diameters not exceeding a few millimeters; this range can be extended by applying certain densitometric correction procedures [35].

In clinical practice the irradiated object does not consist of a homogeneous medium. Therefore, consider an inhomogeneous specimen (of thickness not exceeding L) consisting of various absorbing materials. Let $\mu(x, y, z)$ be the value of the mass attenuation coefficient at point (x, y, z) in the object. Assuming propagation in the z-direction, the number of photons at position (x, y) available to the recording medium is then given by:

$$I(x, y) = I_0(x, y) \cdot \exp(-\beta(x, y)), \tag{II.2}$$

with

$$\beta(x, y) = \int_0^L \mu(x, y, z) \varrho(x, y, z) \, dz \tag{II.3}$$

and $\varrho(x, y, z)$ being the mass density [g/cm^3] of the materials at position (x, y, z). Because of the divergence of the primary X-ray beams, the incident and therefore the transmitted radiation is also a function of the spatial coordinates (x, y). From this point on we will for reasons of simplicity denote the spatial position (x, y) in the projection image by p.

Image intensifier

The image intensifier functions as a radiation frequency converter of the X-ray photons into visible light, while at the same time intensifying the signal [36]. The quality of the output image is determined by its brightness, contrast, resolution, and the uniformity of these measurements across the screen, as well as by the amount of geometric distortion in the image. In addition, adequate image quality should be obtainable at an acceptable exposure rate [37].

The image intensifier is a vacuum tube enclosing a large volume; its walls are made of glass or metal. The input window of modern intensifiers is usually constructed of titanium. The X-ray photons enter through the input window and fall on an input screen, where a visible image is created. An extremely thin semiconductor layer consisting of caesium and antimony is vapor-deposited on the input screen. It absorbs the light emitted by the input screen and transforms it into a corresponding flux of electrons which are emitted into the tube. By means of an appropriately shaped electric field, the electron lens, the 'photo'-electrons are focussed onto the output screen. The electric focussing field accelerates the photoelectrons from a practically negligible initial energy to between 25 and 35 keV at the output screen. As a result of this large potential difference at least 1000 light quanta are generated in the output screen for each photoelectron.

The efficiencies of the three information-converting layers, the input screen, the photocathode and the output screen, as well as the final energy of the photoelectrons, determine the total light flux, or the 'gain'. Another important parameter, the conversion factor G_x, is defined by the luminance, i.e. the light flux per unit area of the output screen, per unit exposure rate at the input, usually expressed in cd $\cdot$ m^{-2} $\cdot$ (mR)$^{-1}$ $\cdot$ sec. or cd $\cdot$ m^{-2} $\cdot$ [0.258 C/kg]$^{-1}$. A modern cesium-iodide image intensifier should have a conversion factor G_x of ≥ 50 for the small mode.

The primary detection of the X-ray quanta occurs in the input screen. To be an efficient converter, it should have the following properties: it must absorb the X-ray photons as much as possible and the interaction must result in the emission of light with a high yield; these characteristics are specified by the detection quantum efficiency (DQE). On the other hand, to achieve a high resolving power the input screen must be a thin layer, which is in contradiction with the requirements for high attenuation of the X-rays. Input screens of modern X-ray image intensifiers consist of evaporated layers of cesium iodide, activated by a small admixture of sodium. This screen material offers a good compromise between adequate spatial resolution and high yield of the conversion of X-ray quanta.

The DQE depends heavily on the X-ray spectrum, i.e. on the kilovoltage of the generating tube. It is therefore customary to state the DQE at a standardized radiation quality, characterized by a half-value layer of 7 mm of aluminum. At this radiation the DQE's of modern image intensifiers lie between 40% and 70%. Current developments aim at maximizing the modulation transfer function (MTF) at a high value of the DQE. Other developments in image intensifiers are directed toward improvements in the photocathode, the electron optics, the output phosphor, tube geometry, construction of the tube housing and the optical coupling.

The brightness intensification is achieved by two phenomena. First, the viewing screen is considerably smaller than the input screen so that a certain amount of brightness amplification is obtained by means of a geometrical reduction of the image area. The second factor contributing to the total gain is the acceleration of the photo-electrons in the vacuumtube.

Image intensifiers are available in a number of sizes from 2″ (5 cm) to 14″ (35 cm) and in single, dual and triple modes. For coronary arteriography the image intensifier should be a cesium-iodide instrument with high resolution used in the 6–7″ mode. Single mode, 6–7″ image intensifiers should provide a resolution through the optical system of not less than 4 lp/mm. Large, multi-mode 9–10″ intensifiers should have a resolution of 3 lp/mm.

The curvature of the input screen of the image intensifier results in a nonlinear geometric distortion (pincushion distortion) and in a nonuniform detection efficiency over the input intensifier screen (vignetting). Due to the last factor the gain of the image intensifier is spatially variant. Various configurations of input screens aimed at minimal geometric and detection efficiency distortions have been developed by the different image intensifier manufacturers. The electro-optical nature of the image intensifier results in an additional image distortion component from optical scattering, referred to as veiling glare (VG). The veiling glare of an intensifying tube is a measure of the contrast obtained for very low frequencies (approximately 1 linepair per cm). To measure the veiling glare in practice, the brightness of the image of a lead strip covering approximately 10% of the input phosphor area is compared to the brightness of the uncovered area. If DI is the light intensity in the dark area below the lead strip and LI the light intensity of the uncovered area, $VG = \dfrac{LI - DI}{LI + DI} \times 100\%$. In a state-of-the-art image intensifier, veiling glare will be $\geq 70\%$.

Together with radiation scatter, veiling glare generates a low spatial frequency component in the image intensified video signal (38). This component non-uniformly biases the black level in video angiography. In general, the presence of X-ray scatter and glare causes a suppression of contrast in the intensified image. A technique using a digital convolution algorithm has been proposed by Shaw et al. to approximate and correct for the scatter and glare (38).

To a first approximation, the luminance $L(p)$ at the output screen can be described by:

$$L(p) = G(p) \cdot (I(p))\gamma_I, \qquad\qquad\qquad (II.4)$$

where $G(p)$ is the image intensifier conversion factor at position (p) and γ_I is the 'gamma' of the image intensifier. Both $G(p)$ and γ_I depend on the quality (energy) of the impinging X-rays. For simplicity, we have omitted the energy-dependence in formule (II.4).

Optics and cinecamera

The image at the output screen of the image intensifier is projected via a 90/10% beam splitter onto the cinefilm in the cinecamera (90% of the light is projected onto the cinecamera and 10% to a coupled video camera). High quality matched optics are vital to image clarity. The MTF of the intensifier and its optics influences the total system resolution.

Most commonly employed 35 mm cinecameras have a rectangular usable film area of 18×24 mm. Since the image presented at the output phosphor of the intensifier is circular, different framing formats are possible; the five most common framing formats are: exact framing, mean diameter overframing, maximum horizontal overframing, subtotal overframing and total overframing (Fig. II.2) [5]. For most cardiac applications, maximum horizontal overframing is preferred; in this mode the diameter of the circle equals the horizontal size of the rectangular film area. The area of the circle is approximately equal to the area of the rectangle; all but about 12% of the available film is used for image display. It provides additional magnification without loss of horizontal field and adapts well to cardiac shape and size.

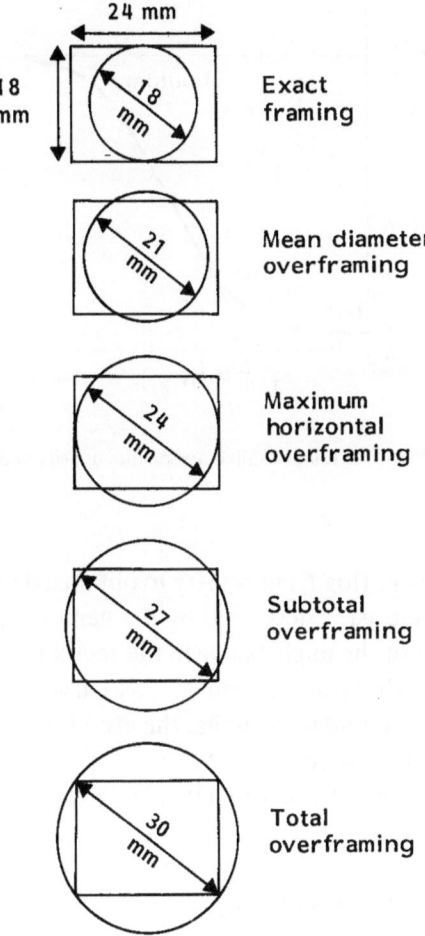

Fig. II.2. Relationship of framing method to field size reduction in cineangiography.

Cinefilm exposure

The cinefilm exposure results after processing in 'opacification' of the film proportional to the amount of absorbed light. The film must be capable of recording a wide range of radiographic densities from air to bone and contrast agents. The sensitivity, contrast and coarseness are three important parameters of a film to be used in cinematography. The response of film exposure is usually expressed graphically as a plot of film density D, defined as the logarithm of the film opacity, versus the logarithm of relative exposure E, the socalled characteristic curve; this curve is also denoted the H and D curve after Hurter and Driffield, who originally devised it in 1890. A typical D vs log E curve is shown in Figure II.3 [39]. An increase in the logarithm of relative exposure (log E) by 0.3 corresponds to a doubling of the exposure. The sensitivity of a film for X-ray cinematography

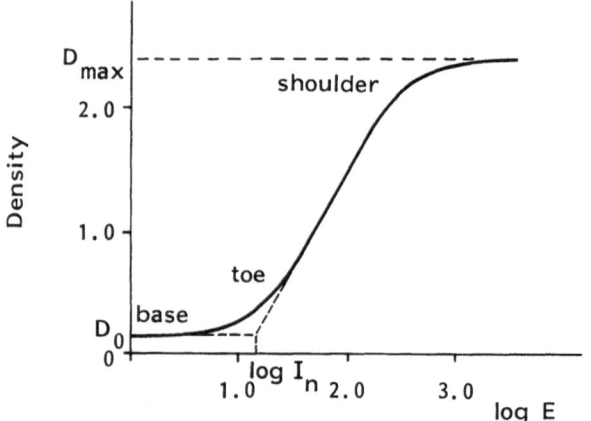

Fig. II.3. Typical curve representing relationship between film density and log exposure (D versus log E curve).

is defined by the exposure (log E) necessary to obtain a density level of 1.0 above the base level. The contrast is described by the gamma γ_F of the film, which is defined by the tangent of the angle between the rectilinear part of the curve and the abscissa. A relatively large portion of this curve is nearly linear and the radiographic exposures should be such that the useful subject contrast falls within this rectilinear part of the curve.

The relationship between the density D(p) and exposure of this linear part the curve can be written as:

$$D(p) = D_0(p) + \gamma_F \log(E(p)/I_n), \qquad (II.5)$$

where $D_0(p)$ is the base density, γ_F the gamma of the film, E(p) the exposure (= L(p) · t with t the film exposure time) and where log I_n is the inertia. I_n is the value of E, where the extension of the rectilinear part of the curve reaches the base density level.

The cinefilm should meet the following criteria:
– Wide latitude
– Low base density (anti-halo layer not colored)
– Strong basis (no damage during use)
– Allows processing at high temperature (hardened emulsion)
– High gradient (1.25–1.30) for the linear part of the D-log E curve; slowly increasing function at the foot and nodding at the shoulder
– Good spectral sensitivity for P20 phosphor
– No coarse grain
– Short drying time
– Available in rolls of 60–90 m
– Reasonable price.

Most modern types of cinefilm on milar basis satisfy these conditions; the Kodak CFE 2711 is in use in our clinic. The contrast and base density of corresponding products from Agfa Gevaert and Illford can hardly be distinguished from those of the Kodak film. More sensitive films show, in general, a larger grain.

Cinefilm processing

To obtain a good quality and reproducible angiographic cinefilm product, the complete film processing chain from film development to film projection must be a stable process. Improper cine processing and excessive quantum mottle are the two most important factors that degrade cinefilm image clarity. Successful cine processing is a meticulous, professional business, that must be given careful attention for day-to-day operation. To achieve a sufficient degree of stability, a great many modifications have been applied to commercially available products in our institute; in addition to that, a number of control procedures were set up.

In our institute the technical quality of an image is based on the average density and the contrast in the image. An image is judged optimal if the mean density equals 0.82 and the range of density levels is in between D 0.2 and D 1.8. A negative that is exposed and developed such that the density levels are within this range, still shows details in the darkest areas (does not saturate in the black portions) and differences can be visualized in the brightest areas. It will be clear that these minimal and maximal density levels can only be distinguished visually, if the density range of the cineprojector system covers this film range. In general, this requires careful selection and maintenance of the cineprojector.

Film processing unit

The processor should perform its function exactly and reproducable and provide uniform quality throughout each film's width and length. Processing variables are temperature, developer time, degree of agitation and recirculation, and replenishing rate.

Temperature control is one of the most critical variables, since it affects the rate of a chemical reaction. In general, variations of developer temperature greater than $\pm 0.3°$ C ($0.5°$ F) tend to produce a significant density variability that will degrade the value of the film. Development time is also a critical variable; film transport speed variations should not exceed $\pm 5\%$ and should be continuously variable. Agitation is of vital importance in obtaining optimal processing, particularly for film speed, contrast and uniformity. Film surfaces should be constantly bathed with recirculated, replenished and temperature-controlled developer. Finally, replenishment is necessary to maintain the concentration of the processing chemicals. A list of desirable features of a cineprocessor is given in ref. 5.

It has been our experience with a production of approximately 500 m cinefilm per day that it is a very tedious task to obtain a stable chemical process with a standard development machine. Our machine has been furnished with 4 developer baths (volume approximately 22 liters as compared to the 11 liters of the standard 2 baths machines), which results in a good temperature and chemical stability. The machine has an electronic temperature and development speed control and indication. Even with this large volume and with daily regeneration it proved to be very difficult to maintain a stable process. A regeneration system has been developed that replenishes a pre-set dose per unit-length of film. With this system deviations in the development gradient do not exceed ±0.06.

With a commercially available regeneration system, that regenerates per unit of time, it turned out to be almost impossible to achieve such small deviations. The development quality is measured with standard pre-exposed test strips of the same material (and emulsion number) as the type of cinefilm used (see Chapter VII).

The film developer to be used should meet the following criteria:
– Machine processible (high temperature, short processing time and good preservation quality)
– Regenerable
– A linear, not too steep, time-gamma curve
– A linear, not too steep, temperature-gamma curve
– A so-called leveling, fine grained developer
– Good solvability
– Standard availability
– Reasonable price.

On the basis of good time/temperature-gamma curves and good preservation qualities we have selected the Agfa Gevaert Refinal developer; the film is developed at a temperature of 26° C.

The Kodak Xomat Fixer is used as fixer, for the following reasons:
– Large supply available in general X-ray departments
– Good hardening quality
– Short fixation period.

Video system

The video display chain, including a video recording device (e.g. video disk) for replay, allows viewing of the images during catheterization and angiography. This viewing modality is used primarily for catheter placement, patient positioning and image viewing during cine filming; it can also be used for backup purposes in case of unexpected failure of the cinecamera or film development process. A high quality video system with excellent image clarity, signal regulation and minimal lag is recommended. To match the resolution of the cesium-iodide intensifier a 525 or 625 line, 10–15 MHz (−3 dB) bandwidth video camera system and monitor is desirable with a signal-to-noise ratio no less than 45 dB.

For those applications in which maximum horizontal overframing is used for the cinefilm, the video camera scanning area should also be overframed; with present day systems this is usually not the case.

Quality control

In our institute a 21 frames step wedge is pre-exposed on each film cassette with a light source of 510 nm; i.e. each of the 21 frames is exposed homogeneously over the entire area of the cineframe with differences in density between the frames of log 1.5. These 21 quality control cineframes are developed simultaneously with the patient material, so that the film development process is identical for both the calibration frames and the images of the angiographic investigation. The density frames of each film are measured and the gamma-curve plotted. A stability of ±0.06 gradient values is achieved with an electronically controlled development system.

Clinical factors in cineangiocardiography

Although a state-of-the-art X-ray system has the potential of providing highly detailed information about the dynamic morphology of the cardiac chambers and the coronary arterial system a great number of clinical precautions must be taken for obtaining high-quality arteriograms, that are suitable for precise clinical diagnosis and adequate for quantitative analysis.

To be able to quantitate the clinical quality of our routine left ventricular and coronary cineangiograms, an objective scoring system has been developed and applied to a total number of 1700 cinefilms from 900 male and 800 female patients acquired over a period of 1.5 years (40).

The clinical quality for left ventricular angiograms was determined from the following set of parameters:

| | Weighting factor | |
	yes	no
Diaphragm in image? (inspiration)	0	2
Extra systoles during injection?	0	1
Catheter not in inflow track?	0	2
Amount of contrast medium injected <12 cc/s?	0	2
Measuring area photomultiplier incorrectly positioned?	0	1
Overprojection spinal column	0	2

For the objective score of the coronary cineangiograms, the following set of parameters were assessed:

| | Weighting factor | |
	yes	no
Diaphragm in image?	0	2
Catheter not selectively positioned?	0	2
Injectant <3 cc/s?	0	2
Measuring area photomultiplier incorrectly positioned?	0	1
Overprojection spinal column?	0	2
Overall image quality poor? (Subjective interpretation)	0	1

The maximal score that could be obtained for a left ventricular or coronary angiogram was 10.

From the 1700 cinefilms an average score of 7.8 was obtained for the left ventricular cineangiograms and of 7.4 for the coronary cineangiograms. There were no statistically significant differences between the males and females.

A subjective quality of a cinefilm, ranging from 1 to 10, was given by the physician. In general, this score matched well with the technical score, except for effects from extra systoles and too little injected contrast agent.

On the basis of our extensive evaluation studies on the technical quality of cinefilms, four acquisition protocols have been defined in our institute for the different clinical studies. These are:

	Protocol 1	Protocol 2	Protocol 3	Protocol 4
Object	LV	LV	aorta	coronaries
Projection	RAO	LAO	RAO + LAO	RAO + LAO
Focus	0.4 mm^2	0.7 mm^2	0.4 mm^2	0.7 mm^2
Tube current	300 mA	700 mA	400 mA	800 mA

The selected pulse width is 4 msec; for patients with an Obesity Index (= weight − (height − 100)) less than −7 a width of 2 msec is used and for children 1 msec.

The kV of the X-ray generator is set automatically on the basis of the intensity level measured with a photomultiplier within a small measuring area (the dominant) in the center of the field of view.

For the nonstandard projections, such as Cranio-Caudal, Caudo-Cranial and Sagittal Oblique, the position of the measuring area in general does not coincide with the area of average absorption of the object. As a result, the cineframes of these projections have a lower quality than the frames of the standard projections. If the measuring area is superimposed on an area with the highest or lowest absorption, the film will be too light or too dark, respectively.

Since only a single central measuring area is built into our X-ray equipment, a high X-ray quality must be selected for these nonstandard projections, resulting in small absorption differences, small density differences and therefore a large exposure margin on the cinefilm. Much improved image quality could be obtained by measuring the maximal and minimal density levels in the entire field of view and by using that information to control the quality of the X-ray generator; however, such control system is not yet available on the commercial X-ray systems.

References

1. Fredzell G: Equipment for angiocardiography. In: Angiocardiography, Current Status and Future Developments. H Just, PH Heintzen (Eds.). Springer-Verlag, Heidelberg, 1984 (in press).
2. Marhoff P: New developments in video systems: camera tubes and storage devices. In: Angiocardiography, Current Status and Future Developments. H. Just, PH Heintzen (Eds.) Springer-Verlag, Heidelberg, 1984 (in press).
3. Nudelman S: Photoelectronic-Digital Radiology. Past, Present and Future. In: Digital Imaging in Cardiovascular Radiology. P.H. Heintzen, R. Brennecke (Eds.). Georg Thieme Verlag, Stuttgart: 1–14, 1983.
4. Heimann B, Heimann W: Fernsehkameraröhren – Eigenschaften und Anwendungen. Fernseh- und Kino-Technik 32: 341–348, 1978.
5. Friesinger GC, Adams DF, Bourassa MG, Carlsson E, Elliott LP, Gessner IH, Greenspan RH,

Grossman W, Judkins MP, Kennedy JW, Sheldon WC: Optimal resources for examination of the heart and lungs: cardiac catheterization and radiographic facilities. Circulation 68: 893A–930A, 1983.

6. Levin DC, Dunham LR, Stueve R: Causes of cine image quality deterioration in cardiac catheterization laboratories. Am J Cardiol 52: 881–886, 1983.

7. Higgins CB, Schmidt W: Direct and reflex myocardial effects of intracoronary administered contrast materials in the anesthetized and conscious dog: comparison of standard and newer contrast materials. Invest Radiol 13: 205–216, 1978.

8. Higgins CB: Effects of contrast materials on left ventricular function. Invest Radiol 15: S220–S231, 1980.

9. Higgins CB: Overview and methods used for the study of the cardiovascular actions of contrast materials. Invest Radiol 15 (Suppl): S188–S193, 1980.

10. Abrams HL: The opaque media: physiologic effects and systemic reactions. In: Coronary Arteriography: A practical approach. H.L. Abrams (Ed.). Little Brown and Company Boston: 87–110, 1983.

11. Fischer HW, Thomson KR: Contrast media in coronary arteriography: a review. Invest Radiol 13: 450–459, 1978.

12. Gerber KH, Higgins CB, Yuh Y-S, Koziol JA: Regional myocardial hemodynamic and metabolic effects of ionic and nonionic contrast media in normal and ischemic states. Circulation 65: 1307–1314, 1982.

13. Trägårdh B, Lynch PR, Vinciguerra T: Effects of Metrizamide, a new nonionic contrast medium, on cardiac function during coronary angiography in the dog. Radiology 115: 59–62, 1975.

14. Higgins CB: Effects of contrast material on the conducting system of the heart. Mechanism of action and identification of the toxic component. Radiology 124: 599–606, 1977.

15. Bentley K, Henry PD: Spasmogenic effect of angiographic dye on normal and atherosclerotic arteries. Circulation 62 (Suppl III): III–218 (Abstract), 1980.

16. Serur JR, Als AV, Miner-Green N, Paulin S: Comparative effects of three radiographic contrast agents in isolated normal and ischemic canine hearts. Invest Radiol 15: S196–S202, 1980.

17. Griggs DM Jr, Nakamura Y, Leunissen RLA, Kasparian H, Novack P: Effects of radiopaque material on phasic coronary flow and myocardial oxygen consumption. Clin Res 14: 247 (Abstract), 1966.

18. Grainger RG: Osmolality of intravascular radiological contrast media. Br J Radiol 53: 739–746, 1980.

19. Dawson P, Grainger RG, Pitfield J: The new low-osmolar contrast media: a simple guide. Clin Radiol 34: 221–226, 1983.

20. Cumberland DC: Low-osmolality contrast media in cardiac radiology. Invest Radiol 19: S301–S305, 1984.

21. Metrizamide: A non-ionic water-soluble contrast medium. Experimental and preliminary clinical investigations. Acta Radiol (Suppl) 335, Stockholm 1973.

22. Enge I, Nitter-Hauge S, Andrew E, Levorstad K: Amipaque: A new contrast medium in coronary angiography. Radiology 125: 317–322, 1977.

23. Svenson RH: Comparison of the hemodynamic effects of Hexabrix and Renografin-76 following left ventriculography and coronary arteriography. Invest Radiol 19: S333–S334, 1984.

24. Wolf GL: A double-blind clinical comparison of the electrophysiologic adverse effects of Hexabrix and Renografin-76. Invest Radiol 19: S328–S332, 1984.

25. Trägårdh B, Lynch P, Trägårdh M: Coronary angiography with diatrizoate and metrizamide. Comparison of ionic and non-ionic contrast medium effect on coronary blood flow in dogs. Acta Radiol 17: 69–80, 1976.

26. Ovitt T, Rizk G, Frech RS, Cramer R, Amplatz K: Electrocardiographic changes in selective coronary arteriography: the importance of ions. Radiology 104: 705–708, 1972.

27. Selin K, Björk L: Two new contrast media in coronary angiography. Acta Radiol Diagnosis 24:

Fasc I: 37–41, 1983.

28. Mancini GBJ, Bloomquist JN, Bhargava V, Stein JB, Lew W, Slutsky RA, Shabetai R, Higgins CB: Hemodynamic and electrocardiographic effects in man of a new nonionic contrast agent (Iohexol): advantages over standard ionic agents.Am J Cardiol 51:1218–1222, 1983.

29. Bettmann MA, Bourdillon PD, Barry WH, Brush KA, Levin DC: Contrast agents for cardiac angiography: effects of a nonionic agent vs. a standard ionic agent. Radiology 153: 583–587, 1984.

30. Wink K, Heinrich R: Frühe hämodynamische kardiovaskuläre Rückwirkungen eines ionischen niederosmolaren und eines nichtionischen Kontrastmittels. Z Kardiol 73: 628–633, 1984.

31. Brinker JA: Advantages of non-ionic contrast in coronary angiography: a multicenter double-blind randomized trial of iopamidol. J Am Coll Cardiol 5: 502 (Abstract), 1985.

32. Gertz EW, Wisneski JA, Chiu D, Akin JR, Hu C: Clinical superiority of a new nonionic contrast agent (iopamidol) for cardiac angiography. J Am Coll Cardiol 5: 250–258, 1985.

33. Bürsch J, Johs R, Heintzen P: Validity of Lambert-Beer's Law in roentgendensitometry of contrast material (Urografin) using continuous radiation. In: Roentgen-, Cine- and Video-Densitometry: Fundamentals and Applications for Blood Flow and Heart Volume Determinations. PH Heintzen (Ed.). Stuttgart, Georg Thieme Verlag: 81–84, 1971.

34. Heintzen P, Moldenhauer M: X-ray absorption by contrast material using pulsed radiation. In: Roentgen-, Cine- and Video-Densitometry: Fundamentals and Applications for Blood Flow and Heart Volume Determinations. PH Heintzen (Ed.) Stuttgart, Georg Thieme Verlag: 73–81, 1971.

35. Pochon Y, Doriot PA, Rasoamanambelo L, Rutishauser W: Densitometry by polychromatic X-ray beam. In: Angiography, Current Status and Future Developments. H Just, PH Heintzen (Eds.) Springer-Verlag, Heidelberg, 1984 (in press).

36. Hofmann FW: Image intensifiers. In: Angiocardiography, Current Status and Future Developments. H Just, PH Heintzen (Eds.) Springer-Verlag, Heidelberg, 1984 (in press).

37. Lee D, Sourkes AM, Holloway AF, Reed MH: Performance evaluation of image-intensifier tubes. Radiology 138: 455–459, 1981.

38. Shaw CG, Ergun DI, van Lysel MS, Peppler WW, Dobbins JT, Zarnstorff WC, Myerowitz PD, Swanson DK, Lasser TA, Mistretta CA, Dhanani SP, Strother CM, Crummy AB: Quantitation techniques in digital subtraction videoangiography. In: Digital Radiography. WR Brody (Ed.) SPIE, Vol 314: 121–129, 1982.

39. Farnell GC: The relationship between density and exposure. In: The Theory of the Photographic Process. TH James (Ed.). The MacMillan Company, New York.

40. Boer, A den: Image quality of cardiological X-ray cineproducts. Internal Report, Thoraxcenter, Erasmus University and University Hospital Dijkzigt, Rotterdam, The Netherlands, 1978.

62

III. Cardiovascular Angiography Analysis System

Introduction

In Chapter I the limitations of the conventional visual evaluation of the severity of coronary obstructions from 35 mm cineangiograms in terms of the relatively large inter- and intraobserver variations have been documented. Moreover, by this technique the degree of luminal narrowing can only be determined in terms of percentage diameter (%-D) narrowing assessed from one or more views. To evaluate the efficacy of modern therapeutic procedures in the catheterization laboratory [1–3], the effects of vasoactive drugs [4, 5], as well as the effects of short- and long-terms interventions on the regression or progression of coronary artery disease [6–8], an objective and reproducible technique for the assessment of coronary atherosclerosis is seriously needed. Such a technique should at least provide absolute measurements on the minimal diameter and extent of the obstructions, as well as on mean luminal diameters of nonobstructed coronary segments.

In this chapter the basic principles of a new computerized analysis procedure for coronary arterial segments will be presented. These software developments have been carried out on the prototype Cardiovascular Angiography Analysis System (CAAS) at the Thoraxcenter. A commercial version of this CAAS is now available from Pie Data Medical B.V., Maastricht, the Netherlands.

At first the architecture of the Thoraxcenter CAAS will be described, followed by a detailed description of the contour detection and contour analysis procedures with the various options. Finally, the architecture of the Pie Data CAAS will be presented, followed by an explanation of the differences in the data acquisition procedure between the two CAAS systems. The results of a validation study of this technique, as well as the overall short-, medium- and long-term variabilities in the assessment of arterial dimensions from repeated coronary angiographies and computer analyses are presented in Chapter V.

Architecture Thoraxcenter CAAS

The procedures for quantitative analysis of coronary arterial segments have been implemented on the computer (PDP 11/44) based Cardiovascular Angiography Analysis System (CAAS), which runs under the multi-user RSX-11M Operating System (version 4.1) [9–17]. A block diagram of the system is given in Figure III.1.

To analyze a coronary arterial segment in a selected cineframe, the cinefilm is mounted on a specially constructed cine-video converter. The image is projected onto the target of a high resolution video camera via a drum with six different lens systems, which allow for the selection of six different optical magnifications. The video camera is attached to a movable x-y stage, so that any area of interest in the cineframe can be selected with the appropriate manification factor. The center square of the resulting analog video image is digitized in real time in matrix size of 512×512 picture elements (pixels) with a VTE* Digitizer and stored in a display memory. The sampling frequency of the analog-to-digital (A/D) converter equals 15 MHz, which results in square pixels; both the even and odd lines of the 2:1 interlaced video system are utilized. The grey scale resolution of the digital data is 256 levels (8 bits). A recursive digitizing procedure over 8 video frames is used to improve the signal/noise ratio. The digitized video image is displayed on a video monitor via a digital-to-analog (D/A) converter. For purposes of contour detec-

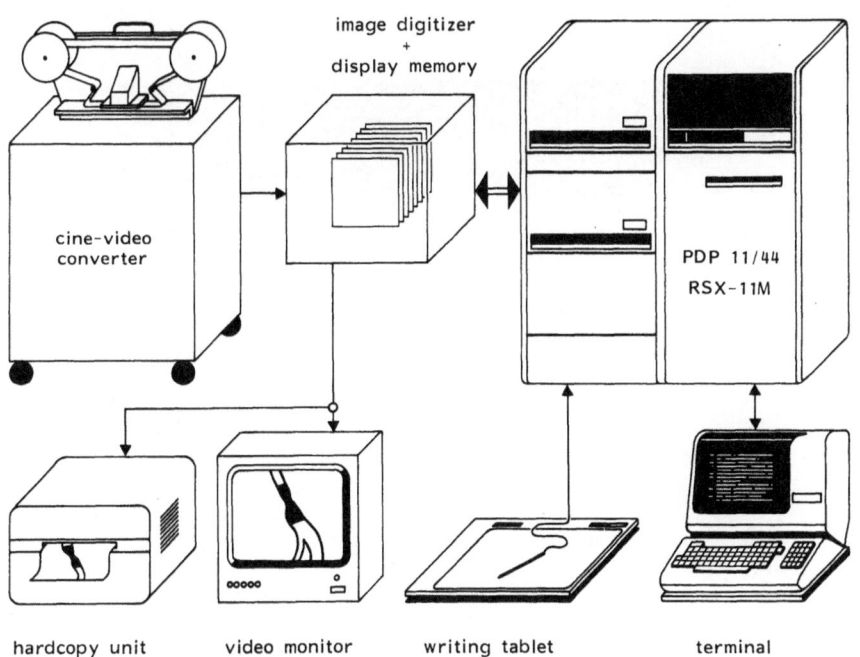

image digitizer
+
display memory

cine-video
converter

PDP 11/44
RSX-11M

hardcopy unit   video monitor   writing tablet   terminal

Fig. III.1. Block diagram of the Cardiovascular Angiography Analysis System.

* VTE Digitalvideo, Braunschweig, Germany.

64

tion, digital image data encompassing a user-selected arterial or catheter segment can be sent to the PDP 11/44 minicomputer for the actual processing of that segment. At several crucial points in the contour detection and analysis procedures user-interaction is possible by means of a writing tablet. A Video Imager is connected to the video monitor for image documentation purposes.

To analyze quantitatively the dimensions of a coronary arterial segment, the following steps are to be performed: (1) computation of the calibration factor by means of the contrast catheter displayed in the image; (2) contour detection of the arterial segment; (3) computation of the diameter function from the detected and pincushion corrected contour positions; (4) if a coronary obstruction is present in the arterial segment, determination of its severity in terms of absolute and relative dimensional parameters, as well as the computation of the pressure gradient over the obstruction at different flows; and (5) if the arterial segment shows no focal obstruction, determination of the mean diameters over one or more user-defined portions of this segment. The different steps will be described in some more detail hereafter using the example of Figure III.2. This image shows a coronary cineangiogram with a focal obstruction in the proximal segment of the left anterior descending (LAD)-artery, digitized in a 512×512 matrix at the optical magnification of 1.

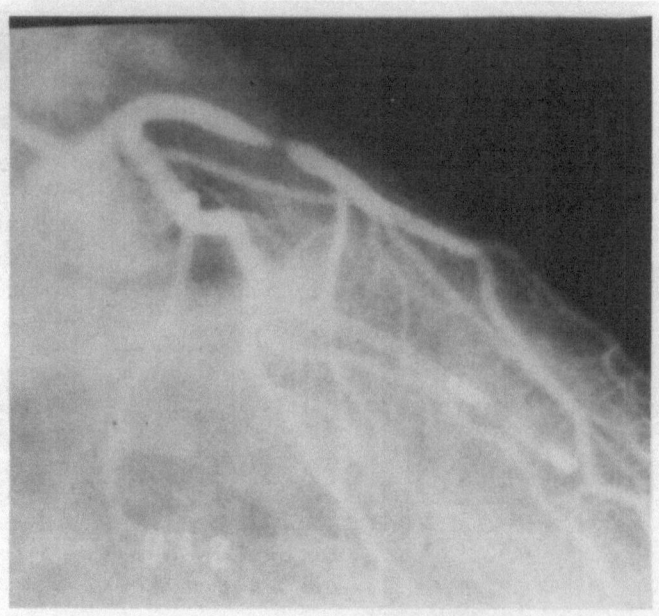

Fig. III.2. Example of left coronary system digitized in a 512×512 matrix at optical magnification of 1.

Cine-video converter

The specially constructed cine-video converter consists of a standard 35 mm film transport mechanism mounted on top of a cabinet (Fig. III. 3). The image is projected downwards into the cabinet onto the target of a 1.5″ vidicon tube of a high resolution video camera via a drum with six different lens systems, which allow for the selection of the desired optical magnification factor from $\frac{1}{\sqrt{2}}$: 1 to 4 : 1 in multiplicative steps of $\sqrt{2}$. Magnification of 1 : 1 is defined such that the projected image of a standard cineframe with dimensions 24×18 mm precisely fills the scanning area of the video camera. The optical chain has been developed such that a homogeneous light response over the scanning area is obtained. The video camera is mounted on a movable x-y stage, so that any area of interest in the cineframe can be selected with the appropriate magnification factor. An electronic circuit controls the amount of light from the halogen projection bulb such that an optimal video signal is obtained independent of the opacity of the cineframe. The cinefilm transport, the selection of the desired optical magnifica-

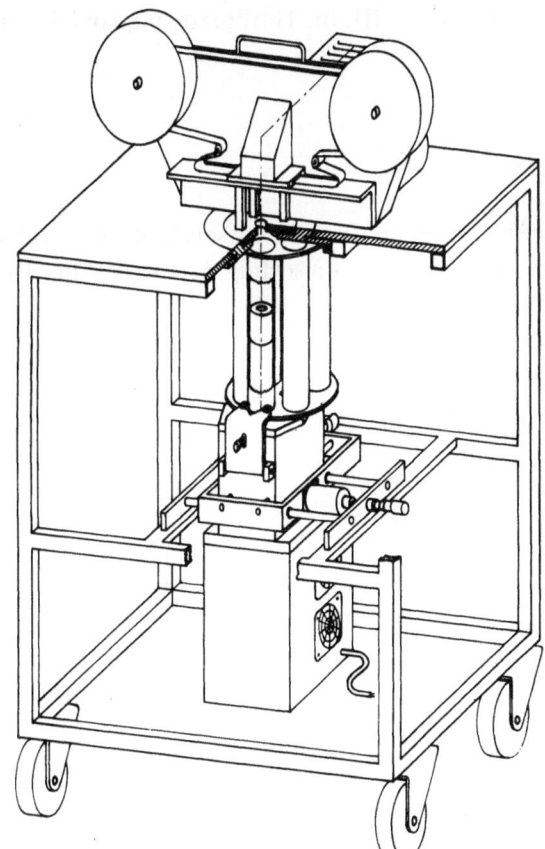

Fig. III.3. Drawing of specially constructed cine-video converter.

66

tion as well as the x-y positioning of the video camera are all under control of the user through the PDP 11/44 host computer.

The improvement in the optical response of this cine-video converter as compared to a conventional set-up, consisting of a standard cinefilm projector (Tagarno 35CX), which was modified with a high resolution transparent screen through which part of the image could be projected onto the target of a video camera, can be clearly demonstrated with the following experiment. A 35 mm cineframe with homogeneous density over the entire field was digitized with both conversion systems. A digitization matrix, defined by 504 horizontal rows and 672 vertical columns, was subdivided into matrices of size 28 × 28. This results in 18 of these submatrices in the vertical direction and 24 in the horizontal direction. For each submatrix the average brightness value of the 28 × 28 pixels was computed and the results displayed in a pseudo three-dimensional representation. Figure III.4a shows the results for the conventional film projection system. The length of a particular bar represents the average brightness level for the corresponding area of 28 × 28 pixels. A hot spot in the center of the image from the light source can be clearly distinguished. This shows that the optical transfer function for this part of the total image chain is rather inhomogeneous. The results for the new cine-video converter are shown in Fig. III.4b. The greatly improved optical response is very clear.

Calibration procedure

Calibration of the diameter data of the vessels in absolute values (mm) is achieved by using the contrast catheter as a scaling device. To this end, a region from the

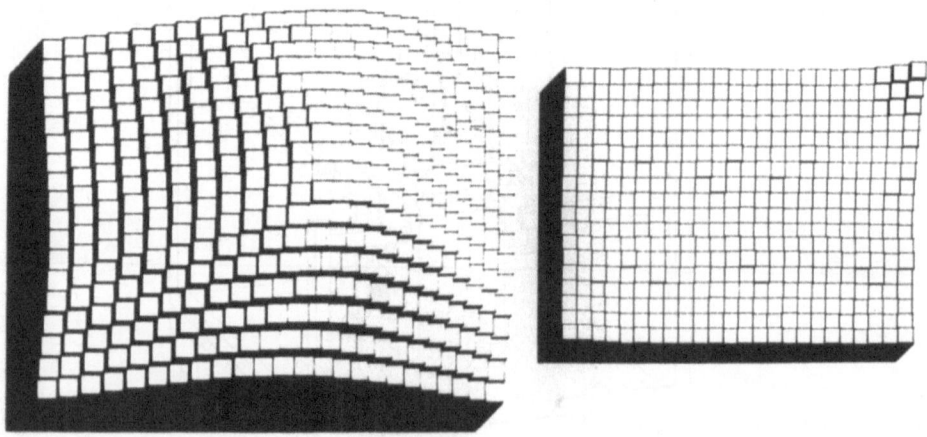

Fig. III.4. Pseudo three-dimensional representation of the optical response of the standard cineprojector-transparent screen-video camera set up (Fig. III.4, left panel) and the cine-video converter (Fig. III.4, right panel).

35 mm cineframe encompassing the catheter is optically magnified with a magnification factor of $2\sqrt{2} : 1$ and digitized. As a next step, the user indicates two positions within the displayed catheter, such that the straight line connecting these positions approximate the local centerline. Subsequently, the contours of this part of the projected catheter are detected in a similar way as will be described for an arterial segment. A priori information is included in the iterative edge detection procedure, based on the fact that the selected part of the catheter is the projection of a circle-cylindrical structure. The positions are detected along the outer edge of the contrast filled catheter. Finally, the contour data are corrected for the pincushion distortion in the image, as will be described in the following section. Fig. III.5 shows the detected contours along a user-defined portion of the contrast catheter of Fig. III.2.

From the detected and corrected contour positions a mean diameter value is determined in pixels, so that the calibration factor in mm/pixel can be computed from the known size of the catheter.

For documentation purposes the part of the catheter used for calibration is displayed in the 1:1 digitized cineframe. Fig. III.6 shows the superimposed square at the catheter; the sequence number of the cineframe that was used for the calibration is also displayed, as well as the name and extension number of the computer file where all the quantitative data for this particular analysis are stored.

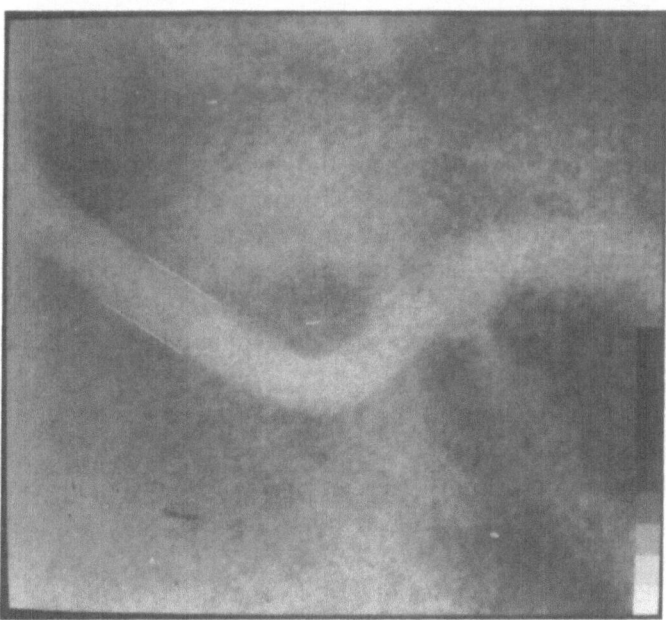

Fig. III.5. Detected contours along a user-defined portion of the contrast catheter.

68

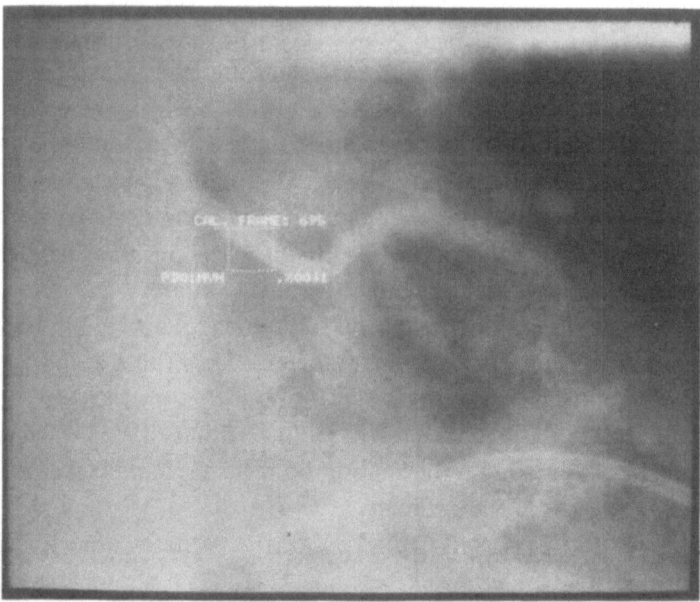

Fig. III.6. Following the catheter calibration procedure a square is superimposed in the 1:1 digitized cineframe to define the analyzed portion of the catheter.

Pincushion correction

It is well known that particularly the older types of image intensifiers introduce a geometric distortion, the pincushion distortion. This results in a position dependent magnification of an object. These differences need to be corrected for if: (1) absolute diameter measurements are to be derived from the coronary cineangiograms; and (2) relative obstruction measurements are to be derived with reference and/or obstruction positions outside of the central region of the image. Since a high accuracy video camera with minimal geometric distortion is used in the cine-video converter, it is assumed that the total nonlinear distortion present in the video image originates from the image intensifier, i.e. the video system introduces no additional distortion. To correct the contour data, the following procedure has been implemented.

Since the distortion cannot be described by a simple analytical function, a cineframe of a cm-grid placed against the input screen of the image intensifier is used to assess the distortion. The cm-grid consists of copper wires embedded in a perspex tablet in x and y directions at distances of exactly 1 cm. A software algorithm has been developed that allows for the fully automated detection of the intersections of the wires in the 1:1 projected cineframe. Under the assumption that the 1 cm square in the center of the cineframe is not distorted, for each detected intersection a corresponding corrected position can be determined. Next, for each intersection position a correction vector is determined on the basis of the actual and calculated ideal positions. For a given point in the image which does not coincide with one of the displayed intersection positions, a correction vector can be determined by means of a bilinear interpolation between the correction vectors of the four neighboring intersection points. Fig. III.7 shows a cm-grid with the correction vectors for each intersection position superimposed. The reference square is indicated by the three markers in the center of the image.

Since the x, y positions of the video camera stage are precisely known, as well as the precise different optical magnifications, these correction data can be applied to the detected contour positions of the catheter and of an arterial segment at the corresponding magnifications. In this way each point of the detected contours can be corrected for the pincushion distortion.

For each image intensifier installed in a catheterization laboratory, the corresponding correction vectors can be stored on computer disk for retrieval at the time of analysis of a cinefilm obtained with that particular image intensifier. Computation of the correction vectors, therefore, is only necessary at regular intervals, for example, each 6 months, or immediately following the installation of a new image intensifier.

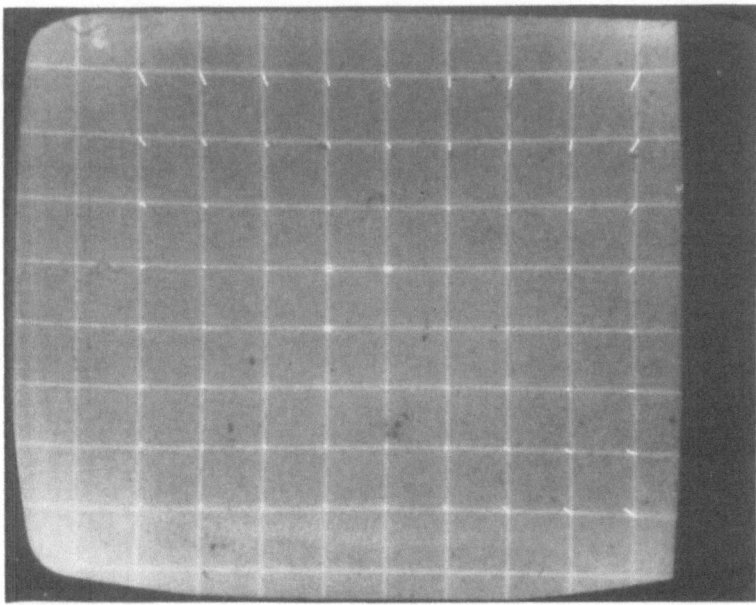

Fig. III.7. Cm-grid with the correction vectors for each intersection point superimposed. The three markers in the center of the image denote the reference square.

Contour detection of arterial segment

Following the calibration procedure, the cine-video converter returns to the initial state with the original image (1:1 magnification) displayed on the video monitor. For the quantitative analysis of a coronary segment a magnification factor of 2:1 is usually chosen. With the writing tablet the user indicates the region encompassing the selected arterial segment to be magnified. Figure. III.8 shows this particular step in the analysis procedure. The + sign near the obstruction in the proximal part of the LAD denotes the center position of the region to be magnified optically, while the four corners of this region are defined by the dots. An administrative data block has been superimposed in the upper portion of the image; the different items will be filled in at a later stage (see Figures III.9 and III.14).

The center coordinates of the selected region are sent to the cine-video converter, the x-y stage moves towards the defined center position and the appropriate lens is selected. The optically magnified image is digitized, stored in an image memory and displayed on the video monitor.

The contour detection procedure requires the user to indicate a number of center positions in the arterial segment to be analyzed (Fig. III.9). These center positions do not need to coincide with the true centerline of the artery; the only requirement is that the interpolated straight lines remain within the arterial

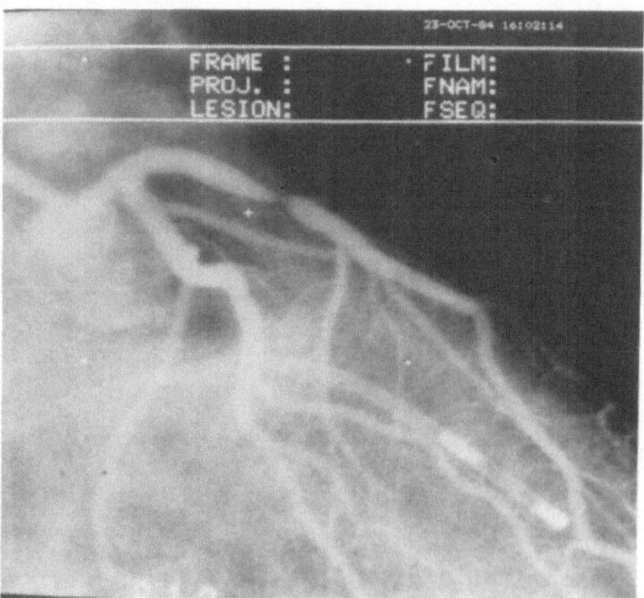

Fig. III.8. Cineframe with center position (+) and corners (.) of region to be magnified optically with factor of two.

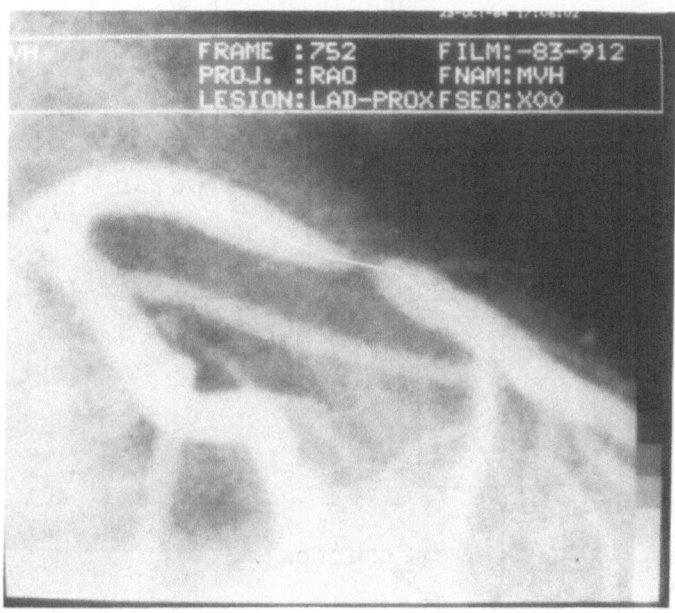

Fig. III.9. Optically magnified region of figure III.8 encompassing the segment of the proximal LAD-artery to be analyzed and the user-defined centerline.

boundaries. For the purpose of standardized analysis of coronary segments, the beginning and end points of the centerline should always coincide with clearly recognizable branch points of that particular segment, such as those defined by the American Heart Association [18].

A smooth continuous curve, the tentative centerline, is generated through these points by means of an interpolation and smoothing procedure. The centerline determines regions of interest of size 96×96 pixels encompassing the arterial segment to be transferred to the host computer for subsequent analysis (Fig. III.10). The first position of the centerline defines the first region, while subsequent regions are defined by the local direction of the centerline and the maximally allowed width of the artery. To decrease spatial fluctuations due to quantum noise the digital data are smoothed spatially with a 5×5 median filter. The resulting brightness data are subsequently transformed logarithmically; as a result, image contrast in the bright parts of the image (inside the vessels) is compressed and in the dark parts (near the boundaries) stretched. Also, the transformed data more closely agree now with the irradiated object thicknesses within the arterial segments.

Contours of the arterial segment are determined on the basis of the weighted sum of first and second derivative functions applied to the digitized brightness information using minimal cost criteria.

The basic principles of the edge detection technique can be clarified with Fig.

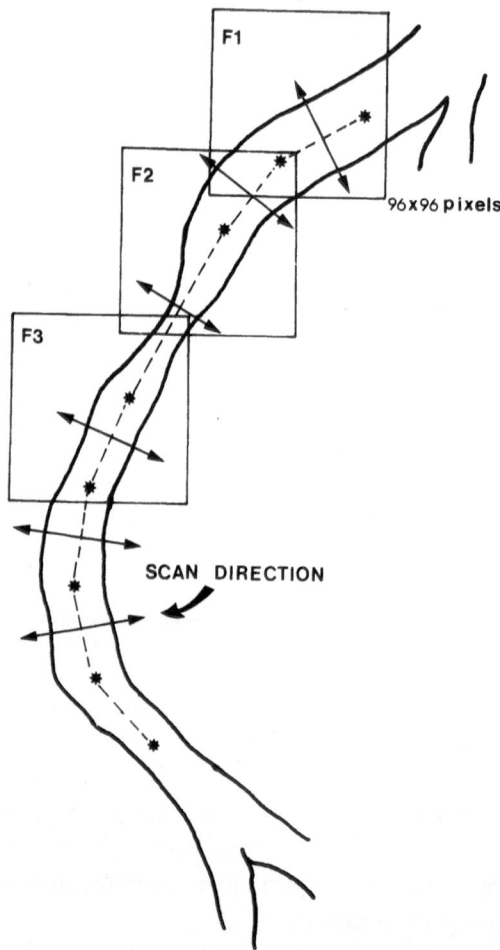

F1

96×96 pixels

F2

F3

SCAN DIRECTION

Fig. III.10. This drawing of a coronary arterial segment illustrates the definition of the regions of interest to be transferred to the host computer. The user indicated the centerline positions (*).

III.11. Fig. III.11a shows the overlapping regions of interest of size 96 × 96 pixels along an Obtuse Marginal branch, which are transferred to the host processor for edge detection purposes. In Figure III.11b a pseudo three-dimensional representation of the digitized brightness information within the region of interest at the location of the obstruction is presented; the brightness information is plotted vertically. The x- and y-directions correspond with the horizontal (from left to right) and the vertical (from top to bottom) directions, respectively in Fig. III.11a. The coronary artery can be recognized as a mountain ridge with a dip at the position of the obstruction. The brightness profile along one particular scanline within this region, perpendicular to the local centerline direction, is plotted in Fig. III.11c. By computing the weighted sum of the first and second derivative values for each point along this scanline, the lower function is obtained. From this example it is clear that the positions with maximal derivative values left and right

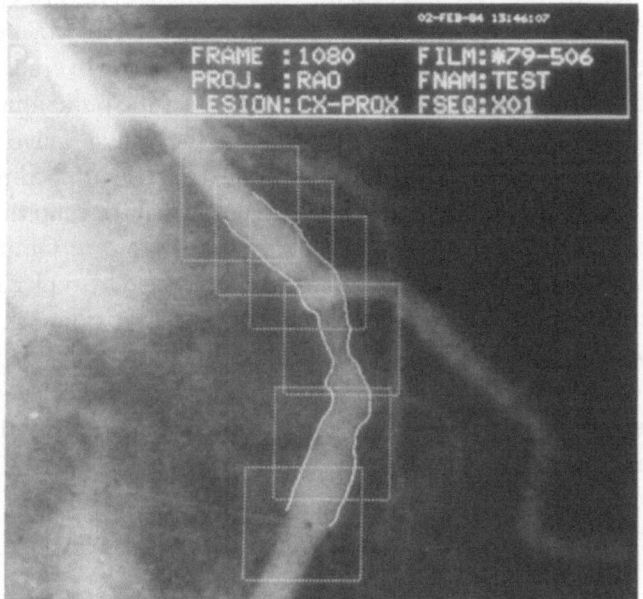

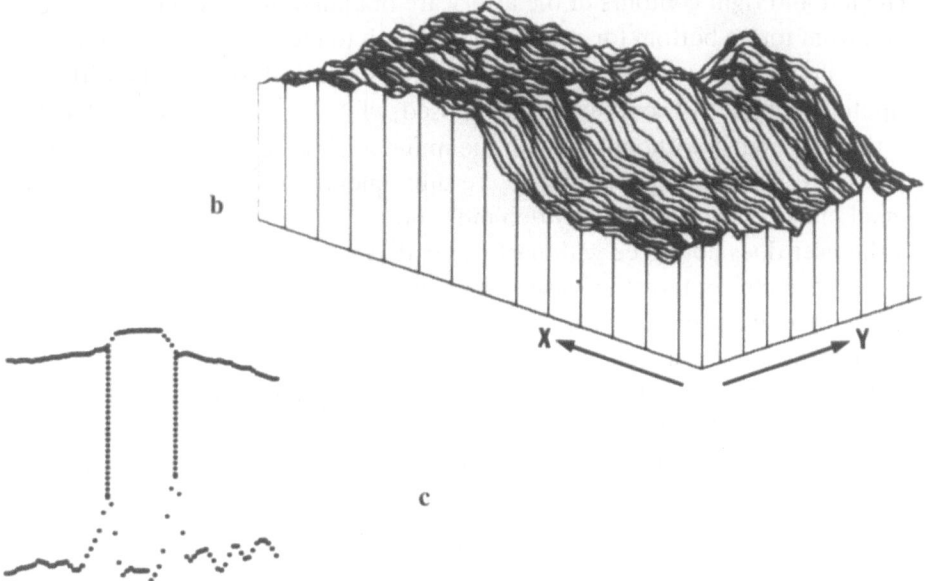

Fig. III.11. Basic principles edge detection technique. Fig. III.11a shows the overlapping regions of interest of size 96 × 96 pixels along the Obtuse Marginal branch, which are transferred to the host processor for edge detection purposes. In Fig. III.11b the digitized brightness information within the region at the site of the obstruction is presented in a pseudo three-dimensional manner. The brightness profile (upper curve) along one particular scanline and the derivative function (lower curve) are shown in Fig. III.11c.

of the center position correspond with the edge positions of the artery. This figure is only intended to illustrate the edge detection process. In practice, the edge positions are not determined per individual scanline, but an overall contour path is searched for through all the derivative functions of the sequential scanlines.

In the implemeted edge detection procedure, the digital image data are re-sampled along the scanlines perpendicular to the local centerline directions. The resampled data are stored in a matrix g in such a way that the centerline forms the center column of this matrix. The resampled matrix for the Obtuse Marginal branch is given in Fig. III.12a. These data are smoothed by replacing each row with the average of this row and its two neighboring rows. For each point of the matrix the one-dimensional gradient (first difference) of the intensity values as well as the change in this gradient (second difference) are calculated. A cost function C is defined as the inverse of the weighted sum of the gradient and the gradient-change values, g' and g'', respectively:

$$C = (\alpha g' + (1-\alpha)g'') \qquad\qquad (III.1)$$

with α being the weighting factor; a value of $\alpha = 0.5$ has been derived at em-perically.

The left and right contours of the artery are obtained by searching in the cost matrix from top to bottom for a minimal cost path to the left and the right of the center column, respectively. Fig. III.12b gives the transformed data with the computed minimal cost contours superimposed, while Fig. III.12c and Fig. III.12d give the cost matrix without and with the minimal cost contours superimposed, respectively. These contour positions are subsequently transformed back to the original image displayed on the video monitor.

If the user does not agree with part of the detected contours, these positions may be corrected interactively with the writing tablet. Since the centerline positions were initially defined by the user, the contour positions may be slightly dependent on the given centerline positions, particularly at sections with high curvature. To minimize this influence as much as possible, a two step iterative contour detection algorithm has been implemented. To this end, a new centerline is computed defined by the midline of the initially detected and possibly corrected contours. The digital data are resampled again and the minimum cost contour detection algorithm is applied to the new data. For those locations along the contours where the user corrected the initially detected contour positions, a narrow expectation window is defined in the cost matrix. As a result of this precaution, in most cases the contour will now follow the desired path at these locations. However, if the user is still not completely satisfied with the detected contours, manual corrections can be applied again at this stage. The computer registers for both the left- and right- hand contours, the lengths of the arterial segments that were manually corrected after the second iteration, expressed as percentages of the total lengths of the analyzed contour sides. In addition to these

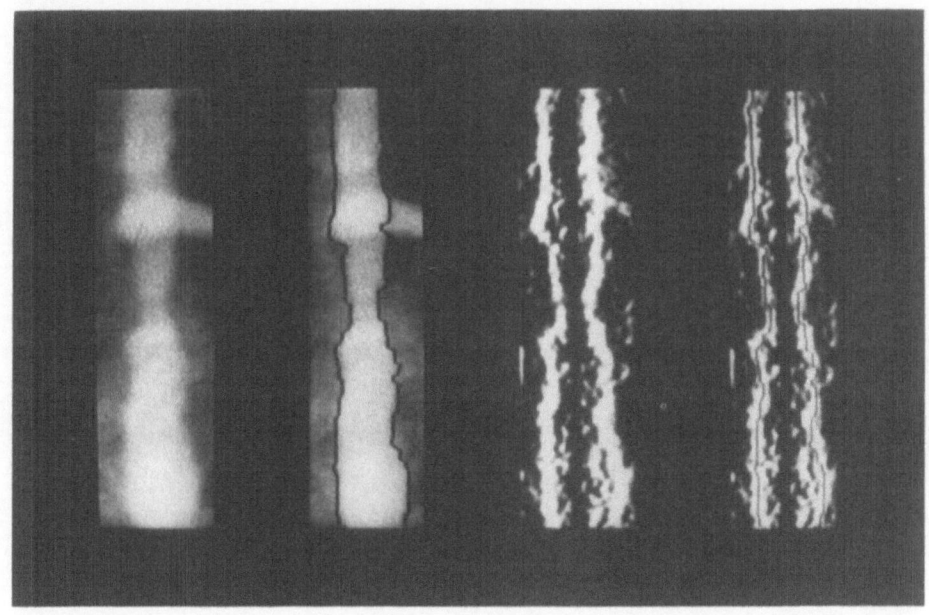

Fig. III.12. Minimal cost contour detection procedure ((a)–(d) from left to right)
(a) Transformed intensity matrix.
(b) Transformed intensity matrix with contours superimposed.
(c) Cost matrix.
(d) Cost matrix with contours superimposed.

values, the mean percentage length of the correction paths for the left- and right-hand contours is provided on the computer printout. Finally, a smoothing procedure is applied to each of the contours, which consists of a least-squared error first degree polynomial fit through the five nearest points on each side of the contour point under consideration. Fig. III.13 shows the retransformed and smoothed contours for the proximal segment of the LAD artery. Before clinically relevant parameters are derived, the contour positions are corrected for the pincushion distortion as described above.

Contour analysis

As a first step, roughness measures are computed for the left and right contour sides. The roughness value R of a particular contour side is defined by the square root of the differences in x,y-coordinates squared between the actual contour and a heavily filtered version of it summed over all the individual contour positions for that contour side; in formula:

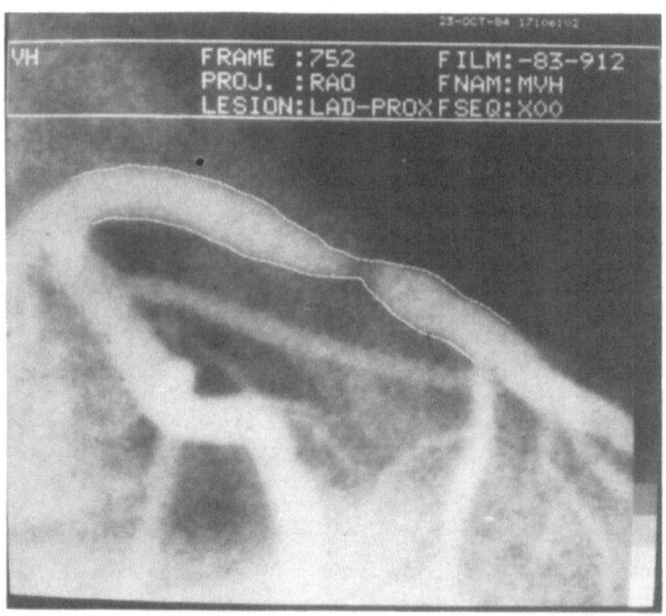

Fig. III.13. Original image of Fig. III.9 with detected contours superimposed.

$$R = \sqrt{\sum_{i=1}^{N} [(x_i - xF_i)^2 + (y_i - yF_i)^2]}, \tag{III.2}$$

where N represents the number of contour positions, (x_i, y_i) the x, y-coordinates of the actual contour and (xF_i, yF_i) the x, y-coordinates of the filtered contour.

These roughness values are measures for the irregularities of the detected luminal contours, i.e. measures for diffuse atherosclerosis. In addition to the edge roughness values for the left- and right-hand contours, a mean edge roughness is computed. For the contours of Fig. III.13 the following roughness data were computed:

Edge roughness right-hand contour : 0.18 mm
Edge roughness left-hand contour : 0.15 mm
Mean edge roughness : 0.16 mm

Next, subsegmental data are computed for the analyzed arterial segment. To this end, the entire segment is divided into an integer number of subsegments, with lengths of approximately 5 mm. In each subsegment, the minimum, maximum and mean diameter values, as well as the standard deviation are calculated. For the contours of figure III.13 the following subsegmental data were computed:

	Subsegments					
	1	2	3	4	5	6
Minimum diam	3.56	3.82	3.19	1.29	1.29	3.72
Maximum diam	3.94	4.14	4.24	3.16	4.22	4.22
Mean diam	3.73	3.96	3.92	2.30	2.94	3.93
Standard deviation	0.12	0.09	0.35	0.61	1.02	0.16

Finally, before any dimensional data are computed, a curvature analysis of the entire segment is performed, resulting in a curvature value, expressed in units. For the proximal LAD-segment a curvature value of 22.31 units was obtained. The clinical relevance of this parameter has not been established at this point.

Assessment severity of coronary obstruction

From the contours of the arterial segment corrected for pincushion distortion the diameter function $D(i)$, calibrated in absolute mm, is determined by computing the distances between corresponding contour points to the left and right of the centerline. From the minimal value D_m of the diameter function and the mean diameter value D_r at a user-indicated reference position, the percentage diameter reduction is computed as:

$$\%\text{-D stenosis} = (1 - \frac{D_m}{D_r}) \cdot 100\%. \tag{III.3}$$

The position with minimal diameter value is detected automatically, but can be changed interactively by the user if more than one focal obstruction is to be processed within the arterial segment. The mean diameter D_r is computed as the average of 11 diameter values in a symmetric region with center at the user-defined reference position. For the example of figure III.13 the final result of the procedure for the obstruction in the proximal-LAD segment is illustrated in figure III.14. For this example the following quantitative measurements were obtained:

Segmental location of obstruction	:	604
Extent obstruction	:	11.89 mm
Reference diameter	:	3.92 mm
Obstruction diameter	:	1.29 mm
Reference area	:	12.10 mm²
Obstruction area	:	1.31 mm²
Diameter stenosis	:	67%
Area stenosis	:	89%

The segmental location of an obstruction is a four-digit number with the first two digits describing the actual arterial segment according to the definitions by the American Heart Association [18], and the last two digits the number of the subsegment, in which the minimal diameter value is measured. In this example, the number 6 refers to the proximal segment of the LAD-artery, and the number 04 means that the minimal obstruction diameter was measured between approximately 1.5 and 2.0 cm from the starting point of the proximal segment of the LAD. The percentage area-reduction (% A-sten) was computed assuming circular cross sections for the obstruction and reference positions.

The diameter function is shown in the lower portion of the image; the calibra-

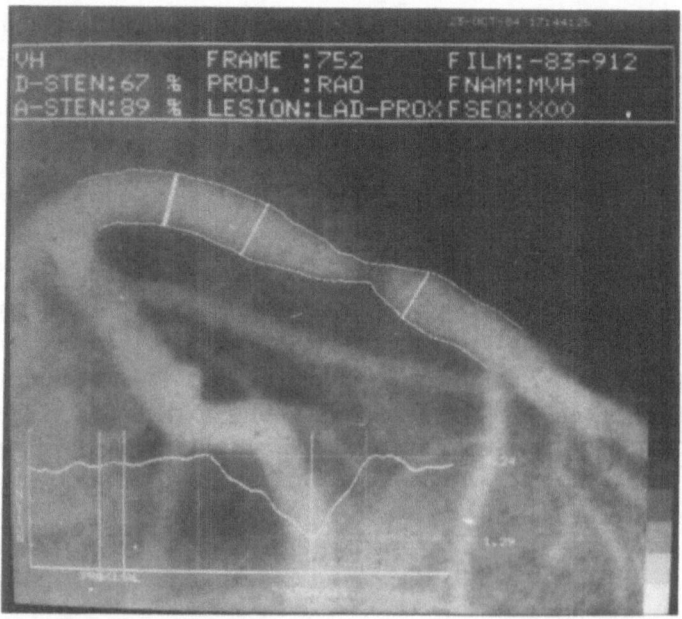

Fig. III.14. Computer output of analyzed lesion. A percentage diameter reduction of 67% with respect to the user-defined reference region was found.

ted diameter values in mm are plotted along the ordinate and the centerline positions from the proximal to the distal part along the abscissa. The reference position was defined proximal of the obstructive lesion as indicated in the diameter function by the shaded vertical bar. The central reference position is also marked in the artery by a straight line connecting the opposing contour sides.

The extent of the obstruction is determined from the diameter function $D(i)$ on the basis of curvature analysis and expressed in mm [12]. This procedure is nearly identical to the one described by Rosenfeld [19]. The extent of the stenotic lesion is indicated in the diameter function by the two dotted lines and in the arterial segment by the two lines on each side of the obstruction connecting opposite contours. The proximal and distal boundaries of the obstruction may be changed interactively.

It is clear from the above that the computed percentage diameter narrowing of an obstruction may depend heavily on the selected reference position. In arteries with a focal obstructive lesion and a clearly normal proximal arterial segment, the choice of the reference region is straightforward and simple. However, in cases where the proximal part of the arterial segment shows combinations of stenotic and ectatic areas, the choice may be very difficult. To minimize these variations, we have implemented an alternative method to express the severity of a coronary obstruction, which is not dependent on a user-defined reference region. This technique is denoted interpolated $\% - D$ stenosis measurement; details have been published elsewhere [12].

The basic idea behind this technique is the computer estimation of the original diameter values over the obstructive region (assuming there was no coronary disease present) based on the diameter function [20]. To this end, a first degree least squares polynomial is determined through all the diameter values outside of the obstructive region; this polynomial allows the vessel to taper. Next, the polynomial is translated upwards until 80 percent of the diameter values are below the polynomial. The resulting polynomial values are then assumed to be a measure for the normal size of the artery at the corresponding points; this polynomial function is denoted reference diameter function. For the interpolated technique with an assumed first degree polynomial reference diameter function to be valid, it is again important, that selected arterial segments do not exceed the boundaries of the recommended standardized coronary segments [18]. The size of a parent vessel beyond one or more major branches changes according to the formula [21]:

$$(D_{\text{Parent}})^3 = (D_{\text{Branch 1}})^3 + (D_{\text{Branch 2}})^3 + (D_{\text{Branch 3}})^3 + \ldots \qquad \text{(III.4)}$$

On the basis of the proximal and distal centerline segments and the reference diameter function, the reference contours over the obstructive region are determined in the following way. Vessel midpoints for the proximal and distal positions are found by averaging the coordinates of the left and right contour

positions. For the obstructive region the vessel midpoints are obtained by interpolation between the proximal and distal vessel midpoints with a second degree
polynomial. The left and right reference contours are then obtained by centering
the reference diameter value for that position perpendicular to the local direction
of the midline in each point. The resulting reference contours for the arterial
segment of Fig. III.13 are presented in Fig. III.15. Following this approach the
reference diameter is taken as the value of the reference diameter function at the
minimal position of the obstruction. The interpolated percentage diameter stenosis is then computed by comparing the minimal diameter value at the obstruction with the corresponding value of the reference diameter value.

The difference in area between the estimated boundaries and the detected
contours is a measure for the 'atherosclerotic plaque', expressed in mm^2; this area
has been marked in Fig. III.15. In addition, this interpolated technique allows the
assessment of the symmetry of the lesion in a given view with respect to its
centerline. The symmetry measure is given as a value between 0 and 1, with 1
representing a concentric lesion and 0 the most severe case of asymmetry or
eccentricity.

For the example of Fig. III.15 the following quantitative measurements were
obtained:

Segmental location of obstruction	:	604
Extent obstruction	:	11.89 mm
Reference diameter	:	4.12 mm
Obstruction diameter	:	1.29 mm
Reference area	:	13.36 mm^2
Obstruction area	:	1.31 mm^2
Area plaque	:	16.79 mm^2
Symmetry measure	:	0.89
Diameter stenosis	:	69%
Area stenosis	:	90%

Mean diameter arterial segment

To measure the mean diameter in mm over an arterial segment, the user indicates
the starting and end positions of this segment. Arterial branch points are often
used for these segmental boundaries. The length of the analyzed segment plus the
standard deviation of the diameter measurements with respect to the mean
diameter value are also provided. An example for the proximal part of the LAD-
segment is given in Fig. III.16. For this particular example, the following parameters were computed:

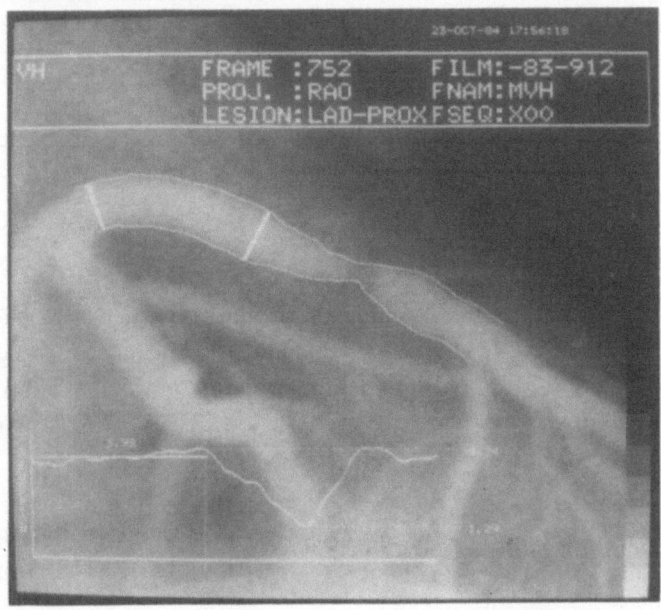

Fig. III.15. The detected contours together with the reference contours for the lesion of Fig. III.13. An interpolated percentage diameter reduction of 69% resulted.

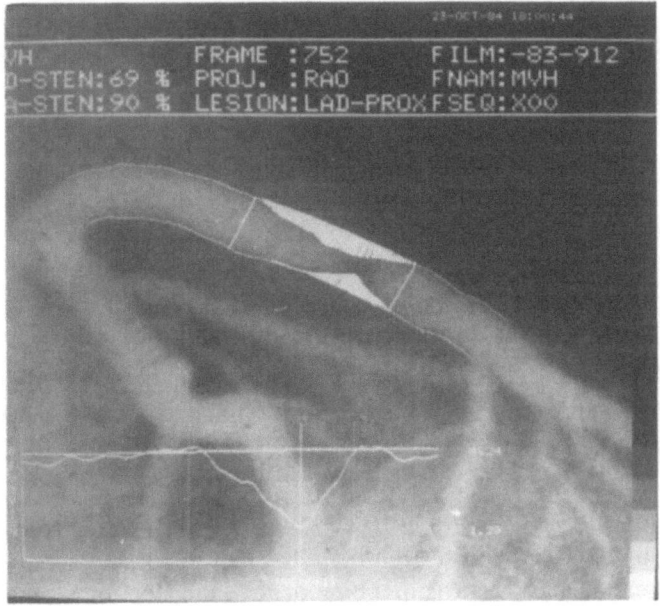

Fig. III.16. For the proximal 12 mm of the analyzed segment a mean diameter of 3.93 mm was found.

Mean diameter	:	3.93 mm
Length segment	:	12.26 mm
Standard deviation	:	0.19 mm

Hemodynamic parameters coronary obstruction

On the basis of the available contour data of a coronary obstruction, the following hemodynamic parameters are computed: Poisseuille resistance, turbulent resistance at flows of 1, 2 and 3 ml/sec, the resulting pressure gradients and finally the inflow and outflow angles of the obstructive region [22–27]. These parameters have been defined as follows:

$$\text{Poisseuille resistance Rpois} = \frac{Cl \cdot (\text{extent obstruction})}{(\text{obstruction area})^2} \left[\frac{mmHg \cdot sec}{ml}\right],$$

where $Cl = 8 \cdot \pi \cdot$ (blood viscosity), with blood viscosity = 0.03 [g/cm · sec].

$$\text{Turbulent resistance Rturb} = C2 \cdot \left(\frac{1}{\text{obstruction area}} - \frac{1}{\text{normal distal area}}\right)^2 \left[\frac{mmHg \cdot sec^2}{ml^2}\right],$$

where $C2 = \frac{\text{blood density}}{0.266}$ with blood density $\approx 1.0 [g/cm^3]$.

The theoretical pressure gradient is then computed by:

$$\text{Pgrad} = Q(\text{Rpois} + Q \cdot \text{Rturb})$$

with Q the mean coronary blood flow [ml/sec].

To be able to compare these theoretical values with the pressure values as measured with a tipmanometer proximal and distal of an obstruction during the catheterization, we have modified the pressure gradient formulas by correcting the obstruction cross-sectional area for the cross section of the catheter; a typical value for such cross section is $0.64 mm^2$ [28].

The inflow angle of a coronary obstruction is defined by the average slope of the diameter function over the section bounded by the position of the minimal obstruction diameter and the proximal boundary of the stenotic segment. Likewise, the outflow angle is defined by the average slope of the diameter function between the position of the minimum obstruction diameter and the distal boundary of the stenotic segment. For the LAD obstruction used in this chapter for demonstration purposes the following hemodynamic values were obtained:

Flow (ml/sec)	Not corrected for catheter cross section			Corrected for catheter cross section (0.64 mm²)		
	Rpois	Rturb	Pgrad (mmHg)	Rpois	Rturb	Pgrad (mmHg)
1	5.26	1.77	7.03	20.20	7.60	27.81
2	5.26	3.54	17.60	20.20	15.21	70.82
3	5.26	5.32	31.71	20.20	22.81	129.04

Inflow angle $= 20.0$
Outflow angle $= 35.3$

Analysis time coronary cineangiogram

The total time required for the analysis of a single coronary segment from a cineframe can be subdivided into the following components:

(i)	Mounting the cinefilm on the cine-video projector	1 min.
(ii)	Completion of the administrative data as requested by the computer program	2 min.
(iii)	Cinefilm-transport to selected cineframe (computed for an average frame displacement of 1200 frames, with film transport speed of 20 frames/s.)	1 min.
(iv)	Optical magnification $(2\sqrt{2}x)$ catheter, iterative contour detection catheter segment (including manual definition centerline positions and pincushion correction) and return of lens-system of $1:1$ magnification	2 min.
(v)	Optical magnification (2x) coronary segment and first iteration contour detection (including manual definition centerline positions and possibly corrections to detected contour)	2 min.
(vi)	Second iteration contour detection (including pincushion correction)	$1^1/_2$ min.
(vii)	Quantitative analysis severity coronary obstruction:	
	– User-definied %-D stenosis	$^1/_2$ min.
	– Interpolated %-D stenosis	1 min.

At the average, the total time necessary for the analysis of a single obstruction in a cineframe in terms of user-defined %-D stenosis is approximately 10 min. To analyze a second arterial segment in the same cineframe requires an additional $4^1/_2$ minutes. In this case time bins i, iii and iv do not apply, while the time for the

84

administrative data (ii) is reduced to $\frac{1}{2}$ min. The other items v through vii remain unchanged.

Pie Data CAAS

The basic components of the commercially available Pie Data CAAS are a cinefilm digitizer, a Pie Data video image processor (VIP 500), an LSI 11/73 minicomputer with terminal, which runs under the multi-user RSX-11M Operating System (Version 4.1), a writing tablet and the identical application software package as on the Thoraxcenter CAAS [29]. A block diagram of this system is shown in Fig III.17. A Video Imager is used for documentation purposes. The entire system, except for the cinefilm-digitizer, has been integrated conveniently in a computer operating desk. A photograph of the Pie Data CAAS is presented in Fig. III.18.

Cinefilm digitizer

The cinefilm digitizer consists of a standard cineprojector (Tagarno 35 CX), with a field-installable modification package for high resolution digitization of a selected cineframe. The modification package consists of a film guiding system, a specially developed optical chain and a high resolution CCD digital camera. The film guiding system ensures optimal flatness of the selected cineframe to be digitized. The optical chain has been designed for homogeneous light distribution

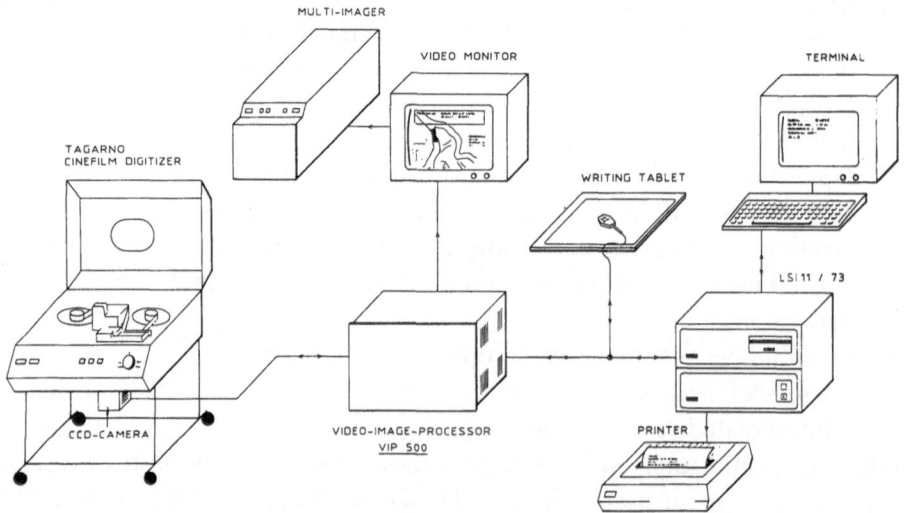

Fig. III.17. Block diagram of the Pie Data CAAS.

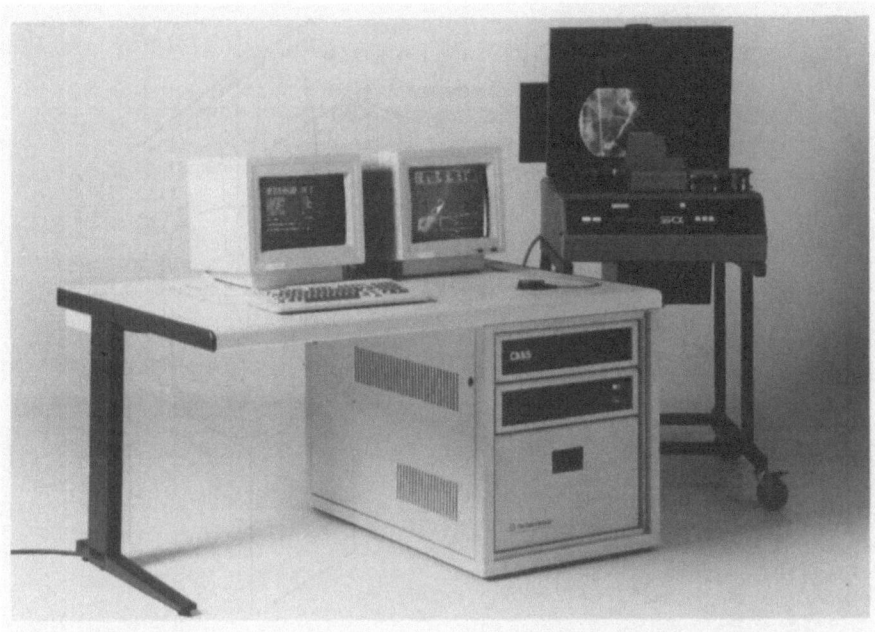

Fig. III.18. Photograph of the Pie Data CAAS.

over the cineframe to be digitized and a high resolution response of the cinefilm (Fig. III.19).

The monochromatic light source consists of an array of LED's optimally suitable for high resolution imaging and densitometric analysis of the cinefilm. Any area of 6.9×6.9 mm in a selected cineframe (size 18×24 mm) can be digitized by the CCD-camera with a resolution of 512×512 pixels (13μm/pixel at the face of the CCD-array) with 8 bits of grey levels. Effectively, this means that the entire cineframe of size 18×24 mm can be digitized at a resolution of 1329×1772 pixels. The concept of the Pie Data cinefilm digitizer differs basically from that of the cine-video-converter used in the Thoraxcenter prototype system. However, the resolution and quality of the digitized subimages used for contour detection and analysis are nearly identical, so that both systems perform equally well. The transportation of the cinefilm and the automated adjustment of the intensity of the light source, such that the density distribution in a subimage is optimally recorded, are remotely controlled by the LSI 11/73 minicomputer. The VIP 500 has two $512 \times 512 \times 12$ bits memories and software routines for general purpose image processing.

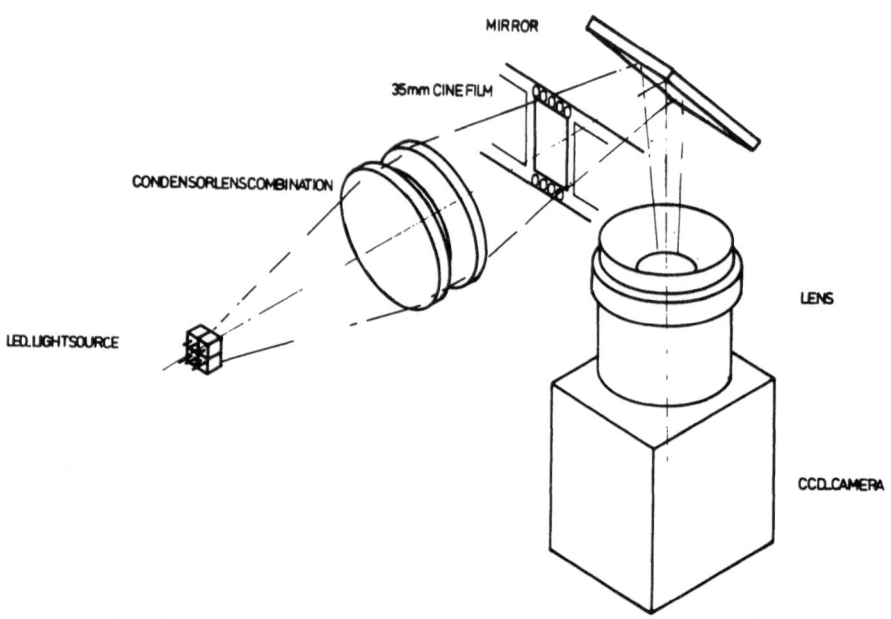

Fig. III.19. Drawing of specially developed optical chain on Tagarno 35CX cineprojector for high resolution imaging.

Data acquisition procedure

Due to the basic differences between the video-based digitizer of the Thoraxcenter CAAS and the digital camera approach in the Pie Data CAAS, the image acquisition procedure for the latter is also different. This new procedure is described briefly in the following paragraphs.

As soon as the user has decided from visual inspection of the projected film which cineframe needs to be analyzed quantitatively, the film is advanced automatically over 20 frames so that the given cineframe is positioned correctly in the new imaging chain. Initially, the center square of this frame with size of 13.9×13.9 mm is digitized at a resolution of 1024×1024 pixels, reduced in size to a matrix of 512×512 pixels and stored in a display memory of the video processor. If this region-of-interest does not contain the desired structure, the user may reposition this matrix of 1024×1024 pixels over the projected image by means of the writing tablet; as a result, any region-of-interest in the cineframe can be digitized in a convenient manner. The reduction in resolution to a matrix of 512×512 pixels is acceptable at this point, since the only function of this image is to allow the user to select subimages encompassing a catheter segment or the arterial segment of interest for subsequent quantitative analysis.

These subimages of size 512×512 pixels can be selected in the displayed overall image with the writing tablet. Such subimage is then redigitized at the original resolution (13 μm/pixel) and stored in the video processor for subsequent contour detection and analysis in an identical manner as described for the Thoraxcenter CAAS.

References

1. Serruys PW, Booman F, Troost GJ, Reiber JHC, Gerbrands JJ, Brand M van den, Cherrier F, Hugenholtz PG: Computerized quantitative coronary angiography applied to percutaneous transluminal coronary angioplasty: advantages and limitations. In: Transluminal Coronary Angiography and Intracoronary Thrombolysis. Coronary Heart Disease IV. M Kaltenbach, A Grüntzig, K Rentrop, WD Bussmann (Eds.), Springer-Verlag, Berlin: 110–124, 1982.
2. Serruys PW, Wijns W, Brand M van den, Ribeiro V, Fioretti ML, Simoons ML, Kooijman CJ, Reiber JHC, Hugenholtz PG: Is transluminal coronary angioplasty mandatory after successful thrombolysis? Br Heart J 50: 257–265, 1983.
3. Wijns W, Serruys PW, Brand M van den, Reiber JHC, Suryapranata H, Hugenholtz PG: Progression to complete coronary obstruction without myocardial infarction in patients who are candidates for Percutaneous Transluminal Angioplasty: A 90-Day Angiographic Follow-Up. In: Prognosis of Coronary Heart Disease – Progression of Coronary Arteriosclerosis. H Roskamm (Ed.), Springer-Verlag, Berlin 190–195, 1983.
4. Serruys PW, Hooghoudt TEH, Reiber JHC, Slager C, Brower RW, Hugenholtz PG: Influence of intracoronary nifedipine on left ventricular function, coronary vasomotility, and myocardial oxygen consumption. Br Heart J 49: 427–441, 1983.
5. Serruys PW, Lablanche JM, Reiber JHC, Bertrand ME, Hugenholtz PG: Contribution of dynamic vascular wall thickening to luminal narrowing during coronary arterial vasomotion. Z Kardiol 72: 116–123, 1983.
6. Arntzenius AC, Barth JD, Bruschke AVG, Buis B, Gent CM van, Houtsmuller UMT, Kempen-Voogd N, Kromhout D, Reiber JHC, Strikwerda S, Velde EA van der, Wezel LA van: Preliminary report on coronary lesions and serum lipids before and after 2 years dietary intervention in 22 patients. In: Atherosclerosis VI. FG Schettler, AM Gotto, G Middelhoff, AJR Habenicht, KR Jurutka (Eds.) Springer-Verlag Berlin 187–196, 1983.
7. Arntzenius AC, Velde EA van der, Reiber JHC, Kempen N, Gent CM van, Houtsmuller UMT, Kromhout D, Buis B: The Leiden Intervention Trial: diet, serum lipids and coronary atherosclerotic lesion growth. J Am Coll Cardiol 3: 549 (Abstract), 1984.
8. Barth JD, Reiber JHC, Hugenholtz PG, Birkenhäger JC, Arntzenius AC: Does thyroid metabolism, independently of lipids, play a role in regression of coronary atherosclerosis? J Am Coll Cardiol 3: 550 (Abstract), 1984.
9. Booman F, Reiber JHC, Gerbrands JJ, Slager CJ, Schuurbiers JCH, Meester GT: Quantitative analysis of coronary occlusions from coronary cine-angiograms. Comp in Card: 177–180, 1979.
10. Gerbrands JJ, Reiber JHC, Booman F: Computer processing and classification of coronary occlusions. In: Pattern Recognition in Practice. ES Gelsema, LN Kanal (Eds.), North Holland Publishing Company: 223–233, 1980.
11. Reiber JHC, Booman F, Gerbrands JJ, Troost GJ: Objective characterization of coronary obstructions from cineangiograms with single and multiple views. Proc 2nd Int Conf on Visual Psychophysics and Medical Imaging. CC Jaffe (Ed.) IEEE Cat No 81 CH 1676–6: 11–17, 1982.
12. Kooijman CJ, Reiber JHC, Gerbrands JJ, Schuurbiers JCH, Slager CJ, Boer A den, Serruys PW: Computer-aided quantitation of the severity of coronary obstructions from single view cineangio-

grams. First IEEE Comp Soc Int Symp on Medical Imaging and Image Interpretation. IEEE Cat No 82 CH1804-4: 59–64, 1982.

13. Reiber JHC, Gerbrands JJ, Booman F, Troost GJ, Boer A den, Slager CJ, Schuurbiers JCH: Objective characterization of coronary obstructions from monoplane cineangiograms and three-dimensional reconstruction of an arterial segment from two orthogonal views. Applications of Computers in Medicine MD Schwartz (Ed.) IEEE Cat No TH0095-0: 93–100, 1982.

14. Reiber JHC, Gerbrands JJ, Kooijman CJ, Troost GJ, Schuurbiers JCH, Slager CJ, Boer A den, Serruys PW: Computer-aided analysis of coronary obstructions from monoplane cineangiograms and three-dimensional reconstruction of an arterial segment from two orthogonal views. In: Physical Techniques in Cardiovascular Imaging. MD Short, DA Pay, S Leeman, RM Harrison (Eds.) Adam Hilger Ltd., Bristol: 173–188, 1983.

15. Reiber JHC, Kooijman CJ, Slager CJ, Gerbrands JJ, Schuurbiers JCH, Boer A den, Wijns W, Serruys PW: Computer assisted analysis of the severity of obstructions from coronary cineangiograms: a methodological review. Automedica 5: 219–238, 1984.

16. Reiber JHC, Kooijman CJ, Slager CJ, Gerbrands JJ, Schuurbiers JCH, Boer A den, Wijns W, Serruys PW, Hugenholtz PG: Coronary artery dimensions from cineangiograms; methodology and validation of a computer-assisted analysis procedure. IEEE Trans Med Imaging, MI-3: 131–141, 1984.

17. Reiber JHC, Serruys PW, Kooijman CJ, Wijns W, Slager CJ, Gerbrands JJ, Schuurbiers JCH, Boer A den, Hugenholtz PG: Assessment of short-, medium- and long-term variations in arterial dimensions from computer-assisted quantitation of coronary cineangiograms. Circulation 71: 280–288, 1985.

18. Austen WG, Edwards JE, Frye RL, Gensini GG, Gott VL, Griffith LSC, McGoon DC, Murphy ML, Roe BB: A reporting system on patients evaluated for coronary artery disease. Report of the Ad Hoc Committee for Grading of Coronary Artery Disease, Council on Cardiovascular Surgery. American Heart Association, 1975. Circulation 51–2, no 4: 7–40, 1975.

19. Rosenfeld A, Johnston E: Angle detection on digital curves. IEEE Trans Comput C-22: 875–878, 1973.

20. Crawford RW, Brooks SH, Selzer RH, Barndt R Jr, Beckenbach ES, Blankenhorn DH: Computer densitometry for angiographic assessment of arterial cholesterol content and gross pathology in human atherosclerosis. J Lab Clin Med 89: 378–392, 1977.

21. Hutchins GM, Miner MM, Boitnott JK: Vessel caliber and branch-angle of human coronary artery branch-points. Circ Res 38: 572–576, 1976.

22. McMahon MM, Brown BG, Cukingnan R, Rolett EL, Bolson E, Frimer M, Dodge HT: Quantitative coronary angiography: measurement of the 'critical' stenosis in patients with unstable angina and single-vessel disease without collaterals. Circulation 60: 106–113, 1979.

23. Kirkeeide R, Wüsten B, Gottwik M: Computer assisted evaluation of angiographic findings. In: Thrombose und Atherogenese. Pathophysiologie und Therapie der arteriellen Verschlusskrankheit. K Breddin (Ed.), Verlag Gerhard Witzstrock, Baden-Baden/Köln/New York: 414–417, 1981.

24. Brown BG, Bolson EL, Dodge HT: Arteriographic assessment of coronary atherosclerosis. Review of current methods, their limitations, and clinical applications. Arteriosclerosis 2: 2–15, 1982.

25. Gould KL, Kelley KO: Physiological significance of coronary flow velocity and changing stenosis geometry during coronary vasodilation in awake dogs. Circ Res 50: 695–704, 1982.

26. Gottwik MG, Siebes M, Kirkeeide R, Schaper W: Hämodynamik von Koronarstenosen. Z Kardiol 73 (Suppl. 2): 47–54, 1984.

27. Siebes M, Lenzen H, Gottwik M, Schlepper M: Influence of geometric errors in quantitative angiography on the evaluation of stenotic hemodynamics. Comp Cardiol: 385–388, 1983.

28. Wijns W, Serruys PW, Brand M van den, Zeegers E, Kooijman CJ, Reiber JHC: Transstenotic pressure gradients obtained during coronary angioplasty are useful but artefactual measurements. Circ 70 (Suppl. II): II–299 (Abstract), 1984.
29. Reiber JHC, Kooijman CJ, Slager CJ, Ree EJB van, Kalberg RJN, Tijdens FO, Plas JFAN van der, Frankenhuyzen J van, Claessen WCH: Taking a quantitative approach to cine angiogram analysis. Diagnostic Imaging, 87–89, April 1985.

IV. Contouromat – A hard-wired left ventricular angio processing system

General description

The Contouromat is a hard-wired electronic system designed for operator-assisted automated analysis of left ventricular cineangiograms [1, 2]. It has been interfaced with the PDP 11/44 minicomputer of the CAAS via an asynchronous serial communication line. A block diagram of the system is shown in Fig. IV.1.

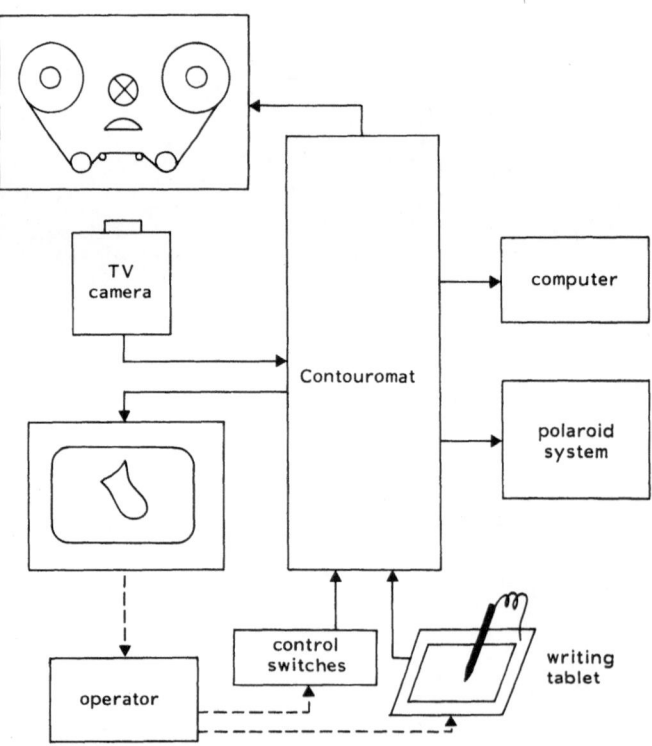

Fig. IV.1. Block diagram of the left ventricular contour analysis system, the Contouromat.

The cinefilm is mounted on a Vanguard-projector system which can be rotated with respect to a video camera mounted underneath the projector. The optical magnification factor is about 0.7, so that the entire cineframe is projected within the boundaries of the scanning area of the video tube, irrespective of the rotation of the cineprojector. The analog video signal is sent to the Contouromat for subsequent contour detection. The projected image is displayed on a video monitor for visual feedback; detected contours plus control functions to be discussed later can be superimposed in the image.

Based on our experiences with earlier versions of the Contouromat, the following specifications were defined at the time when the final prototype was being developed:

(1) The system must be operator interactive; the final decision as to the accuracy of the detected contour is up to the operator. This also requires that the detected contour be superimposed onto the original video image.
(2) It should permit manual interventions in the contour detection process in real time.
(3) All manual interventions should be centralized to facilitate operations. For this purpose the writing tablet was selected.
(4) Time required to detect a single contour must be as short as possible, to allow for the analysis of a left ventricular cineangiogram over a complete cardiac cycle within an acceptable time period.
(5) Total operating time per analyzed cineframe must be considerably shorter than the time required for conventional manual tracing.

The contour detection techniques have been implemented in the Contouromat with analog circuitry, i.e. the video image is not digitized and there is no processor in the apparatus to execute digital image processing algorithms. The advantage of this approach is that the contour detection occurs in real time, i.e. at a rate of 50 fields/s.

Operator-interaction with the system has been made possible with two control switches and a writing tablet. One of the two control switches allows the operator to turn superimposed contours on and off from the video image; this facilitates comparing the detected contour positions with the boundaries of the contrast-filled left ventricular structure. The second control switch is the transport command to the cinetransport system. As soon as the operator has accepted the contours for a particular cineframe, a transport command may be given to transmit the contour data to the computer and to forward the next frame; during this time the contours are turned off from the video image. Half a second after the next cineframe has been displayed on the video monitor, the newly detected contours are superimposed in the display. This half second delay allows the operator to inspect the original unprocessed image briefly before contour data are superimposed.

A special writing tablet, consisting of an x-y controlled sheet of resistive foil, has been implemented in the operator console for real-time user-interaction with the detected contours. The position of the conducting writing pen on the tablet is displayed in the video image by means of a white dot. Specific functions which can be performed with the writing tablet will be described in more detail in the section Basic techniques.

Fig. IV.2 is an example of a video converted cineframe as it is displayed on the video monitor. The Vanguard projector has been rotated in such a way that the long axis of the ventricle is about perpendicular to the video scan direction. In this way there can never be more than two contour points on a video line, which simplifies the hardware edge detection algorithm. In addition, with such orientation the density changes on a videoline at the left ventricular boundaries will at the average be maximal, which improves the reliability of the edge detection procedure. From a large series of left ventricular cineangiograms in the RAO-30° view analyzed with the Contouromat, the mean and standard deviation of the applied rotation was found to be $50° \pm 6°$. Since the system is not very sensitive for small rotational changes, a fixed rotational angle of approximately 50° has been shown to be suitable in more than 90% of our routine cineangiograms.

Two data acquisition modes have been implemented, MAXI-cine and MINI-cine. For the assessment of global and regional left ventricular ejection fraction ànd regional wall motion as a function of time, sequential cineframes must be

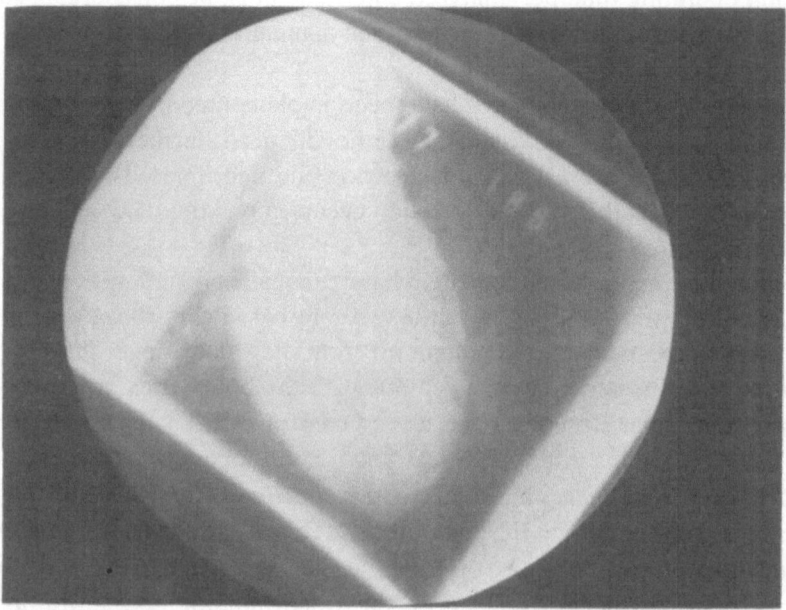

Fig. IV.2. Left ventricular cineangiogram rotated such that long axis is about perpendicular to video scanlines.

analyzed, requiring the use of MAXI-cine. However, if one is only interested in global and regional ejection fraction data derived from the end-diastolic (ED) and end-systolic (ES) cineframes, then the MINI-cine mode is selected. In this mode, the ED- and ES-contours can either be detected automatically with the Contouromat in the corresponding cineframes or traced manually with the writting tablet of the CAAS.

In the following section the basic techniques of the Contouromat will be described. Subsequently, the left ventricular data acquisition procedures in the MAXI- and MINI-cine modes will be explained, followed by a discussion of the MAXI- and MINI-data analysis procedures.

Basic techniques

In this section the basic techniques implemented will be described briefly [1]. Figure IV.3 represents a block diagram of the Contouromat in terms of hardware functional modules. First, the synchronization pulses are clipped from the incoming video signal; the remaining video signal is low-pass filtered, and the dc-level restored in the video preprocessing unit. Contour points are defined by comparing the preprocessed video signal with a dynamic reference voltage derived from the same video signal. Basically, this dynamic reference voltage is constructed from the output signal of an analog extrapolation filter, sample-and-hold voltage levels and analog probability functions defined by the information (D/A-conversion) from different memories as described in the following paragraphs. The sampling moment for the sample-and-hold level on each line is determined by the control logic and depends on the coordinates of the detected contour point on the previous videoline. The algorithm is initialized by the two starting points at the aortic valve, to be defined by the operator in the first cineframe to be analyzed. The sum of the probability functions influences the probability of finding a contour point within a period of the videoline.

The control logic synchronizes the information from:

(1) The writing tablet memory that contains the two starting point positions at the aortic valve and operator-defined correction data.
(2) A contour memory in which the coordinates of the detected contour in the previous cineframe are stored in coded format. This memory has been shown to be very useful, since there exists a high correlation between contours derived from successive cineframes. At each transport command this memory is filled with the last contour data accepted by the operator.
(3) A contour memory in which the coordinates of the detected contour in the previous video field are stored in coded format. At each field synchronization pulse, this memory is refreshed with the detected contour from the previous video field. The recurrent use of this contour as a predictor for the

94

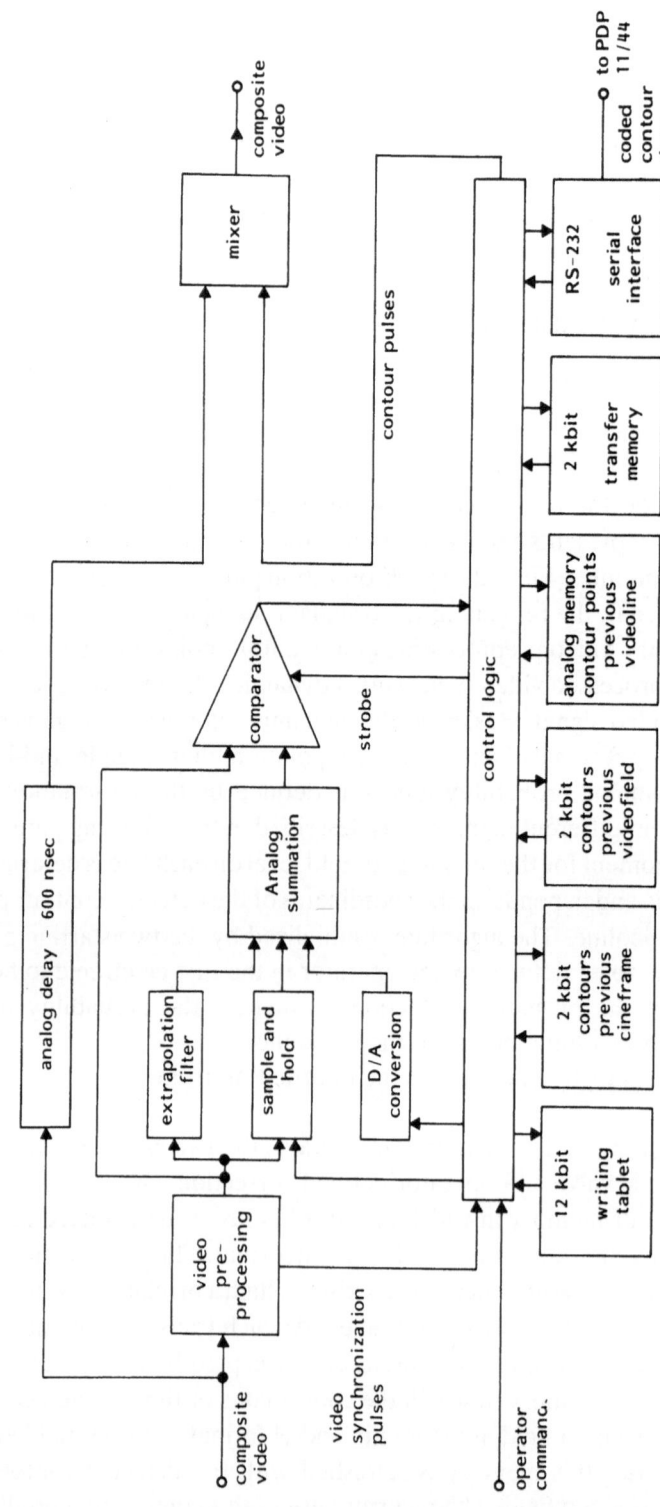

Fig. IV.3. Basic functional modules comprising the Contouromat.

next one greatly stabilizes the detection process, since contour positions only change very little between two successive video fields. The overall effect of this memory is a kind of two-dimensional filtering.

(4) A small analog memory that provides the positional information of the contour point on the previous videoline. This position defines the timing of an expectation window during which period the video comparator is enabled (strobe). This principle can be applied successfully since there is a high degree of coherency between contour points on successive videolines.

At the edges of the comparator output signal contour pulses are generated, and mixed into the delayed video signal. The delay time of 600 nsec compensates for the time required by the detection system to find a contour point and for the delay-time of the low-pass filter in the video preprocessor.

After the operator has accepted the detected and corrected left ventricular contours in a particular cineframe and given the transport command for the following cineframe, the coded data in the contour memories are copied into two 1 kbit transfer memories during the vertical synchronization period of the video signal. Subsequently, the data are transmitted serially (RS-232 serial interface) to the host computer (PDP 11/44) and checked for missing codes. In case a transmission error has been detected, the transmission procedure is automatically repeated until the data have been received correctly.

Left ventricular data acquisition procedure (MAXI-cine)

To analyze a series of cineframes with the Contouromat, the MAXI-cine data acquisition software package must be called.

The acquisition package requests the user to enter on the computer terminal demographic data of the left ventricular cineangiogram to be processed. The following items must be provided:

---

1. Film ID
2. Patient name
3. Date of catheterization
4. Cinefilm speed (fr/s)
5. Film sequence number of first cineframe to be processed
6. Film sequence number of last cineframe to be processed
7. Heart rate at the time of LV cineangiography
8. Body surface area of patient (BSA in m^2)
9. Name of operator Contouromat
10. Calibration method to be used: sphere or cm-grid

Calibration of the left ventricular angiogram can be performed on the basis of either a radiopaque sphere or the cm-grid filmed at the level of the heart of the patient after the catheterization procedure. The calibration procedure is the first step in the left ventricular data acquisition procedure. Figure IV.4 is an example of a filmed sphere with the contours as detected by the Contouromat superimposed in the image. The same contour detection technique as used for the LV-angiograms is applied to this image; the exact procedure will be clarified later for the left ventricular boundaries. In this case with the sphere, the left- and right-hand starting positions were defined at the top of the circle, close to each other. From these contour data, the diameter of the displayed circle can be computed in pixels. The true volume of the sphere being 100 ml and thus the true diameter being 5.7 cm, the calibration factor in units mm/pixel can be computed.

The other calibration possibility with the cm-grid is illustrated in Fig. IV.5. In this example the 4×4 cm square in the center of the image was selected for the computation of the calibration factor. The two starting points were positioned at the left and right upper positions of the square, respectively and the vertical boundaries were drawn manually with the writing tablet of the Contouromat. Again, by measuring the distance between the left and right contour positions and comparing this with the true distance of 4 cm, the calibration factor expressed in mm/pixel is computed.

In our institute, the sphere calibration technique is used almost exclusively.

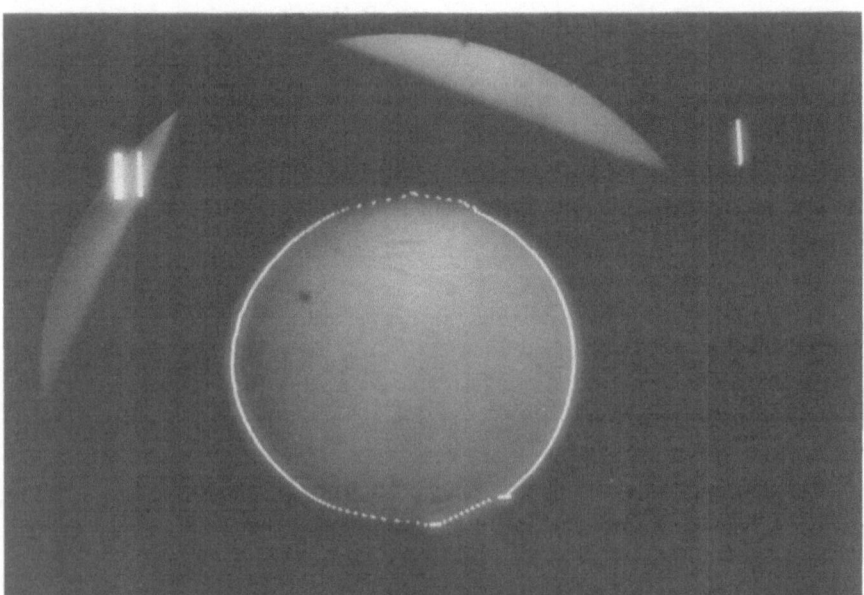

Fig. IV.4. Example of radiopaque sphere filmed at the level of the heart of the patient following the catheterization procedure with the detected contours superimposed.

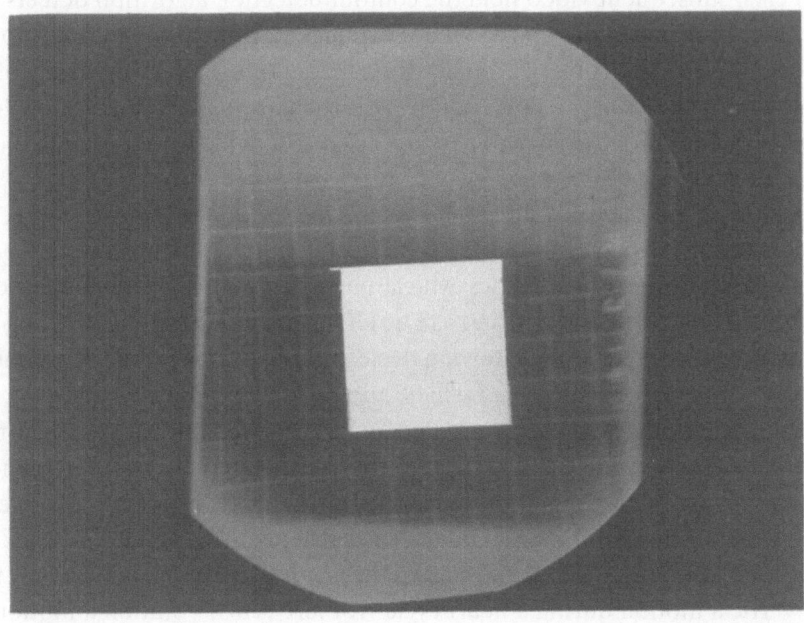

Fig. IV.5. Example of cm-grid filmed at the level of the heart of the patient following the catheterization procedure, with the contours encompassing a 4 × 4 cm square in the center of the field superimposed.

Following this calibration procedure, the user searches for the first left ventricular cineframe to be analyzed.

After the first frame to be analyzed has been displayed on the video monitor, the user rotates the cineprojector such that the long axis is approximately perpendicular to the video scan direction. In this first frame the aortic valve plane must be defined interactively. To this end, the operator places the pen on the writing tablet and moves the displayed pen position to the left-hand side of the aortic valve. In this context, left and right are defined with respect to the structure as the reader observes it on the video image or photograph; i.e. left is at the infero-posterior side of the left ventricle and right at the anterior side. As soon as the correct position has been reached, the pen is lifted from the tablet and the last indicated position is stored in digital format in the writing tablet memory, thus defining the position of the first starting point. In each subsequent video field these x, y-coordinates are read from memory; from this position on, the contour detection algorithm searches for the left contour. Similarly, a second starting point is defined with the position located at the right-hand side of the aortic valve; this point initializes the detection algorithm for the right contour. Between the two starting points a straight line is automatically interpolated simulating the aortic valve plane (Fig. IV.6). At the apex of the left ventricle the left- and right-hand contours meet and the contour detection procedure is automatically terminated. In each subsequent video field the contour detection algorithm detects the left- and right-hand borders on the video scanlines starting at the defined aortic valve positions, i.e. the contours are detected in real time with a frequency of 50 fields/s. During the contour detection in a particular video field, the contour information from the previous video field is used as a guide for the search in the current field (Fig. IV.6).

Repositioning of the starting points is possible with the writing tablet by moving the displayed pen positions to one of the two stored starting points. At the moment the pen position coincides with a particular starting point, this point tracks the displayed pen position and can be left at any new position by lifting the pen again from the tablet. When moving the left-hand starting point the y-coordinate of the right-hand starting point will be adjusted accordingly. In this way, the simulated aortic valve can be translated in vertical direction over a certain distance without changing the direction of the interpolated aortic valve plane.

This simple correction procedure has been shown to be very effective in correcting the position of the simulated aortic valve plane over a cardiac cycle. It has been our experience, that in most cases the aortic valve plane makes only this kind of vertical motion during a heart cycle. If there is also rotational motion of the valve, the right-hand starting point can be adjusted separately without influencing the position of the left-hand starting point, i.e., the right-hand starting point can be rotated over 360° around the left-hand starting point.

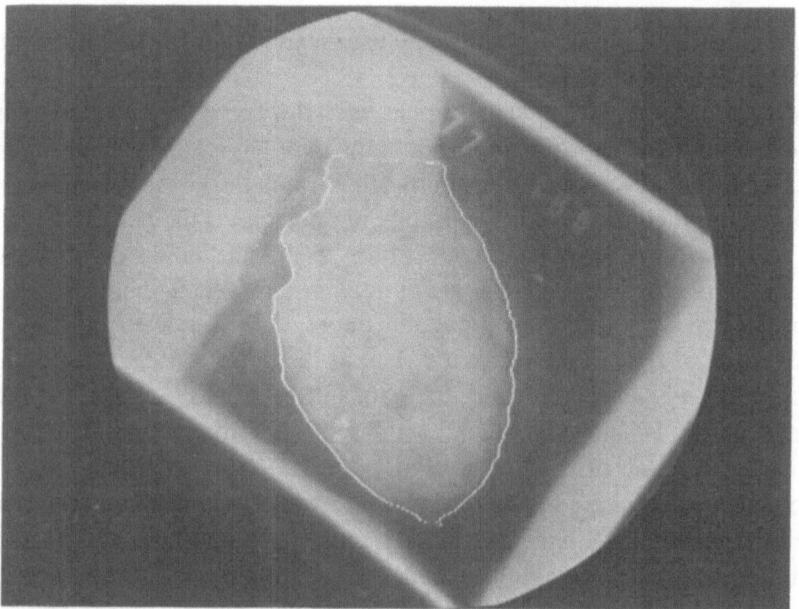

Fig. IV.6. The angiogram of Fig. IV.2 with the detected contours superimposed. The operator only needed to define the two aortic valve starting positions.

If locally the detected left ventricular outline does not coincide accurately with the actual left ventricular outline (Fig. IV.7a), the operator may correct the contour interactively. To this end, the user places the pen on the tablet and moves the displayed dot to the upper part of the area where the problems occur without crossing the detected outline. The correction procedure is started as soon as the pen position crosses the detected outline; from thereon all subsequently drawn positions are stored in the writing tablet memory with the limitation of one correction position per videoline and per contour side. Termination of the correction is achieved by merely lifting the pen from the writing tablet. The writing tablet interface does not differentiate between odd and even fields. The operator-drawn stored data are read out continuously from the writing tablet memory and an analog probability function is applied to the detection algorithm at those positions. As a result, the manually drawn positions can only force the old contour towards a more correct outline, if the video signal around those places satisfies the requirements for stable automatic contour detection. If the operator draws the curve completely wrong, the detection algorithm will not be able to detect this new outline.

From the moment correction data have been stored in memory, these data will be used in each following video field to adjust the detection algorithm. The system does not wait until the complete path has been drawn: the correction procedure works in real time. By watching the displayed contour on the monitor the operator can decide instantaneously, whether to continue with the correction or to stop in case the problematic areas has been passed. In the lower left or right corner of the video image a marker is superimposed, which indicates that a pen correction for the left or right contour path is stored in the writing tablet memory, respectively. Since these correction data will be erased as soon as a film transport command is given, this type of correction is called 'soft' correction, in contrast with the 'hard' correction to be described in one of the following paragraphs. Figure IV.7b shows the corrected contour of Fig. IV.7a. For clarity, the part of the contour where corrections were applied has been emphasized with the short white markers next to it.

As soon as the operator agrees with the detected contours, a film transport command is given and the following cineframe is displayed. At the trigger of the command pulse, the last detected contours are stored in coded format in a contour memory consisting of two 1 kbit shift registers, one for the left contour and one for the right contour; in addition, the soft correction positions are erased from the writing tablet memory. The starting point positions are not erased and thus can be used again for the following cineframe. If necessary, these two points can be repositioned as described earlier. The data in the contour memory are read out continuously and another probability function is applied to the edge detection algorithm at the corresponding positions. This means that the data from the previous contour are used as a priori information to guide the search for the new contour positions in the current cineframe. In this manner, the corrections given

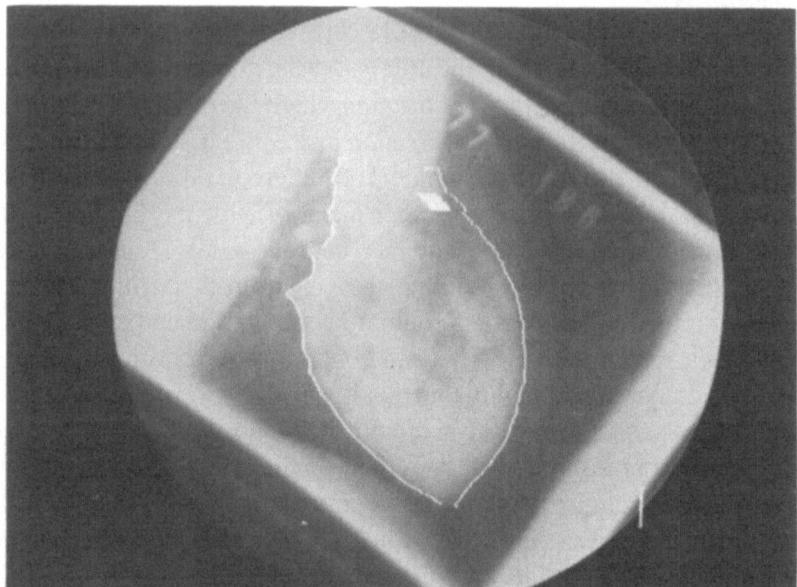

a

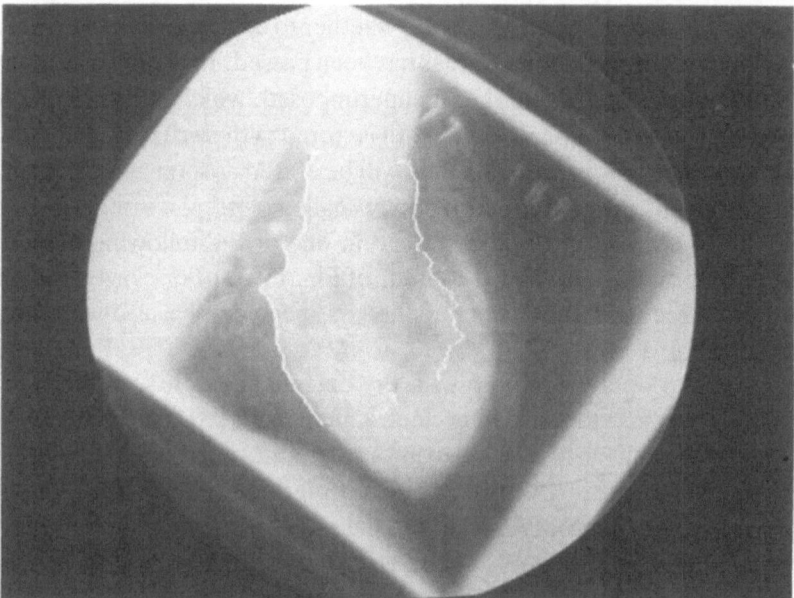

b

Fig. IV.7. Due to an inhomogeneous contrast distribution, the Contouromat initially failed to detect the proper outline in this image (Fig. 7a). The image of Fig. IV.7b demonstrates how a small correction was sufficient to obtain the correct outline. The video lines at which the contour positions were corrected have been labelled with the short horizontal bright lines.

in the previous frame are applied indirectly in the current cineframe, however with a lower weight.

If local detection problems are expected to occur in a large number of successive frames which would require manual corrections in each of these frames, it is possible to apply a so-called hard correction which is not erased when the film is transported to the next cineframe. Such a correction is obtained by first crossing the simulated aortic valve plane with the displayed pen position and then correcting the outline in the usual way as described above for the soft correction. Hard corrections overwrite soft corrections in the writing tablet memory and vice versa, with the limitation that either a soft or a hard correction can be applied to a contour point, but not both. Similarly as implemented for the soft corrections, hard correction markers are displayed in the lower corners of the video image. The hard correction markers can be distinguished from the soft correction markers by their width; the hard correction markers are wider. Hard corrections can only be erased by crossing the corresponding markers with the pen. Soft corrections are erased: (1) when transporting to the following cineframe; and (2) similarly as for the hard corrections by crossing the corresponding markers. This last possibility can be used conveniently, when the operator wants to inspect once more the detected contour without the influence of corrections.

With the tools described above, all the cineframes over a cardiac cycle can be analyzed in a very user-friendly manner.

Left ventricular data acquisition procedure (MINI-cine)

In the MINI-cine mode, only the ED- and ES-left ventricular contours are determined and stored in computer file. This can be done with the Contouromat or manually with the writing tablet of the CAAS. These two possibilities will be described separately.

Automatically detected ED- and ES-contours

In this mode the calibration procedure is identical to the one described for the MAXI-cine mode. Following data calibration, the end-diastolic cineframe is searched for and the Vanguard projector is again rotated such that the long axis of the left ventricle is approximately perpendicular to the video scanlines. The contours are detected automatically following the scheme as described for the first frame of a series of frames in the MAXI-cine mode. As soon as the operator agrees with the detected and possibly corrected outlines, the contour data are sent to the host computer and the end-systolic cineframe is selected. Since a priori information cannot be used in this case for the delineation of the ES-boundaries, the user essentially follows the same procedure as for the ED-cineframe. That is, the aortic starting points are repositioned and if necessary manual corrections are applied to the detected outlines. As soon as the operator agrees with the ES-outlines, the contour data are sent to the computer and the data acquisition procedure is terminated.

Manual tracking ED- and ES-contours

In the entirely manual acquisition procedure, the user selects the cineframe with the calibration sphere and the ED- and ES-cineframes on a Tagarno projector or similar device. For each of these frames (s)he draws with a pencil the outlines of the projected structures on a sheet of paper and places this sheet on the writing tablet of the CAAS. After the demographic data have been entered on the computer terminal, the actual computer acquisition procedure starts. The size of the calibration sphere is determined by requesting the user to indicate three points along the drawn boundary of the sphere. On the basis of these three pairs of x, y-coordinates, the computer program computes the equation of a circle going through these points and displays this circle on the video monitor. These data are then converted to the format as defined by the Contouromat and transferred to the appropriate file. As a next step, the user tracks the pencil-drawn ED- and ES-boundaries. Again these data are converted into Contouromat format and transferred to the file. The acquisition procedure is terminated and the left ventricular analysis program can be executed.

Left ventricular data analysis procedure (MAXI-cine)

For the quantitative analysis of left ventricular contour data detected with the Contouromat, the user calls the data analysis program and requests to use the data stored in the disk file of a particular left ventricular study. As a first step, the left ventricular contour data stored in coded format are decoded and displayed on the video monitor. From these data, instantaneous left ventricular volume and the time-derivative of LV-volume (dV/dt) are computed and displayed on the video monitor of the CAAS. Volume is computed following Simpson's rule, corrected for the angiographic overestimation (3) according to the regression equation:

$$V_{true} = 0.72 \times V_{measured} - 4.7\,ml, \tag{IV.1}$$

and normalized for body surface area and therefore expressed in units of ml/m^2. The LV-volume data are smoothed by determining for each data point the least squared error fit of a straight line through that point and the two neighboring volume values. The slope of this last regression line represents dV/dt, expressed in l/min/m^2. An example of the volume and dV/dt-plots is given in figure IV.8. The instantaneous volume and dV/dt data are also printed on the LV report on the line printer of the computer system.

The user is now requested to indicate the frame numbers of the end-diastolic and end-systolic frames, defined as those frames with maximal and minimal volume, respectively and the frame representing the time of aortic valve opening (Fig. IV.8). This moment occurs usually between 40 msec and 80 msec after end diastole and can be recognized from the dV/dt-plot by the distinct notch in dV/dt followed by a rapid decrease in LV-volume. This point in time closely corresponds with the moment of peak dP/dt, which is usually considered to be the actual moment of the beginning of the ejection phase [4, 5].

From the left ventricular volume data over the systolic period, global LV ejection fraction (EF), stroke index (= EDV-ESV [ml/m^2]), and total cardiac index (= stroke index × heart rate [l/min/m^2]) are computed. The end-diastolic and end-systolic contours are displayed on the computer video monitor with the

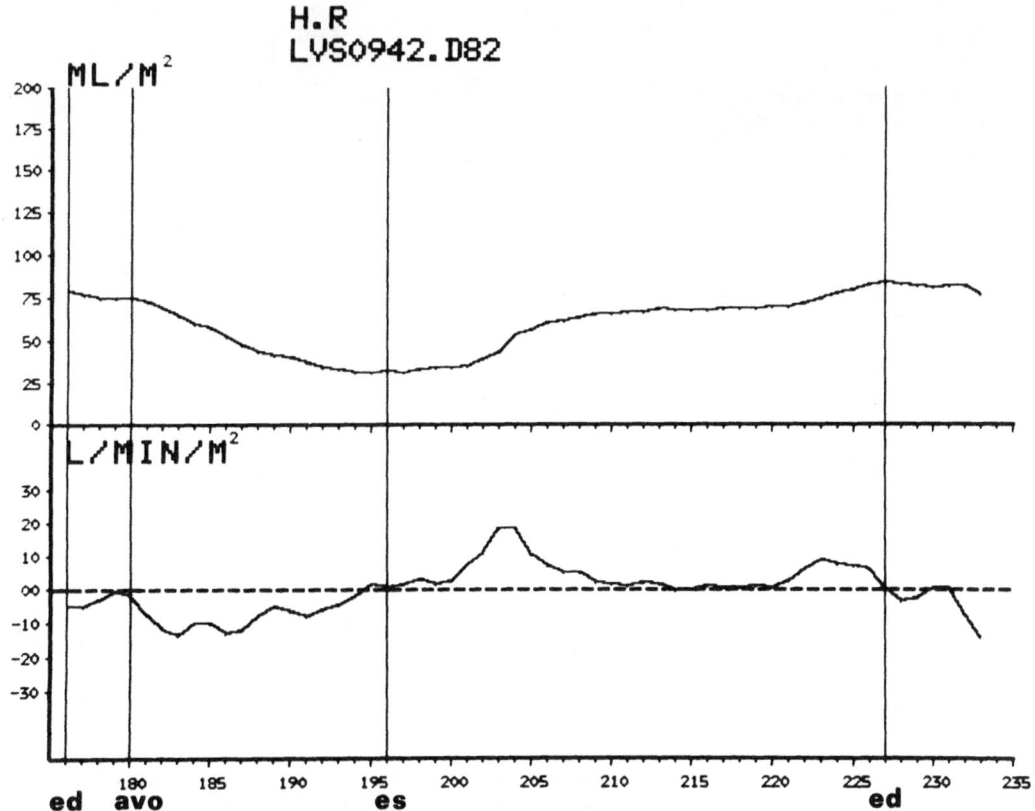

Fig. IV.8. Graphic display of the time course of left ventricular volume, normalized for body surface area, and its time-derivative. Vertical lines indicate the end-diastolic frames (no.'s 176 and 227), the end-systolic frame (no. 196) and the moment of aortic valve opening (frame no. 180), respectively.

values for EDV (end-diastolic volume), ESV (end-systolic volume), EF, heart rate (HR), stroke volume (SV), total cardiac index (TCI) and body surface area (BSA) (Fig. IV.9).

Next, the computer generates a system of coordinates along which regional left ventricular wall motion is determined (Fig. IV.9). This method to analyze left ventricular wall motion is based on the endocardial landmark trajectories as previously established in a group of normal individuals [6–9]; this model is described in more detail in Chapter XI. Over a full cardiac cycle, starting at end diastole, instantaneous segmental wall displacement is determined in twenty segments, ten along the anterior and ten along the infero-posterior wall. Instantaneous regional wall velocity is calculated as the first-derivative of the instantaneous displacement function after a three-point smoothing function has been applied to the displacement data. From the instantaneous displacement and velocity data, the following parameters are computed for each segment and printed on the LV report:

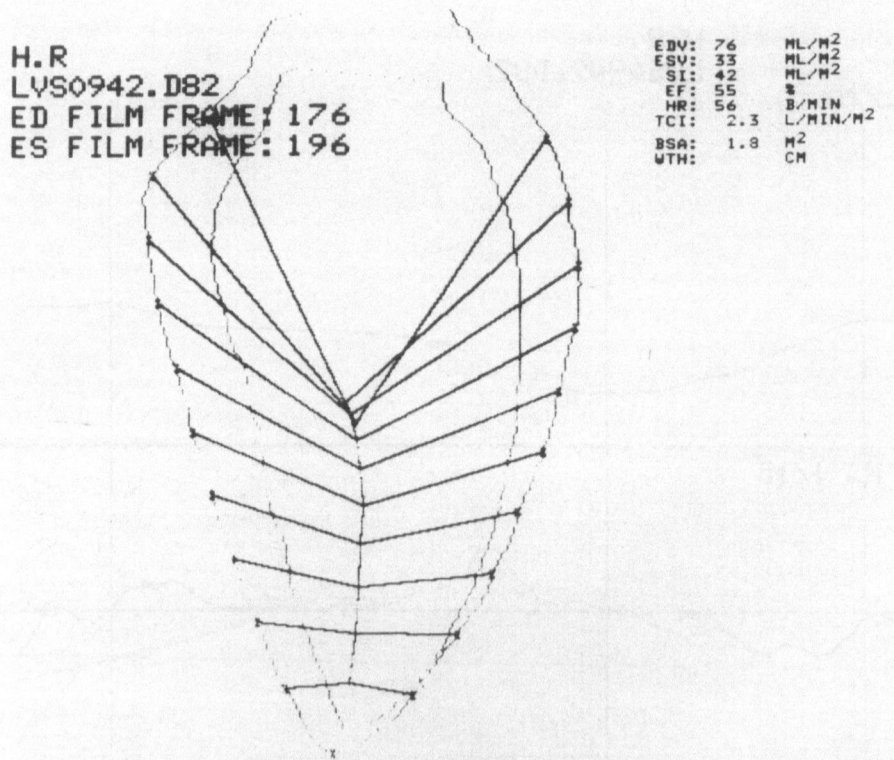

Fig. IV.9. Example of the computer output showing the end-diastolic and end-systolic contours of the 30° RAO angiogram in their relative proportions and place. The corresponding volume data, ejection fraction and other parameters are displayed in the upper right corner. Left ventricular segmental wall motion is determined along a system of coordinates derived from the endocardial landmark trajectories in normals, and is studied in twenty separate segments, ten in the anterior and ten in the infero-posterior wall.

1. Effective mean systolic displacement (cm)
2. Average systolic displacement (cm)
3. Maximal displacement (cm)
4. Delay, moment of maximal displacement with respect to end systole (ms)
5. Mean systolic velocity (cm/s)
6. Mean diastolic velocity (cm/s)
7. Mean ejection velocity (cm/s)
8. Maximal systolic velocity (cm/s)
9. Delay, moment of maximal systolic velocity to end systole (ms)
10. Maximal diastolic velocity (cm/s)
11. Delay, moment of maximal diastolic velocity to end systole (ms)

To eliminate the influence of the pre-ejection period on mean systolic velocity, left ventricular segmental wall velocity is determined during the actual ejection period, i.e. between the selected moment of aortic valve opening and end systole. In addition, the mean systolic circumferential fiber shortening rate (cm/s) is computed for the ten corresponding anterior and infero-posterior sites and printed on the LV report.

The user may now choose from a number of different composite plots:

A. Composite anterior displacement-versus-time plot
B. Composite infero-posterior displacement-versus-time plot
C. Composite anterior velocity-versus-time plot
D. Composite infero-posterior velocity-versus-time plot
E. Composite CREF plot
F. Composite anterior CREF-versus-time plot
G. Composite infero-posterior CREF-versus-time plot

These different plots will be described briefly in the following paragraphs.

The displacement plots for the anterior and infero-posterior sites are very helpful in the analysis of the time course of left ventricular contraction. Figures IV.10a and 10b show the displacement curves for the ten anterior and the ten infero-posterior segments of the left ventricular study of Fig. IV.9, respectively. A late inward motion of the anterior segments no's 5–10 and the infero-posterior segments no's 17–19 following the moment of minimal left ventricular volume (frame 196 in Fig. IV.8) can be readily appreciated.

Figures IV.11a and IV.11b show the instantaneous velocity plots for the ten anterior and the ten infero-posterior sites, respectively of Fig. IV.9.

A very important parameter for the evaluation of regional left ventricular performance has been shown to be the regional contribution to global ejection fraction (CREF). For all 20 segments the CREF-values are derived from systolic wall displacement data and left ventricular long axis shortening. To this end, the end-diastolic lumen – from the level of the mitral valve edge to the apex – is divided into ten slices of equal height, each corresponding to two opposite segments of the model (Fig. IV.12). Each slice is divided into two halves by the left ventricular axis of symmetry. The volume of each half-slice in the end-diastolic situation is computed according to the formula:

$$\tfrac{1}{2} \cdot \pi \cdot R_{ED}^2 \cdot \frac{L_{ED}}{10} = \frac{1}{20} \cdot \pi \cdot R_{ED}^2 \cdot L_{ED} \tag{IV.2}$$

where R_{ED} is the end-diastolic radius of a particular slice and L_{ED} the end-diastolic left ventricular long axis length extending from base to apex.

During systole the volume of a particular half-slice decreases mainly as a consequence of the decrease of radius which is determined by the x-component (x) of the displacement vector (d) (Fig. IV.13), and only slightly by left ventricular long axis shortening. A 14-percent long axis shortening, as previously assessed from normals, was applied to the end-systolic calculations (6–9). Therefore, the volume of each half-slice at end systole is computed according to the formula:

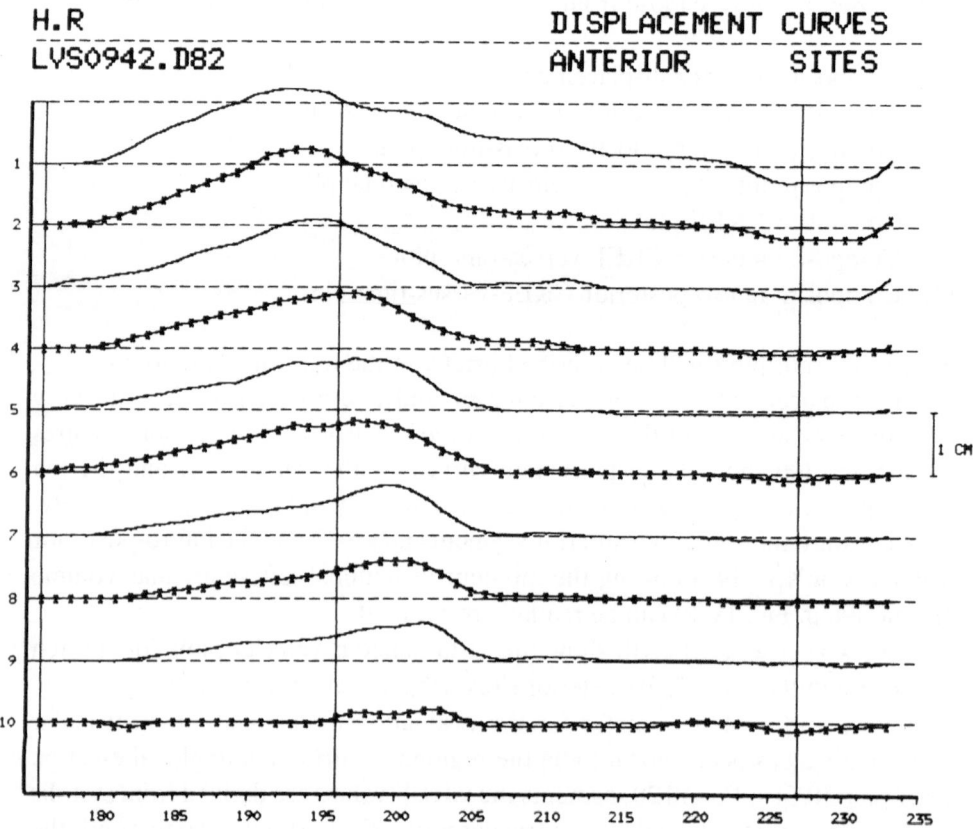

Fig. IV.10a.

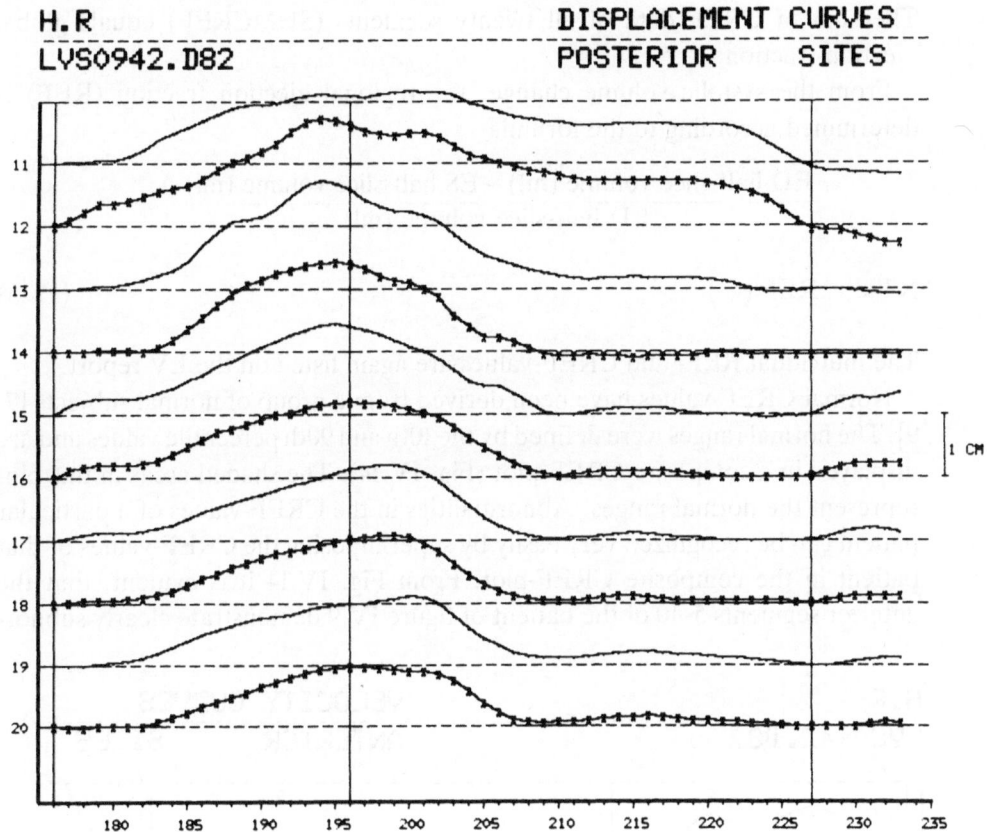

Fig. IV.10b.

Fig. IV.10. Instantaneous left ventricular segmental wall displacement in the ten anterior segments (Fig. IV.10a) and in the ten infero-posterior segments (Fig. IV.10b) for the study of figure IV.9. Note the marked differences in the moments of maximal inward displacement for the various segments with respect to end systole being defined by the frame with the smallest left ventricular volume (Fig. IV.8). The vertical scale (displacement of 1 cm) is indicated in the graphs.

$$\tfrac{1}{2} \cdot \pi \cdot R_{ES}^2 \cdot \frac{0.86 \cdot L_{ED}}{10} = 0.043 \cdot \pi \cdot R_{ES}^2 \cdot L_{ED}, \tag{IV.3}$$

where R_{ES} is the end-systolic radius of a particular slice. Finally, the CREF is defined as the change of volume during ejection of a particular segment normalized for left ventricular end-diastolic volume:

$$\frac{\text{ED half-slice volume (ml)} - \text{ES half-slice volume (ml)}}{\text{global left ventricular end-diastolic volume (ml)}}$$

$$\times 100 = \text{CREF} \ (\%) \tag{IV.4}$$

108

The sum of CREF data of all twenty segments (SUMCREF) equals global ejection fraction.

From the systolic volume change, the regional ejection fraction (REF) is determined according to the formula:

$$\frac{ED\ half\text{-}slice\ volume\ (ml) - ES\ half\text{-}slice\ volume\ (ml)}{ED\ half\text{-}slice\ volume\ (ml)}$$

$$\times 100 = REF\ (\%) \tag{IV.5}$$

The individual REF- and CREF-values are again listed on the LV report.

Normal CREF-values have been derived from a group of normal subjects [7, 9]. The normal ranges were defined by the 10th and 90th percentile values and are displayed in a composite CREF-plot (Fig. IV.14). The shaded areas in this plot represent the normal ranges. Abnormalities in the CREF-values of a particular patient can be recognized very easily by superimposing the CREF-values of that patient in the composite CREF-plot. From Fig. IV.14 it is evident, that the anterior segments 5–10 of the patient of figure IV.9 demonstrate clearly subnor-

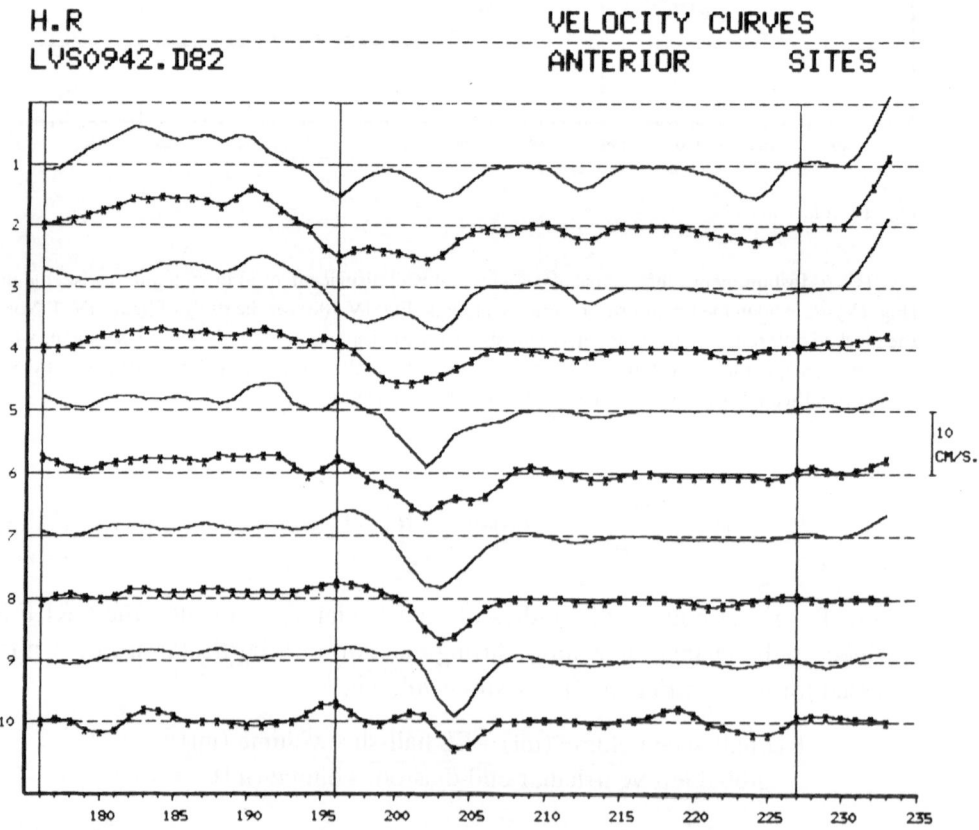

Fig. IV.11a.

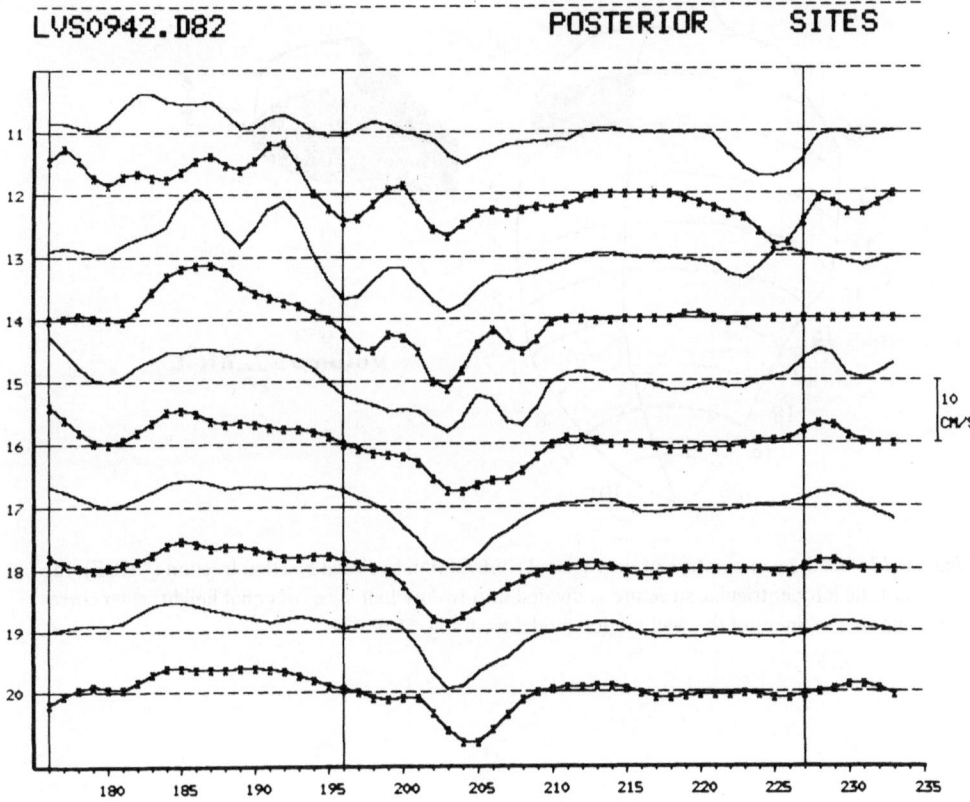

Fig. IV.11b.

Fig. IV.11. Instantaneous velocity curves for the ten anterior (Fig. IV.11a) and the ten infero-posterior sites (Fig. IV.11b) of Fig. IV.9. The vertical scale (velocity of 10 cm/s) is indicated on the graphs.

mal contribution to the global ejection fraction; marginally subnormal responses are found for the infero-posterior segments no's 17–20.

For purposes of comparing the quantitative results with those provided by the usual visual interpretation, the left ventricular boundary has been divided into a

Table IV.1. Assignment of left ventricular segments 1–20 to five anatomical regions.

Regions	Segments	Normal CREF-ranges
Antero-basal	1, 2, 3, 4, $1/_2 \times 5$	14.4–25.4
Antero-apical	$1/_2 \times 5$, 6, 7, 8, $1/_2 \times 9$	10.1–17.3
Apical	$1/_2 \times 9$, 10, 20, $1/_2 \times 19$	2.5–6.3
Postero-basal	11, 12, 13, 14, $1/_2 \times 15$	15.7–25.4
Postero-apical	$1/_2 \times 15$, 16, 17, 18, $1/_2 \times 19$	10.6–18.2

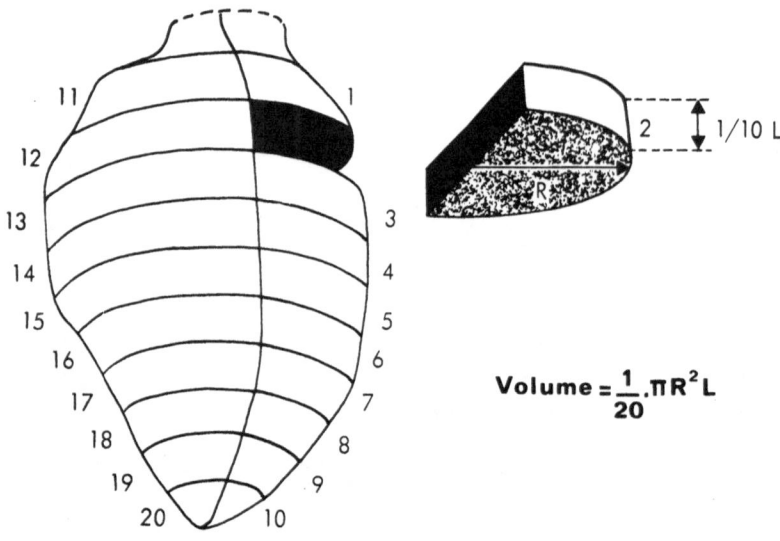

Fig. IV.12. For the computation of the regional contribution to global ejection fraction (CREF), the end-diastolic left ventricular structure is divided into twenty half-slices of equal height, each corresponding to a segment of the wall motion model from Fig. IV.9.

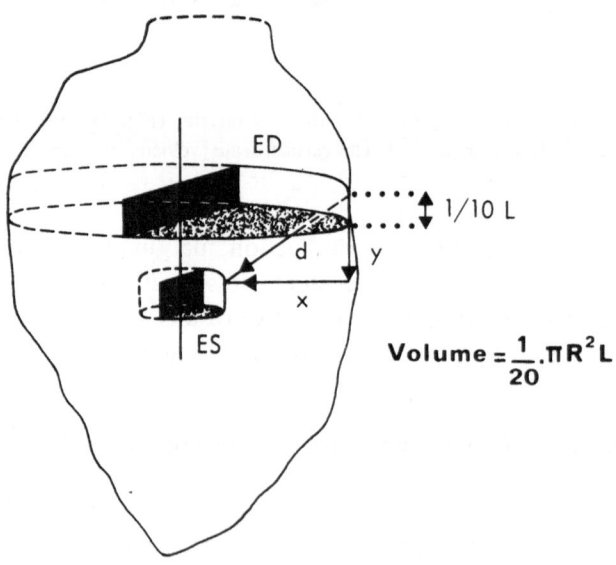

Fig. IV.13. The regional contribution to global ejection fraction (CREF) is determined from the systolic decrease of volume of the half-slice which corresponds to a particular wall segment. The systolic volume change is mainly a consequence of the decrease of radius (R) of the half-slice, which is expressed by the x-component (x) of the displacement vector (d).

total of five anatomical regions, denoted antero-basal, antero-apical, apical, postero-basal and postero-apical. The segments assigned to these regions are listed in Table IV.1. The corresponding normal ranges of the CREF-values for these regions are given in this table as well. These ranges are also displayed in Fig. IV.14, preceded by the letter N. The global CREF-values for this particular patient study, denoted in Fig. IV.14 by the large characters in these five regions, show again subnormal responses for the antero-apical and apical segments.

It was described above how the CREF-values were derived from the ED- and ES-contours. It will be clear, that instantaneous CREF-plots can also be derived by applying the same procedure to the individual left ventricular contours. This is realized by computing for each segment at a particular point in time t the corresponding half-slice volume according to the following formula:

$$\text{half-slice volume at time t:} \quad \frac{1}{20} \cdot \pi \cdot R^2(t) \cdot L_{ED}, \tag{IV.6}$$

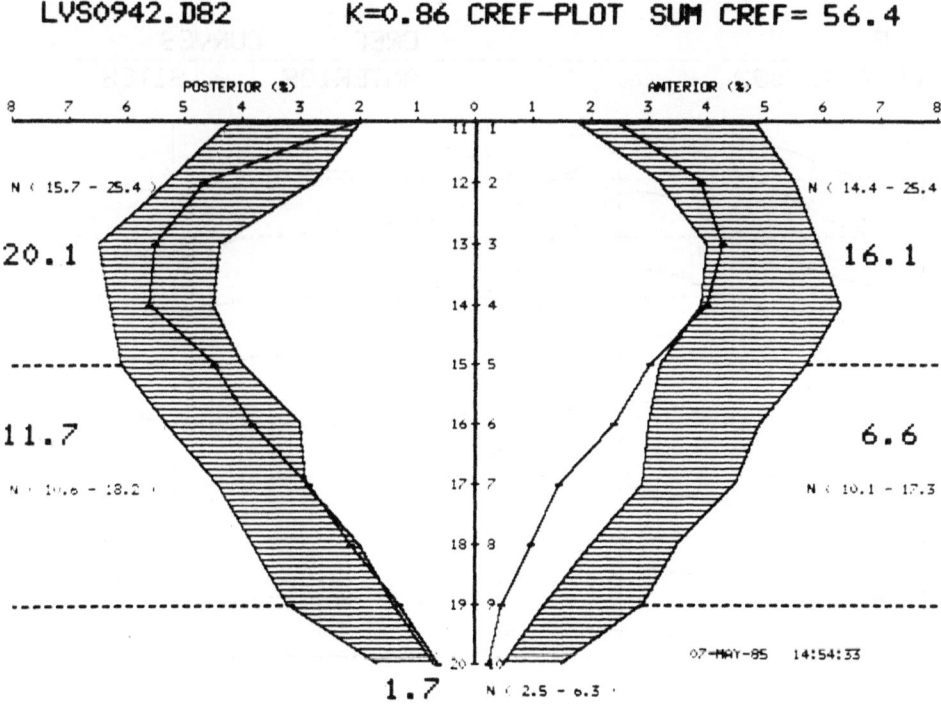

Fig. IV.14. Composite CREF-plot with normal ranges for the CREF-values of the twenty segments (hatched areas). The individual anterior and infero-posterior CREF-values of the patient of Fig. IV.9 have been superimposed in this plot and connected by straight lines. This particular patient demonstrates subnormal contribution to global ejection fraction in the anterior segments no's 5–10, and marginally subnormal responses in the infero-posterior segments no's 17–20.

where R(t) is the radius of a particular slice at time t.

Although the ventricular longitudinal shortening is also a function of time, a constant length L_{ED} equal to the end-diastolic length has been assumed, since the true instantaneous shortening is unknown. The instantaneous CREF-value for a particular slice is then defined by:

$$\frac{\text{ED half-slice volume (ml)} - \text{half-slice volume at time t (ml)}}{\text{global left ventricular ED-volume (ml)}} \times 100 =$$

$$= \text{instantaneous CREF (\%)} \tag{IV.7}$$

The instantaneous CREF-plots for the anterior and infero-posterior sites are given in Figures IV.15a and IV.15b, respectively. These plots basically show the same responses as the displacement plots.

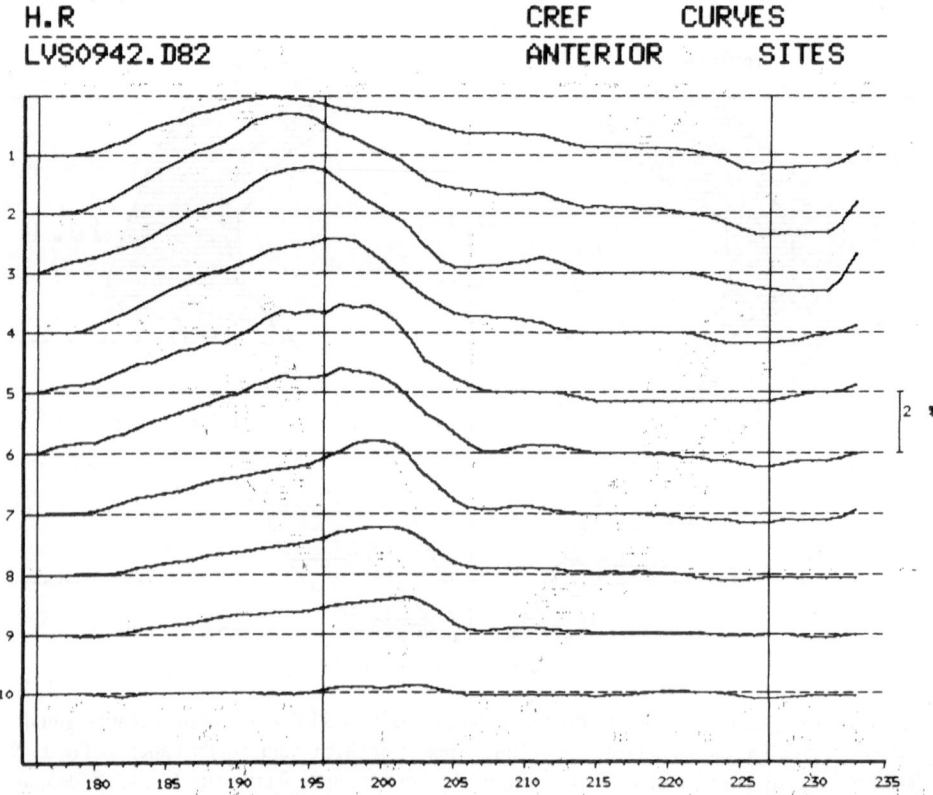

Fig. IV.15a.

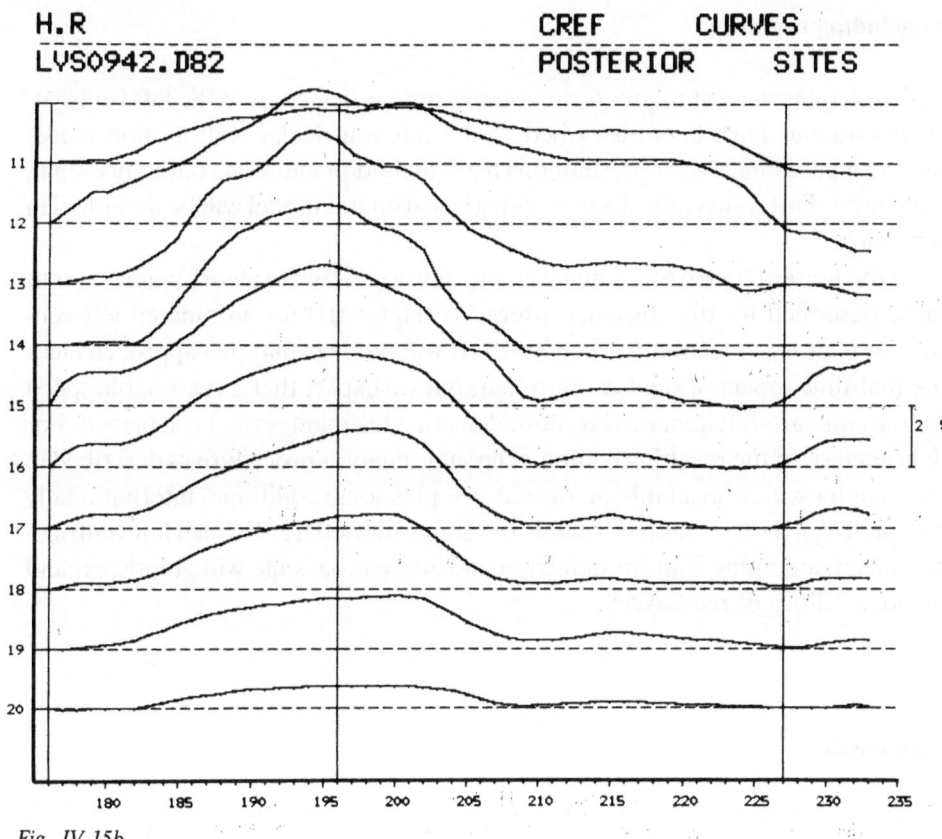

H.R   CREF   CURVES
LVS0942.D82   POSTERIOR   SITES

Fig. IV.15b.

Fig. IV.15. Instantaneous anterior (Fig. IV.15a) and infero-posterior (Fig. IV.15b) CREF-plots.

Left ventricular data analysis procedure (MINI-cine)

When the MINI-cine analysis procedure is executed, the ED- and ES-contours are displayed on the video monitor together with the various derived parameters as shown in Fig. IV.9. The postero-basal reference position for the LV-model, being the mitral valve fornix, is defined automatically [9] and marked in the ED-contour; the user is requested to agree with this position or to correct it interactively. Next, the left ventricular wall motion model is generated and finally, the composite CREF-plot in the format of Fig. IV.14 is generated.

In this mode the following parameters are printed on the LV report for the anterior and infero-posterior segments:
1. Systolic displacement (cm)
2. Mean systolic velocity (cm/s)
3. Mean systolic circumferential fiber shortening (cm/s)
4. REF-values
5. CREF-values

Concluding remarks

In this chapter the techniques for real-time contour detection of the left ventricular boundaries have been described, and a left ventricular wall motion model based on anatomical data presented. This wall motion model is routinely used in our center. Different clinical applications based on this model will be described in this book.

At the present time work is underway to develop software algorithms similar to those described for the coronary arteries (Chapter III) for automated left ventricular contour detection on the CAAS. It will be clear that this approach lacks the real-time aspect of the Contouromat, but we expect that a reasonable speed for the software-implemented contour detection techniques can be achieved. For data analysis of the resulting contours the same analysis procedure as described in this chapter will be available on the CAAS, plus some additional internationally accepted wall motion models, such as the Stanford-model [10]. Such left ventricular cineangiographic contour detection and analysis package will greatly expand the possibilities of the CAAS.

References

1. Slager CJ, Reiber JHC, Schuurbiers JCH, Meester GT: Contouromat – A hard-wired left ventricular angio processing system. I. Design and application. Comp Biomed Res 11: 491–502, 1978.
2. Reiber JHC, Slager CJ, Schuurbiers JCH, Meester GT: Contouromat – A hard-wired left ventricular angio processing system. II. Performance evaluation. Comp Biomed Res 11: 503–523, 1978.
3. Heintzen PH, Brennecke R, Bürsch JH, Lange P, Malerczyk V, Moldenhauer K, Onnasch D: Automated video-angiocardiographic image analysis. Comp Cardiol: 67–75, 1974.
4. Wallace AG, Skinner NS, Jr, Mitchell JH: Hemodynamic determinants of the maximal rate of rise of left ventricular pressure. Am J Physiol 205: 30–40, 1963.
5. Mason DT, Braunwald E, Covell JW, Sonnenblick EH, Ross J, Jr: Assessment of cardiac contractility. The relation between the rate of pressure rise and ventricular pressure during isovolumic systole. Circulation 44: 47–58, 1971.
6. Slager CJ, Hooghoudt TEH, Reiber JHC, Schuurbiers JCH, Booman F, Meester GT: Left ventricular contour segmentation from anatomical landmark trajectories and its application to wall motion analysis. Comp Cardiol: 347–350, 1979.
7. Hooghoudt TEH: Computer analysis of left ventricular cineangiograms. Thesis, Erasmus University Rotterdam, 1982.
8. Slager CJ, Hooghoudt TEH, Reiber JHC, Schuurbiers JCH, Verdouw PD, Hugenholtz PG: Left ventricular wall motion as derived from endocardially implanted radiopaque markers and from contrastangiograms. In: Ventricular Wall Motion. U. Sigwart, P.H. Heintzen (Eds.). Georg Thieme Verlag, Stuttgart/New York: 150–159, 1984.
9. Slager CJ, Hooghoudt TEH, Serruys PW, Schuurbiers JCH, Reiber JHC, Verdouw PD, Hugenholtz PG: Quantitative assessment of regional left ventricular motion. J Amer Coll Cardiol 7, No. 2, 1986.

10. Alderman EL, Schwarzkopf A, Ingels NB, Daughters GT, Stinson EB, Sanders WJ: Application of an externally referenced, polar coordinate system for left ventricular wall motion analysis. Comp Cardiol: 207–210, 1979.

V. Validation quantitation techniques of coronary and left ventricular cineangiograms

Introduction

In Chapter III the CAAS computer-assisted analysis system for the assessment of coronary artery dimensions from 35 mm cineangiograms was described. This system allows the delineation of the boundaries of user-selected coronary arterial segments by means of automated edge detection algorithms. Absolute diameter measurements can be obtained by using the intracardiac catheter as a scaling device; detected contour positions of both the analyzed catheter and the arterial segment are corrected for pincushion distortion in the images. Various parameters can be obtained for the description of the severity of a coronary obstruction, such as minimal obstruction diameter, extent of the obstruction and percentage diameter narrowing with respect to a user-defined or a computer-defined reference diameter. Mean diameter values over user-defined lengths can be obtained for nonobstructed coronary segments.

The Contouromat was described in Chapter IV. This system allows operator-assisted analysis of the boundaries of the left ventricular cineangiograms over a complete cardiac cycle. Global and regional data on the ejection fraction can be derived, as well as data on regional wall displacement and velocity.

It is the purpose of this chapter to: (1) present the results from a validation study on the accuracy and precision of the coronary contour detection technique; (2) present data on the variability of the coronary analysis procedure; (3) discuss the overall short-, medium- and long-term variabilities of repeated coronary angiography ànd computer analysis; and (4) provide data on the reliability and success of the implemented techniques for left ventricular boundary detection.

A. Accuracy and precision contour detection technique

To determine the accuracy and precision of the contour detection process, cinefilms of nine perspex models of coronary arteries with circular cross sections

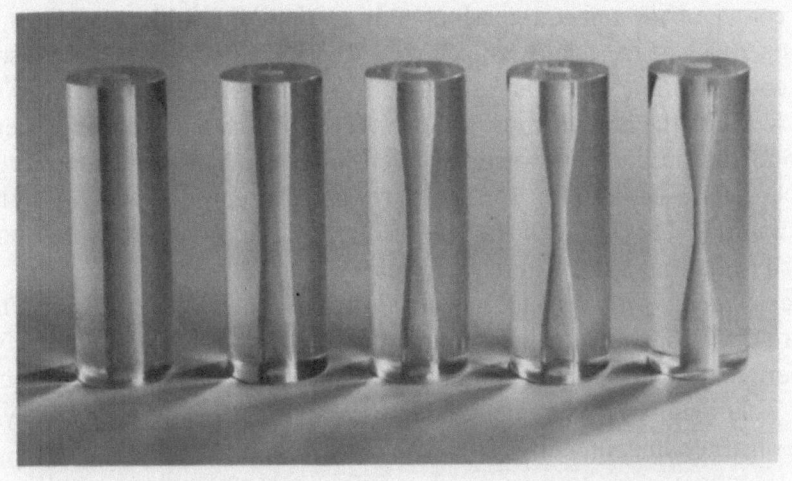

Fig. V.1. Photograph of five perspex models.

filled with contrast medium were analyzed. Figure V.1 is a photograph of five of these perspex models, while figure V.2 is a cineframe of four of these models filled with a 50% concentration of contrast medium. Absolute dimensions of the models were known with an accuracy of ±0.01 mm. The percentage diameter narrowing for this set of models ranged from 0% to 70%. The models were filmed

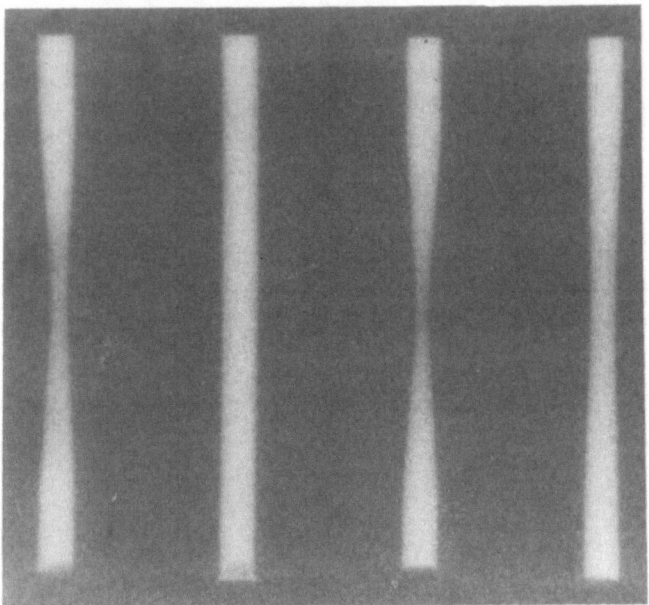

Fig. V.2. Cineframe of the four models filled with contrast medium.

in the center of the image intensifier field-of-view under 10 cm of water with various settings of the quality (range 60–110 kV) of the X-ray system; also different concentrations (50% and 100%) of the contrast agent (Urografin-76[R*]) were used. For the obstructions in the models, the diameter reduction percentages and the absolute obstruction dimensions were measured following the described analysis procedure. The accuracy was defined by the average difference of the computed results with the true values and the precision by the pooled standard deviation of the differences.

For each model with a given concentration of the contrast agent the mean and standard deviation of all the measurements at the various kV-levels of the X-ray tube were determined (Tables V.1 and V.2). The overall accuracy and precision for the %-D stenosis measurements equaled 2.00% and 2.68%, respectively, and for the obstruction diameters $-30\,\mu$m and $90\,\mu$m, respectively.

Table V.1. Measured %-D stenosis versus true %-D stenosis (mean ± s.d.) for the nine perspex models.

True %-D stenosis	Measured %-D stenosis	
	Contrast agent concentration 100%	Contrast agent concentration 50%
0	0.92 ± 1.90	3.33 ± 3.41
20	21.83 ± 2.04	21.83 ± 2.48
25	25.33 ± 3.14	26.33 ± 1.21
40	42.33 ± 3.27	43.17 ± 4.12
50	51.50 ± 3.27	54.83 ± 2.93
60	61.33 ± 1.51	62.50 ± 1.76
62.5	63.33 ± 2.42	64.67 ± 3.27
70	70.50 ± 1.97	73.33 ± 2.25

Table V.2. Measured versus true obstruction diameters (mean ± s.d.) for nine perspex models.

True size in mm	Measured size in mm	
	Contrast agent concentration 100%	Contrast agent concentration 50%
5	4.90 ± 0.10	4.97 ± 0.12
4	3.95 ± 0.10	3.94 ± 0.09
3	2.99 ± 0.09	3.00 ± 0.11
2	1.97 ± 0.11	1.98 ± 0.09
1.5	1.50 ± 0.06	1.50 ± 0.10

* Schering AG, Berlin, Germany.

B. Variability data analysis procedure

The variability of repeated analysis of cineangiograms was assessed from a total of 13 end-diastolic cineframes of 13 routinely performed coronary angiographies. These cineframes were analyzed twice by one technical analyst with a median time interval of 28 days. In each cineframe one coronary obstruction was analyzed, as well as a number of coronary segments showing no focal obstruction. As a result, a total of 13 coronary obstructions and 25 nonobstructed segments were analyzed twice. The mean difference and standard deviations of the repeated measurements as well as the overall mean values of the parameters are presented in Table V.3. These data show that with the exception of the interpolated reference diameter measurement and the mean diameter of nonobstructed segments no significant differences were found between the repeated measurements. The standard deviation of absolute measurements was less than 0.12 mm. The variabilities in the %-D stenosis measurements for the user-defined and interpolated procedures were 2.74% and 3.94%, respectively.

C. Overall variabilities of repeated coronary cineangiography and computer analysis

Knowledge of overall variabilities of repeated coronary cineangiography and computer analysis is necessary to be able to determine whether an observed change in the dimensions of a coronary arterial segment due to a given interven-

Table V.3. Variability in measurements various parameters of coronary arterial segments from repeated analysis of 13 cineframes. A total of 13 coronary obstructions and 25 nonobstructed coronary segments were analyzed twice. n.s. = nonsignificant.

	Overall mean value	Mean diff.	p-value	s.d. diff.
Calibration factor (mm/pixel)	0.096	0.0003	n.s.	0.002
User-defined Reference (N = 13)				
Obstruction diam. (mm)	1.52	0.00	n.s.	0.10
Reference diam. (mm)	2.97	0.005	n.s.	0.12
%-D stenosis (%)	48.40	0.23	n.s.	2.74
Extent (mm)	8.42	−0.38	n.s.	1.89
Interpolated Reference (N=13)				
Reference diam. (mm)	2.87	−0.10	<0.004	0.10
%-D stenosis (%)	47.90	−2.08	n.s.	3.94
Nonobstructed segments (N = 25)				
Mean diam. (mm)	2.42	0.07	<0.005	0.11
Length segment (mm)	17.72	0.02	n.s.	0.97

tion is statistically significant. In this context, various situations must be distinguished. First of all, the effect of a selective injection of contrast medium on arterial dimensions must be studied under identical X-ray system settings (short-term variability). Secondly, the question must be posed what the variability in arterial dimensions is during one particular catheterization session with a relatively long time, for example 1 hour, between contrast injections, during which time other observations may be performed (medium-term variability). Thirdly, what are the worst case changes in arterial dimensions between long term observations, for example over a period of several months (long-term variability)?

Material to study the short-, medium- and long-term variabilities in the acquisition and analysis of coronary cineangiograms were obtained from three different intervention studies. The patient material will be described in more detail below. For all studies, cineframes to be analyzed were selected at end diastole, if possible. In cases of overlap of a particular segment to be analyzed with other vessels, the frame was selected at another instant in time near end diastole. The user-determined beginning and end points of the major coronary segments were standardized according to the definitions by the American Heart Association [1].

Statistical analysis

The results from the various studies were analyzed for significant differences using Student's t-test for paired values (border of significance: $p = 0.01$).

Short-term (5 min.) variability

The short-term variability was defined by the variability in measured arterial dimensions from repeated acquisition and analysis of coronary cineangiographies taken 5 min. apart with unchanged geometry of the X-ray system. Data were collected from 12 patients catheterized for suspected coronary artery disease. Two patients had normal coronary arteries, there was one patient with one vessel disease, six patients had two vessels obstructed and three patients had three vessel obstructions.

A total of 36 coronary segments was selected for quantitative angiographic analysis; eight were stenotic in nature, and 28 were normal. In addition to measuring the various parameters of the obstructions for the 8 stenotic segments, the mean diameters of 7 pre-stenotic and of 4 post-stenotic portions were determined, resulting in a total of 39 measurements for the mean diameters of nonobstructed portions of the coronary arterial system. Two baseline coronary angiograms (C1, C2) were performed five minutes apart. The second control angiogram (C2) was carried out to study the effect of the contrast agent itself on the arteries. The patient's position was kept unchanged in relation to the X-ray equipment during both angiograms. All arteriograms were obtained via the Sones technique and recorded on Kodak 35 mm cinefilm at the rate of 50 frames per second. An ionic contrast medium, Urografin-76^R, was injected at a flow of 3 ml/s with a Medrad injector. Peak systolic pressure remained constant during both control cineangiograms.

Since the views were unchanged during the repeat angiographies, calibration was only performed for the first set of angiograms.

The data on the short-term variability (5 min.) as assessed from the two control cineangiograms (C1, C2) are presented in Table V.4. For the obstruction diameters a small, nonsignificant increase of 0.05 mm (3.01%) was found between the repeat angiographies with a standard deviation of the differences of 0.34 mm. As a result of the contrast injection, 4 obstructions showed a decrease in the minimal obstruction diameter and the 4 other obstructions an increase. The user-defined reference diameters, all taken proximal of the obstructions, showed an average nonsignificant decrease by 0.1 mm with a standard deviation of 0.17 mm. At the average, the severity of the stenoses expressed in terms of user-defined %-D narrowing decreased by 2.46% with a standard deviation of 8.01%; in 3 of the cases the percentage narrowing increased, in the other 5 cases it decreased. The variabilities by the interpolated technique in the reference diameter (0.21 mm) and %-D stenosis (8.30%) were slightly higher than the values obtained by the user-defined technique; the mean differences in these parameters were also nonsignificant.

For the total of 39 nonobstructed segments, a small, nonsignificant decrease in mean diameter of 0.005 mm (0.18%) was found with a standard deviation of 0.16 mm; the average length of the segments was 11.37 mm. Seventeen segments

Table V.4. Short-term variabilities in measurements various parameters of coronary arterial segments for the two control cineangiograms (C1, C2); difference values are computed as C2–C1. n.s. = nonsignificant.

	Overall mean	mean diff.	p-values	.d. diff.
User-defined reference (N = 8)				
Obstruction diam. (mm)	1.66	+0.05	n.s.	0.34
Reference diam. (mm)	3.33	−0.10	n.s.	0.17
%-D stenosis (%)	46.50	−2.46	n.s.	8.01
Extent (mm)	6.60	+0.50	n.s.	1.31
Interpolated reference (N = 8)				
Reference diam. (mm)	3.17	+0.02	n.s.	0.21
%-D stenosis (%)	44.90	−0.90	n.s.	8.30
Nonobstructed segments (N = 39)				
Mean diam. (mm)	2.82	−0.005	n.s.	0.16
Length segment (mm)	11.37	−0.33	n.s.	1.36

122

showed an increase in the mean diameter, while the other 22 segments showed a decrease.

These data show that the short-term variability in the obstruction diameter (s.d. = 0.34 mm) is about twice the variability of measurements at nonobstructed portions of the segments (reference diameter (s.d. = 0.17 mm) and mean diameter of nonobstructed segments (s.d. = 0.16 mm)). These last two variability measures are about 50% higher than the values obtained from repeated analysis of cinefilms alone (Table V.3).

Medium-term (1 hour) variability

As part of a pharmacological intervention study, we have assessed the 1 hour variability in the measurements of coronary arterial segments with repeated coronary angiography and analysis. Eleven patients were studied according to the following protocol. At first, coronary angiography was performed in the control state (angio 1). The geometry of the X-ray gantry and the kV, mA of the X-ray generator were acquired on-line with each angiographic procedure [2]. Immediately, thereafter, the first metabolite of Molsidomine[R]* (Sin 1) was administered in the left main stem and 2 min. thereafter, coronary angiographies were obtained in the same multiple views to study the immediate effect of the drug on the dimensions of the coronary arteries (angio 2) [3]. One hour later these angiographies were repeated to assess the long lasting effect of the drug (angio 3). A fourth angiographic procedure (angio 4) was carried out following a second intracoronary administration of the drug to see whether further dilatation could be achieved by a 2nd administration. Since other observations were performed during the 1 hour period, the X-ray system had to be repositioned in a projection corresponding as much as possible to the projection used during the first two angiographies. For these purposes, the angular settings of the X-ray gantry and the various height levels were readjusted according to the values documented with the on-line registration system. All arteriograms were obtained via the Judkins technique and recorded on Kodak 35 mm cinefilm at a rate of 25 frames per second. For this study, a nonionic contrast medium, Omnipaque[R]* *, was injected manually. By comparing the arterial dimensions from angio's 2 and 4, we can assess the medium-term variability, when standardization of the angio procedure is attempted (including 'control' of the vasomotor tone). Each analyzed cineframe was separately calibrated on the basis of the displayed contrast catheter. Pincushion distortion was corrected for as described. A total of 16 coronary obstructions were analyzed, as well as 90 nonobstructed segments.

The overall mean values and the variabilities in the X-ray gantry settings are

*   Cassella, Frankfurt am Main, Germany
* * Nyegaard, Oslo, Norway

Table V.5. Variability in X-ray gantry settings with repeated cineangiographies (N = 25 views). n.s. = nonsignificant.

	Overall mean value	Mean diff.	p-value	s.d. diff.
Rotation U-arm (degrees)	31.2	0.3	n.s.	4.2
Rotation pat./C-arm (degrees)	26.4	0.3	n.s.	2.2
Isocenter-Image Intensifier distance (cm) (IID)	22.6	1.1	n.s.	3.0
Focus-Isocenter distance (cm) (FID)	72.8	−0.3	n.s.	0.8
Object-Isocenter distance (cm) (OID)	5.3	0.2	n.s.	1.4

presented in Table V.5. The angular variability computed from the absolute differences of angular settings was less than 4.2 degrees. The variability in the various positions of image intensifier and X-ray source was less than 3.0 cm. There were no significant differences between the repeated X-ray system settings. These results show that the X-ray system settings can be reproduced quite accurately in routine clinical practice.

The mean differences in the measured parameters from angio's 2 and 4 were all nonsignificant (Table V.6). The overall mean values were computed from angio

Table V.6. Medium-term variabilities in measurements various parameters of coronary arterial segments from repeated coronary angiographies and analysis. Angiograms 2 and 4 were performed immediately following administration of a vasodilatory drug. Time between angio's 2 and 4 was approximately 1 hour (see text). n.s. = nonsignificant.

		Angio 4–2		
	Overall mean	Mean diff.	p-value	s.d. diff.
Calibration factor (N = 25)				
(mm/pixel)	0.094	−0.001	n.s.	0.002
User-Defined Reference (N = 16)				
Obstruction diam. (mm)	2.13	0.00	n.s.	0.22
Reference diam. (mm)	3.57	0.06	n.s.	0.28
%-D stenosis (%)	41.30	0.75	n.s.	8.09
Extent (mm)	6.28	−0.15	n.s.	2.03
Interpolated Reference (N = 14)				
Reference diam. (mm)	3.32	0.05	n.s.	0.15
%-D stenosis (%)	38.10	1.21	n.s.	7.23
Nonobstructed segments (N = 90)				
Mean diam. (mm)	3.05	0.07	n.s.	0.24
Length segment (mm)	14.03	−0.03	n.s.	1.02

2. The medium-term variabilities in the obstruction diameters are 35% lower than those for the short-term study, while the variabilities in mean diameter and user-defined reference diameter increased by 50% and 65%, respectively. The variability in the interpolated reference diameter decreased by 29% with respect to the 5 min. study.

Long-term (90 days) variability

Out of a group of 153 patients planned for percutaneous transluminal coronary angioplasty (PTCA), a subgroup of 26 PTCA candidates was selected having two good quality cineangiograms performed in a number of standard views and therefore suitable for paired analysis of the stenotic lesions [4]. The first film was the diagnostic angiogram, while the second measurements were obtained from the PTCA-film, immediately prior to the actual PTCA-procedure. At the time of the angiographic investigations, no attempt was made to standardize on inspiratory level, volume and rate of injection of the contrast agent, nor on technical characteristics of the X-ray system. More importantly, the vasomotor tone in both conditions was unknown and neglected. These data therefore represent the worst case changes in arterial dimensions between long-term observations. The median delay between the diagnostic and the PTCA angiogram in these patients was 90 days (range 1–250 days). The median %-D stenosis of the obstructions for this group as assessed from the diagnostic angiogram was 66.2 percent (range 53%–83%).

No significant differences were observed in the mean values of the obstruction and reference diameters, as well as of percentage diameter stenosis (Table V.7). This suggests that no detectable progression or regression of atherosclerotic lesions had occurred over the period of 90 days. These paired data provide some insight in the total variability of the cineangiographic procedure and the computer analysis under worst-case circumstances, since no special care had been taken to reduce the potential sources of variability (X-ray system settings, vasomotor tone, etc.).

Table V.7. Long-term variabilities in measurements various parameters of coronary obstructions.

	Overall mean	Mean diff.	p-value	s.d. diff.
(N = 26)				
Obstruction diam. (mm)	1.25	0.00	n.s.	0.36
Extent (mm)	10.04	0.62	n.s.	4.34
Interpolated Reference				
Reference diam. (mm)	3.72	−0.13	n.s.	0.66
%-D stenosis (%)	66.19	−1.92	n.s.	6.52

Under these uncontrolled conditions the variations in absolute measurements were 0.36 mm for the obstruction diameter and 0.66 mm for the interpolated reference diameter, and 6.5 percent for the interpolated %-D stenosis.

D. Discussion evaluation data CAAS

We feel that we have developed a computer-based system that facilitates an objective and reproducible approach to the assessment of coronary artery disease. The system combines a number of important features: (1) a region of interest in a selected cineframe encompassing the arterial segment to be analyzed is optically magnified and video converted by means of a specially constructed x-y controlled cine-video converter; (2) a highly reliable edge detection algorithm has been developed; (3) the boundary information is corrected for magnification and distortion in the images; (4) absolute values of clinically important parameters of lesion severity can be assessed in a reliable manner; and (5) the analysis procedure has been designed in a user-friendly manner such that a technical analyst can work with it following a short training period.

Technical characteristics

Since large changes in underlying background densities may occur in a cineframe, it is of great importance that a cineframe is illuminated homogeneously over the entire image. Only then it is possible to fully utilize the dynamic range of the video camera and as a result digitize the optical density changes at the arteries with a maximum number of grey levels. The optical path of the cine-video converter has been designed for such a homogeneous response; this plays not only a role for accurate edge detection purposes, but even more so for implementation of densitometric analysis techniques. This homogeneous response can be demonstrated with the experiment described in Chapter III.

The edge detection algorithm is based on the weighted sum of first- and second-derivative functions. From our experience and those of others, it is well known that positions defined by the maximal response of first-derivative criteria lie within the projected arteries [5]. On the other hand, due to the limited frequency response of the entire X-ray/cine/video chain, the maximal response of second-derivative functions will result in detected positions outside of the arterial lumen. Therefore, the weighted sum of first- and second-derivative functions provides an accurate definition of the arterial lumen. The weighting factor has been derived at empirically and has been validated with the perspex models. Great advantage of the minimal cost contour detection algorithm is the fact that the edge positions are not determined per individual scanline, but an overall minimal cost path is computed. Side branches and other disturbing structures therefore only have minimal influence on the contour path.

For those parts along a detected arterial segment, where the observer does not agree with the automatically detected boundaries, manual corrections by means of the writing tablet are possible. If the manual correction is performed after the first iteration of the edge detection procedure, a narrow expectation window is defined in the cost matrix for the corrected scanlines, which allows the system to find an optimal path within these limits during the second iteration. It has been our experience, that in almost all cases the contour will then follow the desired path at these locations. Advantage of this approach is that the final contour will still be based on the available edge information within the limitations set by the user. This type of correction may be designated as 'soft' correction. In those situations, where the soft correction still does not result in the desired contour after the second iteration, the user may apply a final 'hard' correction. The computer registers for both the left- and right-hand contours, the lengths of the arterial segments that were manually corrected, expressed as percentages of the total length of the analyzed contour sides. In addition, the mean percentage length of the correction paths for the left- and right- hand contours is provided on the computer print-out.

Thanks to the ease with which detected contours can be corrected, even films of relatively poor quality can be analyzed. However, it will be clear that with increasing user-interaction, the inter- and intra-variabilities in the results from an analysis will also increase.

From the evaluation study with the perspex models it may be concluded that the detected edge positions closely approximate the true positions. For the absolute minimal obstruction diameters the values for the overall accuracy and precision were $-30\,\mu m$ and $90\,\mu m$, respectively. This $30\,\mu m$ accuracy compares favorably with the accuracy ranges of $59–137\,\mu m$ for the method recently published by Spears et al. [6].

Strictly speaking, the calibration factor computed from a single view is only applicable for objects in the plane of the analyzed catheter segment parallel to the image intensifier input screen. The change in magnification for two objects located at different points along the X-ray beam axis is about 1.5% for each centimeter that separates the objects axially with the commonly used focus-image intensifier distances. For coronary segments lying in other planes corrections to the calibration factor could be determined from a second, preferably orthogonal, view. However, if one is only interested in the changes of sizes of coronary segments as a result of long or short term interventions, acceptable results can be obtained from single plane views. For these situations one must make sure that for the repeat angiogram the X-ray system is positioned in exactly the same geometry as during the first angiogram. Although the calibration factor used for a particular segment is then only an approximation of the true calibration factor, the same systematic error will be present for the first and the repeat angiogram.

It has been our experience, that the size of the catheter as specified by the manufacturer often deviates from the true size, especially for disposable catheters. If the manufacturer cannot guarantee narrow ranges for the size of the catheter, e.g. ± 0.05 F, it should be measured following the catheterization with a micrometer. For a 5.5 F tip of a Sones-catheter, a deviation by 0.05 F will result in an error in the computed calibration factor by 0.9%.

Sources of error in angiographic and analysis procedures

The quality of both the coronary angiographic procedure and the computer analysis procedure are hampered by various sources of variations. In the angiographic data acquisition procedure the following sources of variation can be distinguished: (i) differences in the angles and height levels of the X-ray gantry with respect to the patient at the time of repeated angiography; (ii) differences in vasomotor tone of the coronary arteries; (iii) variations in the quality of mixing of the contrast agent with the blood; and (iv) deviations in size of the catheter as listed by the manufacturer with the true size.

Variations in the data analysis procedure are caused by: (v) quantum noise in the images; (vi) electronic noise contributions in the analog video images; (vii) quantization errors in the analog-to-digital conversion; (viii) the effects of resampling the data along scanlines through the square grid of the digital data; (ix) observer variations in the definition of center positions within the catheter and the selected arterial segment, (x) possible manual corrections to the detected contours; (xi) selection of reference positions; and (xii) manual definition of starting and end points in nonobstructed arterial segments for measurement of overall mean diameter value.

To obtain reliable quantitative results from coronary cineangiograms, these variations should be minimized as much as possible, which requires a number of precautions to be taken. We have developed a number of approaches towards such a standardization. By registering the X-ray system settings on-line with a microprocessor system, differences in the angiographic projections can be minimized at the time of repeat angiography (Table V.5). The variations in vasomotor tone of the arteries can be minimized by the administration of a vasodilatory drug immediately prior to the coronary angiography. Unknown deviations in size of the catheter can be circumvented by measuring the actual size following the catheterization procedure with a micrometer.

The variations in density levels in the cinefilm due to quantum noise can be reduced by filtering the image data. The electronic noise contributions are reduced by recursive digitization of the images. The iterative approach in the edge detection algorithm results in a reduction of the variations due to the causes listed under items viii through x. It has been our experience that the position of a reference point can be reproduced quite accurately by proper documentation of the analysis data on polaroid photo's or on X-ray sheets by means of a Video

Imager (Table V.3). Similarly, the reproducibility of the manual definition of the starting and end points of arterial segments can be improved by making use as much as possible of anatomical landmarks, such as bifurcations (Table V.3).

Variabilities of acquisition and analysis procedures

Repeated analysis of the set of 13 coronary cineangiograms has shown that the variability of the data analysis procedure is excellent. No significant differences were found between the repeated measurements, while the standard deviation of the differences of absolute measurements was less than 0.12 mm. When one wants to specify the reproducibility of a coronary analysis system, this standard deviation of the differences of replicate absolute measurements is the parameter of choice, since it does not depend on arterial size. The variabilities for the user-defined and interpolated procedures were 2.74% and 3.94%, respectively. These data show that the smallest variations were obtained with the user-defined method, whereby a 'normal' reference diameter position must be defined by the user. However, at the expense of a small increase (+ 1.2%) in the variability, the percentage diameter stenosis measurements can be automated with the interpolated analysis procedure. In addition, this interpolated approach provides data about the area of the 'atherosclerotic plaque' and the lesion's eccentricity in a given view. Crawford et al. have demonstrated that such angiographic assessment of the atherosclerotic plaque correlated with the cholesterol content of the corresponding human arterial specimen [7]. Another, very practical, advantage of the use of the interpolated technique is that for the analysis of repeated angiograms, knowledge about the exact location of a reference, either proximal or distal to the stenosis, is not required [4, 8].

From the tables V.4, V.6 and V.7, the mean differences and standard deviations of the differences in the obstruction and interpolated reference diameters, as well as in the interpolated %-D stenosis have been summarized in table V.8 for the short-, medium- and long-term studies. It may be concluded from all studies that the mean differences in absolute diameters are below 0.13 mm. The variabilities in the obstruction diameters for these three types of studies vary from 0.22 mm for the medium-term study to 0.36 mm for the least-controlled long-term study. Likewise, the variabilities in the interpolated reference diameter are the smallest for the medium-term study (0.15 mm) and the largest for the long-term study (0.66 mm). The long-term study clearly demonstrates that the variabilities in absolute dimensions increase if no special care is taken to reduce the potential sources of variability. Possible reasons for the variabilities from the medium study being smaller than those from the short-term study are: (1) controlled vasomotor tone and; (2) possibly the use of a nonionic versus ionic contrast medium. Bentley and Henry, investigating the effect of Renografin-76 (1689 mosmol/l) on animal arteries, demonstrated that the angiographic dye in concentrations not exceeding those during angiography exert potent, dose- and time-dependent vasomotor effects [9]. In addition, in vivo experiments have shown that intracoronary injection of ionic, hyperosmolar and hyperviscous contrast media produce direct myocardial depression, followed by a reflex effect, adrenergically mediated, which potentially could effect the vasomotor tone of the arteries [10]. Bentley et al. have demonstrated that these deleterious effects can be prevented by the use of nonionic, iso-osmotic angiographic dye [11] (such as Omnipaque^R) and therefore may account for the observed decrease in variability measures, although this last hypothesis has not yet been demonstrated.

The variabilities in the interpolated %-D reduction are all of the same order of magnitude ranging from 8.30% for the short-term study to 6.52% for the long-term study. Therefore, an upper limit of 8.30% for the variability in interpolated %-D stenosis from repeated angiography and analysis can be defined. The mean differences are less than 1.92%.

The data from Table V.8 also make clear that the variabilities in the obstruction diameters with repeated angiographies and analysis are 2.2 to 3.6 times greater than those from repeated analysis alone, and 1.5 to 6.6 times greater for the interpolated reference diameters. This is due to the various sources of variation in the data acquisition procedure described earlier. Alderman et al. found an increase in variabilities in absolute sizes with a medium-term study compared to repeated analysis alone by a factor of 3 [12]; we found an increase by a factor of 1.5 to 2.2. In their study identical calibration factors, computed from the geometry of image intensifier and X-ray source, were used for the initial and repeat angiographies. This means that their actual variations in arterial size would be greater than the ones reported, if the calibration factor was also assessed repeatedly from the catheter, as was done in our study.

Thus from our data it may be concluded, that the biological variations are a source of major concern and that further attempts towards standardization of the angiographic procedure are seriously needed.

Table V.8. Summary of the mean and standard deviations of the differences in the absolute diameter measurements and in interpolated percentage diameter-stenosis for the short-, medium- and long-term studies.

	Mean diff.			s.d. diff.		
	Short term	Medium term	Long term	Short term	Medium term	Long term
Obstruction diam. (mm)	0.05	0.00	0.00	0.34	0.22	0.36
Ref. diam. (mm) (Interpolated)	0.02	0.05	−0.13	0.21	0.15	0.66
Interpolated %-D stenosis	−0.90	1.21	−1.92	8.30	7.23	6.52

E. Performance evaluation Contouromat

Goals of this performance evaluation were the determination of the average processing time per cineframe, the percentage of frames that require one or more manual corrections, the average number of corrections per corrected frame and the effect of a correction expressed as a percentage of calculated volume.

For the performance evaluation of the automated left ventricular contour detector 29 left ventricular angiograms in RAO projection were used [13]. These films were selected from our clinical files of left ventricular angiograms on the basis of: (1) technically correct films; and (2) absence of extra systoles. Contrast quality was not a selection criterion. Reasons to call a film technically incorrect included: (1) the apex not being completely shown on angiogram due to mispositioning of left ventricle; and (2) projected patient identification on angiogram interfered with left ventricular shadow. (This identification method has been changed now.)

The evaluation was performed by two observers; one did the actual processing of the angiograms, whereas the other kept notes of the applied corrections and the time involved. For these purposes the left ventricular contour was divided into 8 segments as shown in Fig. V.3. These segments were designated: mitral, postero-basal, diaphragmatic, postero-papillary, postero-apical, antero-apical, antero-lateral, and antero-basal. Corrections to the starting points SPI and SPII were also taken into account; SPI was always positioned at the junction of the mitral and aortic valves and SPII at the junction of the anterior endocardial outline and the aortic valve.

The evaluation study of a particular patient film was started at the first completely contrast-filled end-diastolic frame after the start of the contrast injection and was continued over one or two cardiac cycles depending on image quality. Before the cardiac cycles were processed the film was played back and

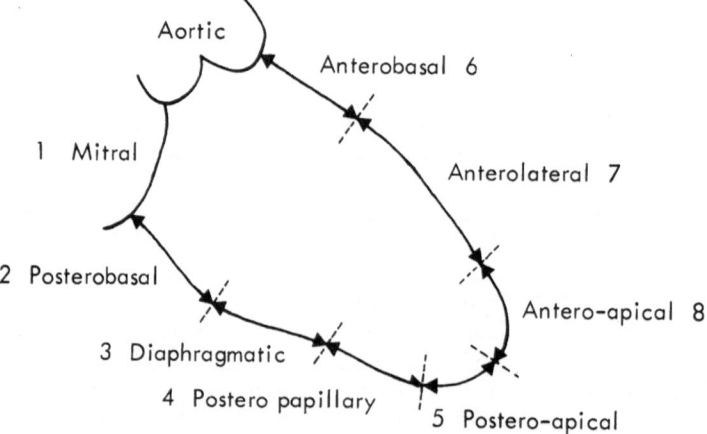

Fig. V.3. For evaluation purposes the left ventricular outline was divided into eight segments.

forth several times at normal speed to select the first end-diastolic frame to be processed, and to give an overview of the movement of the left ventricular chamber and the possible occurrence of double contours, to be discussed later. For each cineframe the frame number was noted. When corrections were necessary every corrected segment was listed with the sequence number of the correction as well as the new volume of the corrected left ventricular chamber determined on-line with a special-purpose calculator [14]. The new volume which was calculated after each correction provided a quantitative measure of the effect of the applied correction; the percentage change in the volume determined the relative effect of the correction. A positive change means that the volume of the corrected left ventricular chamber was larger than before the correction and a negative change indicates a smaller volume after correction. Three percentage classes were distinguished: (A) less than or equal to 5%, (B) less than or equal to 15% and greater than 5% and (C) greater than 15%. For every ten processed frames the total processing time was noted.

Average processing time per cineframe

In 17 of the 29 films the quality was such that the left ventricular contour could be processed automatically over two cardiac cycles. The other 12 films were processed only over one cardiac cycle, since contrast in the second cycle was so low that most of the contours would need extensive operator-controlled corrections.

The first results to be discussed will be the processing times per frame for the double- and single-cycle films. For every 10 processed cineframes the processing time and total number of corrections over these 10 processed frames were determined. For the double-cycle films the processing time per 10 frames as a function of the number of corrections in these 10 frames for all the processed series of ten frames is shown in Fig. V.4a. Applying linear regression analysis on these data yielded the following function for the regression line:

$$T_{10} = 29 + 6 \ N_{10}, \tag{V.1}$$

where T_{10} is the average processing time in seconds over 10 frames and N_{10} the number of corrections over these 10 frames. Assuming that each frame in a series of 10 frames has the same probability of requiring one or more corrections, the average processing time T per frame was

$$T = 2.9 + 6 \ N \ sec, \tag{V.2}$$

where N is the number of applied corrections per frame. The correlation coefficient of the regression analysis was 0.82.

For the one-cycle films the data are shown in figure V.4b. Applying the same kind of analysis as described above, the average processing time for the single-cycle films was

$$T = 4.5 + 6.7\,N \text{ sec.} \tag{V.3}$$

The correlation coefficient was 0.76. When comparing the expressions (V.2) and (V.3) it clearly shows, as is to be expected, that the processing time per frame of the lower quality one-cycle films is longer than for the two-cycle films for the same number of corrections per frame. There is only a 10% difference in the slope of the regression lines.

Percentage of cineframes requiring one or more manual corrections

An important parameter in the performance evaluation is also the percentage of frames requiring a correction as a function of the phase in the cardiac cycle for both the double and single cardiac cycle films. The results are shown in Fig. V.5a and V.5b, respectively. For this purpose, the cardiac cycle was divided into 8 sample periods and all obtained data from the processed angiograms were normalized with respect to this partition. For each time segment, the number of

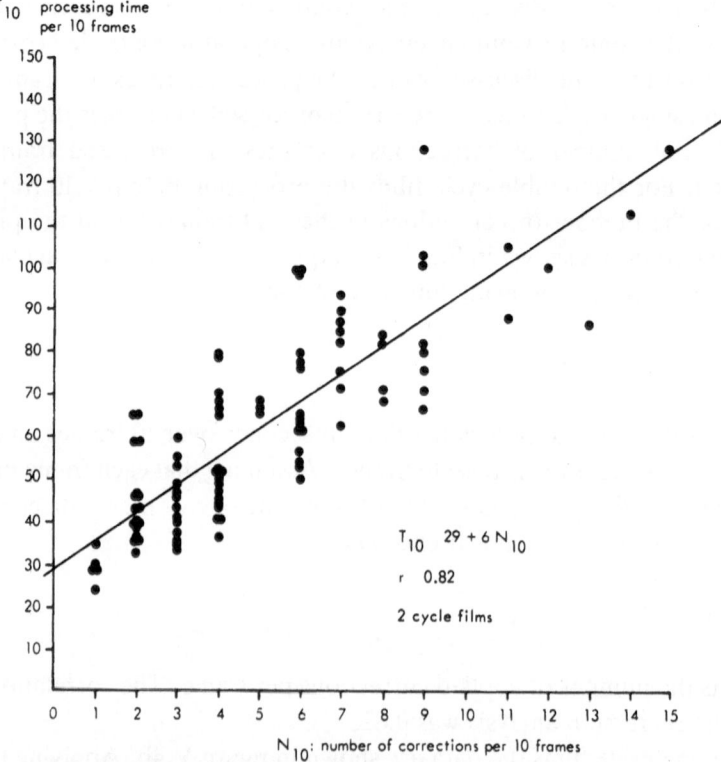

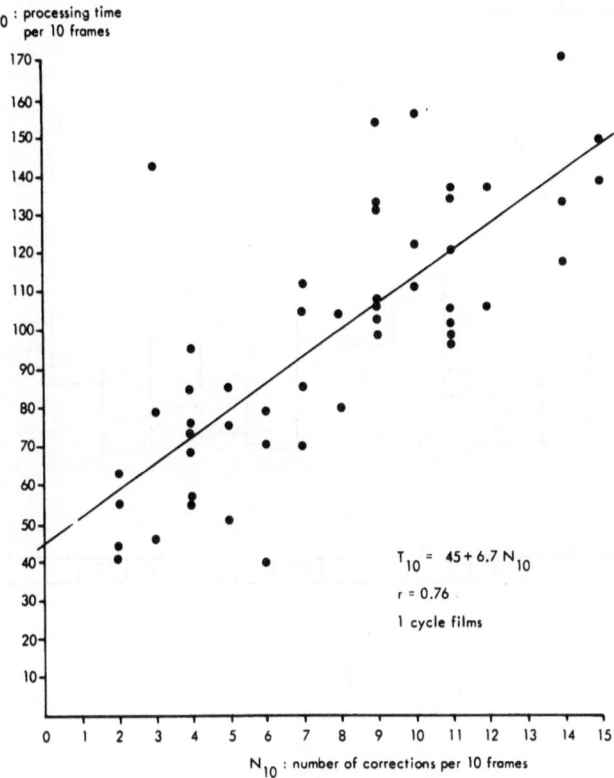

T_{10} : processing time per 10 frames

$T_{10} = 45 + 6.7\, N_{10}$

$r = 0.76$

1 cycle films

N_{10} : number of corrections per 10 frames

Fig. V.4. The processing time T_{10} per 10 consecutive frames is plotted as a function of the number of corrections N_{10} in these frames.
(a) $T_{10} = 29 + 6\,N_{10}$ sec for the double-cycle films.
(b) $T_{10} = 45 + 6.7\,N_{10}$ sec for the single-cycle films.

corrected and uncorrected frames was determined and the number of corrected frames expressed as a percentage of the total number of frames processed within this time slice. A processed frame was marked as a corrected frame, if one or more corrections were necessary for that frame. The data for the double-cycle films shown in Fig. V.5a will be described first. The shape of the correction curve for both cycles is similar.

At end diastole the required number of corrections was minimal at 21.5%. Going from end diastole to end systole the number of corrections increased very often as a result of the occurrence of 'double' contours. In this phase of the cycle the mixture of blood and contrast agent is squeezed from between the deep infoldings of the papillary muscles and trabeculae carnea. The decreasing amount of contrast agent in these areas results in low contrast areas, where it is impossible to draw a definite outline, i.e., at the outside of the infoldings as indicated by the previous frames or to make a sudden jump to the inner boundary. The distances over which such a part of the contour must travel in only a few consecutive frames can be relatively large; however, the applied frame memory in the contour

134

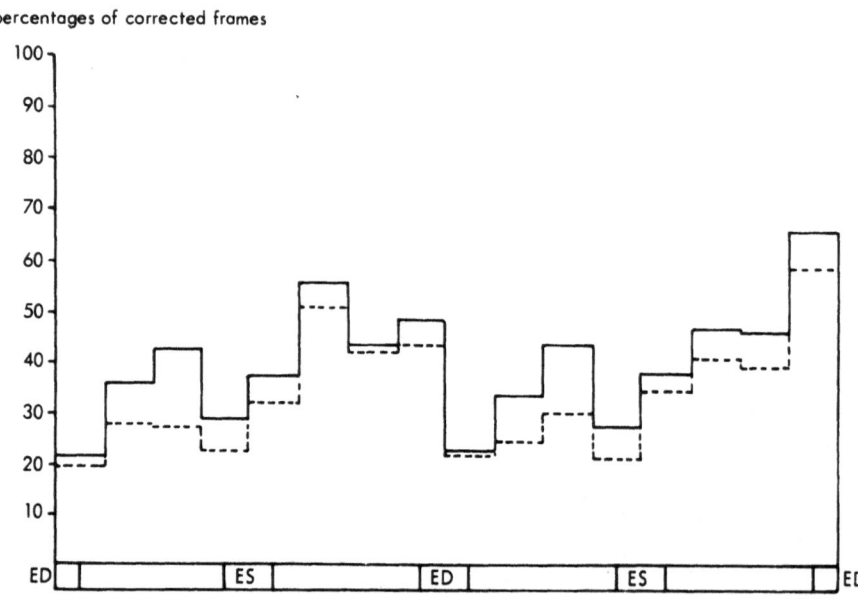

percentages of corrected frames

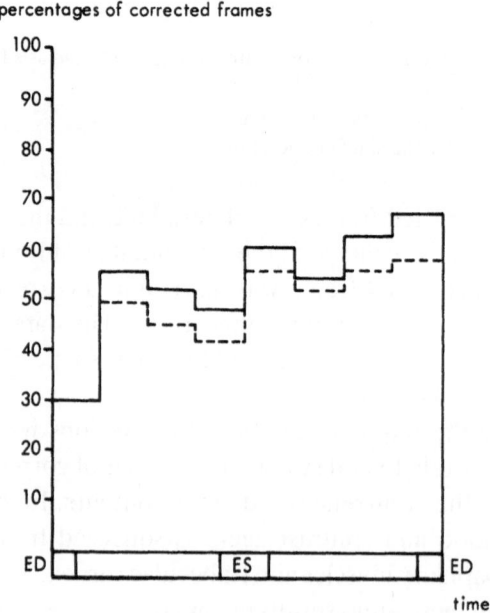

percentages of corrected frames

Fig. V.5. The percentages of the frames that require one or more corrections are given as a function of the phase in the cardiac cycle. (a) The percentage are given for the double-cycle films. (b) The percentages are given for the single-cycle films. For the meaning of the dashed lines, see text.

detector does not allow these large steps thus requiring manual corrections. As all the contrast agent is squeezed from between the deep infoldings the double contours do not occur anymore and the number of corrections decreases. Other possible reasons for corrections have been described in detail elsewhere [13].

After end systole the percentage of corrected frames increased again as during the filling phase new blood entering the left ventricle dilutes the contrast agent and disturbs the homogeneity of mixing. This very often results locally in contrast 'holes', again requiring corrections. The average percentage of corrected frames over two cardiac cycles during the contraction phase was 36.7% and during the filling phase 46.8%; the minimum at end diastole was 21.5% for the first cycle and 21.9% for the second cycle and the maximum during the filling phase 55.7% for the first cycle and 65.2% at the end of the second cycle. A repositioning of one or both starting points was also defined as a correction, although it has not the function of correcting an erroneous automatically detected contour. If we delete the starting point corrections from the counting then the percentage of corrected frames is indicated in figure V.5a with the dashed line. The average percentage over the two cycles was now 23.5% during the contraction phase and 40.4% during the filling phase.

Figure V.5b shows the results for the single-cycle data. Because the image quality of these frames was lower than of the double-cycle films the percentage of corrected frames is higher as expected. The average percentage of corrected frames during the contraction phase was 43.4% and during the filling phase 59.9%; if we exclude again the starting points corrections from the counting the percentage were 38.3% and 55.4%, respectively.

Average number of corrections per corrected cineframe and volume effects of corrections

From the obtained evaluation data it is straightforward to calculate the average number of corrections per frame. For the double-cycle angiograms this amounts to 0.5 ± 0.3 (mean $\pm$ s.d.) and for the single-cycle angiograms to 0.8 ± 0.4.

Taking only the corrected frames from the complete set of frames, the average number of corrections per corrected frame will be of interest, as well as the percentages of starting point corrections and the percentages of minor ($\triangle V \leqslant 5\%$ volume change), medium ($5\% < \triangle V \leqslant 15\%$) and large ($\triangle V > 15\%$) corrections. These last three types of corrections will be denoted types A, B, and C, respectively. The results of the double- and single-cycle films are shown in Table V.9. In both cases the average number of corrections per corrected frame was approximately 1.5. In 45.2% of the total number of corrections in the double-cycle films and in 55.4% in the single-cycle films the corrections had an effect of less than 5% volume change. The percentages medium and large volume corrections (volume changes $\triangle V$ of $5\% < \triangle V \leqslant 15\%$ and $\triangle V > 15\%$, respectively) were for the

Table V.9. For the double- and single-cycle films the number of corrections per corrected frame is given, as well as the percentages of the types A, B, and C corrections as differentiated according to the resulting volume changes and the percentages of starting point corrections.

	Double-cycle angiograms	Single-cycle angiograms
Number of corrections/corrected frame		
(mean ± s.d.)	1.4 ± 0.2	1.5 ± 0.2
Type A: $\triangle V \leqslant 5\%$	45.2%	55.4%
Type B: $5\% < \triangle V \leqslant 15\%$	25.9%	22.4%
Type C: $\triangle V > 15\%$	8.4%	11.6%
SPI, SPII	20.5%	10.6%

double-cycle studies 25.9 and 8.4%, and for the single-cycle studies 22.4 and 11.6%, respectively.

The corrections can also be differentiated according to the particular segment along the left ventricular contour and the phase in the cardiac cycle. These data for the two-cycle films have been presented in detail elsewhere [13].

For both the double- and single-cycle films it will be of interest to determine for each contour segment the percentage of frames calculated over all corrected frames which required a correction for that particular segment. These results are shown in Fig. V.6a for the double-cycle films and in Fig. V.6b for the single-cycle films. The percentages are also distinguished into type A, B, and C corrections.

It follows from Fig. V.6a that the segments which required most corrections were the mitral segment, the postero-basal, the diaphragmatic and the antero-basal segments. Type C corrections only occurred regularly for the antero-basal area.

Because of the movement of the aortic valve plane along the long axis, the SPI corrections also have a high percentage of occurrence. If we compare Fig. V.6b to Fig. V.6a, it becomes clear that for the single-cycle films additional negative corrections were necessary for the diaphragmatic and postero-apical regions, as well as the antero-lateral and antero-apical regions. The maximal positive percentage occurred for the antero-basal region; the percentage of type C corrections was also maximal for this region.

F. Discussion evaluation data Contouromat

The performance evaluation made clear that there are a few often reoccurring situations that generally require operator-controlled corrections to the auto-mated detected left ventricular contours. These were: (1) interference of the image with diaphragm or ribs; (2) occurrence of double contours during the contraction phase when the mixture of blood and contrast agent is squeezed from

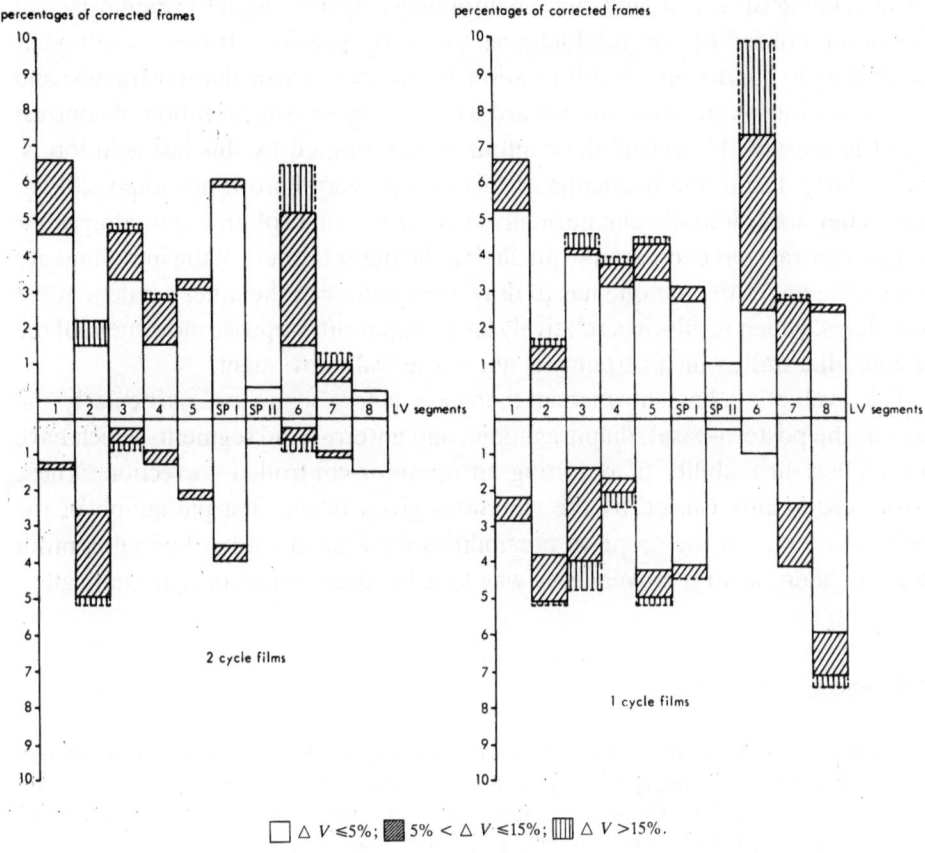

percentages of corrected frames   percentages of corrected frames

2 cycle films

1 cycle films

$\square \; \Delta V \leqslant 5\%$; ▨ $5\% < \Delta V \leqslant 15\%$; ▥ $\Delta V > 15\%$.

Fig. V.6. The percentages of corrected frames for the eight defined segments and the two starting points; the percentages are distinguished into types A, B, and C as defined in the text.
(a) The data for the double-cycle films.
(b) The data for the single-cycle films.

between the deep infoldings of the papillary muscles and trabeculae carnea; and (3) occurrence of contrast holes during the filling phase by incomplete mixing of the contrast agent. The double contours that often occur during the contraction phase not only pose problems to the automated contour detector, but really are a fundamental problem in the tracing of the true left ventricular outline and consequent calculations of left ventricular volumes. The errors which occur when estimating left ventricular volume by the ellipsoid and Simpson's rule models have been reported by Santomore et al. [15]. Due to the deep infoldings of the papillary muscles and trabeculae carnea the cross-sectional areas are not circular.

For purposes of studying the movement of the endocardial left ventricular wall during the contraction phase accurately, one is confronted with the question on where to draw the outline. There are two possibilities for the detection of the outlines in the few frames of the contraction phase during which the contrast agent is being squeezed out from the infoldings: (1) the contour is memorized at the outer border of the infoldings as given by previous frames; contrast is decreasing to almost zero at this location during these particular few frames; and (2) the contour is chosen more inward where a higher concentration of contrast agent is present. However, the contour as determined by this last solution is, particularly during the beginning of this period, very hard if not impossible to find. Therefore, initially one normally chooses the first solution, but after a few frames contrast has decreased so much that the outer borders of the infoldings are not visible anymore and one has to draw the contour at the inner borders of the infoldings, which results in a relatively large 'apparent' stepwise movement of the endocardial wall, which certainly is not a true wall movement.

The evaluation has shown that there are a few segments, particularly the mitral, the postero-basal, diaphragmatic, and antero-basal segments which have the highest probability of requiring an operator-controlled correction. These errors are mainly caused by the situations given in the first paragraph of the discussion. Within the scope of possibilities for a practical hard-wired contour detector there is no relatively easy way to solve these problems automatically.

References

1. Austen WG, Edwards JE, Frye RL, Gensini GG, Gott VL, Griffith LSC, McGoon DC, Murphy ML, Roe BB: A reporting system on patients evaluated for coronay artery disease. Report of the Ad Hoc Committee for Grading of Coronary Artery Disease, Council on Cardiovascular Surgery, American Heart Association, 1975. Circulation 51-2, No. 4: 7–40, 1975.
2. Boer A den: A microprocessor system for on-line registration of the X-ray system settings. Internal Report, Thoraxcenter, 1982.
3. Schultz W, Wendt T, Scherer D, Kober G: Diameter changes of epicardial coronary arteries and coronary stenoses after intracoronary application of SIN 1, a Molsidomine metabolite. Z. Kardiol. 72: 404–409, 1983.
4. Wijns W, Serruys PW, Brand M van den, Suryapranata H, Kooijman CJ, Reiber JHC, Hugenholtz PG: Progression to complete coronary obstruction without myocardial infarction in patients who are candidates for percutaneous transluminal angioplasty: a 90-day angiographic follow-up. In: Prognosis of Coronary Heart Disease – Progression of Coronary Arteriosclerosis. H. Roskamm (Ed.). Springer-Verlag, Berlin/Heidelberg/New York/Tokyo: 190–195, 1983.
5. Hawman EG: Digital boundary detection techniques for the analysis of gated cardiac scintigrams. Optical Engineering 20: 719–725, 1981.
6. Spears JR, Sandor T, Als AV, Malagold M, Markis JE, Grossman W, Serur JR, Paulin S: Computerized image analysis for quantitative measurement of vessel diameter from cineangiograms. Circulation 68: 453–461, 1983.
7. Crawford DW, Brooks SH, Selzer RH, Barndt R, Beckenbach ES, Blankenhorn DH: Computer densitometry for angiographic assessment of arterial cholesterol content and gross pathology in human atherosclerosis. J Lab Clin Med 89: 378–392, 1977.
8. Serruys PW, Lablanche JM, Reiber JHC, Bertrand ME, Hugenholtz PG: Contribution of dynamic vascular wall thickening to luminal narrowing during coronary arterial vasomotion. Z Kardiol 72: 116–123, 1983.
9. Bentley K, Henry PD: Spasmogenic effect of angiographic dye on normal and atherosclerotic

arteries. Circulation 62: III–218 (Abstract), 1980.

10. Higgins CB, Schmidt W: Direct and reflex myocardial effects of intracoronary administered contrast materials in the anesthetized and conscious dog: comparison of standard and newer contrast materials. Invest. Radiol. 13: 205–216, 1978.

11. Bentley KI, Clark M, Henry PD: Angiographic dye relaxes canine coronary artery by a non-osmotic mechanism. Amer J Cardiol 47: 407 (Abstract), 1981.

12. Alderman EL, Berte LE, Harrison DC, Sanders W: Quantitation of coronary artery dimensions using digital image processing. In: Digital Radiography. WR Brody (Ed.). SPIE, Vol 314: 273–278, 1982.

13. Reiber JHC, Slager CJ, Schuurbiers JCH, Meester GT: Contouromat – A hard-wired left ventricular angio processing system. II. Performance evaluation. Comp Biom Res 11: 503–523, 1978.

14. Slager CJ, Reiber JHC, Schuurbiers JCH, Meester GT: Contouromat – A hard-wired left ventricular angio processing system. I. Design and application. Comp Biol Res 11: 491–502, 1978.

15. Santamore WP, DiMeo FN, Lynch PR: A comparative study of various single-plane cin-eangiocardiographic methods to measure left-ventricular volume. IEEE Trans Biomed Eng BME-20: 417–421, 1973.

VI. Assessment of dimensions and image quality of coronary contrast catheters from cineangiograms

Summary

In the quantitative assessment of coronary arterial dimensions from coronary cineangiograms, the contrast catheter is usually used as a scaling device, requiring the definition of the boundaries of a portion of the catheter by semi- or fully-automated contour detection procedures. The image quality of the X-ray radiated catheter is dependent upon the catheter material, the concentration of the contrast agent in the catheter and the kilovoltage of the X-ray source. The effects of these variables on the image quality and on the accuracy of the measurements of the sizes of the filmed catheters were studied for four different catheter materials: woven dacron (wd), polyvinylchloride (pv), polyurethane (pu) and nylon. The following parameters were studied: measured size, image contrast and average brightness gradient along the edges of the displayed catheters. The average differences of the angiographically measured size with the true size for the wd, pv, pu and nylon catheters were +0.2%, −3.2%, −3.5% and +9.8%, respectively. The image contrast at various fillings of the catheters was roughly identical for the wd, pv and pu catheters, but significantly lower for the nylon catheter. Image gradient was highest for the wd catheter, followed by the pv and pu catheters, and lowest for the nylon catheter.

From these data it may be concluded, that the woven dacron catheter is most suitable for quantitative coronary angiographic studies. The polyvinylchloride and polyurethane catheters perform about equally well, but slightly less than the woven dacron catheter. The nylon catheter should not be used for such quantitative studies.

Introduction

Coronary contrast catheters have been used increasingly for calibration purposes in the quantitative assessment of coronary arterial dimensions [1–7]. However, until today no extensive study has been performed on the accuracy of these measurements from coronary cineangiograms; nor has the effect of catheter material, contrast filling of the catheter, and kV-setting of the X-ray source on image quality of the irradiated catheter and thus on the accuracy of measurements been studied. It is the purpose of this chapter to describe the results of such an evaluation study on four different materials, filmed at various settings of the quality of the X-ray system and filled with various concentrations of contrast agent and with water and air.

Methods

Mid-portions of the four contrast catheters were taped on a block of acrylate (Perspex) with dimensions $10 \times 10 \times 10$ cm. The height of the X-ray table was adjusted such that the catheters could be filmed in the isocenter of the X-ray system. Five different fillings were used for the catheters: (1) only air inside; (2) filled with water; and filled with three different concentrations of a contrast agent (Urografin-76^R)* : (3) 370 mg I/cc (100% concentration); (4) 185 mg I/cc (50% concentration); and (5) 92.5 mg I/cc (25% concentration). Each situation was filmed at four different kilovoltages, ranging from 55–81 kV. For calibration purposes, a cm-grid was filmed on top of the acrylate block after the catheter measurements had been performed.

The cinefilms were analyzed with the Cardiovascular Angiography Analysis System (CAAS). The calibration factor for the study was determined by manual definition of three pairs of points on neighboring vertical lines of the cm-grid in the center of the image with the writing tablet. The calibration factor was thus expressed in mm/pixel. The catheter segments were analyzed with an optical magnification of $2\sqrt{2}$. The boundaries of a portion of a given catheter were detected automatically with the coronary artery detection algorithm over a length of approximately 1 cm (Fig. VI.1).

From the analyzed portion of a contrast catheter the following parameters were measured:

(1) Mean diameter (mm)
(2) Average brightness level along centerline in catheter (B. cath)
(3) Average background brightness level (B. bkgr), measured 10 pixels (≈ 0.6 mm) outside of the detected contours.
(4) Difference between B. cath and B. bkgr, being a measure for image contrast
(5) Average value of the weighted sum of first and second gradient functions for the left-hand side contour positions (GRAD(L))
(6) Average value for the weighted sum of first and second gradient functions for the right-hand side contour positions (GRAD(R)).

* Schering AG, Berlin, Germany

142

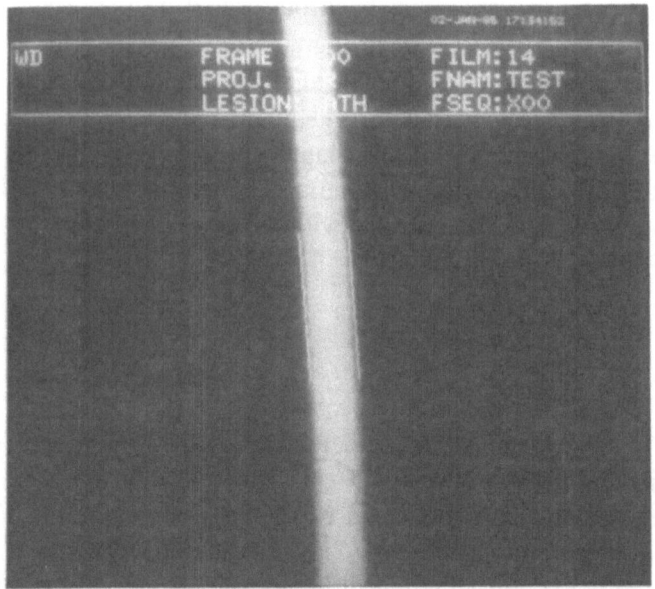

Fig. VI.1. Example of detected contours along a portion of one of the contrast catheters.

Materials

Four catheters fabricated from different materials were used for this study:

A. woven dacron, Sones 7F catheter*
B. polyvinylchloride, Judkins 7.3F catheter* *
C. polyurethane, Femoral – Left Coronary 8F catheter* * *
D. nylon, Alvaflo Judkins 7F catheter* * * *

The true sizes of the catheters were measured with a micrometer.

Figure VI.2 shows the brightness distribution along a scanline across an analyzed catheter segment perpendicular to the centerline direction for each of the four catheter materials filled with 100% contrast agent and with air. In each graph the pixel positions along the scanline are plotted along the horizontal axis and the brightness levels along the vertical axis. From these eight graphs the differences in image contrast between the various materials can be appreciated, as well as the differences in the brightness distribution for a particular segment filled with 100% contrast agent or with air.

*   USCI Int., Inc., Billerica, Mass., USA.
* *   Cook Inc., Bloomington, Indiana, USA.
* * * Cordis Corp., Miami, Florida, USA.
* * * * Mallinckrodt GmbH, Grossostheim, West Germany.

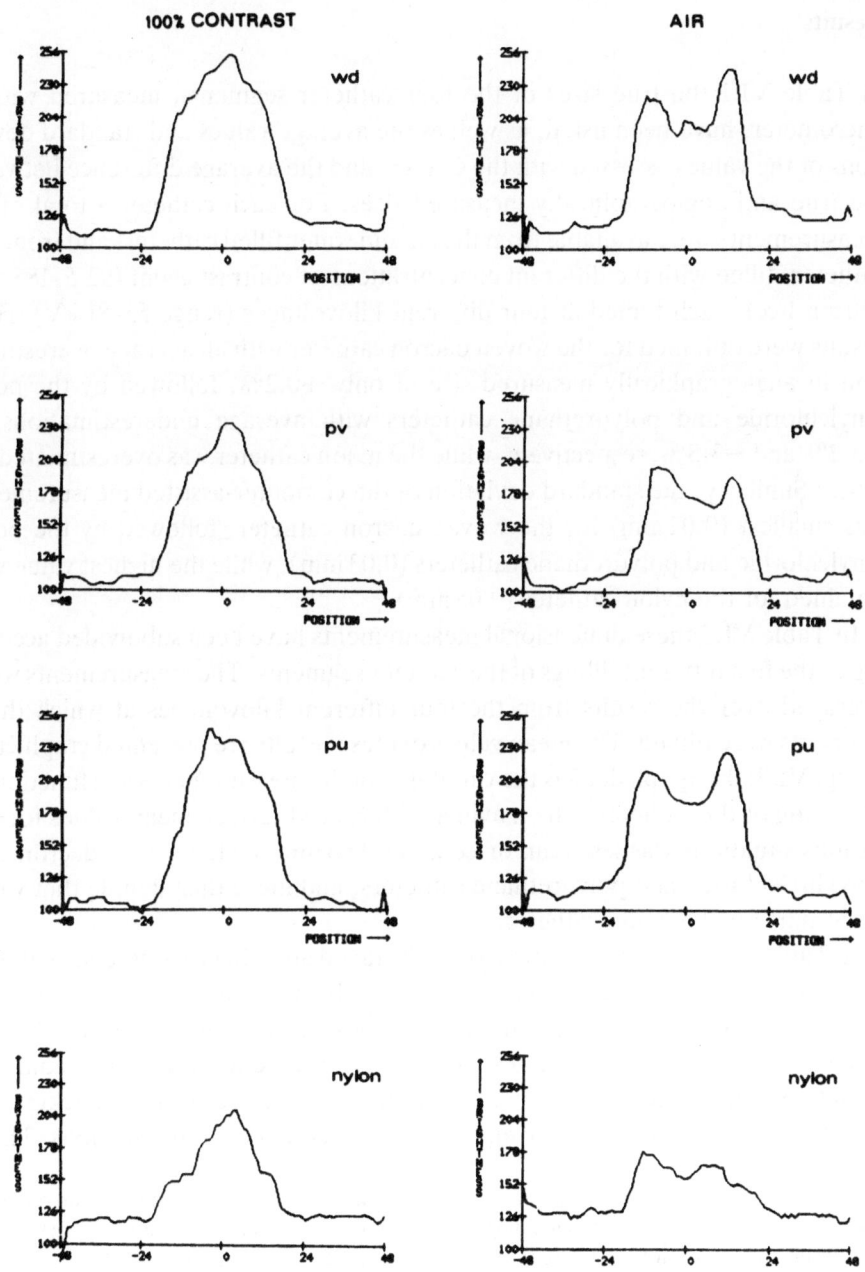

Fig. VI.2. Examples of brightness distribution along scanlines perpendicular to the centerline directions for the four different catheters, filled with 100% contrast agent (left column) and with air (right column). The vertical order of the graphs represent the different materials (from top to bottom): woven dacron (wd), polyvinylchloride (pv), polyurethane (pu) and nylon, respectively. In each graph the pixel positions along the scanline are plotted along the horizontal axis and the brightness levels along the vertical axis.

Results

In Table VI.1 the true sizes of the four catheter segments, measured with a micrometer, have been listed, as well as the average values and standard deviations of the values assessed with the CAAS, and the average difference between the true and angiographically measured sizes. For each catheter a total of 20 measurements were available from the air and water filled catheters and from the catheters filled with the different concentrations of contrast agent (92.5, 185 and 370 mg I/cc), each filmed at four different kilovoltages (range 55–81 kV). Best results were obtained for the woven dacron catheter with an average overestimation in angiographically measured size of only +0.2%, followed by the polyvinylchloride and polyurethane catheters with average underestimations of −3.2% and −3.5%, respectively, while the nylon catheter was overestimated by 9.8%. Similarly, the standard deviation of the computer-assisted measurements was smallest (0.02 mm) for the woven dacron catheter, followed by the polyvinylchloride and polyurethane catheters (0.03 mm), while the highest value was obtained for the nylon catheter (0.05 mm).

In Table VI.2 these dimensional measurements have been subdivided according to the five different fillings of the catheter segments. The measurements were averaged over the results from the four different kilovoltages at which these segments were filmed. The mean values of these results are presented graphically in Fig. VI.3; this graph depicts the variability of the measurements as a function of the filling of the catheter. The maximal difference between mean values for the various situations was less than or equal to 0.04 mm for the woven dacron, the polyvinylchloride and polyurethane catheters, and more than double that value (0.09 mm) for the nylon catheter.

In Table VI.3 the image contrast of the X-rayed and filmed catheters, averaged over the four kilovoltage-measurements, have been listed for the four catheters according to the five different fillings. Image contrast was defined by the difference of the average brightness level along the centerline of the analyzed catheter segment and of the average brightness level measured in the background at a distance of 10 pixels (≈ 0.6 mm) from the defined contour positions. These

Table VI.1. Comparison of true sizes of catheter segments with angiographically measured dimensions, averaged over the five different fillings (air, water, contrast medium concentrations of 92.5, 185 and 370 mg I/cc), each at four different kilovoltages (range 55–81 kV) (mean ± s.d.).

	True size (mm)	Angiographically measured size (mm)	Average difference (%)
Woven dacron	2.35	2.35 ± 0.02 (0.9%)	+0.2%
Polyvinylchloride	2.44	2.36 ± 0.03 (1.3%)	−3.2%
Polyurethane	2.62	2.53 ± 0.03 (1.2%)	−3.5%
Nylon	2.25	2.46 ± 0.05 (2.0%)	+9.8%

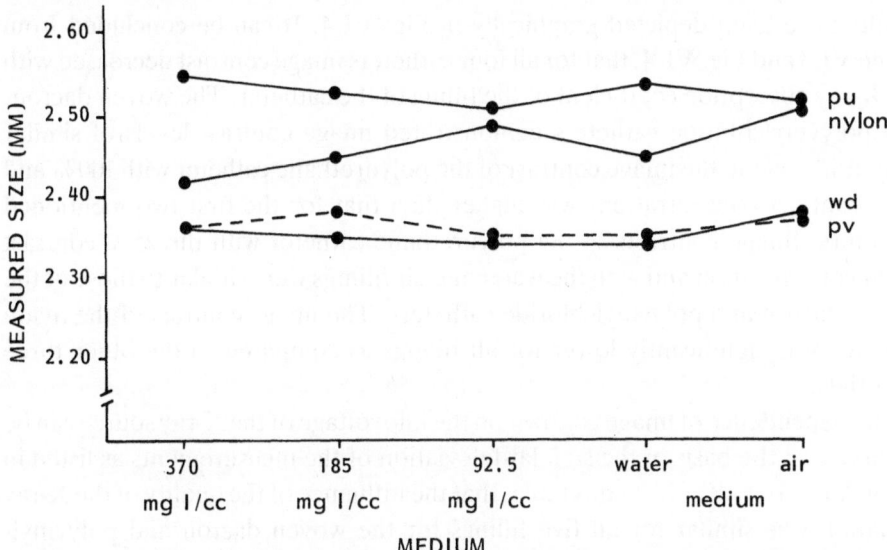

Fig. VI.3. This graph depicts the variability of the angiographically measured catheter size as a function of the filling of the catheter. Each measurement point represents the mean value of four measurements of the catheter at four different kilovoltages of the X-ray source.

Table VI.2. Mean values and standard deviations of the angiographically measured catheter dimensions for the five different fillings of the segments. Measurements were averaged over the four different kilovoltages at which these segments were filmed.

	Measured size (mm)				
	370 mg I/cc	185 mg I/cc	92.5 mg I/cc	water	air
Woven dacron	2.36 ± 0.02	2.35 ± 0.02	2.34 ± 0.01	2.34 ± 0.03	2.38 ± 0.01
Polyvinylchloride	2.36 ± 0.02	2.38 ± 0.02	2.35 ± 0.02	2.35 ± 0.04	2.37 ± 0.02
Polyurethane	2.55 ± 0.02	2.53 ± 0.03	2.51 ± 0.06	2.54 ± 0.04	2.52 ± 0.03
Nylon	2.42 ± 0.08	2.45 ± 0.05	2.48 ± 0.03	2.45 ± 0.02	2.51 ± 0.04

Table VI.3. Mean values and standard deviations (in parentheses) of the measured image contrast for the four catheters at the various fillings of the catheters. Measurements were averaged over the four different kilovoltages at which these segments were filmed. Therefore, the standard deviation is a measure for the influence of the quality (kV) of the X-ray radiation on image contrast.

	Image contrast				
	370 mg I/cc	185 mg I/cc	92.5 mg I/cc	water	air
Woven dacron	83.6 (9.6)	75.6 (12.8)	73.7 (11.3)	64.0 (8.9)	63.0 (9.7)
Polyvinylchloride	82.3 (11.0)	77.3 (13.0)	71.9 (12.7)	64.1 (9.9)	58.0 (9.1)
Polyurethane	100.4 (22.3)	87.8 (23.7)	75.0 (21.4)	63.7 (17.7)	62.5 (18.6)
Nylon	55.8 (12.3)	52.1 (9.3)	48.4 (8.3)	26.4 (2.0)	21.8 (1.1)

results have been depicted graphically in Fig. VI.4. It can be concluded from Table VI.3 and Fig. VI.4, that for all four catheters image contrast decreased with the X-ray absorption coefficient of the filling of the catheter. The woven dacron, and polyvinylchloride catheters demonstrated image contrast levels of similar magnitude, while the image contrast of the polyurethane catheter with 100% and 50% contrast concentrations was higher than that for the first two mentioned catheters. Image contrasts of the polyurethane catheter with the 25% contrast agent concentration and with the water and air fillings were similar to those of the woven dacron and polyvinylchloride catheters. The image contrast of the nylon catheter was significantly lower for all fillings as compared to the other three materials.

The dependence of image contrast on the kilovoltage of the X-ray source can be observed on the basis of the standard deviation of the measurements as listed in Table VI.3. It is clear from this table, that the influence of the quality of the X-ray radiation was similar for all five fillings for the woven dacron and polyvinyl-chloride catheters. The kilovoltage-dependence for the polyurethane catheter was roughly twice as high for all five fillings. On the other hand, the contrast filled nylon catheter showed a dependence again approximately equal to that of the woven dacron and polyvinylchloride catheters, with an absolutely lowest vari-ability for the nylon catheter filled with water and air.

Finally, we have measured along each detected contour side the average brightness gradient along the contour, defined by the weighted sum of first and second gradient values assessed from the edge detection algorithm; the unit of

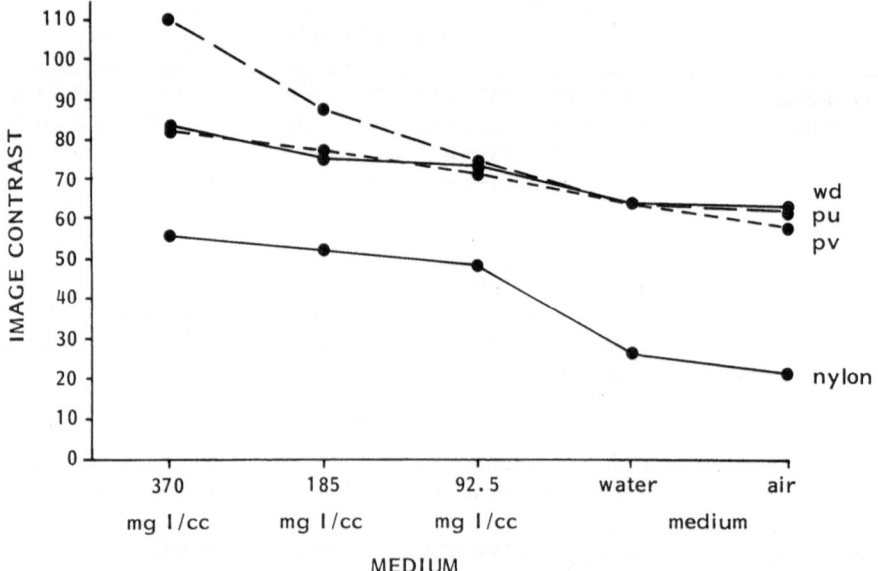

Fig. VI.4. This graph shows image contrast for the four catheter materials as a function of the filling of the catheter. Each measurement point represents the mean value of four measurements of the catheter at four different qualities (kV-level) of the X-ray radiation.

this parameter is brightness level difference (gradient) per pixel. As a result, for each analyzed catheter segment, an average left gradient value (GRAD(L)) and an average right gradient value (GRAD(R)) were obtained. At the average, the differences between the GRAD(L) and GRAD(R)-values were nonsignificant. In Table VI.4 the average gradient values for the four catheters, averaged over the four kV measurements and over the left and right contour sides, are presented for the five different fillings. These results are again depicted graphically in figure VI.5.

It is clear from Fig. VI.5, that the highest gradient levels were obtained with the woven dacron catheter, followed by the polyvinylchloride and polyurethane catheters; the nylon catheter again showed the poorest results. For all catheter materials the brightness gradient increased with decreasing X-ray absorption coefficient of the filling of the catheter.

The standard deviations of the measurements listed in Table VI.4 are a measure for the influence of the quality of the X-ray radiation (kV-level X-ray source) on the gradient level. It is apparent, that two conclusions may be drawn: (1) for the woven dacron, polyvinylchloride and polyurethane catheters the standard deviations increased with decreasing X-ray absorption coefficients for the contrast filled catheters; and (2) for all four materials the highest values of the variations were measured for the water and air-filled catheters.

Discussion

To evaluate the efficacy of modern therapeutic procedures in the catheterization laboratory [9–11], the effects of vasoactive drugs [12, 13], as well as the effects of short and long term interventions on the regression or progression of coronary artery disease [14], absolute coronary artery dimensions must be assessed from

Table VI.4. Mean values and standard deviations (in parentheses) of the average image gradient at the detected contour positions for the four catheter materials at the various fillings of the catheters. Measurements were averaged over the four different kilovoltages at which these segments were filmed. Therefore, the standard deviation is a measure for the influence of the quality (kV) of the X-ray radiation on the image gradient.

	Average grad.				
	370 mg I/cc	185 mg I/cc	92.5 mg I/cc	water	air
Woven dacron	14.9 (1.4)	16.4 (2.4)	18.1 (3.2)	19.4 (3.0)	19.1 (3.5)
Polyvinylchloride	10.5 (1.5)	11.6 (2.0)	12.7 (2.0)	13.4 (2.9)	12.7 (2.0)
Polyurethane	10.9 (2.3)	12.2 (3.0)	12.2 (2.8)	13.0 (4.0)	13.1 (3.6)
Nylon	5.4 (1.7)	6.4 (1.7)	7.4 (1.4)	7.6 (2.3)	7.9 (1.4)

148

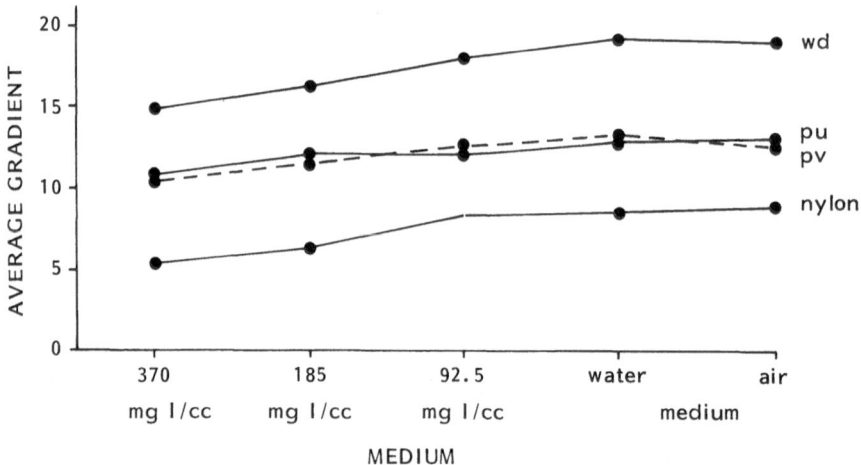

Fig. VI.5. Average brightness gradient at the detected contour positions for the four catheter materials as a function of the filling of the catheter. Each measurement point represents the mean value of four measurements of the catheter at four different qualities (kV-level) of the X-ray radiation.

the repeat coronary cineangiograms with high accuracy [6]. Moreover, it has been shown recently that the minimal cross-sectional area of an individual coronary obstruction is the best predictor of its physiological significance [15, 16]. To this end, a calibration procedure must be available to assess these absolute values from the analyzed cineframes. For these purposes, the size of the contrast catheter visible in these images has been used most frequently (Chapter X). The critique of applying the calibration factor computed from a single view to objects not lying in the plane of the analyzed catheter segment parallel to the image intensifier input screen and possible solutions to this problem have been discussed in Chapter V.

For a coronary contrast catheter to be acceptable for quantitative coronary angiographic studies, it must fulfill a number of criteria:

(1) The standard deviation of a series of measurements as performed in this study, that is with different fillings of the contrast catheter and filmed with different X-ray qualities, must be lower than a certain absolute threshold, for example 0.03 mm, being 0.1 F.
(2) The lowest image contrast measured during such an evaluation study must be higher than a certain threshold.
(3) The average gradient measured during the evaluation study must be above a lower threshold value.

The following critique must be made with respect to the three points mentioned above.

Ad 1.
It is possible that the evaluation study for a given catheter shows that the standard deviation of the measurements is equal to or below the threshold of 0.03 mm, but that a systemic error is observed in the mean values of these measurements. The polyvinylchloride and polyurethane catheters used in this study show such a response. If this is the case, then the systemic error may be corrected for in the coronary analysis software package for this given type of catheter. This means that such correction factors must be available for the different types of catheters to be used in a quantitative coronary angiographic study.

Ad 2.
In this comparative study on the image quality of different catheter materials, the measured image quality has been computed in terms of digitized brightness levels. It will be clear that such values are dependent on the illumination of the analyzed cineframes. The four catheter segments used in this study were analyzed under identical levels of image illumination. However, a general applicable threshold level for the image quality cannot be derived from our data. A better measure would be to describe the image quality of a catheter segment in terms of absolute optical density differences in the cineframes, requiring a densitometric analysis of the cinefilm.

Such techniques are under development in our center (Chapter VII). For these purposes we have designed a cinefilm-sensitometer, that allows the exposure of the first 21 frames of a cinefilm with a light source having the same color temperature as the output screen of the image intensifier. These calibration frames are exposed according to an exponential function:

$$E(n) = k \cdot (\sqrt{2})^{-n}$$

with $E(n)$ being the exposure level and n the frame sequence number ($0 \leqslant n \leqslant 20$). These frames are processed photographically simultaneously with the rest of the coronary cineangiogram, so that the film development process is identical for both the calibration frames and the clinical or experimental cineframes. As a first step in the analysis procedure for one or more cineframes of a given cinefilm, these calibration frames are digitized and stored in the computer. On the basis of these calibration data, for each point in a coronary or catheter cineframe the absolute density level can be computed from the measured brightness level, under the restriction that the illumination of the cinefilm remains constant over the calibration and analysis periods.

Ad 3.
Similarly as described under ad 2, the average gradient levels in this study are not generally applicable for the purpose to define a threshold level. However, as soon as the measurements can be described in terms of absolute density levels, an absolute threshold level can be defined.

150

On the basis of our evaluation data we may conclude that the woven dacron catheter is most suitable for quantitative coronary angiographic studies. The polyvinylchloride and polyurethane catheters perform about equally well, but slightly less than the woven dacron catheter. The nylon catheter should not be used for these studies.

References

1. Brown BG, Bolson E, Frimer M, Dodge HT: Quantitative coronary arteriography. Estimation of dimensions, hemodynamic resistance, and atheroma mass of coronary artery lesions using the arteriograms and digital computation. Circulation 55: 329–337, 1977.
2. Selzer RH, Blankenhorn DH, Crawford DW, Brooks SH, Barndt R: Computer analysis of cardiovascular imagery. Proceedings of the Caltech/JPL Conference on Image Processing Technology, Data Sources and Software for Commercial and Scientific Applications, Pasadena, Nov. 3–5: pp. 1–20, 1976.
3. Ledbetter DC, Selzer RH, Gordon RM, Blankenhorn DH, Sanmarco ME: Computer quantitation of coronary angiograms: noninvasive cardiovascular measurements. In: Noninvasive cardiovascular measurements. HA Miller, EV Schmidt, DC Harrison (Eds.) SPIE 167, pp. 17–20, 1978.
4. Smith DN, Colfer H, Brymer JF, Pitt B, Kliman SH: A semiautomatic computer technique for processing coronary angiograms. Comp in Card: 325–328, 1982.
5. Kooijman CJ, Reiber JHC, Gerbrands JJ, Schuurbiers JCH, Slager CJ, Boer A den, Serruys PW: Computer-aided quantitation of the severity of coronary obstructions from single view cineangiograms. First IEEE Comp. Soc. Int. Symp. on Medical Imaging and Image Interpretation, IEEE Cat No 82 CH1804-4: 59–64, 1982.
6. Reiber JHC, Serruys PW, Kooijman CJ, Wijns W, Slager CJ, Gerbrands JJ, Schuurbiers JCH, Boer A den, Hugenholtz PG: Assessment of short-, medium- and long-term variations in arterial dimensions from computer-assisted quantitation of coronary cineangiograms. Circulation 71: 280–288, 1985.
7. Reiber JHC, Kooijman CJ, Slager CJ, Gerbrands JJ, Schuurbiers JCH, Boer A den, Wijns W, Serruys PW, Hugenholtz PG: Coronary artery dimensions from cineangiograms; methodology and validation of a computer-assisted analysis procedure. IEEE Trans Med Imaging MI-3: 131–141, 1984.
8. Reiber JHC, Kooijman CJ, Slager CJ, Gerbrands JJ, Schuurbiers JCH, Boer A den, Wijns W, Serruys PW: Computer assisted analysis of the severity of obstructions from coronary cineangiograms: a methodological review. Automedica 5: 219–238, 1984.
9. Serruys PW, Booman F, Troost GJ, Reiber JHC, Gerbrands JJ, van den Brand M, Cherrier F, Hugenholtz PG: Computerized quantitative coronary angiography applied to percutaneous transluminal coronary angioplasty: advantages and limitations. In: Transluminal Coronary Angioplasty and Intracoronary Thrombolysis. Coronary Heart Disease IV. M Kaltenbach, A Grüntzig, K Rentrop, WD Bussmann (Eds.). Springer-Verlag Berlin: 110–124, 1982.
10. Serruys PW, Wijns W, Brand M van den, Ribeiro V, Fioretti P, Simoons ML, Kooijman CJ, Reiber JHC, Hugenholtz PG: Is transluminal coronary angioplasty mandatory after successful thrombolysis? Br Heart J 50: 257–265, 1983.
11. Wijns W, Serruys PW, Brand M van den, Reiber JHC, Suryapranata H, Hugenholtz PG: Progression to complete coronary obstruction without myocardial infarction in patients who are candidates for Percutaneous Transluminal Angioplasty: A 90-Day Angiographic Follow-Up. In: Prognosis of Coronary Heart Disease – Progression of Coronary Arteriosclerosis. H Roskamm (Ed.). Springer-Verlag Berlin: 190–195, 1983.

12. Wijns W, Serruys PW, Reiber, JHC, Brand M van den, Simoons ML, Kooijman CJ, Balakumaran K, Hugenholtz PG: Quantitative angiography of the left anterior descending coronary artery: correlations with pressure gradient and exercise thallium scintigraphy. Circulation 71: 273–279, 1985.

13. Serruys PW, Hooghoudt TEH, Reiber JHC, Slager C, Brower RW, Hugenholtz PG: Influence of intracoronary nifedipine on left ventricular function, coronary vasomotility, and myocardial oxygen consumption. Br Heart J 49: 427–441, 1983.

14. Serruys PW, Lablanche JM, Reiber JHC, Bertrand ME, Hugenholtz PG: Contribution of dynamic vascular wall thickening to luminal narrowing during coronary arterial vasomotion. Z Kardiol 72: 116–123, 1983.

15. Marcus M, Wright C, Doty D, Eastham C, Laughlin D, Krumm P, Fastenow C, Brody M: Measurements of coronary velocity and reactive hyperemia in the coronary circulation of humans. Circ Res 49:877–891, 1981.

16. Harrison DG, White CW, Hiratzka LF, Doty DB, Barnes DH, Eastham CL, Marcus ML: The value of lesions cross-sectional area determined by quantitative coronary angiography in assessing the physiologic significance of proximal left anterior descending coronary arterial stenoses. Circulation 69: 1111–1119, 1984.

VII. Densitometric analysis coronary cineangiograms

Introduction

Since the luminal cross section at a coronary obstruction is frequently irregular in shape, percentage diameter reduction measured in a single projection is of limited diagnostic value. The hemodynamic resistance of an obstruction is determined to a great extent by the minimal cross-sectional area of the lumen at the obstruction. Computation of the cross-sectional area reduction from the percentage diameter reduction measured in a single view requires the assumption of e.g. circular cross sections, an assumption which hardly ever holds [1, 2]. The resulting error may be reduced by incorporating two orthogonal projections and computing elliptical cross sections. However, with the often occurring eccentric lesions even this last approach provides poor results, as can be shown with the following

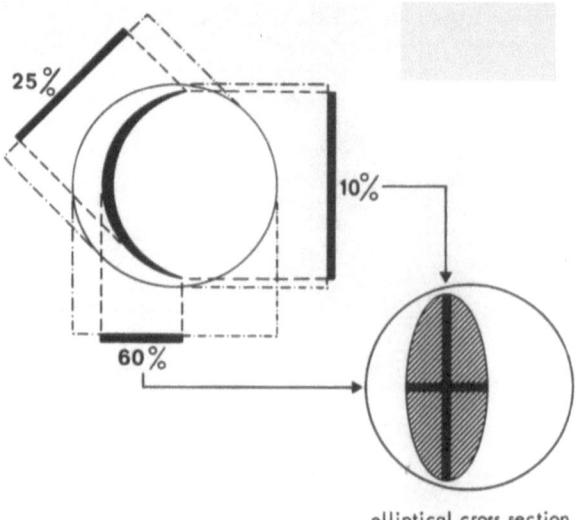

elliptical cross section

Fig. VII.1. Potential errors in the evaluation of the severity of a crescent-like lesion from single and orthogonal views.

example. Fig. VII.1 diagrammatically portrays and depicts the complex problems stemming from a slit-like stenosis having a crescent shape. In cases such as this, even three or more views will not 'provide a faithful portrayal of their severity'[3]. A lateral 'view' of the crescent would suggest a 10% reduction in lumen diameter; a 'left oblique' would yield a 25% narrowing and an 'anteroposterior' would imply a 60% stenosis. Even a technique of quantitating area stenosis from two orthogonal measurements and computing area based on an elliptical model would fail to describe accurately the severity of this lesion [4].

However, some clue to the presence of this grossly asymmetrical lesion will exist, because the density of contrast medium is markedly reduced in that area, even though the caliber seems normal. Unexplained diminution of the opacity of a contrast-filled lumen (density changes) should alert the angiographer to the severity of the luminal narrowing. Therefore, if one could constitute the relationship between the path length of the X-rays through the artery and the brightness values in the digital image, one would obtain the information required to compute the cross-sectional areas from a single view (Fig. VII.2).

It is this particular subject that is referred to as the densitometric analysis technique. To be able to develop and apply such a densitometric technique, knowledge about the characteristics of the different components of the entire X-ray-cine-video chain is required. It is the purpose of this chapter to describe the transfer functions of these components in relatively simple terms and apply the results to two densitometric analysis techniques that we have implemented. The first technique is based on quantitative analysis of the contrast image; this is the most common densitometric procedure. Digitized video brightness levels are transformed into irradiated object thicknesses on a pixel-by-pixel basis by means of mapping functions derived from calibrated homogeneous density images. The second technique is a background subtraction technique requiring a background

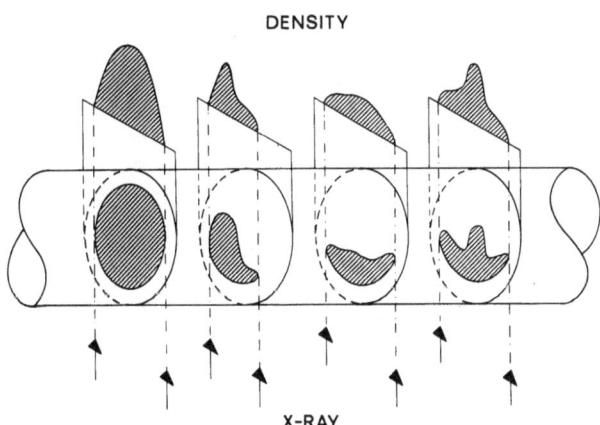

Fig. VII.2. Schematic illustration of the relationship between the irradiated object thickness and the density in the angiographic image.

image taken before the contrast administration and a subsequent contrast image. These two images should be selected at corresponding moments in the cardiac cycles. These two techniques will be illustrated with clinical examples and some preliminary data will be presented. An overview of other densitometric techniques described in the literature is given in Chapter X.

The X-Ray-Cine-Video imaging system

A simple block diagram of the complete X-Ray-Cine-Video chain as it applies to the Thoraxcenter CAAS is shown in figure VII.3. The X-ray system that we have used most frequently for our evaluation studies is a Siemens Cardoscope U placed in one of our catheterization laboratories. The X-ray generator is the Pandoros Optimatic with a kV-controlled loop and the X-ray tube an Optilix with 6° anode angle and foci of 0.4 mm and 0.7 mm. The coronary cineangiograms in the RAO and LAO projections are always produced with the 0.7 mm focus, Cranial Caudal projections with the 0.4 mm focus. A Brilliant 7″ image intensifier with standard optics is used with a ratio 7 grid (50 lp/cm). The cinecamera is an Arritechno 90 with a 100 mm lens used in overframed mode; the film speed for coronary angiograms is usually taken at 25 frames/s. An X-ray documentation system has been developed in our catheterization laboratory, allowing the projection of the geometric parameters of the table and X-ray system and of the generator settings on the first and last frames of an angiographic investigation, respectively [9]. These data are also sent directly to our cath. lab. computer. The Kodak CFE 2711 cinefilm with estar base is developed with the Agfa Gevaert Refinal M developer for 4 min at 26° C; the film gamma equals 1.25 at 550 μm light exposure and the average density 0.82 (Chapter II). Sensitometric and densitometric quality con-

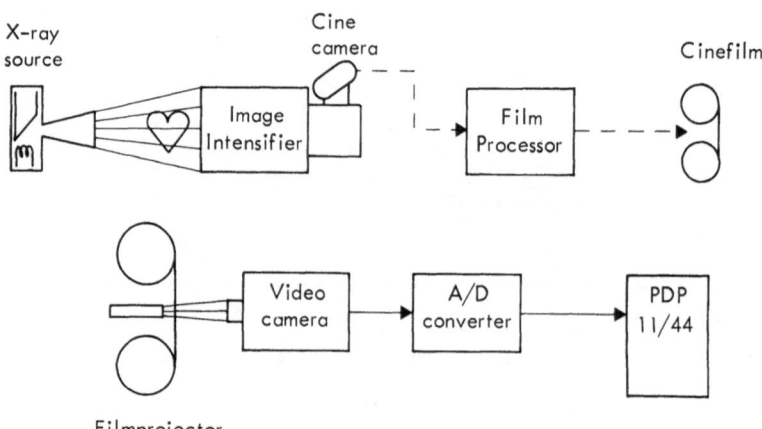

Fig. VII.3. Block diagram of X-ray-cine-video imaging system.

trol of the film development process is performed daily. A special sensitometer has been developed which allows 21 full cineframes covering the entire densitometric range of the film to be exposed on the first portion of the cinefilm before the angiographic investigation is performed.

Constitution of the relationship between path lengths and brightness values requires detailed analysis of the complete imaging system. In a simplified approach, we are only interested in the static properties of the system. Analysis of the static transfer function of each link in the chain reveals that computation of the complete transfer function is very difficult. There is a large number of parameters involved, many of which are spatially variant.

In the following section the transfer functions of the different components in the entire chain will be described in relatively simple terms.

Transfer functions of the different system components

X-ray beam attenuation

The process of X-ray absorption was described in some detail in Chapter II. In general, the absorption process is described by the Lambert-Beer Law:

$$I(E) = I_o(E) \cdot \exp(-\mu \cdot d) \tag{VII.1}$$

with $I_o(E)$ the number of photons of energy E incident on a small area of the absorption medium, $I(E)$ the number of photons transmitted through the object, μ [cm^2/g] the mass attenuation coefficient of the medium and d [g/cm^2] the irradiated mass per cm^2. For an inhomogeneous object (of thickness not exceeding L), consisting of various absorbing materials, formula (VII.1) must be generalized into:

$$I(x,y) = I_o(x,y) \cdot \exp(-\beta(x,y)), \tag{VII.2}$$

with

$$\beta(x,y) = \int_0^L \mu(x,y,z) \cdot \varrho(x,y,z) \, dz \tag{VII.3}$$

In these formulas $\mu(x,y,z)$ is the mass attenuation coefficient at point (x,y,z) in the object, $\varrho(x,y,z)$ the mass density [g/cm^3] and we assume that the X-ray beam is directed into the z-direction. For simplicity, the spatial position (x,y) in the projection image will be denoted by p in the remainder of this chapter; moreover, the energy dependence (E) will also be omitted for the same reason.

Image Intensifier

In Chapter II, the transfer function for the image intensifier was defined by:

$$L(p) = G(p) \cdot (I(p))^{\gamma_I}, \qquad\qquad (VII.4)$$

where $L(p)$ is the luminance at position p of the output screen of the image intensifier, $G(p)$ the conversion factor and γ_I the 'gamma' of the image intensifier.

Cinefilm exposure

The linear part of the function relating the film density D versus the logarithm of relative exposure E can be described by the following relationship (Chapter II):

$$D(p) = D_0(p) + \gamma_F \cdot \log(E(p)/I_n), \qquad\qquad (VII.5)$$

where $D_0(p)$ is the base density, γ_F the gamma of the film, $E(p)$ the exposure ($= L(p) \cdot t$ with t the film exposure time) and where $\log I_n$ is the inertia.

Film digitizer

The developed film is placed on a cinefilm digitizer, either the Thoraxcenter cine-video converter (Fig. III.3) or the Pie Data cine digitizer with the CCD-camera (Fig. III.19) and a selected cineframe projected onto the tube of the video camera or onto the CCD-array, respectively. When the intensity of the projector light is denoted $P_0(p)$, the intensity $P(p)$ of the light transmitted through the film can be described by:

$$P(p) = P_0(p) \cdot 10^{-D(p)} \qquad\qquad (VII.6)$$

The video camera in the Thoraxcenter system is the Sierra Scientific LSV 1.5 R with an RCA 1.5 inch vidicon tube. This camera makes use of the special characteristics of the RCA C23225 camera tube and C23227 deflection system which are designed to work together to provide high resolution and minimum distortion over the entire display area. The resolution in the center area of the target equals 1000 lines/ph (picture height), which corresponds with 33.3 lp/mm on the target and 27.7 lp/mm on the original cineframe. At this resolution the response of the camera equals 10% according to the modulation transfer function (MTF).

Reasons for not having selected a plumbicon with a gamma $= 1$ are the inherent greater noise component, a lower resolution and a decreased sensitivity in the darker areas. The main advantage of the plumbicon tube, its speed, is not important in our application.

The relationship between the signal current I_s of the vidicon and the time-integrated intensity P of the light falling upon the tube can be described by:

$$I_s(p) = (P(p))^{\gamma_v} + i_0(p), \qquad (VII.7)$$

where γ_v is the gamma of the vidicon ($\gamma_v = 0.65$) and i_0 the dark current.

The dark current of the vidicon is spatially variant (greater at the edges) and depends on the ambient temperature. The spatially variant characteristic is called shading which can be compensated for with a shading corrector.

The signal current of the vidicon tube is amplified in the camera electronics and sent as a signal voltage to the analog-to-digital converter. The output signal voltage $V_s(p)$ can thus be written as:

$$V_s(p) = k_1 \cdot (P(p))^{\gamma_v} + V_0(p), \qquad (VII.8)$$

where k_1 is a constant and V_0 the dark voltage.

The CCD-camera in the Pie Data CAAS consists of a linear array of 1728 photodetectors, which can be moved across the image plane of the attached optical system in a total of 2846 steps, forming a two-dimensional matrix of picture elements (Chapter III). Each of these elements is converted into a digital signal of 8 bits per element (256 levels of grey), to produce a high resolution image.

Basically, equation (VII.8) is also valid for the CCD-camera; however, in this case $\gamma_v = 1$.

Analog-to-digital conversion

In the Thoraxcenter CAAS the center square of an analog video image is digitized in real time in matrix size of 512×512 pixels with the VTE digitizer and stored in a display memory (Chapter III). The sampling frequency of the analog-to-digital (A/D) converter equals 15 MHz, which results in square pixels; both the even and the odd lines of the 2:1 interlaced video system are utilized. The grey scale resolution of the digital data is 256 levels (8 bits).

In the Pie Data CAAS any area of size $6.9 \text{ mm} \times 6.9 \text{ mm}$ in a selected cineframe (size 18×24 mm) can be digitized by the CCD-camera with a resolution of 512×512 pixels and stored in an image memory. Also, an area of 13.9×13.9 mm can be digitized at a resolution of 1024×1024 pixels, reduced in size to a matrix of 512×512 pixels and stored in the image memory.

For both digitizing systems the relationship between the digitized grey level V_d and the analog signal V_s can be defined by:

$$V_d(p) = k_2 \cdot V_s(p) \qquad\qquad \text{(VII.9)}$$

where k_2 is constant, if we neglect the quantization error.

Relationship between measured brightness level and object attenuation factor

Now that we have described in mathematical terms the transfer functions of the different system components comprising the X-ray-cine-digitizer chain, the overall relation between the measured brightness level and the object attenuation factor β can be derived. This yields:

$$V_d(p) = k_3(p) \cdot \exp\left(\beta(p) \cdot \gamma_I \cdot \gamma_F \cdot \gamma_V\right) + k_2 \cdot V_0(p) \qquad\qquad \text{(VII.10)}$$

with

$$k_3(p) = \frac{k_1 \cdot k_2 \cdot P_0{}^{\gamma_V}}{10^{\,D_0 \gamma_V} \cdot (G \cdot t/I_n)^{\gamma_F \gamma_V} \cdot I_0{}^{\gamma_I \gamma_F \gamma_V}} \qquad\qquad \text{(VII.11)}$$

In this last expression P_0, G and I_0 are spatially variant. Referring to formula (VII.3), a true object thickness can only be derived from equation (VII.10) if we consider a homogeneous medium with μ and ϱ constants. It should be noted that formula (VII.10) can only be regarded as a first approximation of the entire imaging process, since several factors are not truly constants, but dependent on the X-ray energy distribution, density levels, etc.

Practical applications

With this mathematical background we may attempt to quantitate true luminal narrowing of a coronary stenosis from densitometry. It was mentioned in the introduction, that we have implemented two approaches: i) a transformation technique, whereby the measured density levels in a coronary cineangiogram are mapped into irradiated object thicknesses on a pixel-by-pixel basis; and ii) a gated subtraction technique, whereby a background image in the same phase of the cardiac cycle is subtracted from the actual contrast cineangiogram. These two approaches will be described in the following sections.

Densitometry from contrast image

The densitometric technique to be described attempts to transform the brightness values in the digitized contrast image into calibrated absorption profiles, thus creating the possibility to assess percentage cross-sectional area stenosis from a single view.

The theory behind this densitometric approach is based on the following concepts, which will be described in more detail. For the first part of the chain from the X-ray source to the output of the image intensifier we use the simple relations that were described in this chapter, whereas for the second part from the output of the image intensifier up to the brightness values in the digital image we measure the mapping function on a point-by-point basis.

Let p_c denote a position in the plane of the digitized image which lies within the detected contours of the arterial segment, and let p_b denote a background position just outside of the contours. Let us denote $I(p_c)$ the number of photons at the input screen of the image intensifier at a position corresponding with position p_c in the image plane; similarly $I(p_b)$ can be defined for the background position. The luminances at the output of the image intensifier for these positions are then denoted $L(p_c)$ and $L(p_b)$, respectively.

By approximation, the following relation holds for the X-ray attenuation factor $\beta_2(x,y)$ for a position p_c within a projected coronary arterial segment:

$$\beta_2(p_c) = \beta_1(p_c) + \beta_c(p_c), \tag{VII.12}$$

with $\beta_1(p_c)$ representing the attenuation factor of the position p_c before contrast injection, and $\beta_c(p_c)$ denoting the attenuation factor of the contrast medium in the artery. If a background position p_b is chosen close to p_c, then to a first approximation the following relation is valid:

$$\beta_1(p_b) \approx \beta_1(p_c) \tag{VII.13}$$

Furthermore,

$$I_0(p_c) \approx I_0(p_b) \tag{VII.14}$$

From these definitions and assumptions the following equation can be derived:

$$I(p_c) = I(p_b) \cdot \exp(-\beta_c(p_c)) \tag{VII.15}$$

Under the assumption that the mixing of the contrast agent in the part of the arterial segment to be analyzed is homogeneous and that the mass attenuation coefficient of the contrast-blood mixture is constant, $\beta_c(p_c)$ may be written as:

$$\beta_c(p_c) = \mu \cdot \varrho \cdot d(p_c) \tag{VII.16}$$

with $d(p_c)$ denoting the local thickness of the artery at position p_c. From equations (VII.15) and (VII.16) the thickness $d(p_c)$ can be written as:

$$d(p_c) = k_4 \cdot (\log I(p_b) - \log I(p_c)) \tag{VII.17}$$

with $k_4 = \dfrac{2.30}{\mu \cdot \varrho}$.

From equation (VII.4) the exposures E at positions p_c and p_b at the output screen of the image intensifier can be written as:

$$E(p_c) = t \cdot G(p_c) \cdot (I(p_c))^{\gamma_I} \tag{VII.18}$$

$$E(p_b) = t \cdot G(p_b) \cdot (I(p_b))^{\gamma_I}, \tag{VII.19}$$

where t is the exposure time.
Since $p_c \approx p_b \rightarrow G(p_c) \approx G(p_b)$.
Substituting formules (VII.18) and (VII.19) into (VII.17) and applying the approximations yields:

$$d(p_c) = k_5 \cdot (\log E(p_b) - \log E(p_c)) \tag{VII.20}$$

with k_5 being a constant.
In this simple model all parameters of the source, the absorption process and the image intensifier are mapped into the single unknown constant k_5.

The mapping T from intensities at the output of the image intensifier to brightness values in the digital image is measured on a point-by-point basis.

The mapping T is determined in the following way. The first 21 frames of the cinefilm are exposed homogeneously with a sensitometer having the same color temperature as the output screen of the image intensifier. The calibration frames are exposed according to an exponential function:

$$E(p) = k_6 \cdot (\sqrt{2})^{-n} \tag{VII.21}$$

with n being the frame sequence number ($0 \leq n \leq 20$).
These frames are processed photographically simultaneously with the rest of the coronary cineangiogram, so that the film development process is identical for both the calibration frames and the clinical coronary cineframes. Each of the calibration frames is digitized and stored in the computer. Subsequently, each digitized test frame is divided into 625 subimages of size 20×20; in each subimage the average brightness level is computed. By using all 21 frames this results in a total of 625 local mapping functions each of which is represented by its 21 sample points. Intermediate function values are obtained by linear interpolation. Each of the 625 mapping functions is assigned to the center position of the corresponding 20×20 subimage. The mapping for intermediate positions is obtained by spatial bilinear interpolation. Thus for each position in the image the corresponding

mapping function defines the relation between film exposure levels and the resulting digitized video levels.

The inverse T^{-1} of this mapping must exist to be able to compute the exposures $E(p_c)$ and $E(p_b)$ from the grey levels $V_d(p_c)$ and $V_d(p_b)$ in the digitized image. For position p_c we find:

$$n(p_c) = T^{-1}[V_d(p_c),p_c]$$ (VII.22)

Because of the applied interpolations n may now take on any value between 0 and 20. Equations (VII.21) and (VII.22) yield:

$$\log E(p_c) = k_7 \cdot T^{-1}[V_d(p_c),p_c] + k_8$$ (VII.23)

A similar equation can be defined for the background position p_b.

The brightness values $V_d(p_c)$ and $V_d(p_b)$, in the projected artery and the background, respectively, are now used to compute the length of the absorption path at position p_c by combining (VII.20) and (VII.23) into

$$d(p_c) = k_9 \cdot \{T^{-1}[V_d(p_b),p_b] - T^{-1}[V_d(p_c),p_c]\},$$ (VII.24)

where k_9 is an unknown spatially independent constant. In this way the brightness values in the projected artery can be calibrated in terms of the amount of X-ray absorption. By means of this calibration procedure many nonlinear and spatially variant effects in the filmprocessing and the cine digitizer are taken into account.

Practically, the percentage cross-sectional area reduction of a selected lesion is obtained as follows (Fig. VII.4). When selecting the cineframe for the densitometric analysis of a particular arterial segment, we make sure that the main axis of the segment in 3-D space is reasonably parallel to the projection plane. The contours of the artery are detected automatically as has been described in Chapter III. On every scanline perpendicular to the centerline, a profile of brightness values is measured. This profile is transformed into an exposure profile by means of equations (VII.21) and (VII.22). The background contribution is estimated by computing the linear regression line through the background points directly left and right of the detected contours. Subtraction of this background portion from the intensity profile within the arterial contours according to equation (VII.24) yields the net cross-sectional absorption profile. Integration of this function results in a measure for the cross-sectional area at the particular scanline.

By repeating this procedure for all the scanlines, the relative cross-sectional area function A(i) is obtained. Figure VII.5 shows the clinical case of Chapter III with an obstruction in the proximal LAD in the RAO-projection with the detected contour, the computed diameter function (upper curve) and the densitometric area function (lower curve). The interpolated technique described in Chapter III for the diameter function can also be applied to the densitometric

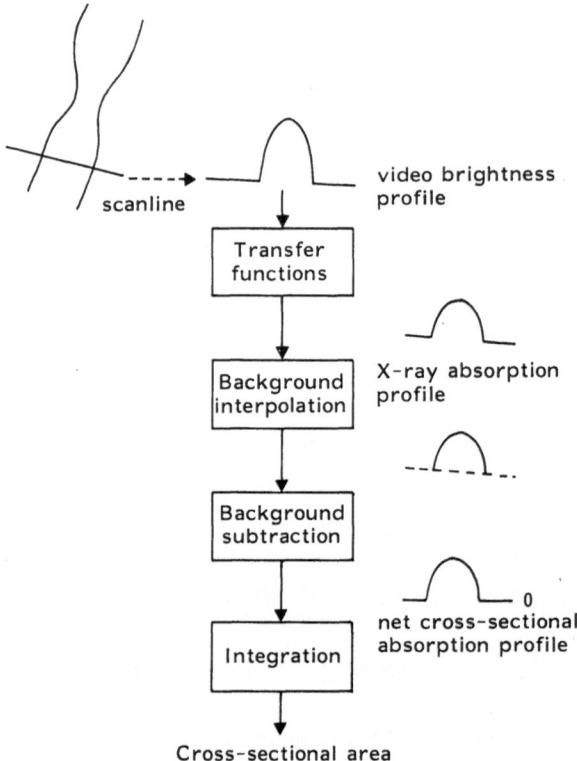

Fig. VII.4. Schematic drawing for determining the cross-sectional area data from the densitometric information within the arterial segment.

area function. For this particular obstruction we found an interpolated percentage diameter reduction of 69% and an interpolated percentage area reduction of 87%. Assuming a model with circular cross sections, a percentage area reduction of 90% would have resulted, thus overestimating the true severity of the obstruction.

A very illustrative example of the clear advantage of this technique as compared to diameter measurements in eccentric lesions is given in Chapter XVII.

Gated subtraction method

The densitometric procedure described above was applied to contrast filled images of the coronary cineangiograms. With that procedure background measurements must be made outside of the vessel. This means that the actual background attenuation factor for a point in an arterial segment can only be approximated by means of a linear interpolation between the background measurements taken left and right of the artery. Particularly when these background levels at both sides of the artery are very different and change relatively strong

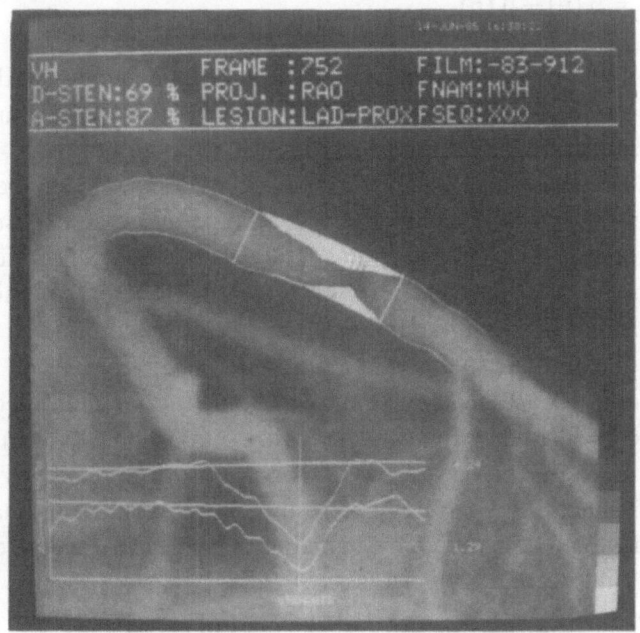

Fig. VII.5. For the obstruction in the proximal LAD the densitometric area function (lower curve) and the diameter function (upper curve) have been computed. An interpolated percentage diameter reduction in this view of 69% is found and an interpolated percentage densitometric area reduction of 87%.

from pixel to pixel due to intervening background structures, then the estimated background level for a position within the vessel may be very different from the actual background level. To come up with a possible solution for such a problem, we have looked at the possibility of subtracting a background image taken before the contrast injection from the contrast-filled image. In the ideal case, an image would then result in which the brightness level at a certain position in a coronary artery would be a measure for the contrast column at this position and in which all areas outside of contrast-filled vessels would have a brightness level equal to zero.

If this procedure provides reliable data, it will be of great interest to apply this technique to nonmagnified images of a coronary arterial system. The resulting subtraction image will then immediately provide information about local defects in arterial cross sections (Ch. IX).

The attenuation factor for X-rays has been defined in equation (VII.3) as

$$\beta(x,y) = \int_0^L \mu(x,y,z)\,\varrho(x,y,z)\,dz.$$ If we distinguish two moments in time, before

and after the contrast injection and define the corresponding attenuation factors by $\beta_1(p)$ and $\beta_2(p)$, respectively, then it is clear that by approximation the following relation holds for a position p within a projected coronary arterial segment:

$$\beta_2(p) = \beta_1(p) + \beta_c(p) \tag{VII.25}$$

with $\beta_c(p)$ denoting the attenuation factor of the contrast medium in the artery. For positions outside of an arterial segment $\beta_2(p) \approx \beta_1(p)$. It must be emphasized that the X-ray settings (kV, mA) must be identical for both situations. Also, the background and contrast images must be taken at corresponding moments in the cardiac cycle and the patient should keep his breath during the exposure of the cinefilm to exclude respiratory motion as much as possible. Since the cinefilm speed is, in general, not in synchrony with the cardiac cycle, the timing of the selected background and contrast images may be off by 20 msec at the most, assuming a regular cardiac rhythm and a film speed of 25 frames/s.

From equation (VII.10) it is clear that logarithmic subtraction is necessary to obtain an image in which the brightness levels are proportional to $\beta_c(p)$. Because an additive term, $k_2 \cdot V_0(p)$ due to the dark current of the scanning device, is present in both images, this term must be subtracted first in these images. The dark current image can be acquired by digitizing an image with the lens cap on the video camera. The subtraction image $V_{d,s}(p)$ yields:

$$V_{d,s}(p) = \ln[V_{d,2}(p) - k_2 \cdot V_0(p)] - \ln[V_{d,1}(p) - k_2 \cdot V_0(p)]$$
$$= \ln[k_{3,2}(p) \cdot \exp(\beta_2(p) \cdot \gamma_I \gamma_F \gamma_v] - \ln[k_{3,1}(p) \cdot \exp(\beta_1(p) \cdot \gamma_I' \gamma_F' \gamma_v']$$

$$= \ln\frac{k_{3,2}(p)}{k_{3,1}(p)} + \ln\frac{\exp[\beta_2(p) \cdot \gamma_I \gamma_F \gamma_v]}{\exp[\beta_1(p) \cdot \gamma_I' \gamma_F' \gamma_v']}$$

$$= \ln\frac{k_{3,2}(p)}{k_{3,1}(p)} + \gamma_I \gamma_F \gamma_v \beta_c(p) + (\gamma_I \gamma_F \gamma_v - \gamma_I' \gamma_F' \gamma_v')\beta_1(p) \tag{VII.26}$$

In formula (VII.26), the subscripts ,1 and ,2 refer to the pre- and postcontrast injection situations, respectively.

In the above derivation we have assumed slight differences in the gamma's, indicated with '. Since $k_{3,2}(p) \approx k_{3,1}(p)$ and $\gamma_I \gamma_F \gamma_v \approx \gamma_I' \gamma_F' \gamma_v'$ equation (VII.26) can be approximated by:

$$V_{d,s}(p) \approx \gamma_I \gamma_F \gamma_v \beta_c(p). \tag{VII.27}$$

This means that for positions within the projection of a coronary arterial segment, the brightness information in the subtraction image is proportional to the attenuation factor of the contrast medium and thus, by assuming homogeneous mixing of the contrast with the blood which results in constant values of μ and ϱ, indeed proportional to the local thickness of the artery.

An example of this procedure applied to a clinical coronary cineangiogram is shown in Fig. VII.6. Figure VII.6a is a coronary cineangiogram of the left coronary arterial system in the RAO-projection of a bypass patient digitized in a 512×512 matrix (optical magnification factor of 1). The corresponding digitized background image is shown in Fig. VII.6b. Applying the described subtraction procedure results in the subtraction image of Fig. VII.6c. The subtraction image has been scaled linearly such that the pixel with the greatest density difference is displayed at brightness level 255; negative numbers have been set to zero. Due to small spatial differences in position in the contrast and background images the catheter and the metal sternal sutures are still visible. These small differences are augmented by the differential nature of the subtraction procedure.

In order to derive from these data the percentage cross-sectional luminal narrowing for a given coronary obstruction, both the lesion and the reference position should ideally be in the same plane parallel to the input screen of the image intensifier and very importantly, a homogeneous mixing of the contrast agent within the artery must be assumed.

Evaluation study

A preliminary validation study has been carried out with cinefilm of four perspex models of coronary obstructions. These models have circular cross sections with proximal and distal reference diameters of 4.0 mm and obstruction diameters of 1.5, 2.0, 3.0 and 4.0 mm, respectively (Fig. V.2). The area reduction percentages

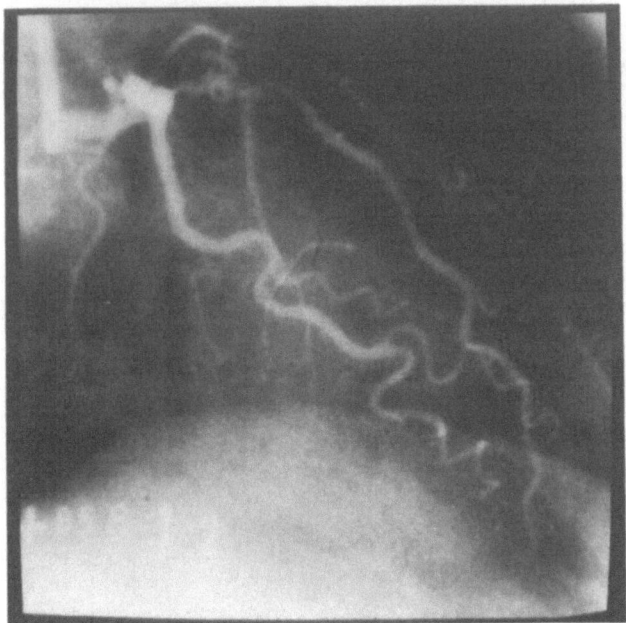

Fig. VII.6a.

166

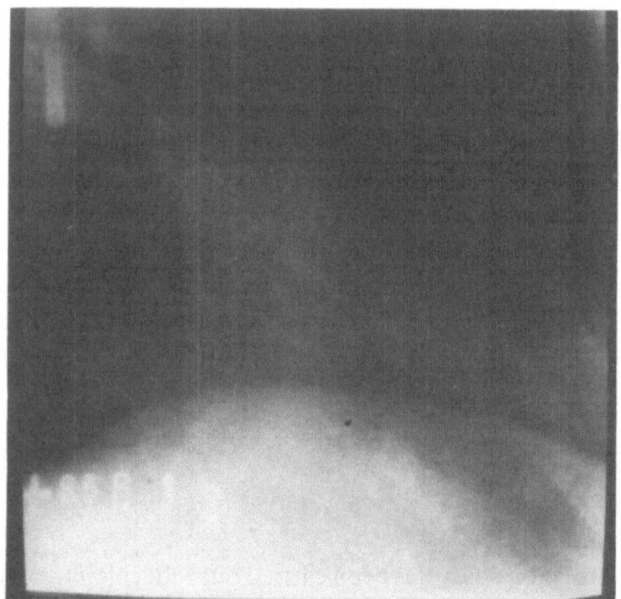

b

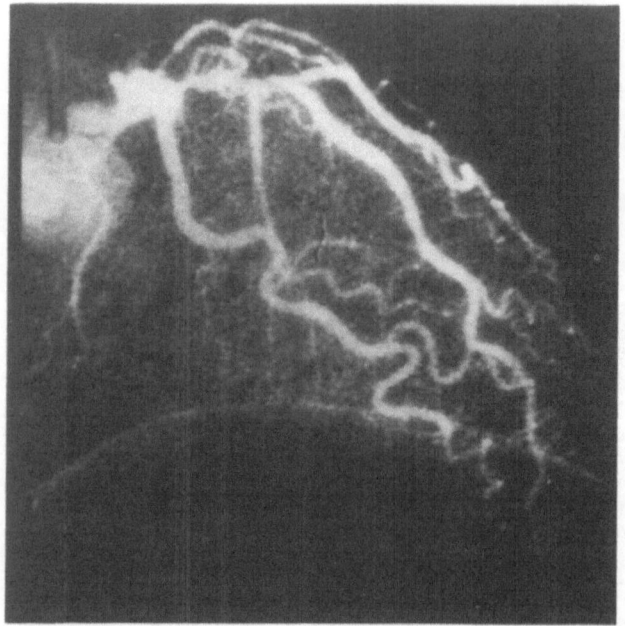

c

Fig. VII.6. Example of subtraction technique applied to coronary cineangiograms. Contrast coronary cineangiogram (Fig. VII.6a), corresponding background image (Fig. VII.6b) and subtraction image (Fig. VII.6c).

Table VII.1. True and measured percentages area-stenosis by densitometric procedures for four perspex models filled with contrast agent.

True %-area stenosis	Measured %-area stenosis		
	Film 1 67 kV	Film 2 74 kV	Film 3 51 kV
86	85	87	85
75	78	72	73
44	44	41	39
0	8	8	4

were measured with the densitometric procedure for various settings of the X-ray system and with different concentrations of the contrast agent (Table VII.1).

These results show that in general there is good agreement between the true and measured percentages area-stenosis. The deviations from the true values for the model with 0% area-stenosis require further investigations.

For the subtraction technique two films were taken of the four perspex models placed next to each other at 70 kV, one film (the background film) with the models filled with water and a second film (the contrast film) with the models filled with contrast agent. The subtraction procedure was carried out as described and percentage area stenosis measured. These results show very close agreement between the true and measured values (Table VII.2).

It is clear that these data can only be regarded as preliminary results obtained from a very small test set. Extension of the validation studies of noncircular models and to postmortem casts [10], at various kV's and concentrations of the contrast agent is being carried out. Also, studying the effects of dynamic flow of blood and contrast agent through the models is being anticipated.

Table VII.2. True and measured percentages area-stenosis by subtraction technique for four perspex models.

True %-area stenosis	Measured %-area stenosis
86	89
75	77
44	43
0	0

168

Concluding remarks

In this chapter the transfer functions of the different components of the entire X-ray-cine-digitizer chain have been described in relatively simple terms. On the basis of the derived formulas two densitometric techniques have been analyzed, i.e. densitometric analysis from a contrast image and the gated subtraction method. For both methods it has been shown how the irradiated object thickness of a coronary arterial segment can be derived from the measured brightness levels in the digitized cineframes. A clinical application of the densitometric technique from contrast images is described in Chapter XVII. An application of the gated subtraction technique is described in Chapter IX.

Densitometric analysis from cinefilm requires a detailed study of the different components in the X-ray-cine-digitizer chain. Special attention must be given to the effect of the selected kV-level of the X-ray system, nonhomogeneous responses of the entire cineframe, the film development process, the characteristics of the light source of the cine digitizer, the scanning system of the digitizer, etc., etc., on the computed object thicknesses. Besides these technical details, angiographic factors must be taken into account as well, such as the homogeneity of the contrast distribution in the vessels, the three-dimensional positions of selected reference and obstruction sites with respect to the image intensifier, etc.

A number of publications have appeared in the literature which neglect most of these potentially disturbing factors mentioned in this chapter [11–15].

References

1. Roberts WC: The coronary arteries and left ventricle in clinically isolated angina pectoris. Circulation 54: 388–390, 1976.
2. Freudenberg H, Lichtlen P: Postmortale Koronarangiographie. In: Koronar-angiographie, P.R. Lichtlen (Ed.). Verlag Dr med D Straube, Erlangen: 341–357, 1979.
3. Gensini GG: Coronary angiography. Futura Publishing Company Inc, New York, 1975.
4. Brown BG, Bolson EL, Dodge HT: Arteriographic assessment of coronary atherosclerosis. Review of current methods, their limitations and clinical applications. Arteriosclerosis 2: 2–15, 1982.
5. Reiber JHC, Gerbrands JJ, Booman F, Troost GJ, Boer A den, Slager CJ, Schuurbiers JCH: Objective characterization of coronary obstructions from monoplane cineangiograms and three-dimensional reconstruction of an arterial segment from two orthogonal views. In: Applications of Computers in Medicine. MD Schwartz, (Ed.). IEEE Cat No TH0095-0: 93–100, 1982.
6. Reiber JHC, Slager CJ, Schuurbiers JCH, Boer A den, Gerbrands JJ, Troost GJ, Scholts B, Kooijman CJ, Serruys PW: Transfer functions of the X-ray-Cine-Video chain applied to digital processing of coronary cineangiograms. In: Digital Imaging in Cardiovascular Radiology. PH Heintzen, R Brennecke, (Eds.). Georg Thieme Verlag, Stuttgart: 89–104, 1983.
7. Reiber JHC, Gerbrands JJ, Kooijman CJ, Troost GJ, Schuurbiers JCH, Slager CJ, Boer A den, Serruys PW: Computer-aided analysis of coronary obstructions from monoplane cineangiograms and three-dimensional reconstruction of an arterial segment from two orthogonal views. In: Physical Techniques in Cardiovascular Imaging. MD Short, DA Pay, S Leeman, RM Harrison

(Eds.) Adam Hilger Ltd, Bristol: 173–188, 1983.

8. Serruys PW, Reiber JHC, Wijns W, Brand M van den, Kooijman CJ, Katen HJ ten, Hugenholtz PG: Assessment of percutaneous transluminal coronary angioplasty by quantitative coronary angiography: diameter versus densitometric area measurements. Am J Cardiol 54: 482–488, 1984.

9. Boer A den: A microprocessor system for on-line registration of the X-ray system settings. Internal Report, Thoraxcenter 1982.

10. Spears JR, Crawford DW, Serur J, Grossman W, Paulin S: A catheterization technique for reproduction of a human atherosclerotic lumen within the dog coronary artery in vivo. Cath and Cardiovasc Diagn 9: 219–229, 1983.

11. Nichols AB, Gabrieli CFO, Fenoglio JJ, Esser PD: Quantification of relative coronary arterial stenosis by cinevideodensitometric analysis of coronary arteriograms. Circulation 69: 512–522, 1984.

12. Collins SM, Skorton DJ, Harrison DG, White CW, Eastham CL, Hiratzka LF, Doty DB, Marcus ML: Quantitative computer-based videodensitometry and the physiological significance of a coronary stenosis. Comp Cardiol: 219–222, 1982.

13. Barth K, Epple E, Irion KM, Faust U, Decker D: Quantifizierung von Stenosen der Herzkranz-gefässe durch digitale Bildauswertung. Erg Bd Biomed Technik 26, 1981.

14. Kishon Y, Yerushalmi S, Deutsch V, Neufeld HN: Measurement of coronary arterial lumen by densitometric analysis of angiograms. Angiology 39: 304–312, 1979.

15. Sandor T, Als AV, Paulin S: Cine-densitometric measurements of coronary arterial stenoses. Cath Cardiovasc Diagn 5: 229–245, 1979.

VIII. 3-D reconstruction of coronary arterial segments from two projections

Introduction

Most efforts in the field of quantitative data extraction from coronary cineangiograms have focused on the development of methods to determine the severity of coronary obstructions in terms of percentage diameter and/or cross-sectional area reduction from single or biplane cineangiograms; a brief overview of the relevant literature in this field is presented in 11. However, if we would be able to determine with a sufficient degree of accuracy the three-dimensional shape and size of coronary arterial segments, an additional number of clinically important parameters would become available. For example, from the three-dimensional data several hemodynamic parameters of the arterial segments may be computed, such as the hemodynamic resistance of an obstruction and the blood flow through the artery after selective administration of a contrast bolus. These data may augment our knowledge in searching for the definition of the 'critical' stenosis. Furthermore, the three-dimensional morphology and particularly the changes over longer periods of time may provide us with detailed information about the presence and development of coronary atherosclerosis.

It is the purpose of this paper to present the basic principles that we have developed and implemented for the three-dimensional reconstruction of an arterial segment from two orthogonal projections. This method is based on the work by Slump on the binary reconstruction of the left ventricle from two orthogonal cineventriculograms [12]. Two versions of this algorithm modified to our specific application will be discussed. The simplest version does not take different noise components in the projection data into account, while a more complex version does. This modified 'noisy' Slump algorithm will be illustrated with a clinical example. The software developed by Onnasch et al. for the reconstruction of the left ventricle has been adapted to the coronary reconstruction problem as well [8, 9]. A preliminary evaluation study on the different reconstruction algorithms will be presented.

171

Problem analysis and overview on pertinent literature

The problem of the three-dimensional reconstruction of a coronary arterial segment can be reduced to a multiple two-dimensional problem by dividing the object into a stack of parallel cross sections. Each two-dimensional cross section consists of one connected region and is reconstructed from its two one-dimensional projections. The thickness of each slice must be taken such that the projections do not change significantly over the slice. Under the assumption that the contrast within the arterial segment is mixed homogeneously, the reconstruction further reduces to a binary problem. Each slice can be represented by a pattern of zero's and one's, with the zero's indicating the positions where there is no contrast and the one's representing the positions belonging to the cross section of the artery. Therefore, we may state our problem as the reconstruction of a binary matrix from its row and column sums. In general, there is no unique solution to this problem. A priori knowledge has to be used to reduce the ambiguity.

There exist only a few publications on the binary reconstruction problem from two projections. Chang and Chow have described a method for the reconstruction of a binary convex symmetric object from two orthogonal projections [2]. Chang shows that if the shape of the slice is convex and one contour position not being an extreme point along the boundary is known, the object can be reconstructed uniquely from two orthogonal projections [3]. However, a cross section of a coronary arterial segment is not convex symmetric, in general, so that this method is not applicable to our problem. Onnasch and Heintzen have described an algorithm for binary reconstruction of the left or right ventricle from two projections that is based on a priori information from an earlier reconstructed spatially adjacent slice and/or from the same slice at another point in time of the cardiac cycle [8, 9]. The method is based on the use of a probability array defined as a product of three factors: the fundamental probability array, which is essentially a normalized product of the two orthogonal density profiles, and two probability arrays which take the similarity of the ventricular slices in space and in time into account. We have implemented this method for the coronary reconstruction problem with one difference, namely that we use slice matrices of 64×64 pixels instead of the 30×30 pixel matrices proposed by Onnasch. Finally, Slump and Gerbrands describe a method for the left ventricular reconstruction application, that basically consists of a minimum cost capacitated network flow algorithm [12]. They state the problem of the reconstruction of a binary slice as the finding of a matrix satisfying the two projections with maximum resemblance to the corresponding temporally or spatially adjacent cross sections. The resemblance criterion is incorporated into the reconstruction process by means of a cost function.

This method, further referred to in this paper by the 'Slump' reconstruction method, has been modified to our particular coronary artery reconstruction problem. New algorithms from the field of Operations Research have been implemented to speed up the reconstruction process.

Basic principles

Under the assumption of homogeneous mixing of the contrast agent in the arterial segment to be reconstructed, we adopt the following discrete model. A slice of the artery is represented by a binary matrix. The matrix elements are '1' for positions that lie within the arterial cross section and '0' for positions outside of it. In this discrete model the two absorption profiles obtained from densitometric analysis of the cineangiograms represent the row and column sums of this matrix (for detailed description of this densitometric procedure see Ch. VII and ref. 11). Therefore, we state our fundamental problem of reconstructing one slice as the reconstruction of a binary matrix from its row and column sums. Let X denote and m∗n matrix with entries $x(i,j) \varepsilon \{0,1\}$. The elements of X are to be determined from the following set of equations:

$$\sum_{j=1}^{n} x(i,j) = \alpha(i) \quad i = 1, \ldots, m$$

$$\sum_{i=1}^{m} x(i,j) = \beta(j) \quad j = 1, \ldots, n \quad \text{(VIII.1)}$$

where $\alpha(i), i = 1, \ldots, m$ are the elements of the vector α containing the row sums of X and $\beta(j), j = 1, \ldots, n$ the elements of the vector β containing the column sums of X.

This set of equations is not independent, since

$$\sum_{i=1}^{m} \alpha(i) = \sum_{j=1}^{n} \beta(j) \quad \text{(VIII.2)}$$

i.e. the total sum of the row projection equals the total sum of the column projection. Thus $m \times n$ variables $x(ij) \varepsilon \{0,1\}$ need to be computed from $m + n - 1$ independent equations, which is an underdetermined problem.

This reconstruction problem can be illustrated with the drawing of Fig. VIII.1 showing a coronary segment to be reconstructed. Given the two orthogonal absorption profiles with the row and column sums $\alpha(i)$ and $\beta(j)$, respectively, the elements $x(i,j)$ belonging to the bottom slice need to be determined.

From combinatorial mathematics the conditions are known for the existence of no, one or more than one solution of this problem. In the ideal case without noise and measurement errors there may be many solutions, and other information has to be used to reduce the ambiguity. On physiological grounds, there must be a strong resemblance between two adjacent cross sections of the artery. We therefore reformulate our problem as the search for a binary matrix satisfying the projections with maximum resemblance to the previously reconstructed adjacent slice. Under practical circumstances, the acquired absorption profile data will be disturbed by noise and measurement errors and no single solution can be found, in general. The effects of these deviations on the reconstruction process will be discussed later on in this paper under noise considerations. For the time being we

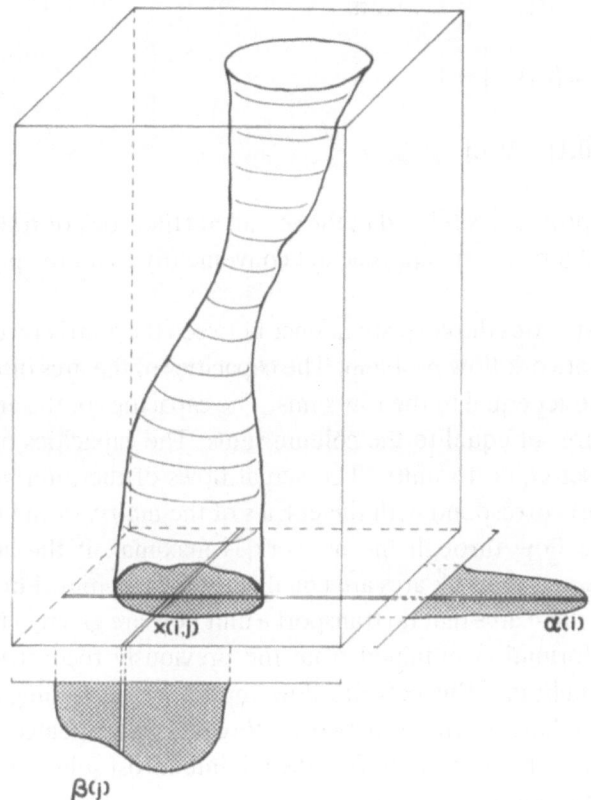

Fig. VIII.1. Illustration of the reconstruction problem. Given the two orthogonal absorption profiles with row and colums sums $\alpha(i)$ and $\beta(j)$, respectively, the elements $x(i,j)$ belonging to the bottom slice need to be computed.

will consider the reconstruction process in the ideal case.

It is attractive to incorporate a resemblance criterion in the reconstruction process directly, which we have achieved by introducing a cost coefficient $c(i,j)$ for every element (i,j) of the matrix, which represents the penalty for assigning that element the value '1' in the reconstruction. A simple example is to set $c(i,j)$ equal to zero if the matrix element (i,j) was element of the arterial cross section in the previously reconstructed slice and equal to one otherwise. The minimum cost solution of the reconstruction problem will then show a high degree of similarity to the previous cross section.

We formulate therefore the following optimization process:

$$\text{Minimize Z with } Z = \sum_{i=1}^{m} \sum_{j=1}^{n} c(i,j) \cdot x(i,j) \qquad \text{(VIII.3)}$$

under the constraints:

174

$$\sum_{j=1}^{n} x(i,j) = \alpha(i) \quad i = 1, \ldots, m \tag{VIII.4}$$

$$\sum_{i=1}^{m} x(i,j) = \beta(j) \quad j = 1, \ldots, n \tag{VIII.5}$$

$$x(i,j) \ \varepsilon \ \{0,1\} \quad \forall \ i,j \tag{VIII.6}$$

This optimization problem is related to the so-called Hitchcock or transportation problem. This problem can be approached conveniently as a flow problem in a direct network.

Figure VIII.2 illustrates the correspondence between the matrix reconstruction problem and the network flow problem. The capacities of the arcs directed away from the source are set equal to the row sums. The capacities of the arcs directed towards the sink are set equal to the column sums. The capacities of the intermediate arcs are set equal to unity. The actual flows of the intermediate arcs (either zero or one) correspond with the entries of the matrix of the reconstruction problem. The flow through the network is maximal, if the actual flows through the source and the sink arcs are equal to their capacities. For simplicity, only those intermediate arcs that do transport a unit flow are given in Fig. VIII.2.

The a priori information obtained from the previously reconstructed cross section can be brought into this network flow approach by assigning cost coefficients to the intermediate arcs in the network. We can then adapt algorithms from the Operation Research literature to find the minimum cost solution at maximal flow through the capacitated network.

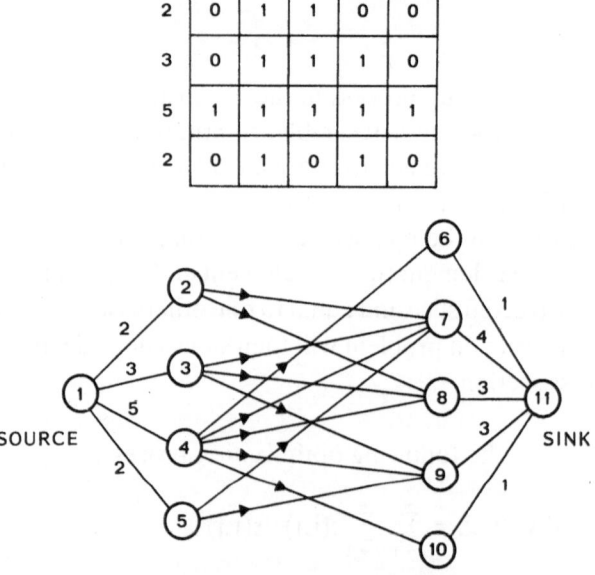

Fig. VIII.2. The matrix reconstruction problem and the network flow approach.

The procedure starts with an algoritm to obtain a feasible flow through the network, i.e. a flow which corresponds with the projection values. As proposed by Slump et al., the maximum flow algorithm of Ford and Fulkerson has been implemented for this purpose [4, 12]. Subsequently, Slump used Klein's (primal method) minimal cost flow algorithm to find the solution to the problem [7]. However, on our minicomputer this would lead to processing times on the order of 5 minutes per slice. Therefore, we have implemented a variant of the (dual method) 'Out of Kilter' algorithm of Ford and Fulkerson. This method has been described in detail by Wagner [14]. Implementation of this algorithm reduced the average processing time of the actual reconstruction step on a PDP 11/34 to approximately 6 sec. per slice.

Cost coëfficient matrix

We now describe a method for obtaining a cost coefficient matrix from the binary matrix that serves as a model of the cross section to be reconstructed. In the work by Slump for the reconstruction of the left ventricle, it was assumed that the area of the model is smaller than the cross section to be determined. It is clear that this assumption is not valid for our application of the coronary arteries with possibly widely varying cross sections along an arterial segment. Therefore, we have extended the procedure for the computation of the cost coefficient matrix such that the cases with slices smaller than the model also can be facilitated.

The implemented procedure can be explained most easily by first looking at the original Slump approach. Initially, all the cost elements within the contour of the model are set to zero. Subsequently, the contour is enlarged iteratively by means of an expansion algorithm. At each iteration the cost of all elements outside of the enlarged contour are increased with 8 and the cost of a new contour position with 8 minus the degree of 8-connectivity with the elements within the contour. This expansion procedure can also be inversed to compute the cost of elements within the contour of the model, so that slices with an area smaller than the model can be reconstructed. Finally, a normalization step is carried out to obtain positive cost values for all the elements in the cost coefficient matrix. An example of the model matrix and the resulting cost coefficient matrix is given in Fig. VIII.3. It should be noted that the 'Out of Kilter' algorithm does not require positive cost values. However, this normalization step has been included to obtain cost values which intuitively suit our understanding of the concept of cost best.

Noise considerations

In the previous sections we have ignored the presence of noise and measurement errors corrupting the projection data. Obviously, this is a gross simplification.

```
0  0  0 │1│ 0  0  0  0  0  0        15 14 12 │ 8│12 14 15 21 23 30
0│1  1  1  1  1│0  0  0  0         13│ 7  6  5  6  7│13 15 22 28
1  1  1  1  1  1  1│0  0  0          8  7  0  0  0  5  7│14 20 23
0│1  1  1  1  1  1│0  0  0         13│ 7  4  0  0  0  6│12 15 22
0  0│1  1  1  1  1  1│0  0         15 12│ 6  0  0  0  6  8│15 21
0  0│1  1  1  1  1│0  0  0         20 14│ 7  4  0  4  7│13 15 22
0  0  0│1  1  1│0  0  0  0         22 15 12│ 6  0  6│12 15 21 23
0  0  0│1  1  1│0  0  0  0         23 20 14 │7  7  7│14 20 23 29
0  0  0  0│1│0  0  0  0  0         28 22 15 13│ 8│13 15 22 28 31
0  0  0  0  0  0  0  0  0  0         30 23 21 15 15 15 21 23 30 36
```

Fig. VIII.3. The model matrix and the computed cost coefficient matrix.

Due to these effects, it is very unlikely that the two measured projections are even consistent. Several noise sources in the entire X-ray-cine-video chain can be distinguished, such as the discrete photon-character of the X-rays itself, the absorption and scatter process of the X-rays through the patient, electronic noise in the image intensifier, film grain noise and electronic noise in the video system, to mention the most important contributions. The resulting deviations in the measured absorption profiles from the true values have serious consequences for the reconstruction method described above. Instead of finding many solutions satisfying the constraints (VIII.4), (VIII.5) and (VIII.6), in general, not a single solution may be found for this problem due to these errors. To be able to compute a 'most probable' solution, the constraints (VIII.4) and (VIII.5) must be softened such that they are no longer inconsistent.

An obvious solution is:

$$\sum_{j=1}^{n} x(i,j) \geqslant \alpha(i) \quad i = 1, \ldots, m \tag{VIII.7}$$

$$\sum_{i=1}^{m} x(i,j) \geqslant \beta(j) \quad j = 1, \ldots, n \tag{VIII.8}$$

Because of the minimization in (VIII.3) the projections of the resulting reconstruction will not deviate much from the measured projections. In the implementation of the Slump method we have used a (mathematically slightly simpler) variant of this approach.

An improved modification of the constraints (VIII.4) and (VIII.5) can be obtained if the noise characteristics are known.

In clinical practice, the X-ray noise contribution is the most severe component. A common assumption in the literature is to model the noise in the measured data as Poisson noise, a custom we follow here as well [6, 13].

Let us assume that the true object thickness at a particular pixel in the coronary cineangiogram is denoted d and that a thickness dm is measured. Then the following is true, if the measurement technique has no systematic error.

expectation E[dm] = d $\qquad$ (VIII.9)

and variance $\sigma^2 (dm) = \gamma^2 \cdot d$ $\qquad$ (VIII.10)

with γ being a constant which is mainly dependent on the X-ray source current.

It has been explained in Chapter VII that the irradiated object thickness is measured as a difference of two absorption profiles, namely (background + artery) − (background). This means that the noise contributions must be added, resulting in a variance:

$$\sigma^2 (dma) = \gamma^2 \cdot (2 \cdot db + da) \qquad (VIII.11)$$

with dma the measured artery thickness, db the true effective background thickness and da the true artery thickness. Also,

$$E [dma] = da \qquad (VIII.12)$$

Equation (VIII.11) is rewritten as:

$$\sigma^2(dma) = \gamma^2 \cdot (da + b), \qquad (VIII.13)$$

where $b(= 2 \cdot db)$ is, to a first approximation, spatially independent.

To reduce the effects of noise on the three-dimensional reconstruction, the image, that contains all the thickness profiles after the densitometric transformation procedure, is filtered with the two-dimensional spatial Tukey-filter [1]. This filter reduces the noise, while preserving the edge information.

For this situation in which the noise contributions are also taken into account, the optimization process as defined by equation (VIII.3) must be solved under the following constraints (instead of the constraints defined by equations (VIII.4)–(VIII.6):

$$\alpha(i) - \gamma \cdot \sqrt{\alpha(i) + b} \leqslant \sum_{j=1}^{n} x(i,j) \leqslant \alpha(i) + \gamma \cdot \sqrt{\alpha(i) + b}, \quad i = 1, \ldots, m \qquad (VIII.14)$$

$$\beta(j) - \gamma \cdot \sqrt{\beta(j) + b} \leqslant \sum_{i=1}^{m} x(i,j) \leqslant \beta(j) + \gamma \cdot \sqrt{\beta(j) + b}, \quad j = 1, \ldots, n \qquad (VIII.15)$$

$$\sum_{i=1}^{m} \sum_{j=1}^{n} x(i,j) = (\sum_{j=1}^{n} \beta(j) + \sum_{i=1}^{m} \alpha(i))/2 \qquad (VIII.16)$$

$$x(i,j) \ \varepsilon \ \{0,1\} \quad i = 1, \ldots, m, \quad j = 1, \ldots, n \qquad (VIII.17)$$

It can be shown that for a given value of b, a minimal value of γ (γ min) can be found such that the equations (VIII.14)–(VIII.17) are satisfied. Subsequently, the minimization process defined by equation (VIII.3) under the constraints (VIII.14)–(VIII.17) can be solved by the Out-of-Kilter algorithm. This procedure is called the 'noisy'-Slump method.

Registration of the two orthogonal projections

So far we have looked at the algorithms to solve the three-dimensional reconstruction problem assuming the necessary information from the two projections of the arterial segment to be reconstructed were available. In this section the acquisition of the projection data and the necessary steps to be taken to register the two projections accurately will be described. A block diagram of the total procedure is shown in Fig. VIII.4.

The data acquisition starts with the user selection of two corresponding orthogonal frames of the arterial segment. Next, the contours of the selected segments in the two projections are detected automatically and the brightness information within the bounded segments transformed into irradiated object thickness as has been described in detail elsewhere [10, 11, Ch. VII]. Calibration of the diameter data occurs as usual on the basis of the contrast catheter visible in the images. For each projection the computed calibration factor can be corrected for the axial distance between the catheter and arterial segments on the basis of the information from the other projection (Chapter V).

Since the object thickness is given in arbitrary units, a relation must be found between this object thickness in one projection and the width in the other projection. This can be assessed from a nondiseased part of the segment; usually the first slice to be reconstructed is used for these purposes. If we assume that the cross section in this part is circular in shape, then the maximal thickness in one projection must correspond with the computed diameter in the other projection. Since these two measurements may be disturbed by noise, we have implemented an optimization procedure to compute from the available thickness data and width of the artery the parameters of a circle not disturbed by noise. The scaling factors are then determined from this ideal circle.

Clinical example

The results from the described reconstruction algorithm can be demonstrated with the following clinical example. Figure VIII.5a shows an optically enlarged part of a cineangiogram of a right coronary artery in the RAO-projection. The automatically detected contours are superimposed in the image. Figure VIII.5b shows the same segment in the LAO-projection, again with the detected contours superimposed. For these two images the brightness information within the bounded segments has been translated into local object thickness and for the

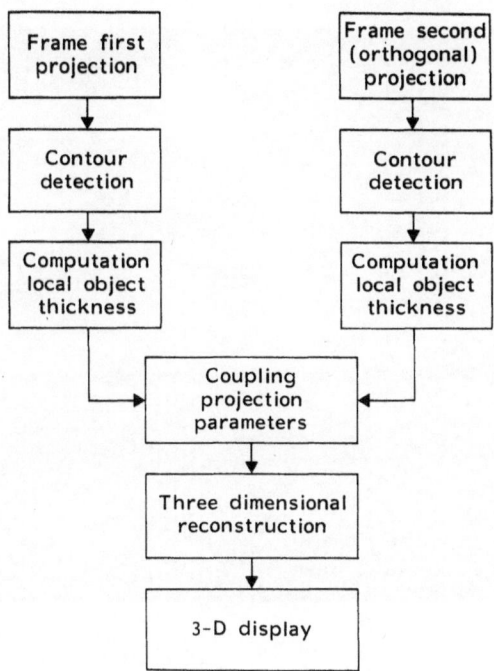

Fig. VIII.4. Flow diagram of the data-acquisition procedure for the three-dimensional reconstruction of a coronary segment.

three-dimensional reconstruction the noisy Slump method has been applied. The three-dimensional representation is given in Fig. VIII.6 for the RAO30 (Fig. VIII.6a), LAO60 (Fig. VIII.6b) and RPO60 (Fig. VIII.6c) views, respectively. For this particular example a total of 155 slices were reconstructed. The display technique is based on the work by Van der Zanden [15].

Preliminary evaluation 3-D reconstruction algorithms

To measure the performance of the three reconstruction algorithms, we have performed two tests:

A. Reconstruction of Perspex Model with Circular Cross Sections

One of our perspex test models was filled with contrast medium and filmed in two orthogonal projections. This model has circular cross sections with diameters ranging from 4.0 mm at the proximal and distal ends to 1.5 mm at the obstruction. For this model 290 slices were reconstructed. For each slice the relative mean error as discussed by Herman was determined [5]. This relative mean error $\bar{R}$ is defined by:

180

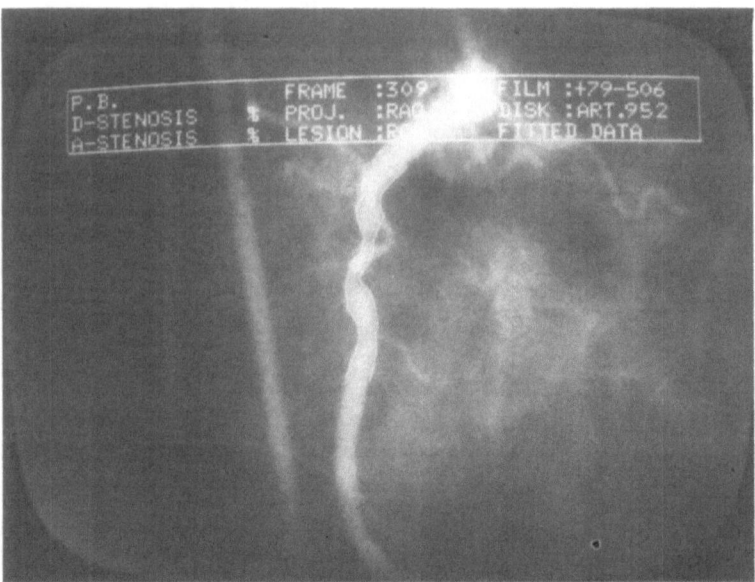

a

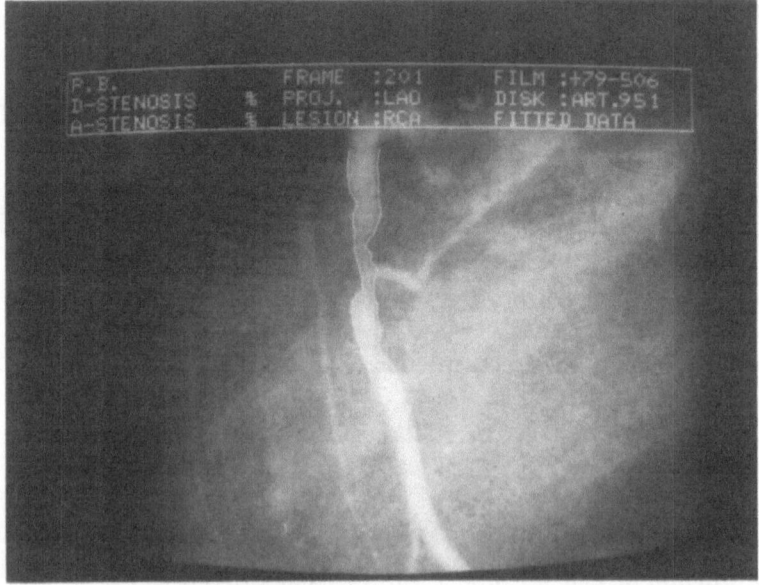

b

Fig. VIII.5. Two orthogonal cineangiograms of a right coronary artery with the detected contours superimposed from which the three-dimensional representations of Fig. VIII.6 are reconstructed (a) RAO-projection, (b) LAO-projection.

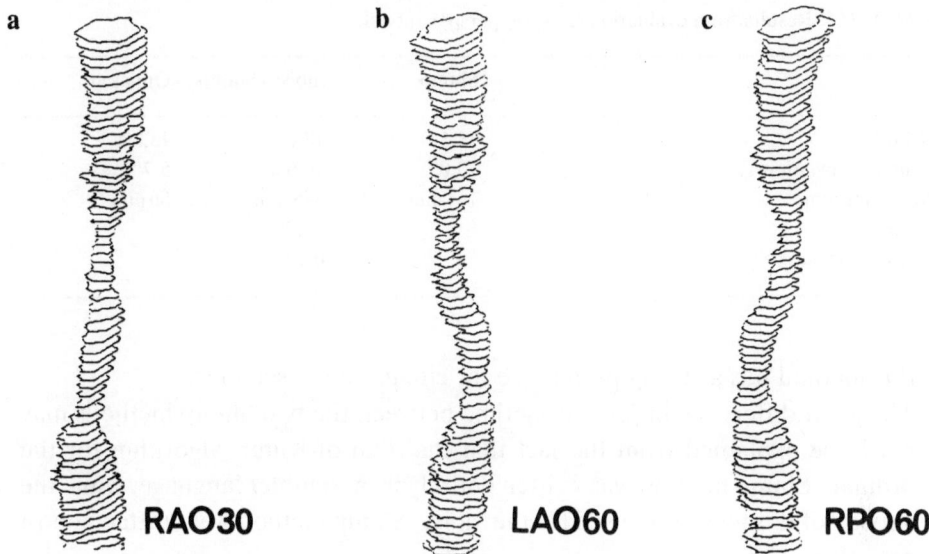

Fig. VIII.6. Three-dimensional representation of obstructed arterial segment reconstructed of Fig. VIII.5, displayed in the RAO30 (Fig. VIII.6a), LAO60 (Fig. VIII.6b) and RPO60 (Fig. VIII.6c) views, respectively.

$$\bar{R} = \frac{\sum\limits_{i=1}^{m} \sum\limits_{j=1}^{n} |x(i,j) - o(i,j)|}{\sum\limits_{i=1}^{m} \sum\limits_{j=1}^{n} o(i,j)} \times 100\% \qquad \text{(VIII.18)}$$

where $o(i,j)$, are the elements of the original binary matrix and $x(i,j)$ the elements of the reconstruction matrix. Finally, from the 290 $\bar{R}$-values, the mean and standard deviation were computed. The results for the Slump, 'noisy' Slump and Onnasch reconstruction algorithms, respectively, are given in table VIII.1, together with the processing time for this model on a PDP 11/34 minicomputer.

A few remarks have to be made when interpreting the results from this evaluation study.

– The processing times in Table VIII.1 include reading the registered absorption profiles from disk, computation cost matrices, the reconstruction itself with display on the video monitor for each slice of the absorption profiles and the reconstructed cross section and finally writing all the results back to disk. The processing times for contour detection, the densitometric procedure and the interactive alignment were not included.

– For the reconstruction following the 'noisy' Slump method the variable b was chosen equal to 2. Further investigations are necessary to determine the influence of this variable on the results.

– The good results for the Onnasch method may be explained from the fact that

Table VIII.1. Results from evaluation study on perspex model.

	Slump	'noisy' Slump	Onnasch
Mean R̃	18.5%	18.0%	13.2%
Standard deviation R̃	10.0%	10.9%	5.7%
Processing time	144 min	355 min	86 min
Mean γ		0.294	
Standard deviation γ		0.134	

this method has a strong preference for circular cross sections.

- The great difference in processing time between the two Slump methods may partly be explained from the fact that the 'Out-of-Kilter' algorithm for the ordinary Slump method was written entirely in Assembler language, while the version of this algorithm used for the 'noisy' Slump method was written almost entirely in Fortran.

B. Reconstruction of artery with noncircular cross sections

Since the true cross-sectional data for the arterial segment of Fig. VIII.5 are not known, another test criterion had to be developed. We have looked at the model-dependency of the different algorithms by reconstructing the segment twice, once starting from the proximal part of the segment and once from the distal part. The difference between these two reconstructions can then be computed. The mean model-dependency $\bar{S}$ for a particular slice is then defined by:

$$\bar{S} = \frac{\sum_{i=1}^{m} \sum_{j=1}^{n} |x1(i,j) - x2(i,j)|}{\sum_{i=1}^{m} \sum_{j=1}^{n} (x1(i,j) + x2(i,j))/2} \times 100\% \qquad (VIII.19)$$

where $x1(i,j)$ denotes the elements for the first reconstruction and $x2(i,j)$ for the second reconstruction. Again the mean and standard deviation of $\bar{S}$ were determined for the 155 slices of Fig. VIII.6. The results are given in Table VIII.2. The following remarks can be made concerning this evaluation criterion:

- In general, the changes in the structure of a nondiseased part of a coronary segment from slice to slice are small, which must result in a small value of $\bar{S}$ for a good reconstruction method. A reconstruction method with a relatively large value of $\bar{S}$ in a nondiseased segment shows instability.
- On the other hand, in practice the mean value of $\bar{S}$ over a stenotic part of a coronary segment must increase for a good reconstruction method, since the method is supposed to use the information from previous slices. In a stenotic segment the two neighboring slices of a particular slice are usually very dif-

Table VIII.2. Results from preliminary evaluation study on reconstructed coronary arterial segments.

	Slump	'noisy' Slump	Onnasch
Mean $\bar{S}$	13.1%	15.9%	9.9%
Standard deviation $\bar{S}$	11.9%	9.3%	10.2%
Processing time	54 min	122 min	34 min
Mean γ		0.684	
Standard deviation γ		0.325	

ferent. Reconstruction methods for which the $\bar{S}$-value does not increase over the stenotic segment as compared to the values over a nondiseased segment apparently use little information from the model and will not give reliable results. It will be clear that this increase in the model-dependency parameter will not occur if the stenotic segment is exactly symmetric in shape and size with respect to the site of maximal obstruction.

– The mean $\bar{S}$-value in Table VIII.2 concerns the entire coronary segment of Fig. VIII.6. Further investigations are necessary to determine the $\bar{S}$-values for the different reconstruction methods over diseased and nondiseased segments.

It is clear that this preliminary evaluation set is too small to draw conclusions about which reconstruction method is to be preferred. We anticipate performing more perspex model studies, including those with irregular cross sections, as well as studies from postmortem coronary casts.

In this chapter the 'noisy' Slump method has been described as an approach towards incorporating the stochastic nature of the imaging process. Naturally, other models may be feasible as well. Recently, Gerbrands and Slump have published another approach based on probability models for the photons emitted by the X-ray source and for the X-ray absorption mechanism [16]. Further developments and evaluation studies are necessary to determine which of these is most suitable for this particular three-dimensional reconstruction problem.

References

1. Bell PR, Dougherty JM: Nonlinear Image Processing Methods. IEEE Trans on Nucl Sci, NS-25: 928–938, 1978.
2. Chang SK, Chow CK: The reconstruction of three-dimensional objects from two orthogonal projections and its application to cardiac cineangiography. IEEE Trans Computers C-22: 18–28, 1973.
3. Chang SK, Wang YR: Three-dimensional object reconstruction from orthogonal projections. Pattern Recognition 7: 167–176, 1975.
4. Ford LR, Fulkerson DR: A simple algorithm for finding maximal network flows and an application to the Hitchcock problem. Canad J Math 9: 210–218, 1957.
5. Herman GT: Two direct methods for reconstructing pictures from their projections: a compara-

184

tive study. Comp Graphics and Image Processing 1: 123–144, 1972.

6. Johnson SA: Total body exposure, pixel size and signal to noise ratio considerations for three-dimensional X-ray attenuation reconstructions: A convolutional derivation of reconstruction photon statistics. In: Reconstruction Tomography in Diagnostic Radiology and Nuclear Medicine. MM Ter-Pogossian, ME Phelps, G Brownell, JR Cox, DO Davis, RG Evens (Eds.) University Park Press, Baltimore: 199–214, 1977.

7. Klein M: A primal method for minimal cost flows with applications to the assignment and transportation problems. Manag Sci 14: 205–220, 1967.

8. Onnasch, DGW: A concept for the approximative reconstruction of the form of the right or left ventricle from biplane angiograms. In: Roentgen-Video-Techniques for Dynamic Studies of Structure and Function of the Heart and Circulation. PH Heintzen, JH Bürsch (Eds.) Georg Thieme Verlag, Stuttgart: 235–242, 1978.

9. Onnasch, DGW, Heintzen PH: A new approach for the reconstruction of the left or right ventricular form from biplane angiocardiographic recordings. Comp Cardiol: 67–73, 1976.

10. Reiber JHC, Gerbrands JJ, Booman F, Troost GJ, Boer A den, Slager CJ, Schuurbiers JCH: Objective characterization of coronary obstructions from monoplane cineangiograms and three-dimensional reconstruction of an arterial segment from two orthogonal views. In: Applications of Computers in Medicine, MD Schwartz (Ed.). IEEE Cat No TH 0095–0: 93–100, 1982.

11. Reiber JHC, Slager CJ, Schuurbiers JCH, Boer A den, Gerbrands JJ, Troost GJ, Scholts B, Kooijman CJ, Serruys PW: Transfer functions of the X-ray-cine-video chain applied to digital processing of coronary cineangiograms. In: Digital Imaging in Cardiovascular Radiology, PH Heintzen, R Brennecke (Eds.). Georg Thieme Verlag, Stuttgart/New York: 89–104, 1983.

12. Slump CH, Gerbrands JJ: A netwerk flow approach to reconstruction of the left ventricle from two projections. Comp Graphics and Image Processing 18: 18–36, 1982.

13. Tanaka E, Iinuma TA: Correction functions and statistical noises in transverse section picture reconstruction. Comput Biol Med 6: 295–306, 1976.

14. Wagner WM: Principles of Operations Research. Prentice-Hall International London, 1975.

15. Zanden J van der: A set of subroutines for masked 3-dimensional plotting with rotations. International Report, Laboratory of Aero- and Hydro-dynamics, Delft University of Technology, 1975.

16. Gerbrands JJ, Slump CH: 3-D Reconstruction of homogeneous objects from two Poisson-distributed projections. Pattern Recognition Letters 3: 137–145, 1985.

IX. Structural analysis of the coronary and retinal arterial tree

Introduction

Main emphasis in earlier chapters has been on the accurate and reproducible assessment of the severity of coronary obstructions from magnified portions of 35 mm cineframes. No attention has been given to the possibilities of frame-to-frame analysis of the entire coronary tree from nonmagnified images for research or diagnostic purposes. If one would be able to determine in a semi- or fully-automated manner the centerlines and boundaries of all major-branches and side-branches of the coronary arterial system in each frame over a complete cardiac cycle, a number of clinically relevant questions could possibly be answered. Among these are:

(1) Automated search for locations of coronary lesions exceeding a certain percentage diameter or area narrowing.
(2) Computer-identification of the anatomy of the coronary tree and automated classification of the tree in one of a number of structure classes.
(3) Research towards the possibly existing relation between the physical configuration of the coronary tree and the presence or development of coronary artery disease.
(4) Assessment of epicardial contraction patterns by using the arterial bifurcations as landmarks.

In this chapter our approaches towards the computer processing of the entire coronary tree implemented on the CAAS will be described. Our software developments have been applied to nonmagnified cineframes digitized with a spatial resolution of 512×512 pixels and 256 grey levels. However, since the pictorial information at the output screen of the image intensifier can also be digitized on-line with progressive or interlaced scan video camera's with the same spatial and temporal resolution, the algorithms will in principle be applicable to such on-line acquisition procedures as well.

The first goal, the automated detection and analysis of coronary obstructions from nonmagnified images requires the processing of only one single image, e.g. the end-diastolic image. Therefore, if one would be able to process selected arterial segments from on-line digitally acquired images with a clinically acceptable speed, then the arteriographist would be provided with immediate diagnostic information during the cardiac catheterization. This means that the procedure must be imbedded in a digital vascular imaging system (on-line CAAS) with the digitized video images obtained directly from the image intensifier (Fig. IX.1). It will be clear that the accuracy of the on-line results will be lower than those from cinefilms, but most probably sufficient for diagnostic decision making. For research purposes requiring maximal accuracy, arterial dimensions must be assessed off-line from cinefilm, thereby allowing for optical magnification of the selected arterial segments.

The three other applications require analysis of all the images over one or more cardiac cycles. Because of the large amounts of data that need to be processed for these applications, only off-line analysis either from cineframes or from digitized video images acquired directly from the image intensifier seems feasible for the time being. Each of the four applications requires the accurate delineation of the

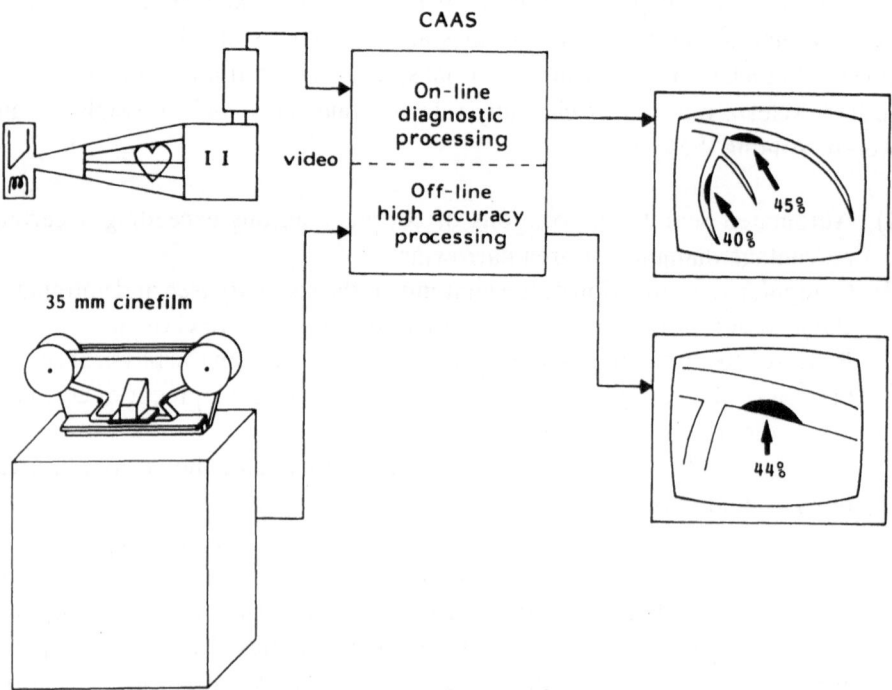

Fig. IX.1. Future developments towards on-line analysis of coronary angiograms with the CAAS will provide diagnostic information about the location and severity of coronary obstructions during cardiac catheterization. For research studies requiring maximal accuracy, off-line processing from cinefilm is required.

projected arterial system in one or more frames. With the permissible exception of the very first frame, we want to apply a relatively simple and, if possible, fully automated segmentation procedure for the subsequent frames of a coronary angiogram.

Following a brief overview of other published approaches towards the delineation of the entire coronary tree, the techniques implemented on the CAAS will be described in this chapter. At first, the segmentation of the coronary tree in the first of a series of frames will be discussed, followed by a description of the approaches towards the frame-to-frame segmentation. On the basis of the detected arterial branches and the derived bifurcation positions, the three-dimensional epicardial motion can be assessed from two orthogonal views, as will be explained thereafter. As a next step, a number of clinical examples will be given. At the end of this chapter it will be demonstrated that the techniques developed for the automated tracing of the centerlines of the coronary arteries, can also be applied successfully to retinal angiograms, providing information about arrival times of fluorescein in the arterial branches and about arterial blood flow velocities.

Overview of other approaches

The first publications on extensive computer processing of nonmagnified coronary angiograms appeared in 1974 from Starmer and Smith [1–3]. Goal of their project was to study the relation between the physical configuration of the coronary tree and the development or presence of coronary artery disease. Studies of the coronary arterial tree and of the changes in length of the arterial segments during a cardiac cycle had been shown to have diagnostic value for coronary artery disease [4, 5]. As a first step, they developed an algorithm for the three-dimensional geometric representation of coronary arterial trees from biplane cineangiograms [1, 3]. Assuming the coronary arteries to be line segments, the algorithm combined two orthogonal representations of the tree into a single unambiguous three-dimensional representation. This procedure was interactive and required the operator to indicate manually the positions of the nodes, i.e. of the bifurcations and of arterial end points in each of the two orthogonal film planes.

As a next step, Starmer and Smith described a method for automating the collection of trees from a biplane projection for a single cardiac cycle [2]. In the first cineframe of a sequence of cineangiograms, a representation of the tree was stored on disk using the manual technique described above. Processing a subsequent frame started by locating the root of the tree on the new frame by means of a bifurcation finder. From the root each path was followed using a primitive ridge-following technique, which was closely guided by the corresponding path from the previous frame (constrained path follower). This ridge-following technique was based on a crude detection of the edges of the artery by finding the maximum and minimum derivatives of smoothed density profiles, defined perpendicular to the local centerline directions; the center of mass between the edge points along a density profile was then recorded as a path point, and used to center the cross-sectional line at the next step. If a path terminated in a bifurcation, the location of this bifurcation on the previous frame was updated, using both information from the current path and an extrapolation of the bifurcation's motion over several preceding frames, and the bifurcation finder was applied to the new prediction. Any paths which originated in the bifurcation were then followed as before. This project was stopped before clinical results could be demonstrated.

Fukui et al. have also described a method for the automated detection of the coronary tree in a coronary cineangiogram with the ultimate goal to derive a three-dimensional representation of the tree [6]. Selected 35 mm cineframes were converted into 256×256 matrices with 256 grey levels by means of an image dissector camera. Their approach is based on two properties of the arteries: (1) arteries are cord-like structures; and (2) the brightness distribution perpendicular to its centerline is unimodal. The procedure starts with the search for parallel segments in a gradient image. After two such segments have been located, the average brightness function measured perpendicular to these segments is tested for unimodality. If the segments satisfy the criteria, the positions with maximal gradient at both sides are defined as arterial positions. Subsequently, the complete arteries are detected by means of a tracking procedure. No data on success scores or validation studies were presented.

Finally, Kindelan and Suarez de Lezo have developed an interactive image processing procedure for the analysis and quantification of coronary obstructions from a computer processed coronary tree [7]. Cineframes were digitized in matrix size of 270×360 pixels with 256 grey levels. The user selects with a cursor on an image display terminal, the origin and end points of an artery. Typically, the contour detection is performed in two steps: (1) local operators are applied in order to locate edge points; and (2) edge-following algorithms are used to connect these edge elements and to build continuous contours. The user can accept the traced contour or reject it, in which case he may change some of the parameters of the algorithm and repeat the procedure until the artery is correctly tracked. Once accepted, the coordinates of the middle line, the width of the artery, and the average grey level at each point, are stored in a file for later processing with a graphic editor. This editor may be used to display the coronary tree, magnify it, link arteries, eliminate portions of arteries, plot the width or grey-level distribution, perform average filtering of those distributions, locate candidate points for coronary obstructions, or compute the percentage diameter or grey level narrowing on those candidate points. It was concluded at the time of publication that the line-detection algorithm still produces too many errors, requiring extensive editing. Also, it seems that the images are digitized too coarsely to provide reliable and clinically relevant results.

For many years Potel et al. have been working on the assessment of three-dimensional left ventricular epicardial wall motion derived from the displacement of coronary bifurcations [8]. Their procedure requires the manual definition of the bifurcation positions from biplane cineframes over two to four cardiac cycles. Several different coordinate systems have been studied for the assessment of epicardial wall motion. They conclude that on an instantaneous basis, almost all (91%) of the true tree-dimensional motion over the entire heart is directed towards (or away from) a single three-dimensional point, the left ventricular center of contraction. Also, viewed in fixed (external coordinates), basal regions appeared to move like a contracting sphere and apical regions moved both towards and around the left ventricular long axis ('wringing').

From the above it is clear that until to date only a few groups have attempted to develop methods towards the automated delineation of the entire coronary tree. Only very preliminary results of the different techniques have been published. Our approaches towards this difficult segmentation problem will be presented below.

Methodology

Preprocessing

In each frame, the arterial system is represented by one connected component, which consists of a number of major-branches and side-branches. The actual brightness levels within the projected arteries depend a.o. on the absorption by the contrast agent and thus on artery size. Arterial segments which are separated in 3-D space may very well show partial overlap in the 2-D projection images. The background is rather nonuniform and may show a number of disturbing structures like the vertebral column, the diafragm, catheters and possibly even metal structures. Segmentation of a frame into arterial structures and background cannot be accomplished by global thresholding techniques or straightforward edge detection. The connectivity of the object justifies the use of sequential tracing procedures, which can easily be made locally-adaptive. In our approach, the disturbing background structures are removed to a large extent by applying a gated background subtraction method. Each frame is corrected by logarithmically subtracting a corresponding background image, which is recorded in the same phase of the cardiac cycle prior to the contrast injection [9, 10, Ch. VII]. If necessary, spatial fluctuations due to quantum noise are decreased by smoothing the subtraction image with an unweighted 3×3 operator.

Segmentation in first frame

Under the assumption of complete and homogeneous filling with the contrast agent, the brightness values within a projected artery in the subtraction images are approximately proportional to irradiated object thicknesses (Chapter VII). For a circle-cylindrical artery with main axis orthogonal to the X-ray beam, this means that the brightness values show maxima in the center of the projected artery. This approximation seems to be applicable in most practical cases, which leads to a segmentation procedure basically consisting of the following steps:

(I)   detection of the tentative centerline of an arterial branch by tracing local brightness maxima;
(II) detection of the contours of the arterial branch using a minimum cost path search algorithm.
(III) detection of possible side-branches, and
(IV) repetition of steps I to III.

These various steps will be described in this section. More detailed descriptions of these procedures can be found in earlier publications [10–14].

For the detection of the tentative centerline of the first major artery, the user defines a starting point in the root of this artery as well as a global starting direction. The tracing procedure is applied to a low-resolution version of the subtracted image, which is obtained by first applying a 5×5 spatial low-pass filter to the image. As a result of this filter operation the spatial frequency band of the image is reduced by a factor of 3. Next, the filtered image is resampled with a sampling distance of three pixel positions in the original image.

For the tracing procedure 8 main search directions are defined (Fig. IX.2a). The direction of the last detected point L with respect to its predecessor defines the current search direction. Three points C1, C2 and C3 are candidate for the next point of the tentative centerline (Fig. IX.2b). These candidate points are the point C2 lying in the current search direction and the points C1 and C3 lying in the two neighboring main directions which have angles of 45° with respect to the

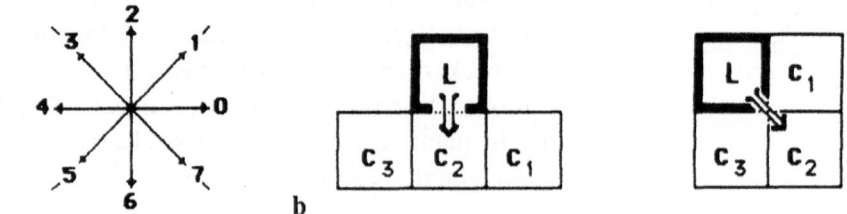

Fig. IX.2. Eight search directions are defined for the tracing procedure (Fig. IX.2a) If L is the last detected tracer position, then three candidate points C1, C2 and C3 are defined. Figure IV.2b shows the positions of the candidate points for two of the eight possible search directions.

current search direction. The forthcoming point of the centerline is selected from among the three candidate points by searching for the maximum average brightness level over a number of pixels in the current search direction and in two other directions which differ by 22.5° from the current direction ('Beam-like forward looking') (Fig. IX.3). The candidate point with the highest average brightness level computed in the corresponding search direction is defined as the next path position. The number of pixels used in the calculation of the average brightness value in a particular direction is dependent on the local diameter of the artery. The length of these search windows must be of the same order as the local arterial diameter. In Fig. IX.3 the search windows are shown for a look-ahead distance of 5 pixels.

The detection of the tentative centerline is achieved piecewise, in subsegments. In each detected subsegment a number of parameters are calculated, such as the local arterial diameter, the mean brightness value within that subsegment and the background brightness value. These parameters are used as a priori information in the detection of the next subsegment. For example, the length of the next subsegment to be traced is set equal to the measured local diameter of the artery. Restrictions set on the change of mean brightness values in subsequent subsegments, on the contrast between object and background and on the minimum local arterial diameter yield criteria that make it possible to check whether the last detected subsegment of the centerline still lies within the artery.

If the centerline has left the artery and entered the background area, or if it has entered a severely obstructed region, the max-tracing procedure stops. A trace-back procedure is then initiated towards the last point of the centerline that still belonged to the normal sized arterial segment. At this point, the user must decide whether the end of the artery has been reached. If this is not the case, a continuation point is searched for at a distance of two times the local diameter of the artery from the last defined point. This search procedure is illustrated in figure IX.4. Along the circumference of a circle with radius equal to two times the local diameter of the artery, the brightness profile in the image is determined. Each local maximum in this brightness profile is a potential position of an artery in the image. The position along the circular path for which the height and width of the brightness peak correspond best with these parameters from the reference posi-

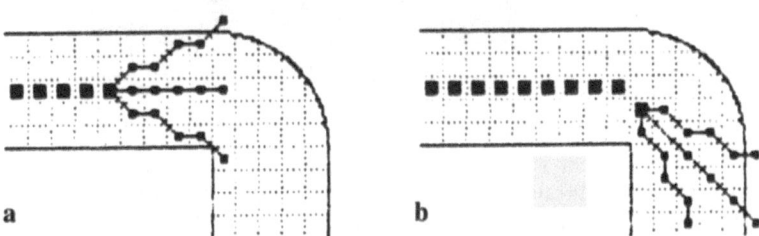

Fig. IX.3. Search windows for a look-ahead distance of 5 pixels.

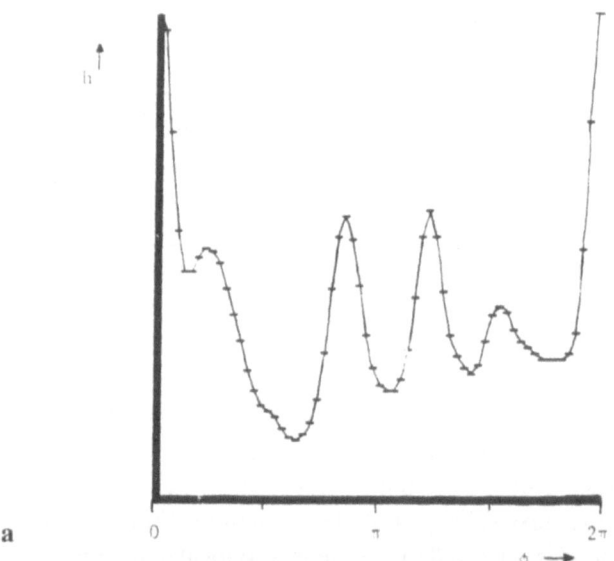

a

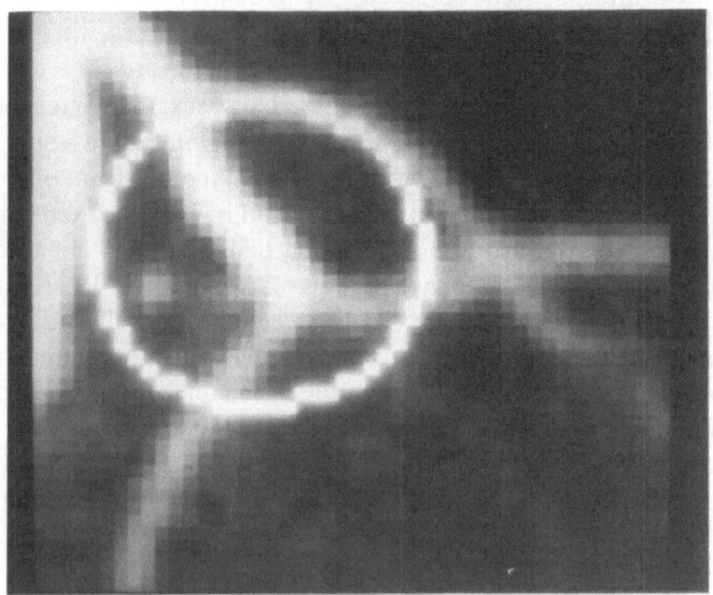

b

Fig. IX.4. To cross the bifurcation, the brightness profile along the circumference of a circle is computed (Fig. IX.4b). The image is scanned at a distance of two times the local diameter of the artery from the last defined point (Fig. IX.4a). The first point of the brightness profile ($\varnothing = 0°$) corresponds with the intersection of the circle with the known centerline.

tion, being the intersection of the circle with the known centerline ($\emptyset = 0°$), is defined as the continuation point for the tracing procedure.

Between the last accepted centerline point and the continuation point a centerline path is defined on the basis of maximal cumulative grey values. Subsequently, the normal max-tracing procedure continues from the continuation point until another error occurs or the end of the artery is reached. The final result of the arterial centerline detection for a relatively complex coronary structure is shown in Fig. IX.5.

Following the max-tracing procedure the contours of the arterial branch are detected in the following way. First, the low-resolution max-tracer path is expanded to a high-resolution path and subsequently filtered to obtain a smooth, continuous curve. Next, the low-pass filtered full resolution image is locally resampled along straight lines perpendicular to the local centerline directions; these lines are denoted scanlines. To each point a cost coefficient is assigned, defined by the inverse of the weighted sum of first- and second- order derivatives. These derivatives are obtained by convolving each scanline with one-dimensional difference operators. The two contours of the arterial segment are obtained by searching in the resulting cost matrix for minimal cost paths, using dynamic programming methods [11, Ch. III].

Side-branches are identified by searching for local maxima in background brightness profiles defined along the boundaries of the detected arterial segment. The complete procedure of max-tracing, edge detection and side-branch detection is then subsequently applied to each of the identified starting points of the side-branches. Results of the entire procedure will be presented in this chapter in the section Applications.

Frame-to-frame segmentation

Following the segmentation of the first frame in which some user-interaction may be required, the subsequent frames should preferably be segmented without any user-interaction. The question arises to what extent information gathered from a given frame can be utilized to guide the segmentation of the next frame. Due to contraction, rotation, etc. of the coronary tree in 3-D space, substantial changes in the projection of the tree may occur in subsequent frames. However, in most practical cases the shape of the object is rather similar in two adjacent frames. This leads to the assumption that an object detected in a given frame may be used to construct a structural model which then guides the segmentation process for the next frame and so on.

Since the actual contour detection process has been shown to be sufficiently reliable, the model is only needed to guide the max-tracer. Furthermore, the model needs to contain just enough information to guide the max-tracer at those locations, where it tends to wander off the right track e.g. at high curvature

194

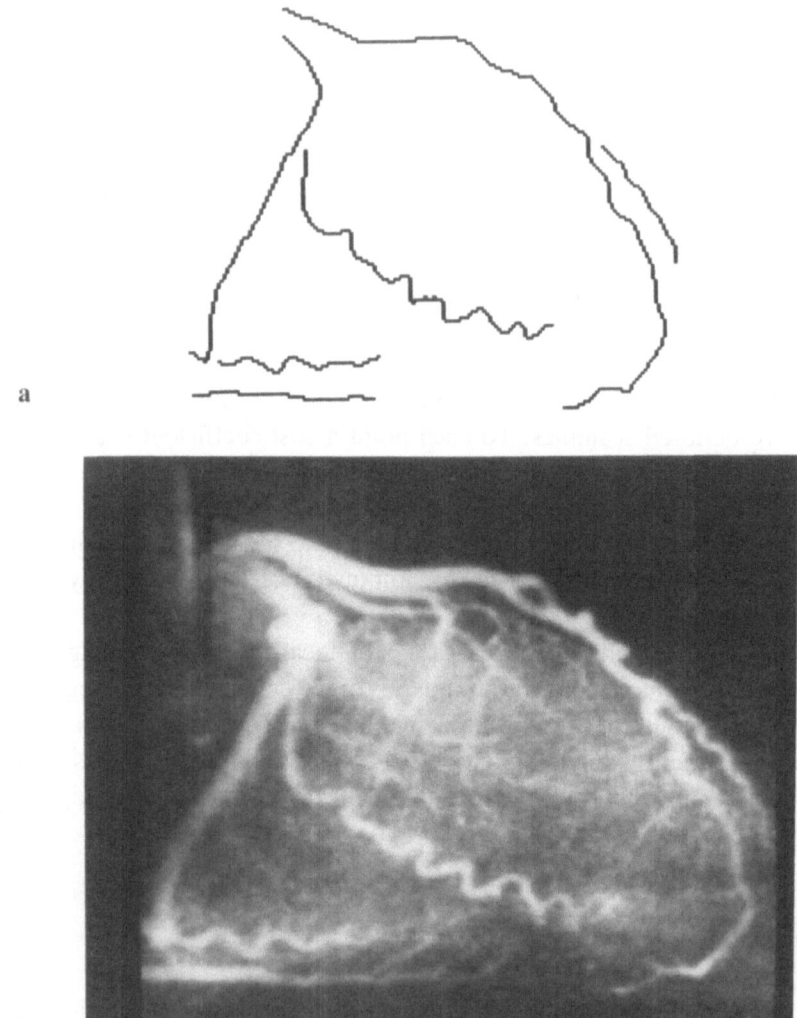

a

b

Fig. IX.5. Result of the centerline detection procedure (Fig. IX.5a) applied to the image shown in Fig. IX.5b.

sections where the max-tracer might proceed into the background and near bifurcations where the max-tracer may choose another branch than the one selected in the previous frame.

The model is constructed in the following way. The coronary tree is represented by a polygonal approximation of the various centerlines representing the coronary branches in the previous frame. In this way the centerline is decomposed into sections (straight line segments). Bifurcations are always identified as breakpoints between sections.

Each time the max-tracer has proceeded a little further in the new frame, the model and the actual path must be matched to detect local scale variations, thus synchronizing model and actual data. Matching of model and data is performed by employing a distance measure for polygonal curves to describe the differences between the model and a newly detected centerline section. The result of the matching is used to specify the expected direction and length of subsequent new centerline sections. Further details will be described in the following section [15].

Guided centerline detection in the frame under consideration is performed by two kinds of guided sequential tracing procedures. The first procedure is a modification of the earlier described tracing routine which follows local image brightness maxima. The other procedure is based on the construction of a maximum cumulative brightness path in locally resampled parts of the image data, in order to detect a centerline more reliably in complex situations.

The guidance procedure is based on the specification of the general search direction for the next section to be detected and the maximum allowable length of this new section. The guiding and tracing procedures are kept in rein by checking whether the newly detected centerline points can be approximated by a single straight line section. The detection process is temporarily halted and matching of centerline and model is re-executed as soon as the approximation fails, so that the current general search direction and the maximum allowable trace length can be updated. In the way described above both narrow and wide, smooth and curved centerlines can be detected reliably. The basic principles of the model and data synchronization will be described in the following section of this chapter.

Figure IX.6 gives an example of the results of the procedure described above. Figure IX.6a shows a digital subtraction image of a right coronary arterial tree with the detected centerline and the centerline from the preceding frame superimposed. For purposes of clarity, these centerlines have been plotted separately in Fig. IX.6b. In the centerline from the preceding frame markers have been defined, representing the end points of centerline sections used in the model synchronization process.

Model/data synchronization

Contraction and relaxation, rotation and translation of the cardiac structures in 3-D space result in local shortening, lengthening, rotation and translation of arterial segments as observed in consecutive projection frames. The model-guided tracing procedure requires that we know at all times which part of the model is applicable. In other words, one must keep track of the position of the max-tracer with respect to the structural model. The simple approach of overlaying the model on the data and applying a minimum euclidean distance criterion between points of the model centerline and the max-tracer path cannot be used here. Even a slight shift results in serious misinterpretations, especially near high curvature sections.

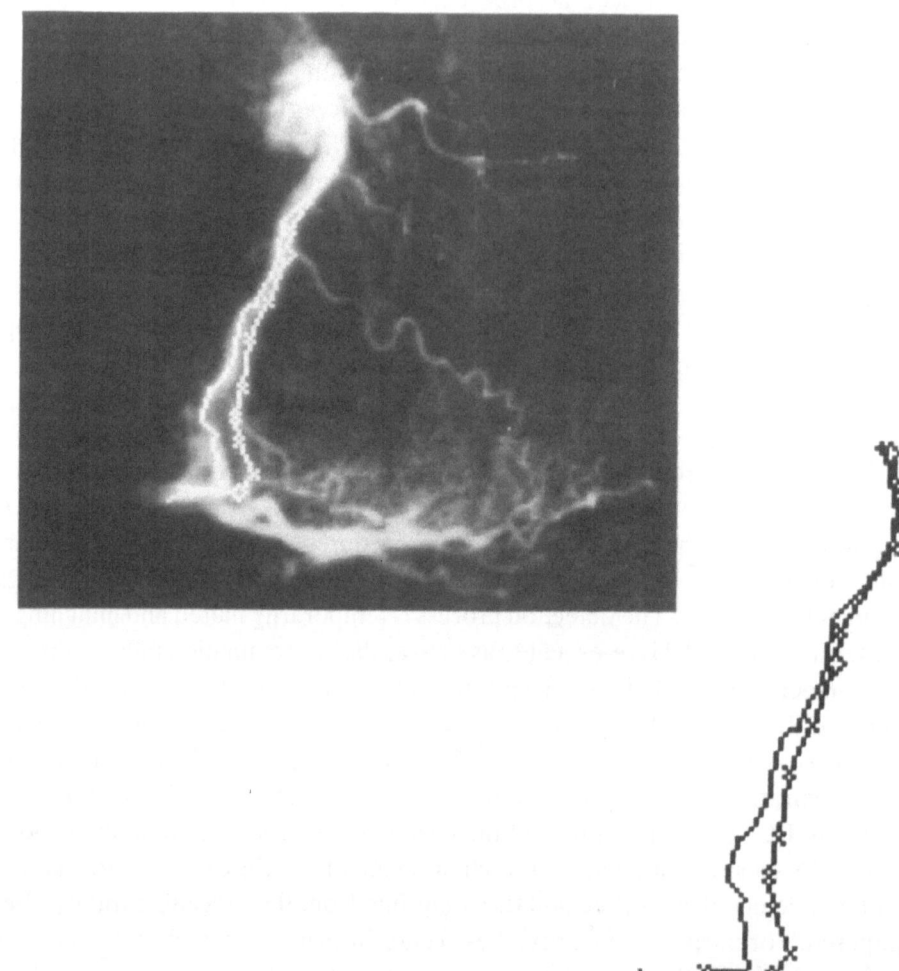

Fig. IX.6. Example of digital subtraction image of right coronary arterial system with centerline detected with the aid of the centerline from the preceding frame (Fig. IX.6a). These centerlines have been displayed separately in Fig. IX.6b.

The method that has been implemented is based on a measure for comparing linearly segmented curves that are geometrically distorted relative to one another. This method was introduced by Burr, who applied the technique to the problem of on-line recognition of handprinted characters [16]. This comparitive procedure makes use of dynamic programming, a technique for finding minimal cost paths in certain weighted networks. When used to match linearly segmented curves, dynamic programming produces section pairs, which have been optimized in the sense that the sum of pairwise differences between curve-sections is minimal under the constraint of connectivity of subsequent sections of model and traced data.

In order to compute the costs for both model and data sections, a geometric distortion measure is introduced, that relies on positional and angular differences between sections of model and data. The angular distance measure D_{ang} is defined by the cross product of two vectors $\vec{A}$ and $\vec{B}$, normalized by the magnitude of vector $\vec{A}$; $\vec{A}$ is always the vector with the greatest magnitude (Fig. IX.7). In formula [16]:

$$D_{ang} = \frac{|\vec{B} \times \vec{A}|}{|\vec{A}|} + 3U(-\vec{B} \cdot \vec{A}) \cdot \frac{|\vec{B} \cdot \vec{A}|}{|\vec{A}|} \qquad (IX.1)$$

This angular distance measure is a good estimate of gross directional error.

The second term in formula (IX.1) is necessary to impose a greater distance measure for opposing vectors. When the projection of $\vec{B}$ onto $\vec{A}$ is negative, a value proportional to $|\vec{B} \cdot \vec{A}|/|\vec{A}|$ is added by means of the unit step function U, defined by:

$$U(t) = 0 \quad (t < 0)$$
$$U(t) = 1 \quad (t \geqslant 0) \qquad (IX.2)$$

The positional distance measure is also based on a cross product; however, for this purpose a third vector $\vec{C}$ is introduced (Fig. IX.8). Vector $\vec{C}$ connects the beginning point of vector $\vec{A}$ with the midpoint of vector $\vec{B}$. The cross term $\dfrac{|\vec{C} \times \vec{A}|}{|\vec{A}|}$ is a measure for the perpendicular distance between the vectors $\vec{A}$ and $\vec{B}$. The positional distance measure D_{pos} is defined by [16]:

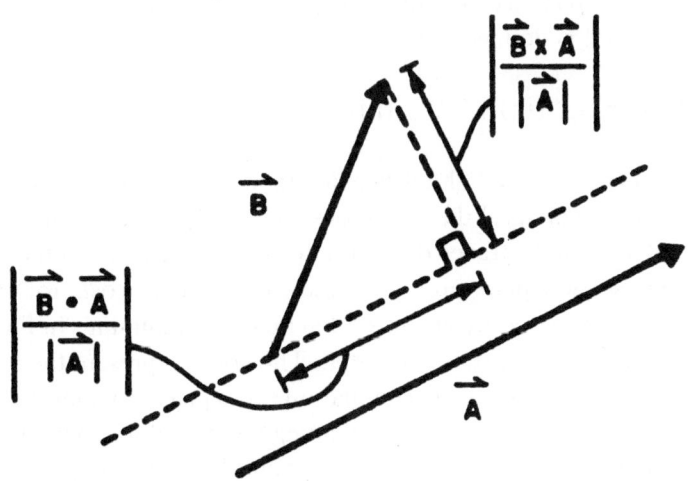

Fig. IX.7. Quantities relating to the angular distance measure D_{ang} between the vectors $\vec{A}$ and $\vec{B}$ ($|\vec{A}| \geqslant |\vec{B}|$).

198

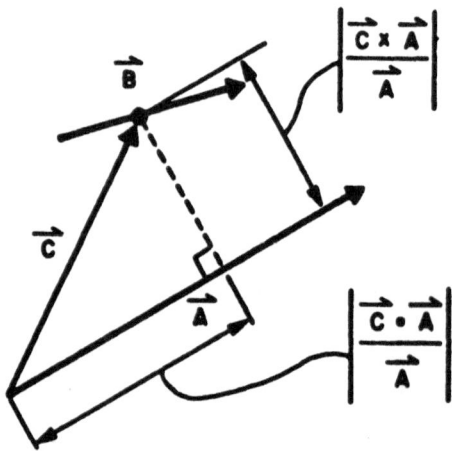

Fig. IX.8. Quantities relating to the positional distance measure D_{pos} between the vectors $\vec{A}$ and $\vec{B}$ ($|\vec{A}| \geqslant |\vec{B}|$).

$$D_{pos} = \frac{|\vec{C} \times \vec{A}|}{|\vec{A}|} + U\left\{ \frac{\vec{C} \cdot \vec{A}}{|\vec{A}|} - |\vec{A}| \cdot \left| \frac{\vec{C} \cdot \vec{A}}{|\vec{A}|} - |\vec{A}| \right| \right\} +$$

$$+ U\left\{ -\frac{\vec{C} \cdot \vec{A}}{|\vec{A}|} \cdot \frac{|\vec{C} \cdot \vec{A}|}{|\vec{A}|} \right\} \tag{IX.3}$$

The two additional terms are added to increase the positional distance measure for two specific cases: (1) the projection of $\vec{C}$ onto $\vec{A}$ is greater than $|\vec{A}|$; and (2) the projection of $\vec{C}$ onto $\vec{A}$ is less than zero.

Finally, the total distance measure D(i,j) between a traced data section s(i) and model section m(j) is defined by:

$$D(i,j) = D_{pos}(i,j) + 2 D_{ang}(i,j). \tag{IX.4}$$

The angular measure is weighted heavier than the positional measure, since angles are more meaningful than positions when distortions occur.

For the matching of the traced data with the model, the costs for the differences of the various section pairs are computed. The sum of costs for subsequent sections is then minimized by means of dynamic programming. In Fig. IX.9 the dynamic programming lattice is illustrated. The nodes represent the costs for the corresponding section pairs. Cost cumulation takes place from left to right along the traced data, and from bottom to top along the model sections. In practice, a number of section pairs (i,j) are exempted from the matching procedure; these pairs have been shaded in Fig. IX.9. It is not useful to try to match section pairs for which the difference in section numbers exceeds a certain value (a difference

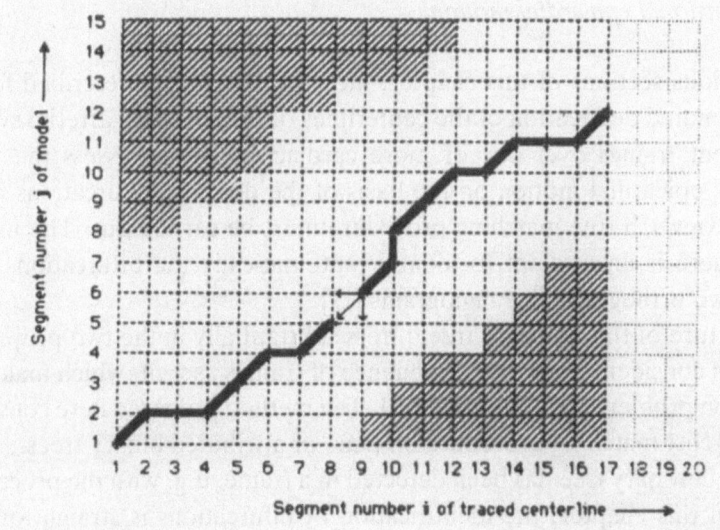

Fig. IX.9. Illustration of the dynamic programming lattice for data sections ($1 \leqslant i \leqslant 17$) and model sections ($1 \leqslant j \leqslant 15$). When the tracing proceeds, new columns with cumulative costs are added, until the end of the model has been reached. The shaded areas represent combinations that are exempted from the matching procedure.

of 8 in Fig. IX.9). The arrows tn the figure denote the section pairs, that may preceed the section pair (i,j) in order to satisfy the constraint for connectivity.

The cumulated cost for section pair (i,j) is defined by:

$$S(i,j) = D(i,j) + \min \{S(i-1,j), S(i-1,j-1), S(i,j-1)\} \qquad (IX.5)$$

under the following constraints:

$$
\begin{aligned}
S(1,1) &= D(1,1) \\
S(i,1) &= D(i,1) + S(i-1,1) \quad i \geqslant 2 \\
S(1,j) &= D(1,j) + S(1,j-1) \quad j \geqslant 2
\end{aligned}
\qquad (IX.6)
$$

When the tracing proceeds into a new section, a new column is added to the dynamic programming lattice and filled with cumulative costs, as shown in Fig. IX.9 with the dotted part of the lattice (last three columns).

To find an optimal match between model and current tracer-data, the minimum cumulative costs are searched for in the last column. A backtrace through the dynamic programming lattice then yields the best match. In this way the best point on the model centerline, corresponding with the current tracer position can be determined.

Three-dimensional epicardial motion

In the previous sections of this chapter, methods have been described for the (semi)-automated delineation of the centerlines of the coronary arterial systems in subsequent frames over one or more cardiac cycles. To assess the three-dimensional epicardial motion on the basis of the detected bifurcations in two orthogonal views, a tree matching procedure must be carried out. The method presented here is an attempt to identify automatically the bifurcations in all frames of two orthogonal cineangiograms [17].

The structure of the coronary tree differs substantially in the two projections and changes considerably over the sequence of frames as well, which makes the identification problem certainly not trival. The method proposed here consists of a minimum-cost matching procedure on pairs of attributed binary trees.

Once the coronary tree has been detected in a frame, e.g. with the procedures described in this chapter, the identification of bifurcations is straightforward. There may, however, also be crossings as arteries of the 3-D coronary tree may very well intersect in the 2-D projections, a problem which will be delt with later. In the absence of intersections of arteries, the construction of a binary tree (in a graph-theoretic sense) is simple, where the nodes correspond with the bifurcations and the arcs with connectivity between bifurcations, i.e., the presence of an arterial segment. The coordinates of a bifurcation are assigned to the corresponding node as attributes or labels.

Given two attributed trees F and G, we can derive G from F by applying specific transformations. There is a penalty assigned to each transformation. The total penalty of the series of transformations which transforms F into G with minimum costs is called the distance between F and G [18]. The following transformations may be distinguished:

(1) Deletion of a node with penalty p
(2) Insertion of an extra node with penalty q
(3) Substitution, where the label of node k of F is changed into the label of node m of G with penalty r.

The use of the transformations is restricted in the sense that if node α is a descendant of node β in the original tree, the image $T(\alpha)$ of α in the transformed tree is a descendant of the image $T(\beta)$ of node β, i.e., the ordering of the nodes is to be preserved.

We have implemented an efficient algorithm to determine the distance between two attributed binary trees. It is, however, not possible to describe this algorithm in detail in the context of this chapter. The algorithm also produces the set of transformations corresponding with the minimum cost solution. Every substitution transformation in this set points to a pair of nodes, one in F and one in G, that correspond. The set of all substitution transformations defines the optimal mapping between F and G, thus solving the bifurcation identification problem.

The tree-matching procedure can be used to identify corresponding bifurcations in two orthogonal projections, as well as in consecutive frames of a single projection. The two orthogonal projections are calibrated to absolute mm by means of the known size of the contrast catheter and corrected for pincushion distortion and for the diverging nature of the X-rays. After this calibration, the vertical coordinates of a bifurcation are essentially identical in both projections. This coordinate is assigned as label to each node, and the penalty of the substitution transformation is set equal to the absolute difference between the labels. For the case of consecutive frames of a single projection, the penalty of the substitution transformation is set equal to the euclidean distance between the positions of the two bifurcations.

When the skeleton does not only contain bifurcations, but intersections as well, there is confusion about how these intersections should be cut to obtain a tree-structure. This is illustrated in Fig.IX.10. For each intersection there are two interpretations.

The trees for both possibilities are examined by means of the minimum cost matching procedure with the orthogonal projection and the optimal solution is selected. If there are more intersections present, all combinations are examined.

The results of the procedure discussed here are illustrated in Figs. IX.11, IX.12 and IX.13. Figure IX.11 shows the locations of a number of bifurcations followed over one cardiac cycle in the RAO- and LAO-projections, Figs. IX.11a and IX.11b, respectively. Figure IX.12 gives the trajectories of a single bifurcation in the two projections. In Fig. IX.13 the distance between a pair of bifurcations is plotted as a function of time (frame number). Notice that these distances are in 3-D and calibrated in mm. From these curves the local epicardial contraction pattern can be assessed.

Applications

Some of the earlier mentioned applications, like the automated classification of the coronary tree and the automated labeling of arterial segments are still only at a very early stage of development. Others, like the computation of epicardial wall motion have been implemented in our laboratory [10], but clinical evaluation studies still need to be performed. The application first mentioned in the introduction, the automated selection of coronary obstructions in nonmagnified im-

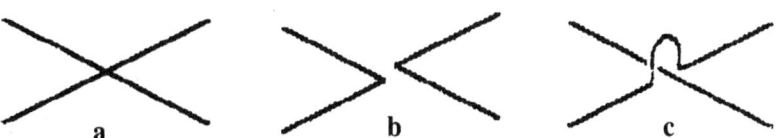

Fig. IX.10. Intersections in the skeleton (a) may be interpreted as (b) or (c).

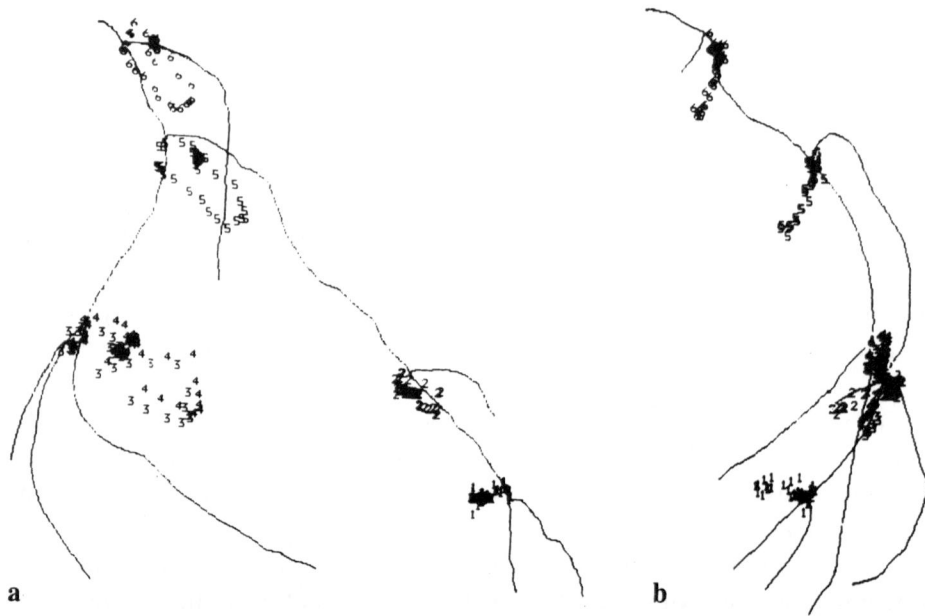

Fig. IX.11. Locations of bifurcations in the RAO- (Fig. IX.11a) and the LAO-projections (Fig. IX.11b) followed over a cardiac cycle.

ages and the determination of the severity in terms of percentage diameter- and densitometric area-stenosis, will be implemented in our catheterization laboratory as soon as an on-line digital vascular imaging system has been installed. An extensive performance evaluation will then be carried out, but preliminary results from routinely obtained cineangiograms are certainly promising. An example of

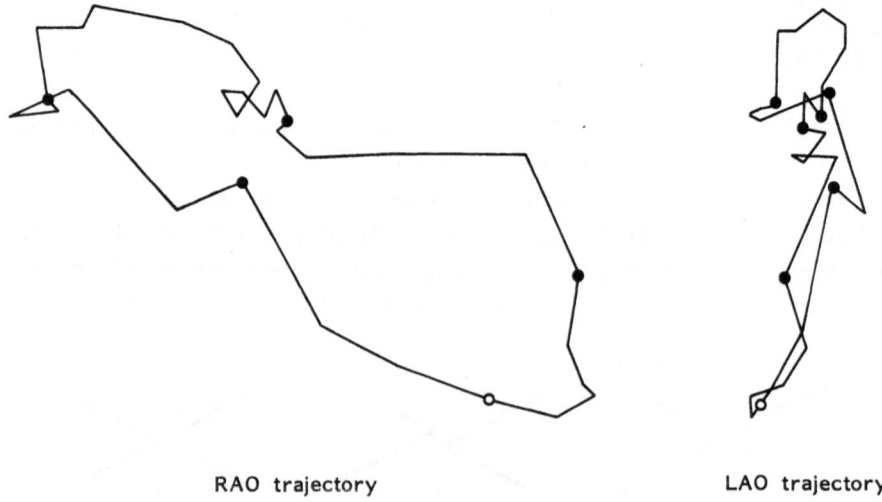

RAO trajectory   LAO trajectory

Fig. IX.12. Trajectories of a single bifurcation in the RAO (left)- and LAO (right)-projections.

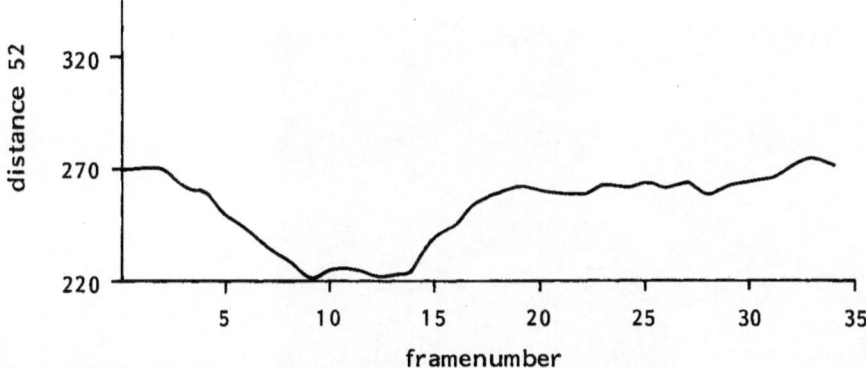

Fig. IX.13. Three-dimensional distance between a pair of bifurcations plotted as a function of time (frame number).

the proposed analysis procedure is presented in the following paragraphs.

Figure IX.14 shows a subtraction image of a right coronary arterial system taken in the RAO-view. The tentative centerline of the right coronary artery as found by the max-tracing routine is displayed in Fig. IX.15, both superimposed in the subtraction image as separately. In the centerline the breakpoints between different sections which are used to guide the max-tracer in the next frame are indicated by the square markers. This centerline is input for the contour detection algorithm, which locates the contours of the artery by searching for minimal cost paths.

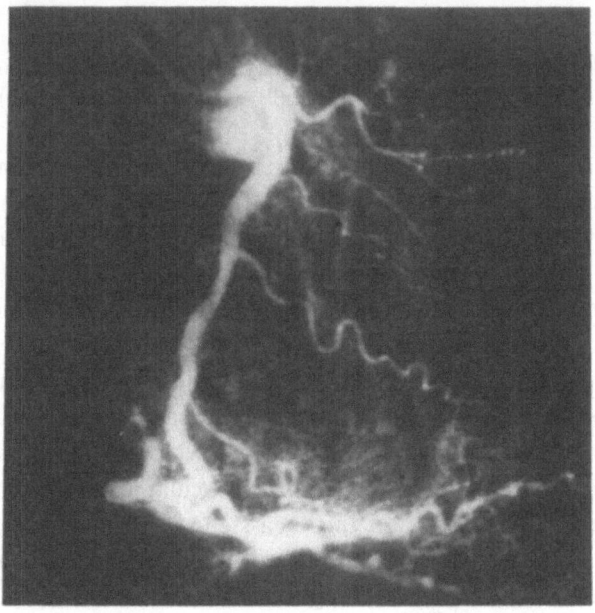

Fig. IX.14. Gated background subtracted image of right coronary arterial system in RAO-view.

204

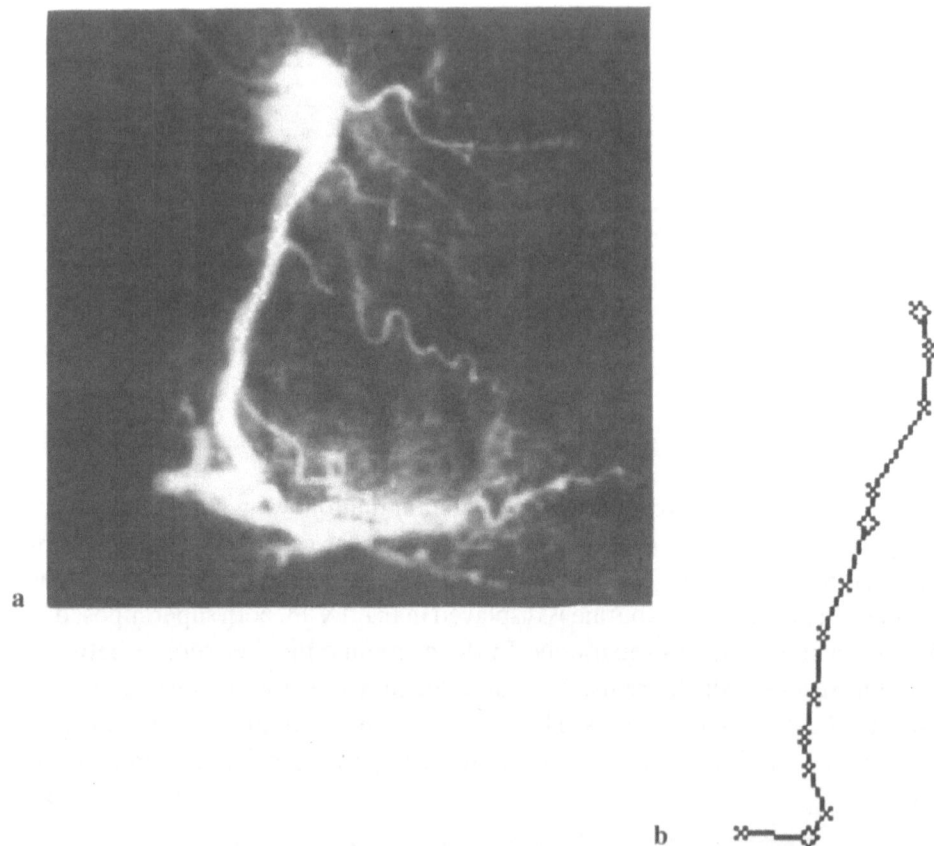

a

b

Fig. IX.15. Detected tentative centerline in right coronary artery together with section breakpoints, both superimposed in the image (Fig. IX.15a) and displayed separately (Fig. IX.15b).

The detected contours of the right coronary artery and of a number of side-branches are shown in Fig. IX.16. In addition, Fig. IX.17 shows the computed diameter and densitometric area functions for the mid-portion of this artery and the patient-data block; the densitometric area function was computed from the brightness information in the arterial segment according to the principles of the gated subtraction technique described in Chapter VII. Two positions for the obstruction were found, one defined by a significant local minimum in the diameter function, the other by a minimum in the area function. The percentages diameter and area stenoses were determined following the interpolated stenosis measurement technique (Ch. III); for this particular example the diameter-stenosis was found to be 37% and the area-stenosis 40%, indicating that the obstruction is eccentric in shape, since the percentage densitometric area-stenosis is significantly smaller than the percentage circular area stenosis (60%). It will be clear that such data will be extremely useful for the cardiologist if it can be provided during the cardiac catheterization procedure.

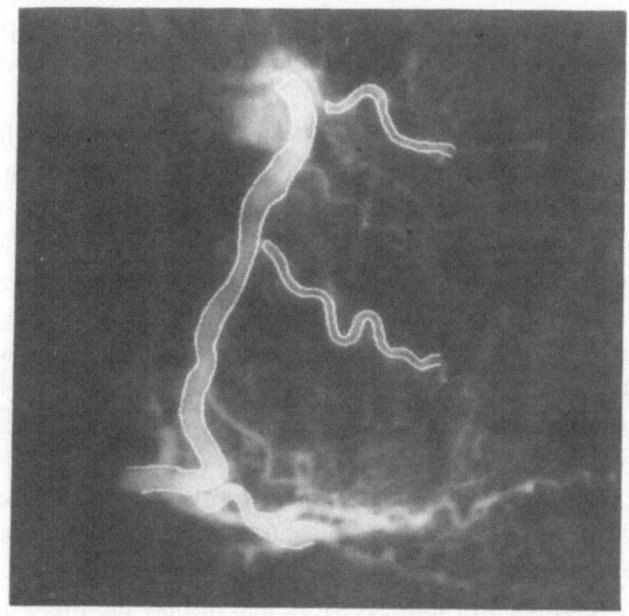

Fig. IX.16. Detected contours of right coronary artery and of a number of side-branches.

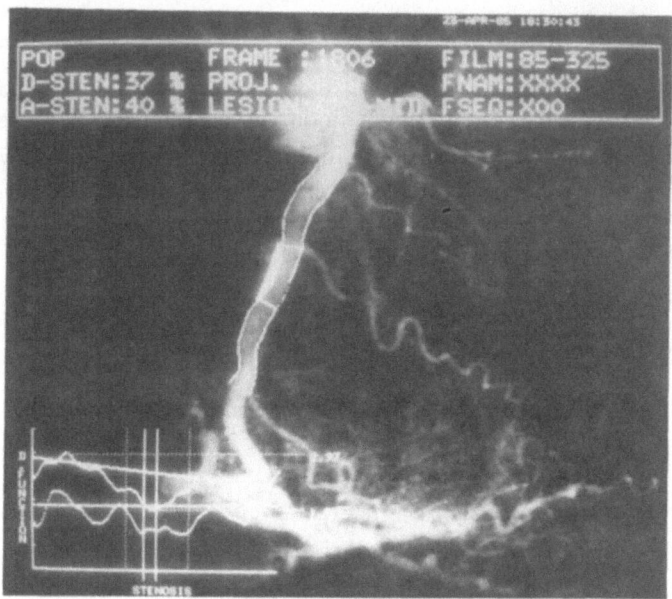

Fig. IX.17. Automated selection of coronary obstruction with computation of percentages diameter- and densitometric area-stenoses by the interpolated technique. The obstruction is eccentric, since the percentage densitometric area stenosis (40%) is significantly smaller than the percentage circular area stenosis (60%).

The accuracy of these percentage diameter stenosis measurements has not been determined as yet, but worst case assumptions show an upper limit of approximately 8%, based on our experiences with the analysis of optically magnified coronary segments.

An example of the outcome of a frame-to-frame analysis of a right coronary tree is given in Fig. IX.18. This figure displays the centerlines of the coronary arteries for a number of consecutive frames during the systolic time-interval.

These data may be used as input, together with similar data obtained from an orthogonal projection, to a procedure for computing epicardial wall motion. Studying the so obtained contraction patterns could result in a classification scheme of coronary tree structures, where each class is homogeneous with respect to the geometrical patterns. Such classification scheme may then be used to validate the hypothesis that there is diagnostic and prognostic value in the geometric configuration of the coronary tree.

In achieving this goal it is necessary to develop techniques for assessing the similarity between coronary trees. A useful utility in obtaining a similarity measure for coronary trees is a cardiovascular database. This database should have the ability to efficiently store, retrieve and display the three-dimensional structure of the coronary trees. In this way, it will be possible to look for pattern similarities by visual methods, to use the results from this classification and for obtaining a similarity measure.

Analysis of retinal fluorescein angiograms

The retinal vessels are the only 'inner' blood vessels than can be observed in a direct optical manner. This optical accessibility is a challenge to those who would like to quantitate the flow of blood in the smaller and smallest blood vessels. Such

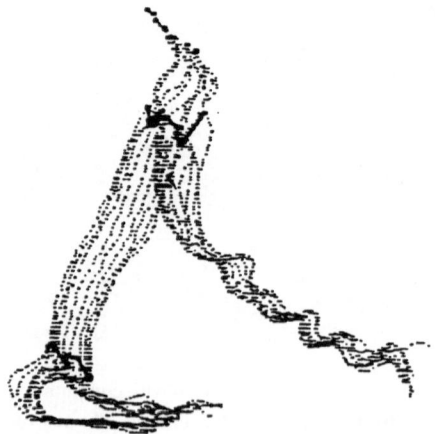

Fig. IX.18. Coronary tree movement during the systolic time-interval.

data would be of great importance in certain diseases, such as diabetes mellitus and hypertension, both for diagnostic purposes and for the measurement of the effect of treatment.

Retinal fluorotachometry (RFT) is a recently developed clinical method for the measurement of retinal blood flow [20–25]. The displacement of a sharp fluorescein dye front in the retinal arteries are recorded on 35 mm cineangiograms. Quantitative analysis of these films may provide the clinican with objective information about the linear flow (= flow velocity) in the retinal arteries.

In an attempt to derive such quantitative data we have applied our techniques for vessel tracing to these retinal images and developed algorithms for the definition of the location of the dye front in the successive frames of a cineangiogram.

The RFT cinerecording of retinal flow

During the acquisition of the RFT cineangiograms, the patient is positioned in front of a RFT retinal cinecamera, and the image of the selected retinal area is focussed on the plane of the film (Fig. IX.19). A bolus of 5 ml of a 10% fluorescein solution is injected into a brachial vein. After about ten seconds (arm to retina circulation time) the photomultiplier detects the arrival of the first trace of fluorescein in the eye and activates the suction cup, which causes an abrupt

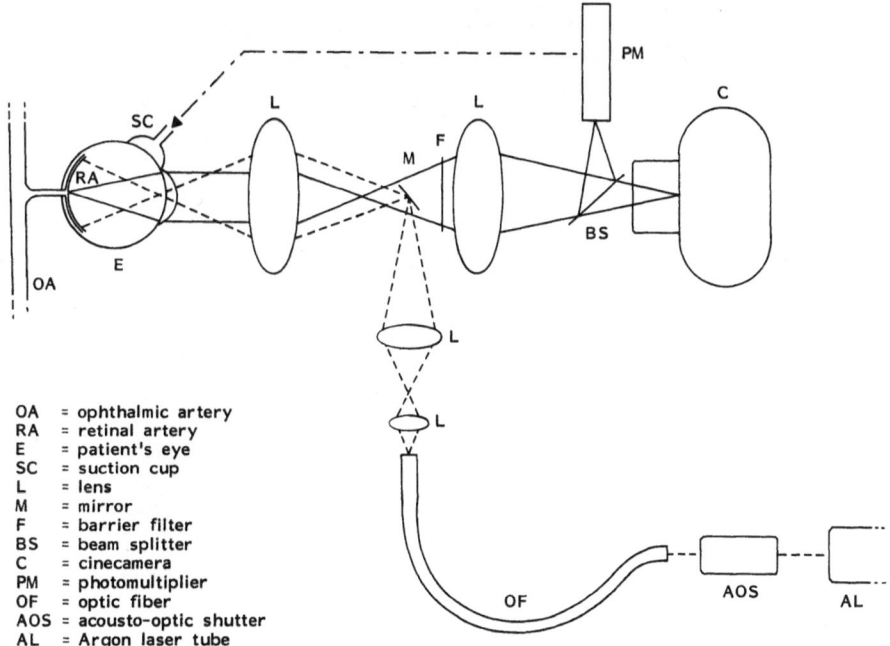

OA = ophthalmic artery
RA = retinal artery
E   = patient's eye
SC = suction cup
L   = lens
M   = mirror
F   = barrier filter
BS = beam splitter
C   = cinecamera
PM = photomultiplier
OF = optic fiber
AOS = acousto-optic shutter
AL = Argon laser tube

Fig. IX.19. Schematic diagram of the RFT retinal cinecamera with the retina of a patient's eye in focus.

elevation of the intra-ocular pressure (IOP) to just above the systolic pressure in the ophthalmic artery, resulting in a cessation of the retinal blood flow. When the concentration of fluorescein in the ophthalmic artery has reached a level at which maximum fluorescence occurs (i.e. 2 seconds later), the elevation of the IOP is discontinued, the retinal blood flow returns to its previous value, and the fluorescein enters the retinal vessels with a sharp dye front. The transposition of this dye front is selectively recorded by high speed cinematography. An Argon laser is used to produce monochromatic (488 nm) light flashes for the excitation of the fluorescein and an interference filter (barrier filter) allows the fluorescence light (520–530 nm) to only reach the film. As a result of this technique, the RFT cineangiograms are accurate recordings of the fluorescein inflow, which reflects the flow of blood serum in the retinal arteries.

Detection of the retinal arterial vessel patterns

The four images in Fig. IX.20 are examples of digitized cineframes acquired during the arterial filling phase; the time between the successive frames is approximately 80 ms. The last frame of such a sequence shows the entire arterial pattern.

Therefore, if we could determine the centerlines of the vessels in this last frame and superimpose these centerlines on the preceding images, the brightness dis-

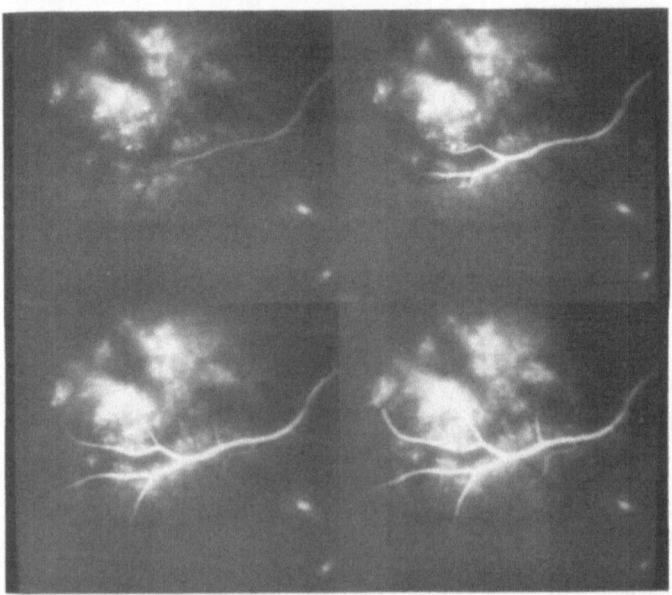

Fig. IX.20. Example of four RFT cineframes acquired during arterial filling phase; time between sucessive images is approximately 80 ms.

tribution along these lines in the sequential images can be measured, providing information about the arrival times of the dye front.

For these purposes, an accurate definition of the centerlines is required. As a first approximation of a centerline, the maxtracer-algorithm described in this chapter can be applied to a low resolution image. Additional possibilities for user-interaction have been implemented, allowing the maxtracer to trace side-branches at bifurcations, so that arrival times can be assessed for all arteries in the image. Following detection of a vessel in the low resolution image, the centerline is determined more accurately in the high resolution image based on this approx-imative information. Thereto, the maxtracer-path is projected onto the high resolution image. Subsequently, the high resolution image is resampled along scanlines, perpendicular to the local centerline directions of the maxtracer-path. The resampled data are stored in a matrix such that the (enlarged) maxtracer-path forms the straight center column of this matrix. A maximum brightness path is determined in this matrix on the basis of a minimum cost algorithm. This path is retransformed to the original high resolution image and filtered. Experiments have shown that this final path follows precisely the actual centerlines of the detected retinal arteries. Figure IX.21 shows the centerlines detected in the last image of Fig. IX.20.

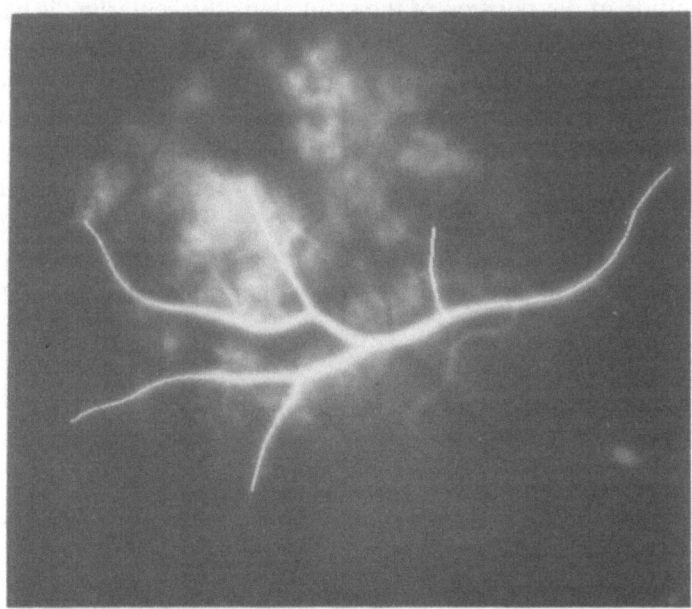

a

210

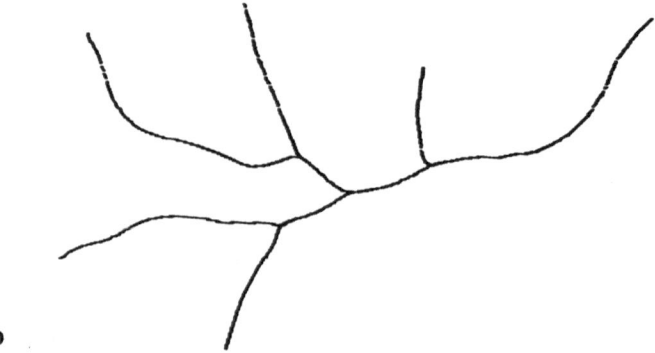

b

Fig. IX.21. Centerlines of retinal arteries, detected from and superimposed in the last image of Fig. IX.20 (Fig. IX.21a) and displayed separately (Fig. IX.21b).

Measurement flow velocities in retinal vessels

To measure the flow velocity of the fluorescein in a retinal artery, the front displacement must be determined as a function of time. The assessment of the front displacement is achieved by the analysis of the brightness curves measured along the centerline of the vessel in the successive images. An example of these brightness curves measured along one of the centerlines of Fig. IX.21 over five frames is given in Fig. IX.22. The increasing brightness levels in the successive images indicate increasing fluorescein concentrations in the blood. The front displacement can be appreciated from this figure.

The definition of the position of the front along the centerline is based on an algorithm involving the brightness curve and its first- and second- derivates. From these front displacements, the flow velocity can be calculated as a function of time if the film speed and the ratio of pixel size to true distance between pixels are known. The film speed for the RFT cineangiogram of Fig. IX.20 was 60 frames/s, yielding a frame-period of 17 ms. This particular experiment was carried out on a monkey having a heart frequency of 120 to 160 beats per minute. As a result, a complete cardiac cycle covers about 20 frames. The relation between pixel size and true distance was about 300 pixel distances per centimeter. From these data,

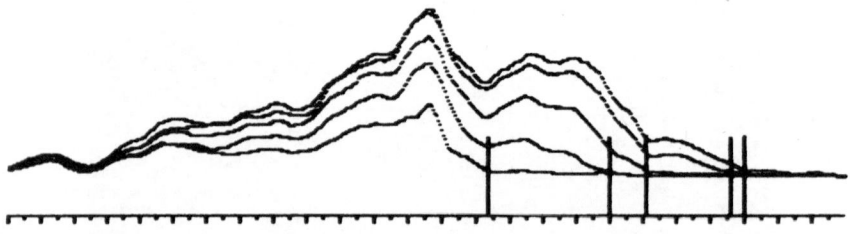

Fig. IX.22. Front displacement in retinal artery of Fig. IX.21.

flow velocity can be readily assessed. If the front displacement between two successive images equals X pixel distances, the flow velocity V equals:

$$V = X \cdot \frac{60}{300} = 0.2 \text{ X cm/s} \tag{IX.7}$$

The results of the flow velocity measurements for two different arteries in the same angiographic investigation are given in Table IX.1. The flow velocities calculated from these data as a function of time are displayed in Fig. IX.23. There is a high degree of resemblance between these two curves. The flow velocity is

Table IX.1. Front displacements and flow velocities for two series of images.

Frame	Front displacement (pixel distance)		Current speed (cm/s)	
	1°meas.	2°meas.	1°meas.	2°meas.
9	–	–	–	–
10	–	30.1	–	6.0
11	–	29.1	–	5.8
12	–	12.1	–	2.4
13	11.0	9.7	2.2	1.9
14	9.3	6.8	1.9	1.4
15	14.1	5.6	2.8	1.1
16	19.3	12.3	3.9	2.5
17	7.1	3.4	1.4	0.7
18	14.4	17.1	2.9	3.4
19	8.0	2.1	1.6	0.4
20	10.1	3.2	2.0	0.6

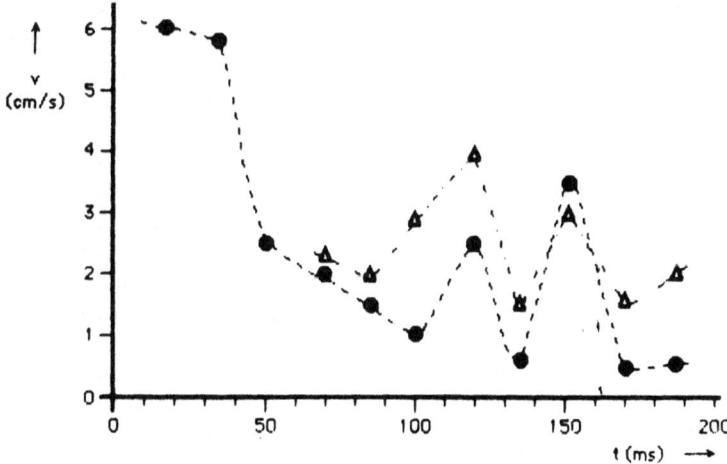

Fig. IX.23. Flow velocities as a function of time.

212

dependent on the instantaneous blood pressure, which is dependent on the phase in the cardiac cycle. Further investigations are necessary to determine the precise relation between the blood flow velocity and instantaneous blood pressure.

Concluding remarks analysis retinal images

Our results in a limited validation study have shown that the arteries could be traced fully automatically without any operator interaction. The procedure for finding the maximal brightness path in the high resolution image resulted in all cases in an excellent approximation of the centerline of the retinal arteries. Extensive validation studies are planned for the near future; furthermore, the advantages and limitations of this technique in clinical practice need to be established.

References

1. Starmer CF, Smith WM: Problems in acquisition and representation of coronary arterial trees. Comp Cardiol: 143–147, 1974.
2. Starmer CF, Smith WM: Computer storage and retrieval of coronary trees. In: Cardiovascular Imaging and Image Processing. Theory and Practice – 1975. DC Harrison, H Sandler, HA Miller (Eds.) SPIE 72: 195–199, 1975.
3. Smith WM, Starmer CF: Computer representation of coronary arterial trees. Comp Biomed Res 9: 187–201, 1976.
4. Kong Y, Morris JJ, McIntosh HD: Assessment of regional myocardial performance from biplane coronary cineangiograms. Am J Cardiol 27: 529–537, 1971.
5. Daughters GT, Ingels NB, Carrera CJ, Wexler L, Smith NTy: Regional myocardial dynamics from single-plane coronary cineangiograms. J Biomech 6: 25–30, 1973.
6. Fukui T, Yachida M, Tsuji S: Detection and tracking of blood vessels in cine-angiograms. Proc 5th Int Conf on Pattern Recognition, Miami: 383–385, 1980.
7. Kindelan M, Suarez de Lezo J: Artery detection and tracking in coronary angiography. In: Digital Image Analysis. S Levialdi (Ed.). Pitman Publishing Inc., Marshfield, Mass: 283–294, 1984.
8. Potel MJ, MacKay SA, Rubin JM, Aisen AM, Sayre RE: Three-dimensional left ventricular wall motion in man. Coordinate systems for representing wall motion direction. Invest Radiol 19: 499–509, 1984.
9. Reiber JHC, Slager CJ, Schuurbiers JCH, Boer A den, Gerbrands JJ, Troost GJ, Scholts B, Kooijman CJ, Serruys PW: Transfer functions of the X-ray-cine-video chain applied to digital processing of coronary cineangiograms. In: Digital Imaging in Cardiovascular Radiology. PH Heintzen, R Brennecke (Eds.) Georg Thieme Verlag, Stuttgart: 89–104, 1983.
10. Gerbrands JJ, Reiber JHC, Scholts B, Langhout G, Kooijman CJ: Structural analysis of the coronary arterial tree. Int. Symp. Medical Imaging and Image Interpretation, ISMIII'82. IEEE Press, Cat No 82 CH1804-4: 54–58, 1982.
11. Gerbrands JJ, Reiber JHC, Kooijman CJ, Rademaker RT: Model-guided segmentation of coronary cine-angiograms. In: Signal Processing II: Theories and Applications. HW Schüssler (Ed.) Elsevier Science Publishers B.V. (North-Holland): 601–604, 1983.
12. Kooijman CJ, Rademaker RT, Gerbrands JJ, Reiber JHC: Developments towards frame-to-frame computer processing of the entire coronary tree. Comp Cardiol: 389–392, 1983.

13. Kooijman CJ, Gerbrands JJ, Reiber JHC, Rademaker RT, Ommeren J van: Developments towards frame-to-frame computer processing of coronary angiograms. Proc Int Symp on Medical Images and Icons, ISMII '84. IEEE Press, Cat No CH2047-9/84: 356–362, 1984.

14. Ommeren J van: Coronary tree detection. Thesis, Information Theory Group, Delft University of Technology, 1984.

15. Meenen RJ van: Detection of the coronary tree in series of digital subtraction images. Thesis, Information Theory Group, Delft University of Technology, 1985.

16. Burr DJ: A technique for comparing curves. Proc IEEE Comp Soc Conf on Pattern Recogn and Image Proc: 271–277, 1979.

17. Langhout G: Structural analysis of the coronary tree from X-ray films. Thesis, Information Theory Group, Delft University of Technology, 1982.

18. Hilditch CJ: Linear skeletons from square cupboards. Machine Intelligence 4, Edinburgh University Press: 413–420, 1969.

19. Lu SY: A tree-to-tree distance and its application to cluster analysis. IEEE Trans Pattern Anal and Mach Intell 1: 219–224, 1979.

20. Schulte AVM: Retinal fluorotachometry. Academic thesis, to be published 1985.

21. Schulte AVM, Jong PT de: Retinal fluorotachometry. Invest Ophthalmol Vis Sci (Suppl.) 25: 7. (Abstract), 1984.

22. Schulte AVM, Reiber JHC, Heuven WAJ van: Retinal fluorotachometry. Invest Ophthalmol Vis Sci (Suppl.) 26: 246 (Abstract), 1985.

23. Schulte AVM: Apparatus for (high-speed) fluorescein angiography. Patent no NO 31727 TM, Dutch Patent Office, The Hague, 1983.

24. Schulte AVM: Apparatus for retinal or choroidal angiography or hematotachography. Patent no. NO 32389 TM, Dutch Patent Office, The Hague, 1984. Patent application no 85200522.2, European Patent Office, The Hague, 1985.

25. Beckmann LHJF, Vlasbloem H, Schulte AVM: Method and apparatus for measuring the flow of blood in the eye. Patent application no 85200558.6, European Patent Office, The Hague, 1985.

X. A methodological review of quantification systems for coronary and left ventricular cineangiograms

Quantitative coronary cineangiography

Introduction

Over the last few years there has been a growing interest in digital processing of coronary angiograms to derive quantitative measures on the severity of coronary obstructions [1]. In general, 35 mm cinefilm has continued to be the medium of choice for registration of the coronary angiograms, because of its inherently high resolution. The various systems employed to date vary to a great extent from manual procedures using a cross-hair measuring system [2], a vernier caliper on magnified (about $3 \times$) projection images of the film [3–7], or an optical magnifying ($6 \times$) device applied to 105 mm photospot film [8] through a computerized manual edge-tracing procedure [9], to methods which employ computer edge detection algorithms to determine luminal diameter values in a two-dimensional projection [10–23]. Several investigators have also employed densitometric procedures in an attempt to derive cross-sectional area measures from single view coronary cineangiograms [24–34]. Finally, methods have been proposed for the three-dimensional reconstruction and representation of coronary arterial segments assessed from two orthogonal views [9, 11, 35, 36]. Table X.1 describes a number of important features of the various published systems, which will be discussed in more detail in the following paragraphs [35].

Cinefilm conversion

Digitization of the brightness information in a selected 35 mm cineframe has been accomplished by various techniques: (1) photometer scanner [10, 11]; (2) linewise scanning with an array of 1024 photodiodes [25]; (3) conversion of an optically magnified portion of the cineframe into a video signal by means of a cine-video projector system [13, 14, 17, 19, 20, 27, 34]; or a high resolution CCD camera [16]. With real-time video digitizers now widely available at affordable prices from various manufacturers, the cine-video conversion approach has been employed most frequently. The simplest cine-video projector system consists of a simple lightbox with a cinefilm transport mechanism and the video camera positioned at various distances from the film. The more complex systems employ different lens systems for optical magnification and allow for manual or computer controlled selection of magnified regions of interest. High resolution video camera's with 1" or 1.5" vidicon tubes have been employed in these systems. The latest development employs a CCD camera, consisting of a high resolution linear array that is moved mechanically over the projected image. In this system a monochromatic light source has been used, that is optimally suitable for high resolution imaging and densitometric analysis of the cinefilm [16].

The pixel widths in the digitized images projected back to the original cine-frame dimensions vary from $10\,\mu$m to $20\,\mu$m for the routinely used magnifications. These accuracies can be achieved with good quality video camera's using standard video systems with the appropriate optical magnification. It has been our experience, that a two-fold optical magnification provides sufficient accuracy for the analysis of coronary arterial segments. At this magnification the pixel size in the digitized video image projected back to actual size at the level of the heart equals approximately 0.1 mm for a 7" image intensifier. This means that for a coronary obstruction with a width of 0.5 mm 5 pixels are available for subsequent contour detection and possibly densitometric analysis.

Contour detection coronary arterial segment

For the computer assisted definition of the boundaries of a selected coronary segment, in general, the following steps can be distinguished:
(1) Definition global centerline of coronary segment,
(2) Edge enhancement,
(3) Contour definition.
The different implementations of these steps will be discussed in some more detail in the following paragraphs.

Definition global centerline
Edge positions of coronary segments in the digitized video images can best be detected along scanlines perpendicular to the local centerline directions of the segment. Therefore, the first step in the contour detection algorithm is the definition of the global trajectory of the centerline.

Selzer et al. require the operator to define a midline estimate for the artery to be analyzed by indicating a few center points along the vessel with a sonic pen [19, 20]. A smoothed continuous path is then calculated from the manual input by angular interpolation over 4 points. Following the fill-in, all points are smoothed over 9 points.

We have implemented a similar approach described in Chapter III; the user indicates by means of a writing tablet a number of centerline positions within the arterial segment, such that the straight line segments connecting consecutive pairs of these points remain within the artery. The corners of this initial centerline are smoothed by means of a first degree least squared error polynomial fit. This centerline will be updated by a new centerline computed from the subsequently detected contour positions and the contour detection procedure is repeated. This iterative approach has been implemented to minimize the influence of the user definition of the center points on the detected contours.

Barth et al. have developed an automated tracking procedure for the centerline; the user only indicates a starting position and a flow direction within the arterial segment of interest [10, 11]. The tracking algorithm apparently stops at the boundary of the matrix; stop criteria have not been published nor data on the performance for arteries with side-branches.

Edge enhancement
Edge enhancement of the digital data is usually based on the application of first or second derivative or difference functions or a combination of these two. The widely used term derivative is, strictly taken, reserved to analog functions. For digital signals or images the term difference or gradient should be used. However, since derivative has been employed in the literature of this particular application most frequently, we will follow this custom where appropriate.

The maximal response of first-derivative operators has been employed by Sanders et al. and Selzer et al. [17–20].

To simplify and speed up the edge enhancement and contour definition procedures both Barth et al., Kooijman et al. and Reiber et al. resample the digital data along straight lines perpendicular to the local centerline directions; these straight lines are denoted scanlines [10, 11, 13, 14, 16]. This stretching procedure has been discussed in Chapter III. Following the approach by Kooijman, for each point of the matrix the one-dimensional gradient of the intensity values as well as the change in this gradient are calculated. Next, a cost function is defined as the inverse of the weighted sum of the gradient and the gradient-change values. The value of a pixel in this cost matrix is a measure for the local edge strength.

Kirkeeide et al. compute the derivative of the one-dimensional grey level scan across the vessel by means of a least squares convolution technique with a quadratic function [23]. Grey scale derivatives have been derived with kernel sizes of 9 to 33 points.

Contour definition
In all published systems with automated contour detection different techniques have been employed for the final contour detection of the arterial segments. The

different techniques will be briefly described in the same order as listed in Table IX.1.

Barth et al. used a correlation technique with 18 to 27 pixels wide edge models, one for the left edge and one for the right edge, to find the positions along the scanlines which correlate best with this model [10, 11]. The contour positions essentially correspond with the maximal 2nd-derivative response of the model.

Kirkeeide et al. define the edge positions at a user-selected threshold (75%–100% of the maximal derivative value) of the grey scale derivative function [23].

In our approach the left and right contours are obtained by searching in the cost matrix from top to bottom for a minimal cost path (satisfying some connectivity constraints) to the left and right of the center column, respectively [13] (see Fig. III.12). Great advantage of this minimum cost contour detection algorithm is the fact that the edge positions are not determined per individual scanline, but that information gathered from all the other scanlines is also taken into account. As a result, this approach is less sensitive to intervening structures such as branches. If the user does not agree with part of the detected contour, these positions may be corrected interactively with a writing tablet.

Sanders et al. determine the positions with maximal first-derivative response along lines perpendicular to manually traced margins to improve on these manually determined positions [17, 18].

Selzer et al. search for positions with maximal first-derivative response along scanlines perpendicular to the local directions of the earlier defined centerline [19, 20]. These positions correspond with the inflection points of the density profiles along the scanlines. It has been our experience that such positions fit the arterial segments too tight; if only the 1st-derivative response is used, certain correction factors should be employed such that the final contour positions are shifted towards the base of the density profile.

Smith et al. do not employ 1st- or 2nd-derivative operators to determine the arterial contours; their approach is based on the selection of a global threshold level following background subtraction [21]. The varying background in the image is removed by sliding a large sphere underneath the surface of the image. If the diameter of the sphere is chosen to be larger than the diameter of the artery, only the background signal will be located by the transformation. This signal is then subtracted to provide a background normalized image. As a final step, a threshold level is determined from this background normalized image that locates the contours of the artery.

In most publications no mention is made of particular procedures to eliminate extraneous detected positions. Experience from our earlier work made clear that certain precautions need to be taken if the contours are determined on a line-to-line basis. That means that one should define, for example, an expectation window for a certain scanline based on the detected position(s) on the previous scanline(s).

Following contour definition, a smoothing procedure is usually applied to each of the detected contour paths, which may consist of a least squared error first degree polynomial fit through a number of nearest points on each side of the edge point under consideration.

Pincushion correction

The pincushion distortion results in selective magnification of an object near the edges of the cineframe as compared to its size in the center of the field. These differences need to be corrected for, if absolute diameter measurements are to be derived from coronary cineangiograms. The standard procedure to assess the degree of distortion present is to film a cm-grid, which is positioned against the input screen of the image intensifier.

A number of approaches to correct for the pincushion distortion have been implemented. Theoretically, the pincushion distortion is radially symmetric about the central X-ray beam, because of the rotational symmetry of the curved input screen and its internal fields. The first method makes the assumption that the distortion is indeed radially symmetric about the center of the image intensifier and that relative magnification can be determined from the distance of the pixel under consideration to the center of the image intensifier. An empirically determined analytical function of the radius is then used to correct for the distortion [9]. The second method is also based on radial symmetry, but relative magnification factors for a single radial line are stored in memory of the computer system. The relative magnification for each distance was obtained by averaging of four values measured in the four quadrants of the cm-grid image. Hence, no analytical function is employed [17, 18]. The third method, which is in use in our center, makes no assumption about the geometrical distribution of the distortion and stores the relative magnifications of all the intersection points of the cm-grid [13, 14, 16] (see Ch. III). For a given point in the image which does not coincide with one of the intersection positions, a correction vector can be determined by means of a bilinear interpolation between the correction vectors of the four neighboring intersection points.

Calibration

To compute absolute sizes of the arterial segment analyzed the calibration factor needs to be determined. Basically, two different approaches are in use for the coronary arteries: (1) analytically from geometric X-ray system parameters; (2) on the basis of the known diameter of the contrast catheter. Following the first approach, the size of an object placed at the center of rotation of the X-ray system (isocenter) can be determined from simple geometric principles from the height levels of X-ray tube and image intensifier. However, for objects above or below the center of rotation a slightly more complicated analysis must be carried out, requiring a second, preferably orthogonal view of the object. The corrections on the calibration factor can be assessed from the distance of the object to the center of the image in the second view [38].

If the known size of the catheter is used for calibration purposes, the computed calibration factor is theoretically only applicable to objects in the plane of the analyzed catheter segment parallel to the image intensifier input screen. However, for coronary segments lying in other planes corrections to the calibration factor can be assessed from other views.

From the above it is clear that for the measurement of truly absolute sizes of coronary segments two views, preferably but not necessarily orthogonal to each other, are required. However, if one is only interested in the changes of sizes of coronary segments as a result of long or short term interventions, good results can be achieved from single plane views. For these situations one must make sure that for the repeat angiogram the X-ray system is positioned in exactly the same geometry as during the first angiogram. This requires registration of the angles and height levels of the X-ray system, preferably on-line with a geometry read-out system. Although the calibration factor used for a particular segment is then only an approximation of the true calibration factor, the same systematic error will be present for the first and the repeat angiogram.

If the catheter is used as a scaling device, the contours of a small segment may be either drawn manually or computer detected by applying similar contour detection principles as used for the coronary segment. In our routine practice, the catheter is magnified optically with a factor of $2\sqrt{2}$:1 and a priori information is included in the iterative edge detection procedure, based on the fact that the selected part of the catheter is the projection of a cylindrical structure. It should be realized that the size of the catheter as given by the manufacturer, in general, will deviate from the true size especially for disposable catheters. Therefore, with long term intervention studies it may be advisable to measure the size of the catheter following the catheterization with a micrometer [Ch. VI].

Contour analysis

From the contours of the analyzed arterial segment, following pincushion correction and calibration, a diameter function can be determined by computing the distances between the left and right edges. From these data a number of parameters may be calculated such as: (1) minimal obstruction diameter; (2) extent of the obstruction; (3) reference diameter; (4) percentage diameter stenosis; (5) percentage area stenosis; (6) area of atherosclerotic plaque; (7) symmetry of the stenosis; (8) hemodynamic parameters of the obstruction [9, Ch. III]; and (9) mean diameter of a nonobstructed coronary segment. Particularly the minimal obstruction diameter is of great importance as it is present to the inverse fourth power in the formulas describing the pressure loss over a coronary obstruction. Moreover, to determine the effect of interventions on the severity of coronary obstructions, one should compute the changes in minimal obstruction diameter and not those in percentage diameter narrowing, as the reference position in general will also be affected by the intervention.

However, as cardiologists have been trained to express the severity and also the changes in severity of an obstruction in terms of percentage diameter narrowing, these values are usually also included in quantitative reports. The usual way to determine percentage diameter stenosis of a coronary obstruction, requires the user to indicate a reference position. In general, the reference diameter is then computed as the average value of a number of diameter values in a symmetric region with center at the user-defined reference position. It is clear that this computed %-D narrowing of an obstruction depends heavily on the selected reference position. In arteries with a focal obstructive lesion and a clearly normal proximal arterial segment, the choice of the reference region is straightforward and simple. However, in cases where the proximal part of the arterial segment shows combinations of stenotic and ectatic areas, the choice may be very difficult. To minimize these variations, alternative methods have been developed which are not dependent on a user-defined reference region [13, 14, 16, 19, 20]. By these methods an estimation of the normal or pre-disease luminal size over the obstructive lesion is obtained on the basis of the computed centerline and the 90th-percentile of the diameter values [19, 20] or on the basis of the proximal and distal centerline segments and a reference diameter function defined by a first degree polynomial through all of the diameter values outside of the obstructive region, followed by a translation to the 80th percentile level [13, 14, 16]; tapering of the vessel to account for a decrease in arterial caliber associated with branches is allowed. By comparing the actual luminal positions at the obstruction with the estimated pre-disease reference contour positions, the area of the atheroslerotic plaque, expressed in mm², can be computed in that particular view. Furthermore, assessment of the symmetry of the obstruction is feasible [14, 16].

The mean diameter of a nonobstructive coronary segment can easily be determined from the diameter data by requesting the user to indicate with a writing tablet, lightpen or similar device the proximal and distal boundaries of the desired segment; the length of the segment in mm is usually also provided. For intervention studies coronary branch points may be used to define the boundaries of the segment, as these can be determined fairly reproducible.

Densitometry

Since the luminal cross section at a coronary obstruction is frequently irregular in shape, percentage diameter reduction measured in a single projection is of limited diagnostic value. The hemodynamic resistance of an obstruction is determined to a great extent by the minimal cross-sectional area. Computation of this cross-sectional area reduction from the percentage diameter reduction measured in a single view requires the assumption of e.g. circular cross sections, an assumption which hardly ever holds. The resulting error may be reduced by incorporating two orthogonal projections and computing elliptical cross sections. However, with the often occurring eccentric lesions even this last approach may yield inaccurate results.

The edge detection techniques described above are based on the measurement of changes in the brightness profiles along scanlines perpendicular to local centerline segments. However, if one could constitute the relationship between the path lengths of the X-rays through the artery and the absolute brightness values in the digital image, one would obtain the information required to compute the cross-sectional areas from a single view. It is clear that a homogeneous mixing of the contrast agent with the blood must be assumed for the measurements to have any meaning.

A simplified block diagram of our complete X-ray/cine/video-acquisition and analysis system is shown in Fig. X.1. By substituting another input device for the video camera, e.g. a photometer scanner or CCD camera, this same block diagram applies to the other described systems as well. Constitution of the relationship between path length and brightness value requires detailed analysis of the complete imaging system. In a simplified approach, we are only interested in the static properties of the system. Analysis of the static transfer function of each link in the chain reveals that computation of the complete transfer function is very difficult. There is a large number of parameters involved, many of which are spatially variant [29].

A few different approaches towards densitometric analysis of selected coro-

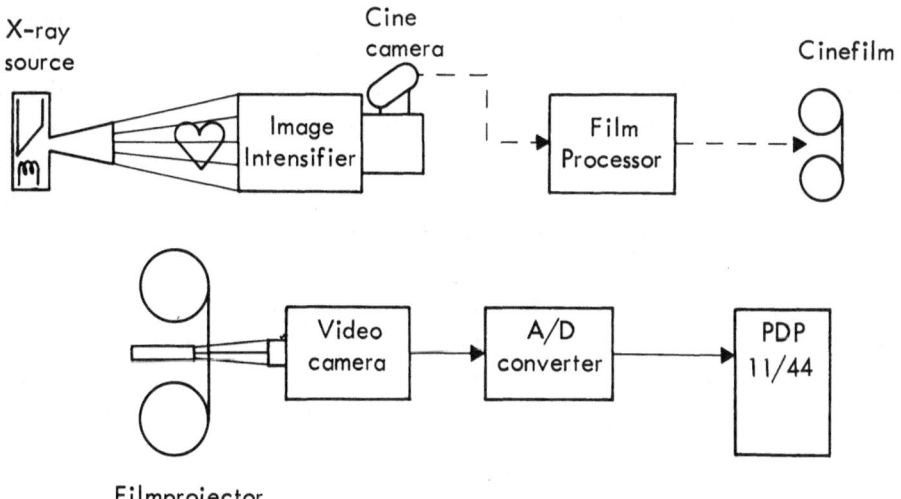

Fig. X.1. Block diagram of X-ray/cine/video-imaging system.

nary arterial segments have been published [24–34]. Most authors assume that the X-ray absorption process, comprising the first part of the imaging chain from X-ray source to the input screen of the image intensifier, can be described by the Lambert-Beer Law. Despite many potential sources of errors in the absorption process (nonmonochromatic X-ray spectrum, beam hardening, scattering, etc.) it has indeed been demonstrated by Bürsch and Heintzen that by the use of appropriate filters and scatter grids the Lambert-Beer Law is applicable for densitometric measurements in clinical studies with a sufficient degree of accuracy [39, 40]. Pochon and Rutishauser have shown that the Lambert-Beer Law is applicable for coronary arteries with diameters not exceeding a few millimeters; this range can be extended by applying certain densitometric correction procedures [28].

For the remaining subsystems of the imaging chain comprising the image intensifier, the cinefilm exposure and development process, and the film sampling process which may be achieved directly by means of a photo-optical read-out system or via video conversion, usually simplified formulas, relating measured video brightness level with the irradiated object thickness, are used neglecting the influence of spatially nonhomogeneous responses [10, 25, 27, 30, 34]. Correction for background levels is mostly achieved by measuring the video brightness levels outside of the vessel and subtracting the interpolated background levels from the measurements within the arterial segment.

We have implemented a more complicated approach in an attempt to correct for spatially variant responses and for the daily variations in the cinefilm processing [29]; for further details see Chapter VII.

A completely different approach has been published by Spears [32, 33]. During patient exposure a series of frames is used to calibrate steps of a rotating wedge against film grey scale. The step-wedge consists of a gradually increasing number of layers of stainless steel tape, such that a total of 15 increments in thickness is obtained. Two such step-wedges are placed about the circumference of a circular non-attenuating gear, which is rotated by a constant tension, spring-driven mechanism under a 6 inch image intensifier perpendicular to the direction of the radiation beam at one revolution per second. The rotation of the circular wedge and film exposure (33 frames/s) are synchronized so that the wedge moves one step per frame. By including a small lung segment during held inspiration in the coronary angiographic field, a motionless region of temporally constant tissue thickness is presented for sequential superimposition of wedge steps. By means of a calibration curve, the relative thickness of contrast medium is expressed in equivalent units of steel thickness. Background contributions underlying the arterial segment are corrected for by assuming a linear change in tissue thickness between vessel edges. For measurement of light intensity in a projected cine-frame a motor driven photocell measures the intensities along selected scanlines one mm in anatomic length. Ratios of planimetered areas under thickness contribution curves can then be used to calculate relative cross-sectional areas.

Three-dimensional reconstruction

Most efforts in the field of quantitative data extraction from coronary cineangio-grams have focussed on the development of methods to determine the severity of coronary obstructions in terms of percentage diameter and/or cross-sectional area reduction from single or biplane cineangiograms. However, if one would be able to determine with a sufficient degree of accuracy the three-dimensional shape and size of coronary arterial segments, an additional number of clinically important parameters would become available. For example, from the three-dimensional data several hemodynamic parameters of the arterial segments, such as the hemodynamic resistance of an obstruction, the pressure drop over the obstruc-tion, local blood flow through the artery, etc., can be assessed with higher accuracy than from the single plane data (Ch. III). These data may augment our knowledge in searching for the definition of the 'critical' stenosis. Furthermore, the three-dimensional morphology and particularly the changes over longer periods of time may provide us with detailed information about the presence and progression or regression of coronary atherosclerosis.

In general, the problem of the three-dimensional reconstruction of a coronary arterial segment can be reduced to a multiple two-dimensional problem by dividing the object into a stack of parallel or nonparallel cross sections. Each two-dimensional cross section consists of one connected region and is to be recon-structed from its two one-dimensional projections. The thickness of each slice must be taken such that the projections do not change significantly over the slice. The simplest approach towards the three-dimensional representation of a vessel segment requires the contour information from 2 orthogonal views to be matched at a point thought to be identical in both [9]. This may be a vessel branch point, a bit of mural calcium, or the point of maximum lumen constriction. The two projected centerlines are then matched along their entire length to construct a three-dimensional centerline with corresponding vessel diameters from the two views. As a result, each cross section is approximated by means of an ellipse.

Barth et al. construct a 3D-representation of a coronary segment from the thickness information assessed from one view using a densitometric procedure by placing for each pixel along a scanline the thickness information symmetrical with respect to this scanline [11]. Asymmetrical cross sections can be obtained by incorporating the thickness information from an orthogonal view; details of this method have not been published as yet.

We have developed a binary reconstruction algorithm for the slice-by-slice reconstruction of the 3D-shape of an arterial segment from two orthogonal projections based on diameter and densitometric data [35, 41, Ch. VIII].

Spears et al. have applied a maximum entropy iterative algorithm to recon-struct the lumen cross section from a set of projection data consisting of the cinedensitometric profiles from 36 radiographic views taken at 10° increments [36]. They have studied the feasibility of reconstruction of coronary luminal cross sections from a small number of cineradiographic views in studies of in vitro model lumena with well-defined geometric shapes. It was concluded that as few as three to five radiographic views may be useful in reconstructing coronary luminal shape.

Concluding remarks

A review has been given on the different methodologies in use for the quantitative analysis of coronary cineangiograms. Unfortunately, the systems could not be compared in terms of accuracy and precision of the analysis procedure, success scores under different image qualities, computation time, etc., since these data were usually not provided in the papers. Most systems are still under development with only a few being applied more or less routinely for clinical studies. From the description of the systems and the parameters listed in Table IX.1 it is clear that there exists a great divergence in the architectures of the image processing systems and in the application software algorithms.

Quantitative left ventricular cineangiography

Various systems have been developed for the quantitative analysis of left ventricular angiograms. These videometry systems can be distinguished into three general categories:
(1) Light-pen computer processing
(2) Analog video processing
(3) Digital image processing
These three categories will be described briefly in the following sections.

Light-pen computer processing

Systems have been developed for the manual tracing of the left ventricular boundaries and subsequent analysis from either cinefilm (off-line) or from analog or digitized video images stored on video tape or disk (on-line).

Off-line processing of left ventricular cineangiograms
One of the first systems that used a computer to automate the determination of volumes of cardiac chambers was reported in 1961 by Baker et al. [42]. This largely mechanical, biplane projection and tracing system can be regarded as a forerunner of modern light-pen computer systems.

The method most frequently used for the analysis of left ventricular cineframes consists of projecting the cineframes onto a plotting table or x–y digitizer. The LV borders are manually traced with a magnetic cursor or with the stylus of a spark-gap digitizing pen, and the resulting x–y coordinates transferred to a desk calculator or computer system for subsequent analysis [43, 44]. For the analysis of biplane ventriculographic images, double cineprojectors with stop-frame capability and precise frame registration have been constructed [45]. In a slightly more complicated design, monoplane cineframes can be projected from underneath a table onto a frosted screen equipped with two linear microphones which respond to the arrival of pulses from a hypersonic pulse generator built at the tip of a freely manipulated pen [46–48]; a timing device determines the x–y coordinates of the pen positions.

On-line processing of left ventricular angiograms
In this category the angiograms, which are available as analog video images acquired from the output of the image intensifier with a video camera, are stored in analog format on a video tape or video disk. These analog images can be retrieved at a later point in time and displayed on a video monitor, or digitized and stored in a computer system for subsequent analysis.

For systems equipped with an analog video tape or disk, the analog images can be retrieved and displayed in stop-action mode on a monitor for subsequent analysis; for these purposes a light-pen interfaced to a digital computer is used most frequently [49–51]. Systems have been developed which allow biplane analog left ventricular angiograms to be displayed side-by-side on the video monitor, so that both contours can be traced in one and the same video image [52–54].

Brennecke et al. have developed a digital system for Roentgen-Video Image Processing [55–57]. The analog video images from the X-ray TV-chain are digitized in real time; an earlier digitized background image can be subtracted. The resulting image is multiplied and clipped, transformed into an analog video image by means of a D/A-converter, and stored on an analog video tape recorder. These recorded images can be retrieved, digitized and stored in a minicomputer for subsequent processing. Similarly as described for their earlier systems, a light-pen is used for operator-interaction, such as endocardial or epicardial contour tracing, in the digitized images.

With state-of-the-art digital radiology systems, the analog video images from the output of the image intensifier are digitized in real time, and stored in memory of a computer system or on a digital disk. Left ventricular contours can be traced manually with a light-pen, joystick or trackball, or detected semi- or fully-automatically.

Analog video processing

Analog video processing systems are characterized by the fact that the left ventricular contours are detected in the analog video images by means of electronic video techniques. Great advantage of this approach is the instantaneous response of detected positions on changes in electronic threshold levels; the processing occurs with a speed of 50 or 60 fields/s. Disadvantage is due to the difficulty of implementing certain edge detection algorithms in hardware, plus the inflexibility of these designs. With digital image processing systems, minicomputers and image processing software packages now widely available at affordable prices, this category is loosing its importance.

One of the first reported systems was by the Mayo Clinic and used a biplane video angiographic system for dynamic measurements of volume and shape of the left ventricle recorded on video tape or video disk recorder [58–62]. A main feature of this system was the so-called video quantizer [58]. An operator-interactive flying-spot scanner assembly was used to improve a replayed video image, such that automated border recognition on the basis of an operator-adjusted video quantizer level was possible. The detected border positions were stored in real time in a digital computer for subsequent processing.

A thresholding technique with constant threshold level was reported in 1970 by Covvey [63]. Single cineframes were scanned with a video camera and, with a special effect circuit, only the region around the left ventricle was selected, while the rest was blanked out. With this constant threshold level, only ventricles in pictures with exceptional image contrast could be recognized.

Another method that used a video quantizer was described by Marcus et al. [64–65]. Left ventricular cineangiograms taken in the RAO view at 60 frames/s were projected with a flickerless projector onto a plumbicon television camera. A second video camera, the key camera, was used by a skilled operator to mask out noncontributing portions of the film and to shade selected areas so that the chamber could be identified. A video planimeter with a variable threshold level was adjusted by the operator so that an accurate fit was obtained between the opacified area of the video planimeter and the area actually visualized.

Finally, the Contouromat described in more detail in Chapter IV, is based on a dynamic thresholding technique, whereby the reference level at which a border point is detected is determined from local sampled video levels on a line-by-line basis [66–69]. The information on detected contour positions at previous video lines, the previous video field as well as the previous cineframe are converted into probability functions superimposed on the dynamic reference level to determine the border point on the current video line.

Digital image processing

With digital image processing systems, the left ventricular edge detection techniques have been implemented in software and are thus applied to digitized left ventricular angiograms. Various types of cameras have been used to digitize cineframes, such as standard video camera, dissector camera, flying spot scanner, etc. Again with the modern digital radiography systems, the digital images are directly available without an intermediate cinefilm step.

In many semi-automatic boundary definition procedures, the user starts with tracing an approximate outline of the ventricular boundary in the first cineframe of a series to be analyzed, by light-pen or similar device, and the system uses this outline as a global guidance to automatically determine the precise boundary. For the following cineframe the detected outline from the previous frame is used as a first approximation for the current one, etc.

Robb developed a computer algorithm that detects the left ventricular contour within a border search interval defined by the contour in the previous frame or by a manually traced approximation of the contour for the first frame [70–72]. Cineframes were digitized by a flying spot scanner in a 512×512 matrix with 64 grey levels. The implemented algorithm assumes that the slope of the contrast transfer function across the image border is approximately zero for background and image areas, and approaches a third-degree polynomial at the border area. Detecting the actual border points thus requires the determination of a third-degree least-squared polynomial that fits the data in the border search interval; the border coordinate is defined by the zero-crossing of the second-derivative of the polynomial.

A threshold method based on statistical principles and heuristics to detect boundaries in radiographic images was reported by Chow and Kaneko [73]. Thirty-five mm cineframes were scanned by a flying spot scanner, converted into a 256×256 array of 16-bit words and stored on a magnetic disk. All the digitized images were first logarithmically transformed and a reference image subtracted from each of these; the reference image was obtained by averaging seven logarithmically transformed images before dye injection. Their fundamental assumption was that the probability distribution of the intensity for any small region of the image consisting solely of the object or background is unimodal. On the other hand, the distribution of a small region containing a boundary is consequently a mixture of two unimodal distributions and is in general bimodal. The valley point in a bimodal histogram therefore determines the threshold that separates object and background. The thresholds were thus set dynamically according to local rather than global characteristics.

Kaneko and Mancini described a method for straight-line approximation of the boundary of the left ventricular chamber from consecutive video- or cineframes, assuming that the boundary on a reference frame is available [74]. This boundary on the reference frame may be defined manually by means of a light-pen, or by more sophisticated automated video processing methods [73]. The previous boundary is divided into a set of segments along which local rectangular regions are set up on the current frame. The boundary on the current frame is then approximated by a set of straight lines, which minimize the square error in each rectangular region with the spatial derivative as its weight.

Tasto developed a guided boundary detection approach, under the assumption that the previous LV boundary is available, either manually drawn or detected semi- or fully-automatically [75, 76]. Cineframes were digitized to 256×256 picture elements with 8 bits accuracy. Then, using the knowledge of the previous boundary and assigning a safety zone around it, a window is constructed, and a new subpicture of 32×32 picture elements is constructed from the fine grid by averaging. Next, to find the current boundary a boundary search range and search directions are constructed around the previous boundary, taking into account two types of prior information: (1) location – the search for the next boundary is restricted to some area around the previous boundary; and (2) direction – only eight search directions at increments of 45° are allowed. For each search path perpendicular to the local direction of the previous contour the gradient function is computed and a point is defined as a new contour point on the basis of a four-feature majority voting scheme, including spatial connectivity and connectivity in time, sizes of the local maxima of the brightness gradient, and sizes of the gradient values one step towards the inside of the ventricle from each local maximum. Finally, three types of postprocessing are applied to each newly found sequence of boundary points, before it is accepted as the actual ventricular boundary: (1) a gap filling operation; (2) a cleaning operation which removes redundant points, loops and bumps; (3) a smoothing operation. They concluded, that the consistency of the algorithm is slightly worse than the consistency of a doctor, but considerably better than the agreement between doctors, engineers and the algorithm.

Later, Tasto described an automated procedure for the definition of the first outline, based on the fact that brightness in the images as a function of time varies much stronger inside the ventricle than outside due to heart contraction and contrast medium fluctuation [76, 77]. A series of successive frames were digitized (256×256) and reduced in size to 32×32 pixels by means of spatial filtering. For each pixel element the average absolute value of the slope of the brightness value versus time was computed (motion value). To separate motion areas from no-motion areas a threshold value was defined by the overall sample mean of the 1024 elements. Following a noise cleaning operation, a binary image of the global ventricular shape was obtained. Finally, the approximate ventricular boundary was found by selecting potential boundary points linewise and columnwise from the center of gravity of the binary picture. To obtain the precise ventricular border in a particular frame an edge detector operator can be applied in conjunction with the global outline.

An approach that differs from previously described works poses the problem of outline or contour extraction as one of minimum cost tree searching [78]. Modestino et al. defined branch costs or metrics which are indicative of the likelihood that a particular branch of the graph lies on the true contour. The branch metrics incorporate both local and global or contextual image information. By this method the outline of the left ventricle plus the aorta are found. A separate algorithm has been developed by Griffith et al. to find the aortic valve and the apex from the entire outline [79]. This is achieved by looking at the amount of 'turn' in the trace at each point along the aorta-ventricle boundary.

A videodensitometric technique for the measurement of left ventricular volume has been described by Trenholm et al. [80]. Left ventricular angiograms were recorded either on video tape or on 16 mm cinefilm; a selected cineframe was converted into video format by means of a vidicon camera. To obtain well-mixed opacified blood into the left ventricle, contrast agent was administered through the right pulmonary artery. A background subtraction technique was applied to a submatrix encompassing the left ventricle in the digitized video image. Subsequently, the video data were preprocessed with a digital low-pass spatial filter. The left ventricular boundary was defined by a simple grey level technique; the critical boundary intensity level was defined as a specified percentage of the mean background intensity level. Applying Lambert-Beer's Law to the left ventricular pixels followed by a summation results in a measure for left ventricular volume. They concluded that the videodensitometric technique with a reduced spatial resolution and 4 bits intensity resolution provides accurate measurements of left ventricular volume; moreover, videodensitometry is the most accurate of single plane techniques (area length and Simpson's Rule).

Clayton et al. have developed a contour detection algorithm for left ventricular angiograms acquired on-line on an analog video disk recorder, which uses a probability product approach [81]. The replayed video images were digitized in a 256×256 matrix with 1024 grey levels. The algorithm consists of four border-defining terms which are combined in a product to represent the likelihood that a particular point along a given line of the digitized matrix should be designated as the border point. The first term in the product, the 'Matched Gradient Filter', employs the concept of spatial differentiation, where the border is assumed to lie in regions of rapidly changing intensity. The second term, the Video Level Predictor, takes into account the brightness profiles at detected border positions on previous video lines. The third, Location term, predicts for a given line the location of the border based on the direction computed from the border positions on the previous two lines. Finally, the fourth, Time Sequence term, predicts for a given line the location of the border in the current video field based upon the border points in the two previous video fields.

Barrett et al. have extended this approach by generating for each of the four terms probability functions based on the contour and video information in a training set [82]. In addition to that, a fifth term, denoted the Quadratic Predictor, has been introduced which is a flexible template or model of the left ventricle constructed from key anatomical features derived from the training set, providing global guidance to the edge detection process. A comparison of hand-traced and computed contours showed over 90% of computer-determined coordinates to lie within the interval of reproducibility for manually traced contours.

Smalling et al. have developed a boundary detection algorithm that relies on two criteria: (1) an intensity gradient criterion; and (2) an absolute intensity criterion [83]. The cineframes were digitized with an image dissector camera in matrix size of 256×304 pixels with 64 levels of grey. Thresholds for both criteria are derived from every 25th line of the first digitized frame in each ventriculogram and thus can be modified on a regional basis. These threshold values are then used to process the rest of the ventriculogram. Since several points on a line satisfying the criteria may be detected, a contour smoothing is subsequently applied to obtain the definite LV contour.

A commercially available analysis system, the Magiscan 2 image analyser, has been developed by Brunt et al. [84, 85]. Left ventricular cineframes are digitized with a video camera at a resolution of $256 \times 256 \times 8$ bits. In the first frame of an angiographic sequence to be analyzed, partial manual initialization is used. To this end, the operator must indicate five reference points: the two margins of the aortic valve, the apex and a position on the inferior and on the anterior wall of the ventricle. From these reference points the program constructs the initial model boundary, which defines a search region; the boundary positions to be detected are forced to lie within this search region. Along the model boundary a total of 72 inital boundary positions with corresponding search directions are defined. The edge detection algorithm is applied along each search direction in turn and incorporates the following criteria: (1) maximal first-derivative of the brightness distribution in the search direction; (2) maximal second-derivative; (3) maximal first-derivative of a cubic fit through the brightness data; (4) fixed fraction between the extremes of the grey levels represented by the fit; (5) extrapolation from the positions of the corresponding boundary points on the previous two frames (if available); and (6) extrapolation from the position of the previous point on the present boundary, using the direction between the equivalent pair of points in the previous frame. The final position chosen along each direction corresponds to a weighted mean of the positions suggested by the individual criteria. Finally, improbably positioned boundary points are removed by repeatedly applying a nonlinear operator to the boundary. In the next frame to be analyzed, the previous boundary is used as a model boundary.

The left ventricular contour detection algorithm developed by Fujita et al. is based on the generation of a gradient image obtained by spatial differentiation of grey levels [86–88]. The cineframes were digitized with a flying spot scanner in matrices of 128×128 pixels with 256 grey levels. The derivative values are modified by two, multiplicative weighting factors, α and β. Alpha is a direction weighting coefficient that prevents the occurrence of abrupt changes in the direction of edge tracing; β is the depth weighting coefficient by which sequential information from remote points can be added. The left ventricular boundary is obtained by selecting points with maximum weighted gradient values. For frame-to-frame analysis boundary information from the preceding frame is incorporated in the edge detection process for the current frame; this has been achieved by adding a constant value to the gradient image of the current frame for positions within an expectation window defined by the preceding contour.

Concluding remarks

From the above it will be clear that various techniques have been developed for the manual, semi- or fully-automated detection of the left ventricular boundaries. Unfortunately, data about the performance of these techniques in terms of accuracy, success score, computation time, etc. again are usually not given in these publications. To our knowledge, none of these automated systems have been perfected to the extent that they are used on a routine basis.

References

1. Brown BG, Bolson EL, Dodge HT: Arteriographic assessment of coronary atherosclerosis. Review of current methods, their limitations, and clinical applications. Arteriosclerosis 2: 2–15, 1982.
2. Gensini GG, Kelly AE, Da Costa BCB, Huntington PP: Quantitative angiography: the measurement of coronary vasomobility in the intact animal and man. Chest 60: 522–530, 1971.
3. Kober G, Spahn G, Spitz P, Becker H–J, Kaltenbach M: Weite der grossen Koronararterien im selektiven Arteriogramm bei Myokardhypertrophie. Verh Dtsch Ges Kreislaufforsch. 38: 191–194, 1972.
4. MacAlpin RN, Abbasi AS, Grollman JH, Eber L: Human coronary artery size during life. A cinearteriographic study. Radiology 108: 567–576, 1973.
5. Feldman RL, Pepine CJ, Curry C, Conty CR: Case against routine use of glyceryl trinitrate before coronary angiography. Br Heart J 40: 992–997, 1978.
6. Rafflenbeul W, Heim R, Dzuiba M, Henkel B, Lichtlen P: Morphometric analysis of coronary arteries. In: Coronary Angiography and Angina Pectoris. PR Lichtlen (Ed). Georg Thieme Publ, Stuttgart: 255–265, 1976.
7. Scoblionko DP, Brown BG, Mitten S, Caldwell JH, Kennedy JW, Bolson EL, Dodge HT: A new digital electronic caliper for measurement of coronary arterial stenosis: comparison with visual estimates and computer-assisted measurements. Am J Cardiol 53: 689–693, 1984.
8. Feldman RL, Pepine CJ, Curry RC, Conty CR: Quantitative coronary arteriography using 105-mm photospot angiography and an optical magnifying device. Cath Cardiovasc Diagn 5: 195–201, 1979.
9. Brown BG, Bolson E, Frimer M, Dodge HT: Quantitative coronary arteriography. Estimation of dimensions, hemodynamic resistance, and atheroma mass of coronary artery lesions using the arteriograms and digital computation. Circulation 55: 329–337, 1977.
10. Barth K, Epple E, Irion KM, Faust U, Decker D: Quantifizierung von Stenosen der Herzkranzgefässe durch digitale Bildauswertung. Erg Bd Biomed Technik 26, 1981:
11. Barth K, Faust U, Both A, Wedekind K: A critical examination of angiographic stenosis quantitation by digital image processing. First IEEE Comp. Soc. Int. Symp. on Medical Imaging and Image Interpretation. IEEE Cat No 82 CH1804–4: 71–76, 1982.
12. Reiber JHC, Gerbrands JJ, Booman F, Troost GJ, Boer A den, Slager CJ, Schuurbiers JCH: Objective characterization of coronary obstructions from monoplane cineangiograms and three-dimensional reconstruction of an arterial segment from two orthogonal views. In: Applications of Computers in Medicine. MD Schwartz (Ed). IEEE Cat No TH0095–0: 93–100, 1982.
13. Kooijman CJ, Reiber JHC, Gerbrands JJ, Schuurbiers JCH, Slager CJ, Boer A den, Serruys PW: Computer-aided quantitation of the severity of coronary obstructions from single view cineangiograms. First IEEE Comp. Soc. Int. Symp. on Medical Imaging and Image Interpretation IEEE Cat No 82 CH1804–4: 59–64, 1982.

232

14. Reiber JHC, Kooijman CJ, Slager CJ, Gerbrands JJ, Schuurbiers JCH, Boer A den, Wijns W, Serruys PW, Hugenholtz PG: Coronary artery dimensions from cineangiograms; methodology and validation of a computer-assisted analysis procedure. IEEE Trans Med Imaging MI–3: 131–141, 1984.

15. Reiber JHC, Serruys PW, Kooijman CJ, Wijns W, Slager CJ, Gerbrands JJ, Schuurbiers JCH, Boer A den, Hugenholtz PG: Assessment of short-, medium- and long-term variations in arterial dimensions from computer-assisted quantitation of coronary cineangiograms. Circulation 71: 280–288, 1985.

16. Reiber JHC, Tijdens FO, Kooijman CJ, Slager CJ, Plas JFAN van der, Frankenhuyzen J van, Ree EJB van, Kalberg RJN, Claessen WCH: A novel approach to the accurate assessment of coronary arterial dimensions from cineangiograms by means of digital imaging techniques. Diagnostic Imaging, April 1985: 87–89.

17. Sanders WJ, Alderman EL, Harrison DC: Coronary artery quantitation using digital image processing techniques. Comp in Card: 15–20, 1979.

18. Alderman EL, Berte LE, Harrison DC, Sanders W: Quantitation of coronary artery dimensions using digital image processing. In: Digital Radiography. WR Brody (Ed.). SPIE Vol 314: 273–278, 1982.

19. Selzer RH, Blankenhorn DH, Crawford DW, Brooks SH, Barndt R: Computer analysis of cardiovascular imagery. Proceedings of the Caltech/JPL Conference on Image Processing Technology, Data Sources and Software for Commercial and Scientific Applications. Pasadena Nov 3–5: 1–20, 1976.

20. Ledbetter DC, Selzer RH, Gordon RM, Blankenhorn DH, Sanmarco ME: Computer quantitation of coronary angiograms. In: Noninvasive Cardiovascular Measurements. HA Miller, EV Schmidt, DC Harrison (Eds.). SPIE Vol 167: 17–20, 1978.

21. Smith DN, Colfer H, Brymer JF, Pitt B, Kliman SH: A semiautomatic computer technique for processing coronary angiograms. Comp in Card: 325–328, 1982.

22. Spears JR, Sandor T, Als AV, Malagold M, Markis JE, Grossman W, Serur JR, Paulin S: Computerized image analysis for quantitative measurement of vessel diameter from cineangiograms. Circulation 68: 453–461, 1983.

23. Kirkeeide RL, Fung P, Smalling RW, Gould KL: Automated evaluation of vessel diameter from arteriograms. Comp in Card: 215–218, 1982.

24. Crawford DW, Brooks SH, Barndt R, Blankenhorn DH: Measurement of atherosclerotic luminal irregularity and obstruction by radiographic densitometry. Invest Radiol 12: 307–313, 1977.

25. Kishon Y, Yerushalmi S, Deutsch V, Neufeld HN: Measurement of coronary arterial lumen by densitometric analysis of angiograms. Angiology 39: 304–312, 1979.

26. Ruhn G, Erikson U, Helmius G, Hemmingsson A: Computerized quantitation of atherosclerosis in an experimental model. Acta Radiologica Diagnosis 23: 621–624, 1982.

27. Collins SM, Skorton DJ, Harrison DG, White CW, Eastham CL, Hiratzka LF, Doty DB, Marcus ML: Quantitative computer-based videodensitometry and the physiological significance of a coronary stenosis. Comp in Cardiol: 219–222, 1982.

28. Pochon Y, Doriot PA, Rasoamanambelo L, Rutishauser W: Densitometry by polychromatic X-ray beam. In: Angiography, Current Status and Future Developments. H Just, P Heintzen (Eds) Springer Verlag, Berlin 1982 (in press).

29. Reiber JHC, Slager CJ, Schuurbiers JCH, Boer A den, Gerbrands JJ, Troost GJ, Scholts B, Kooijman CJ, Serruys PW: Transfer functions of the X-ray-cine-video chain applied to digital processing of coronary cineangiograms. In: Digital Imaging in Cardiovascular Radiology. PH Heintzen, R Brennecke (Eds) Georg Thieme Verlag, Stuttgart: 89–104, 1983.

30. Sandor T, Als AV, Paulin S: Cine-densitometric measurement of coronary arterial stenoses. Cath Cardiovasc Diagn 5: 229–245, 1979.

31. Sandor T, Spears JR, Paulin S: Densitometric determination of changes in the dimensions of

coronary arteries. In: Digital Radiography. WR Brody (Ed) SPIE Vol 314: 263–272, 1982.

32. Spears JR: Rotating step-wedge technique for extraction of luminal cross-sectional area information from single plane coronary cineangiograms. Acta Radiologica Diagnosis 22: 217–225, 1981.

33. Spears JR, Sandor T, Serur J, Paulin S: Computer-aided densitometric evaluation of coronary cineangiograms. In: Radiological Functional Analysis of the Vascular System. FHW Heuck (Ed) Springer-Verlag, Berlin: 195–206, 1983.

34. Nichols AB, Gabrieli CFO, Fenoglio JJ, Esser PD: Quantification of relative coronary arterial stenosis by cinevideodensitometric analysis of coronary arteriograms. Circulation 69: 512–522, 1984.

35. Reiber JHC, Gerbrands JJ, Troost GJ, Kooijman CJ, Slump CH: 3-D Reconstruction of coronary arterial segments from two projections. In: Digital Imaging in Cardiovascular Radiology. PH Heintzen, R Brennecke (Eds). Georg Thieme Verlag, Stuttgart: 151–163, 1983.

36. Spears JR, Sandor T, Kruger R, Hanlon W, Paulin S, Minerbo G: Computer reconstruction of luminal cross-sectional shape from multiple cineangiographic views. IEEE Trans Medical Imaging MI-2: 49–54, 1983.

37. Reiber JHC, Kooijman CJ, Slager CJ, Gerbrands JJ, Schuurbiers JCH, Boer A den, Wijns W, Serruys PW: Computer assisted analysis of the severity of obstructions from coronary cineangiograms; a methodological review. Automedica 5: 219–238, 1984.

38. Wollschläger H, Lee P, Bonzel T, Zeiher A, Just H: Quantitative Koronarangiographie: Neue Vermessungsmethode durch Bestimmung der Vergrösserungsfaktors bei Anwendung der Geometrie biplaner isozentrischer Röntgensysteme. Biomedizinische Technik 29: 53–54, 1984.

39. Bürsch J, Johs R, Heintzen P: Validity of Lambert-Beer's Law in roentgendensitometry of contrast material (Urografin) using continuous radiation. In: Roentgen-, Cine- and Video-Densitometry: Fundamentals and Applications for Blood Flow and Heart Volume Determinations. PH Heintzen (Ed). Georg Thieme Verlag, Stuttgart: 81–84, 1971.

40. Heintzen P, Moldenhauer M: X-ray absorption by contrast material using pulsed radiation. In: Roentgen-, Cine- and Video-Densitometry: Fundamentals and Applications for Blood Flow and Heart Volume Determinations. PH Heintzen (Ed). Georg Thieme Verlag, Stuttgart: 73–81, 1971.

41. Slump CH, Gerbrands JJ: A network flow approach to reconstruction of the left ventricle from two projections. Comp Graphics and Image Processing 18: 18–36, 1982.

42. Baker O, Khalaf J, Chapman CB: A scanner-computer for determining the volumes of cardiac chambers from cinefluorographic films. Am Heart J 62: 797–803, 1961.

43. Cole JS, Brown DD, Glaeser DH: A semiautomated technique for the rapid determination of left ventricular volume from left ventricular cineangiograms. Comp Biom Res 7: 575–589, 1974.

44. Hood WP, Strand EM, Wixson SE, Mantle JA, Smith LR, Zisserman D, Rogers WJ, Russell RO, Rackley CE: Catheterization and angiographic analysis computer applications. Comp in Cardiol: 131–135, 1975.

45. Bove AA, Kreulen TH, Spann JF: Computer analysis of left ventricular dynamic geometry in man. Am J Cardiol 41: 1239–1248, 1978.

46. Brower RW, Meester GT, Hugenholtz PG: Quantification of ventricular performance; a computer-based system for the analysis of angiographic data. Cath Cardiov Diagn 1: 133–155, 1975.

47. Brower RW, Meester GT, Zeelenberg C, Hugenholtz PG: Automatic data processing in the cardiac catheterization laboratory. Comp Progr Biomed 7: 99–110, 1977.

48. Rasmussen D: Computer measurement and representation of the heart in two and three dimensions. In: Cardiovascular Imaging and Image Processing. Theory and Practice – 1975. DC Harrison, H Sandler, HA Miller (Eds.). SPIE 72: 177–182, 1975.

49. Alderman EL, Sandler H, Brooker JZ, Sanders WJ, Simpson C, Harrison DC: Light-pen computer processing of video image for the determination of left ventricular volume. Circulation 47: 309–316, 1973.

50. Alderman EL: Clinical application of a light-pen computer system for quantitative angiography. In: Cardiovascular Imaging and Image Processing. Theory and Practice – 1975. DC Harrison, H

Sandler, HA Miller (Eds.). SPIE 72: 209–216, 1975.

51. Alderman EL, Sandler H, Brooker JZ, Sanders WJ, Simpson C, Harrison DC: Light-pen computer processing of video image for the determination of left ventricular volume. Circulation 47: 309–316, 1973.

52. Heintzen PH, Malerczyk V, Pilarczyk J, Scheel KW: On-line processing of the video-image for left ventricular volume determination. Comp Biom Res 4: 474–485, 1971.

53. Heintzen PH, Malerczyk V, Pilarczyk J: A videometric technique for automated processing of pressure-volume-diagrams. Comp Biom Res 4: 486–492, 1971.

54. Heintzen PH, Brennecke R, Bürsch JH, Lange P, Malerczyk V, Moldenhauer K, Onnasch D: Automated videoangiocardiographic image analysis. IEEE Computer 8: 55–64, 1975.

55. Brennecke R, Brown TK, Bürsch JH, Heintzen PH: A digital system for Roentgen-Video Image Processing. In: Roentgen-Video-Techniques for Dynamic Studies of Structure and Function of the Heart and Circulation. PH Heintzen, JH Bürsch (Eds.) Georg Thieme Publishers, Stuttgart: 150–157, 1978.

56. Brennecke R, Brown TK, Bürsch J, Heintzen PH: Computerized video-image preprocessing with applications to cardio-angiographic roentgen-image series. In: Digitale Bildverarbeitung. HH Nagel (Ed.). Springer-Verlag, Berlin/Heidelberg/New York: 244–262, 1977.

57. Bürsch JH, Radtke W, Rünger T, Moldenhauer K, Hoffmann B, Heintzen PH: Endocardial and epicardial contour detection of the left ventricle by digital angiocardiography. In: Ventricular Wall Motion. U Sigwart, PH Heintzen (Eds.). Georg Thieme Verlag, Stuttgart/New York: 49–57, 1984.

58. Sturm RE, Wood EH: The video quantizer: An electronic photometer to measure contrast in roentgen fluoroscopic images. Mayo Clinic Proc 43: 803–806, 1968.

59. Ritman EL, Sturm E, Wood EH: A biplane roentgen videometry system for dynamic (60/second) studies of the shape and size of circulatory structures, particularly the left ventricle. In: Roentgen-, Cine-, and Video-Densitometry: Fundamentals and Applications for Blood Flow and Heart Volume Determination. PH Heintzen (Ed) Georg Thieme Verlag, Stuttgart: 179–211, 1971.

60. Wood EH, Ritman EL, Sturm RE, Johnson S, Spivak P, Gilbert BK, Smith HC: The problem of determination of the roentgen density, dimensions and shape of homogeneous objects from biplane roentgenographic data with particular reference to angiocardiography. Proc of the San Diego Biomedical Symposium 11: 3–43, 1972.

61. Greenleaf JF, Ritman EL, Wood EH, Frye RL, Robb RA, Johnson SA: Dynamic computer generated displays for study of the human left ventricle. Proc SPIE, Developments in Electronic Imaging Techniques, 32: 111–119, 1972.

62. Ritman EL, Sturm RE, Wood EH: Biplane roentgen videometric system for dynamic (60/sec) studies of the shape and size of circulatory structures, particularly the left ventricle..Am J Cardiol 32: 180–187, 1973.

63. Covvey HD: Measuring the human heart with a real-time computing system. Data Processing Magazine: 27–32, 1970.

64. Marcus ML, Schuette WH, Whitehouse WC, Bailey JJ, Glancy DL: An automated method for the measurement of ventricular volume. Circulation 45: 65–76, 1972.

65. Marcus ML, Schuette WH, Whitehouse WC, Bailey JJ, Douglas MA, Glancy DL: Use of a video system in the study of ventricular function in man. Am J Cardiol 32: 175–179, 1973.

66. de Jong LP, Slager CJ: Automatic detection of the left ventricular outline in angiographs using television signal processing techniques. IEEE Trans Biomed Eng, BME-22: 230–237, 1975.

67. Reiber JHC: Real time detection and data acquisition system for the left ventricular outline. In: Cardiovascular Imaging and Image Processing. Theory and Practice – 1975. DC Harrison, H Sandler, HA Miller (Eds.). SPIE 72: 139–147, 1975.

68. Reiber JHC: Real time detection and data acquisition system for the left ventricular outline. Ph.D. thesis, Stanford Univ. 1975.

69. Slager CJ, Reiber JHC, Schuurbiers JCH, Meester GT: Contouromat – A hardwired left

ventricular angioprocessing system. I. Design and application. Comput Biomed Res 11: 491–502, 1978.

70. Robb RA: Computer-aided contour determination and dynamic display of individual cardiac chambers from digitized serial angiocardiographic film. In: Roentgen-, Cine-, and Video-Densitometry: Fundamentals and Applications for Blood Flow and Heart Volume Determination, PH Heintzen (Ed.) Georg Thieme Verlag, Stuttgart: 170–178, 1971.

71. Robb RA: Computer aided analysis of cardiac dynamics using roentgenographic and videometric techniques. Ph.D. Dissertation, University of Utah, 1971.

72. Wiscomb WK: A hardware system for man-machine interaction in the study of left ventricular dynamics. In: Roentgen-, Cine-, and Video-Densitometry: Fundamentals and Applications for Blood Flow and Heart Volume Determination. PH Heintzen (Ed.) Georg Thieme Verlag, Stuttgart: 165–169, 1971.

73. Chow CK, Kaneko T: Automatic boundary detection of the left ventricle from cineangiograms. Comp Biom Res 5: 388–410, 1972.

74. Kaneko T, Mancini P: Straight-line approximation for the boundary of the left ventricular chamber from a cardiac cineangiogram. IEEE Trans Biom Res, BME-20: 413–416, 1973.

75. Tasto M: Guided boundary detection for left ventricular volume measurements. Proc First Int Joint Conf on Pattern Recognition, Washington DC, 1973.

76. Tasto M, Felgendreher M, Spiesberger W, Spiller P: Comparison of manual versus computer determination of left ventricular boundaries from X-ray cineangiograms. In: Roentgen-Video-Techniques for Dynamic Studies of Structure and Function of the Heart and Circulation. PH Heintzen, JH Bürsch (Eds.) Georg Thieme Publishers, Stuttgart: 168–183, 1978.

77. Tasto M: Motion extraction for left-ventricular volume measurement. IEEE Trans Biom Eng, BME-21: 207–213, 1974.

78. Modestino JW, Kaufman H, Grant C, Griffith R: Digital image processing with application to angiocardiograms. Presented at Eascon, 1974.

79. Griffith RL, Grant C, Kaufman H: An algorithm for locating the aortic valve and the apex in left-ventricular angiocardiograms. IEEE Trans Biom Eng, BME-21: 345–349, 1974.

80. Trenholm BG, Winter DA, Reimer GD, Mymin D, Lansdown EL, Sharma GP: Automated ventricular volume calculations from single plane images. Radiology 112: 299–304, 1974.

81. Clayton PD, Harris LD, Rumel SR, Warner HR: Left ventricular videometry. Comp Biom Res 7: 369–379, 1974.

82. Barrett WA, Clayton PD, Warner HR: Determination of left ventricular contours: a probabilistic algorithm derived from angiographic images. Comp Biom Res 13: 522–548, 1980.

83. Smalling RW, Skolnick MH, Myers D, Shabetei R, Cole JC, Johnston D: Digital boundary detection, volumetric and wall motion analysis of left ventricular cine angiograms. Comput Biol Med 6: 73–85, 1976.

84. Brunt JNH, Taylor CJ, Rowlands DJ: A software based system for geometrical analysis of left ventricular cineangiograms. Comp Cardiol: 437–440, 1979.

85. Brunt JNH, Taylor CJ, Dixon RN: Theory and practice of applying image analysis to angiography. In: Physical Techniques in Cardiological Imaging. MD Short, DA Pay, S Leeman, RM Harrison (Eds.). Adam Hilger Ltd., Bristol: 153–162, 1983.

86. Eiho S, Kuwahara M, Fujita M, Sasayama S, Kawai C: Boundary detection of left ventricle from cineangiocardiograms and analysis of regional left ventricular wall motion. Proc. 6th Conf. Computer Applications in Radiology and Computer/Aided Analysis of Radiological Images. IEEE Cat No 79CH1404-3C: 221–227, 1979.

87. Fujita M, Sasayama S, Kawai C, Eiho S, Kuwahara M: Automatic processing of cineventriculograms for analysis of regional myocardial function. Circulation 63: 1065–1074, 1981.

88. Sasayama S, Fujita M, Nonogi H, Kawai C, Eiho S, Kuwahara M: Quantitative assessment of regional disorders of left ventricular wall motion in patients with coronary artery disease by cineventriculography. In: Ventricular Wall Motion. U Sigwart, PH Heintzen (Eds.) Georg Thieme Verlag, Stuttgart/New York: 62–73, 1984.

Table X.1. Overview of computerized systems for quantitative analysis of coronary cineangiograms.

		Barth	Brown	Collins	Kirkeeide	Kishon	Nichols
1.	Cineflim conversion	photometer scanner; region of interest of size 256 × 256 pixels within 35 mm frame selected and digitized	optical projection; 5 × magnification	images projected at high magnification	cinefilm projection system	linewise scanning with 1024 photodiodes 25 μm apart perpendicular to arterial long axis	Vanguard projector M-35C with video camera attachment (model 1 XR-TV-1)
	Type video camera	–	–	Hamamatsu C1000 video camera	vidicon camera	–	vidicon camera
2.	Computer system and imaging system	PDP 11/40 + image store with pseudo color	PDP 11/45	Portion of optically magnified image digitized into 256 × 256 × 8 matrix	Spatial Data Systems Eyecom II Image Analyzer. Image Analysis on VAX 11/780. Images digitized into 640 × 640 × 8 matrix.	–	MDS-system A². (Nova computer). Image digitized into 512 × 512 × 8 matrix.
3.	Pixel width of digitized image, referred to original cineframe	10 μm	–	–	20–100 μm	25 μm	–
4.	Definition of coronary segment to be analyzed	user indicates starting point + direction within segment; subsequent automated tracking of centerline	user manually traces boundaries of coronary segment on projected image with 0.1 mm resolution	user selects number of scanlines at obstruction and reference point for densitometric analysis	–	user tracks arterial pathway	user selects two rectangular ROI's, two pixels in width across the stenotic and normal segments of the artery.
5.	Edge-definition	2-D info encompassing	manual tracing	user identifies approximate vessel	edge-points defined at user-selected	edge points manually defined	no edge-detection algorithm used.

	1	2	3	4	5
	artery stretched; correlate edge model (18–27 pixels wide) to brightness info along horizontal lines; contour points correspond with max. 2nd-deriv. response of model		edges from density profile and its first-derivative	threshold level of grey scale derivative function, computed by least squares convolution technique with a quadratic function	on densitometric curve at sharp rise above background level
6. Pincushion correction?	no	yes, assuming distortion being radially symmetric; relative magnification computed with empirically determined analytical function of radius	no	no	no
7. Method of calibration to convert measurements to absolute sizes	analytically from geometric X-ray system parameters	catheter manually traced in biplane views	catheter segment analyzed in same manner as for arterial segment	—	on basis of radiopaque markers spaced 1 cm apart on catheter.
8. Single/biplane analysis of coronary segment?	single	biplane	single	single	single
9. Correction for differential magnification between catheter and arterial segments from biplane views possible?	no	yes	no	no	no

	Barth	Brown	Collins	Kirkeeide	Kishon	Nichols
10. Reference for %-D stenosis measurement	user-defined	user-defined	user-defined	–	user-defined	user-defined
11. Densitometry	analytically using basic formulas describing imaging chain	no	along density profile within the vessel, logarithm of grey level computed and background corrected by subtraction of logarithm of average background grey level	no	scanner reads optical density levels from cinefilm	videodensity of cinefilm is linearly proportional to amount of contrast medium
12. Basis for computation cross-sectional narrowing	integrated thickness profiles from densitometry	eliptical cross sections from biplane contour data	integrated density levels	–	integrated density levels	integrated density level in rectangular ROI corrected for background videodensity measured in 2 ROI's (each 2×2 pixels) positioned adjacent to the end of the arterial ROI's
13. 3-D reconstruction	from 1 view thickness info per slice placed symmetrically with respect to scanline; symmetric corrections if 2nd view available	assuming elliptical cross sections using contour information from biplane views	no	no	no	no

	Reiber	Sanders	Sandor/Spears	Selzer	Smith
1. Cinefilm conversion	computer controlled cine-video projector system with optical magnifications of 0.7, 1.0, 1.4, 2.0, 2.8 and 4.0;	cine-video projector system with optical magnifications of 1, 3.7 and 7; motor controlled x-y positioning of lens turret and video camera;	cine-video projector system with interchangeable optics	cine-video projector system with optical magnifications of 1, 2.5, 3.7; motor controlled x-y positioning of lens turret and video camera;	video camera positioned such that region of interest in 35 mm frame is scanned
Type video camera	1.5" vidicon camera	1" vidicon camera	1" vidicon camera	vidicon camera	–
2. Computer system and imaging system	PDP 11/44 + VTE Image Digitizer with storage for 8 $512 \times 512 \times 8$ matrices	HP2100 + DeAnza model 5524 Image Digitizer with storage for 3 $480 \times 512 \times 8$ matrices	VAX 11/780 + EyeCom Picture Analyzer	PDP 11/45 + DeAnza IP 5500 Image Array Processor	Cyto-computer
3. Pixel width of digitized image, referred to original cineframe	15 μm (2.0× optical magnification)	13 μm (3.7× magnification)	10–20μm	15.6 μm (2.5 × magn.) or 10.6 μm (3.7 × magn.)	–
4. Definition of coronary segment to be analyzed	user indicates number of center points within coronary segment	user manually traces boundaries of coronary segment	curve fitting to a series of midpoints located between edges in horizontal camera scans	user indicates number of center points approximating the vessel path	centerline determined automatically in binary image following background subtr. and user-selection of brightness threshold
5. Edge-definition	contour path determined in cost matrix based on weighted sum of 1st- and 2nd-deriv. functions; 2 iterations	max 1st-deriv. of density profiles perpendicular to initially manually defined margin	automatically at base or max. slope of optical density profiles	max. intensity gradient (1st-deriv.); 2 iterations	user-defined threshold following local background subtraction

	Reiber	Sanders	Sandor/Spears	Selzer	Smith
6. Pincushion correction?	yes; intersection points of cm-grid detected automatically; correction vector computed for each pixel	yes; relative magnification factor for each radial distance stored; assessed from cm grid	no	no	no
7. Method of calibration to convert measurements to absolute sizes	automated edge detection of catheter segment; optical magnification 2.8	object size determined from 2 orthogonal views (isocenter) on the basis of X-ray system geometry	no absolute measurements	edge detection of catheter segment	catheter segment analyzed in same way as for arterial segments
8. Single/biplane analysis of coronary segment?	single or biplane	single or biplane	single	single	single
9. Correction for differential magnification between catheter and arterial segments from biplane views possible?	yes	yes	no	no	no
10. Reference for %-D stenosis measurement	–user-defined –interpolated technique for estimation 'normal' vessel diameters (tapering vessel allowed)	user-defined	user-defined	computer-lumen technique for estimating 'normal' vessel diameters (allows tapering vessel)	proximal normal segment
11. Densitometry	21 homogeneously exposed density frames generated on each patient film for conversion density levels to arterial thickness	no	rotating step wedge technique for conversion density levels to arterial thickness data	yes, details unknown	no

XV. Quantitative Assessment of regional left ventricular function: enclosed wall landmark motion

12.	Basis for computation cross-sectional narrowing	−nondensitometric: circular cross sections from single plane contour data −densitometric: integrated thickness profiles from densitometry	circular (single plane) or elliptical (biplane) cross sections from contour data	planimetric area determination under thickness distribution curves	unknown	circular cross sections from single plane contour data
13.	3-D reconstruction	from 2 orthogonal views using contour and densitometric information	program from Brown	−	no	−

XI. Quantitative Assessment of regional left ventricular function: endocardial landmark motion

Summary

In this study the hypothesis is tested that the motion patterns of small anatomical landmarks, which can be recognized along the left ventricular endocardial border in contrast angiocardiograms, reflect the motion of the endocardial wall. To validate this hypothesis, minute metal markers were inserted into the endocardium of eight pigs with a novel retrograde transvascular approach. Marker motion was subsequently recorded with roentgen cinematography and compared with the motion of the landmarks along the endocardial contours detected from the contrast ventriculograms with the Contouromat. Linear regression analysis of the directions of the systolic metal marker trajectories and of the endocardial landmark trajectories yielded a correlation coefficient of r = 0.86 and a SEE of 10.3⁰. Landmark pathways were also measured in 23 normal human left ventriculograms. From this human study it was concluded, that normal left ventricular endocardial wall motion during systole as observed in the 30° RAO view is characterized by a dominant inward transversal motion of the opposite anterior and infero-posterior walls and a descent of the base towards the apex. The apex itself is almost stationary. Based on these observations a widely applicable mathematical model for left ventricular wall motion was developed.

Introduction

Although contrast angiography provides detailed information about the left ventricular endocardial boundaries, quantitative manual analysis of contrast ventriculograms has not been able to reveal the actual pathways of specific sites on the endocardium. In animals, these pathways can easily be followed with endocardially implanted metal clips and roentgencinematography [1–3]. For obvious reasons, these endocardial markers were never inserted in humans, although midwall and epicardial motion have been studied in humans with surgically implanted metal markers [4–7]. However, major differences exist, both in extent and direction, between the motion of neighboring endocardial, midwall and epicardial sites as the wall thickens [1, 8]. Therefore, none of these methods can provide an accurate description of endocardial motion. The Contouromat allows the detection of small landmarks along the left ventricular contrast border, which can be followed throughout the cardiac cycle by analysis of consecutive frames of the cineangiogram. In this study, the hypothesis that these landmarks actually represent the temporal motion of specific anatomical sites has been validated with the information from minute 'harpoons' injected into the endocardium of piglets. By comparing the mean systolic pathways of these artificial landmarks with those occurring naturally, their usefulness could be substantiated. Subsequently, the landmark trajectories in normal human individuals as assessed from left ventricular cineangiograms were determined and a widely applicable mathematical model for the description of human left ventricular wall motion was derived.

Materials and methods

The first study group consisted of eight anesthetized pigs with a weight of 24 ± 3 kg (mean $\pm$ s.d.). Left ventricular pressures were monitored with tip-micromanometer catheters. A 7F Gorlin pacing catheter was introduced into the coronary sinus. A fixed heart rate at 10 bpm above resting heart rate was maintained during the study. Left ventriculography was performed during injection of 0.75 ml/kg Urographin 76* at a rate of 12 ml/s through an 8F angio catheter. The opacified ventricles were filmed in the left lateral projection at a rate of 50 frames per second. During angiography artificial respiration was stopped to exclude extracardiac motion. After the acquisition of a technically satisfactory cineangiogram, specific sites of the endocardial wall were marked with small metal darts or 'miniharpoons'. For this purpose a springloaded insertion device (Fig. XI.1) attached to the tip of a flexible catheter with tip steering facilities* * was used. The combination of the sharp barbed hook and a blunt body guarantees an excellent fixation of the marker with minimal damage to the myocardium and an accurate delineation of the endocardium. In each pig five markers were inserted along the anterior and infero-posterior walls of the left ventricle in a pattern outlining the ventricular cavity as seen in the left lateral projection (Fig. XI.2). In order to detect possibly occurring myocardial injury due to the insertion procedure, the ECG and left ventricular pressure were monitored continuously. Once marker insertion was completed, a second left ventricular angiogram was taken with identical X-ray geometry and with the respirator turned off. A

---

* Schering A.G., Berlin, Bergkammer, G.F.R.
* * Muller Guide System and Variflex 7F catheter, USCI, Billerica, USA.

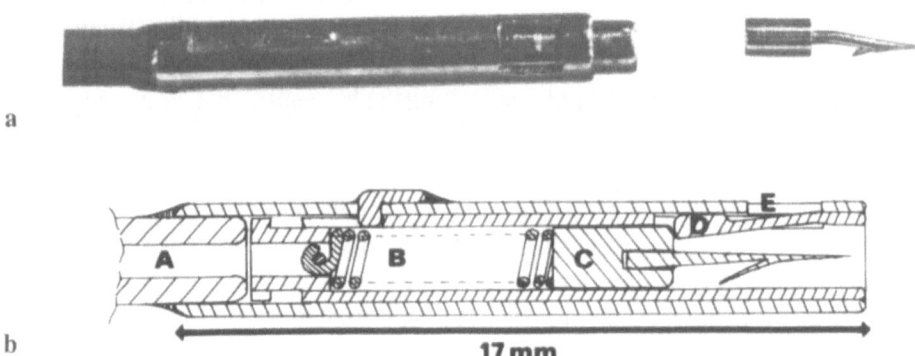

a

b

17 mm

Fig. XI.1. Schematic drawing and photograph of spring loaded metal marker insertion device attached to the tip of a 7F catheter. The inner tube – including trigger lever D – is advanced by manual injection of saline into the catheter A, thus releasing metal marker C.

centimeter grid was filmed for calibration purposes. An interval of at least 30 minutes was observed between the consecutive angiograms.

The second study group consisted of 23 individuals, submitted to a diagnostic heart catheterization because of suspected heart disease, who appeared to have no hemodynamic or angiocardiographic abnormalities. Patients were studied after an overnight fast without premedication; all drugs which might influence left

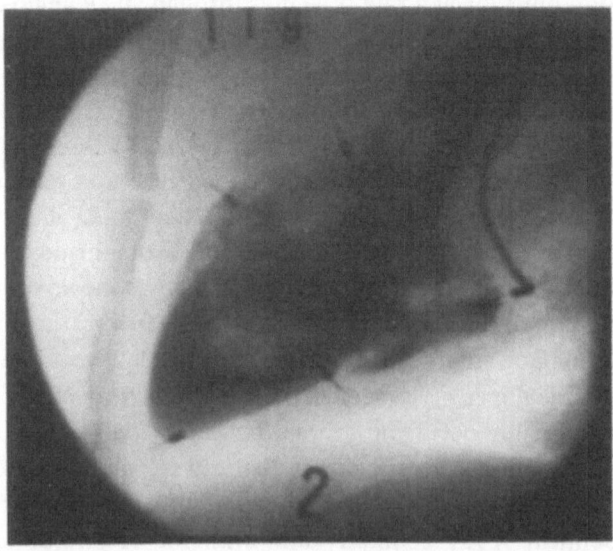

Fig. XI.2. End-diastolic frame from pig left ventricular angiogram with metal markers outlining the left ventricular cavity as seen in the left lateral projection.

ventricular contractile function were discontinued at least 24 hours prior to the study. Left ventricular cineangiography was performed at resting heart rate, during injection of 0.75 mg/kg Urographin 76 at a rate of 16–18 ml/s. The 30° RAO projection of the opacified ventricle was filmed at a rate of 40–80 (typically 50) frames per second. During angiography care was taken to maintain a steady position of the patient with regard to the X-ray equipment, while respiratory motion was prevented by suspended respiration. For calibration purposes a centimeter grid was filmed at midthoracic level.

The endocardial outlines of both the human and pig contrast angiograms were determined on a frame-by-frame basis with the Contouromat (Chapter IV). In each frame left ventricular volume was determined according to Simpson's rule [9]. End diastole and end systole were defined as the moments of maximal and minimal left ventricular volume, respectively. The detected contours of all systolic frames were displayed on a video monitor and collectively recorded on a single 8.3×10.8 cm Polaroid photograph. The contours were displayed as detected from the cineframes, i.e. a fixed external reference system was employed [10]; translational and/or rotational 'correction' procedures were not applied. On this contour-graph small landmarks at varying sites along the left ventricular contrast border can be traced over substantial parts of the systolic period. However, the information may be partially obscured by the overlap of successive contours. To eliminate such superimposition, a 'shift' procedure was applied to the detected contours [11]. An example of such a set of superimposed and shifted contours is shown in Fig. XI.3a. After photographic enlargement of the shifted contours, the various pathways of these landmarks were traced manually (Fig. XI.3b). Subsequent interpolation between neighboring pathways (Fig. XI.3c) and correction for the previously added shift yielded a set of actual systolic trajectories projected onto the original frame of reference (Fig. XI.3d).

The pig contrast cardioangiograms obtained after metal marker implantation were projected onto a sheet of paper. The end-diastolic and end-systolic contours were drawn manually and the positions of the markers indicated. In subsequent calculations the curved systolic landmark and marker trajectories were represented by straight vectors connecting the end-diastolic with the end-systolic positions of these trajectories, respectively.

For subsequent quantitative analysis a nonindexed rectangular coordinate system was defined on the basis of the end-diastolic contour. The origin coincided with the end-diastolic apex, defined as the point at maximal distance from the superior aspect of the aortic valve [12]. A basal transverse axis, extending from the mitral valve fornix to a point on the opposite anterior wall, was constructed, such that an isosceles triangle with its vertex at the ventricular apex arises (Fig. XI.4). The ventricular long axis was defined as the median of this triangle through the vertex; the y-axis of the coordinate system coincides with this line.

To be able to compare the landmark pathways of ventricles with different shapes and sizes, a normalization procedure was carried out. As a first step ten

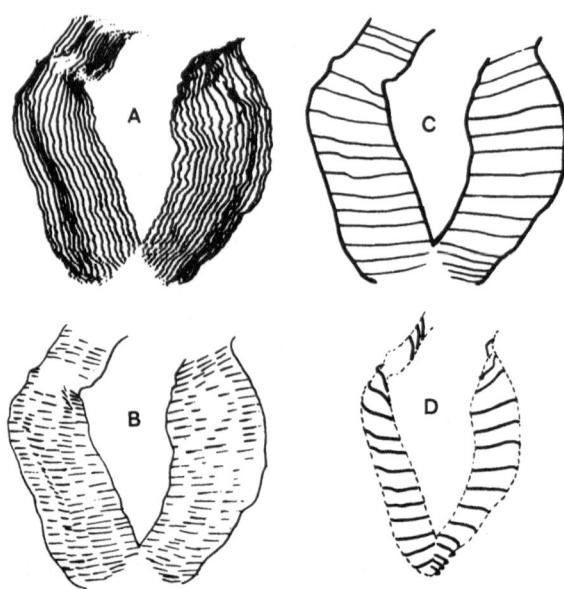

Fig. XI.3a. Results from automated frame-by-frame analysis of the endocardial contours over the systolic period from a left ventricular cineangiocardiogram; subsequent contours have been shifted artificially in horizontal directions.

Fig. XI.3b. Pathways of small anatomical landmarks along the left ventricular contrast border were analyzed, resulting in a pattern of trajectories.

Fig. XI.3c. Interpolation between neighboring pathways allows the definition of a set of trajectories covering the entire systolic period.

Fig. XI.3d. Correction for the previously added shift yields the actual endocardial landmark motion with respect to the original frame of reference.

equidistant points were defined along the long axis. Lines through these points with a direction perpendicular to the long axis defined a total of twenty intersection points with the end-diastolic contour (Fig. XI.4). These twenty points were defined as the end-diastolic starting points of new pathways with magnitude and direction obtained by interpolation of the results from the previously mentioned neighboring landmarks along the endocardial border. For both the human and pig ventricles, left ventricular dimensions were normalized such that for each study group the end-diastolic long axis lengths became equal to the mean value. As a result of this procedure, corresponding starting points had equal y-coordinates, but still different x-coordinates. Finally, the (normalized) systolic trajectories of corresponding starting points were shifted parallel to the x-axis, such that the starting points coincided with the mean value of the individual x-coordinates (Fig. XI.5).

Finally, the individual pathways were decomposed into their x- and y-components, expressed as $\triangle x$ and $\triangle y$ with respect to the defined coordinate system. The direction of each pathway was defined by the acute angle between the pathway and the x-axis, in formula:

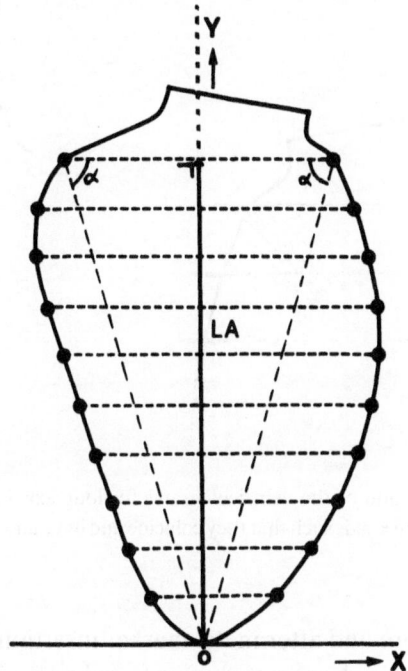

Fig. XI.4. The median of an isosceles triangle with its vertex at the ventricular apex and its base extending from the mitral valve fornix, defines the y-axis of the applied rectangular coordinate system. Left ventricular long axis length (L) is defined by the distance from base to apex. A total of 20 end-diastolic starting points, generated at equidistant y-levels are defined for the assessment of pathways of the endocardial landmarks.

$$\alpha = \text{arc tg} \frac{|\triangle x|}{\triangle y} \qquad \qquad \text{(XI.1)}$$

Using linear regression analysis, the extent and direction of the metal marker pathways, defined by $\triangle x_{metal}$, $\triangle y_{metal}$ and α_{metal}, were compared with the nearest corresponding endocardial landmark pathways, defined by $\triangle x_{endo}$, $\triangle y_{endo}$ and α_{endo}. Statistical analysis was performed with the paired t-test of Student (border of significance: $p = 0.05$).

Results

Endocardial wall motion in pigs

The mean and standard deviations (s.d.) of the hemodynamic variables left ventricular end-diastolic volume (LVEDV), ejection fraction (EF), end-diastolic pressure (LVEDP) and peak dP/dt (peak rate of change of pressure), as well as

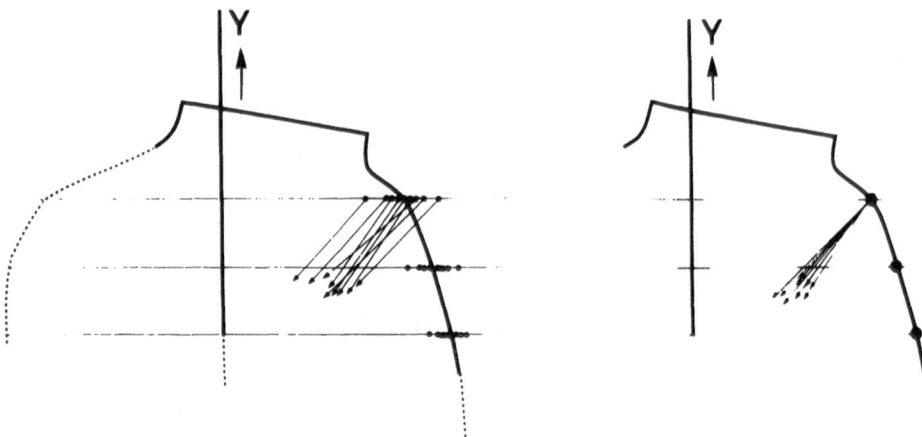

Fig. XI.5. After normalization of the ventriculograms for long axis length, corresponding starting points were shifted along the x-axis such that they coincide and have an x-coordinate equal to the mean x-value.

heart rate (HR), before and after metal marker insertion are presented in Table XI.1. The hemodynamic changes were not found to be significantly different.

Following the experiment the areas of the myocardium where marker insertion had taken place were inspected visually. No substantial damage such as hemorrhage or cardiac rupture was observed.

In Fig. XI.6 the normalized systolic pathways of the endocardial landmarks of each individual pig (1a – 8a) are shown, with the systolic pathways of the implanted metal markers of the same ventricles (1b – 8b). Comparison of the x- and y-components of corresponding pathways of endocardial landmarks ($\triangle x_{endo}$ and $\triangle y_{endo}$) and of metal markers ($\triangle x_{metal}$ and $\triangle y_{metal}$) resulted in correlation coefficients of r = 0.74 and r = 0.86, respectively with the linear regression equations given by:

Table XI.1. Hemodynamic data before and after metal marker implantation in 8 pigs.

	Control	Markers implanted	Statistical significance
LVEDV [ml]	28.5 ± 5.2	29.4 ± 6.7	n.s.
EF [%]	61.4 ± 14.2	56.3 ± 12.0	n.s.
LVEDP [kPa]	1.4 ± 0.3	1.1 ± 0.5	n.s.
pk dP/dt [kPa/s]	230 ± 37	191 ± 52	n.s.
HR [bpm]	88 ± 5	87 ± 3	n.s.

Abbreviations: LVEDV, left ventricular end-diastolic volume; EF, ejection fraction; LVEDP, left ventricular end-diastolic pressure; HR, heart rate; bpm, beats per minute; n.s., not significant at a p-value of 0.05 (Student t-test).

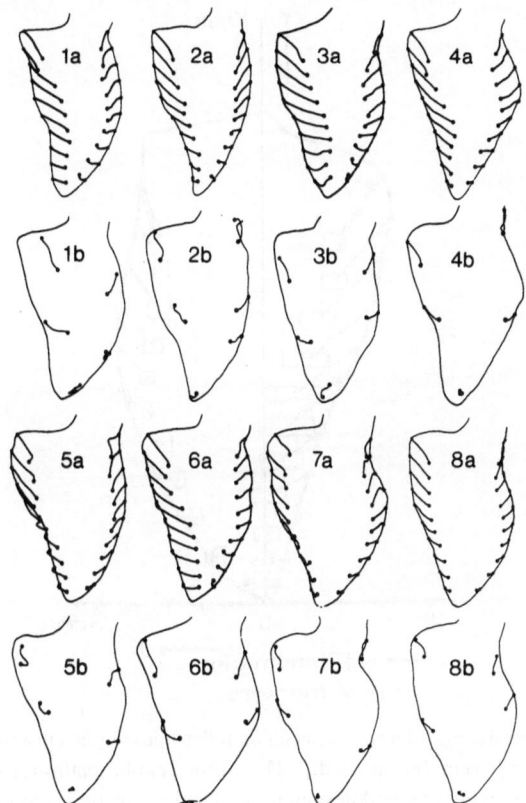

Fig. XI.6. Normalized left ventricular systolic pathways of the endocardial landmarks of each individual pig (1a–8a). In Figs 1b–8b the systolic pathways of the implanted metal markers in the same pig ventricles are shown.

$$|x_{endo}| = 0.16\,\text{cm} + 1.2|x_{metal}|; \tag{XI.2}$$
$$y_{endo} = -0.13\,\text{cm} + y_{metal}, \tag{XI.3}$$

These results are based on a total of 41 pairs of data. The relation between the directions of the endocardial landmark pathways and those of the metal marker pathways was similarly evaluated.

$$\alpha_{endo} = 0.86\alpha_{metal} - 2.9°,$$
$$r = 0.86, \text{SEE} = 10.3°, N = 33 \tag{XI.4}$$

In this last comparison the apical segments were excluded as the displacements of these segments are characterized by such short trajectories, that accurate assessment of α is almost impossible.

Figure XI.7 shows the normalized shape of the end-diastolic left ventricular contours of the eight animals with the mean systolic pathways of the endocardial landmarks and their standard deviations, as well as the mean pathways of the metal markers. Left ventricular long axis length was $7.3 \pm 0.4\,\text{cm}$ (mean $\pm$ s.d.).

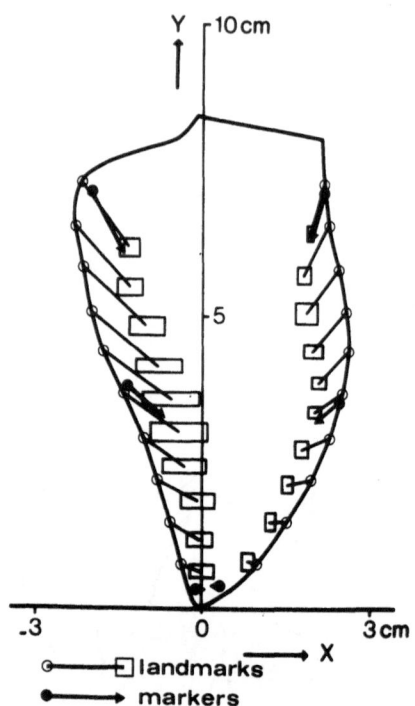

Fig. XI.7. Mean normalized shape of left ventricular end-diastolic contours in 8 pigs. Left ventricular long axis length is 7.3 ± 0.4 cm (mean $\pm$ s.d.). The mean systolic pathways of the endocardial landmarks are shown with their standard deviations in x- and y-directions represented by means of rectangles, as well as the mean metal marker pathways.

Endocardial wall motion in humans

The normalized starting point positions which define the normalized shape of the end-diastolic left ventricular contour with the mean and standard deviation of their x-coordinates in the 23 normal human subjects are presented in Fig. XI.8. Left ventricular long axis length was 8.3 ± 1.3 cm (mean $\pm$ s.d.). The mean systolic landmark pathways and their standard deviations are presented in Fig. XI.9. The points of intersection of the mean pathways extending from the ten pairs of opposing starting points are depicted in figure XI.10a; the x- and y-coordinates of these intersection points are given as well. For the second pair taken from the apex position, no point of intersection could be found within the ventricular cavity because of an almost parallel course of the opposite trajectories. The results shown in Fig. XI.10a can be formulated mathematically, so that for any point of an end-diastolic contour the approximative mean direction of motion can be calculated. Let L be the length of the end-diastolic long axis, (x_a, y_a) the coordinates of a point along the anterior wall and (x_i, y_i) the coordinates of a point along the opposite infero-posterior wall such that $y_a = y_i = y$. Then, to a first approximation, the coordinates (x_p, y_p) of the point towards which both opposite

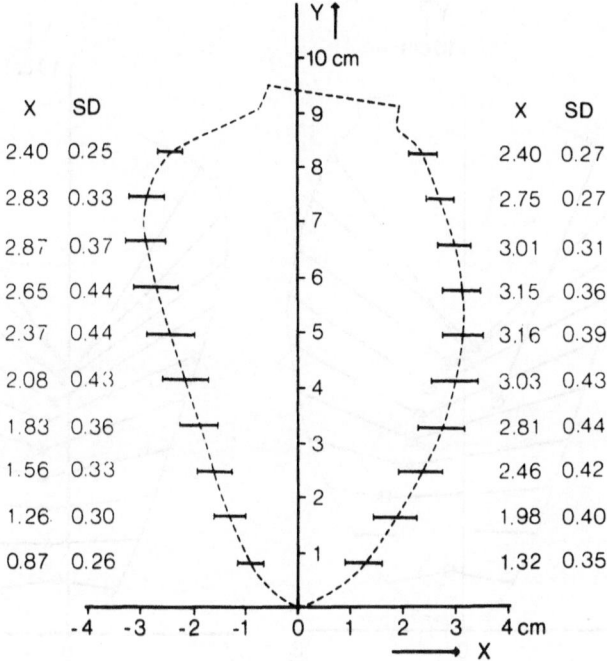

X	SD		X	SD
2.40	0.25		2.40	0.27
2.83	0.33		2.75	0.27
2.87	0.37		3.01	0.31
2.65	0.44		3.15	0.36
2.37	0.44		3.16	0.39
2.08	0.43		3.03	0.43
1.83	0.36		2.81	0.44
1.56	0.33		2.46	0.42
1.26	0.30		1.98	0.40
0.87	0.26		1.32	0.35

Fig. XI.8. Normalized shape of the end-diastolic left ventricular contour of 23 normal human subjects. Dimensions are expressed in cm; left ventricular long axis length is 8.3 ± 1.3 cm (mean ± s.d.).

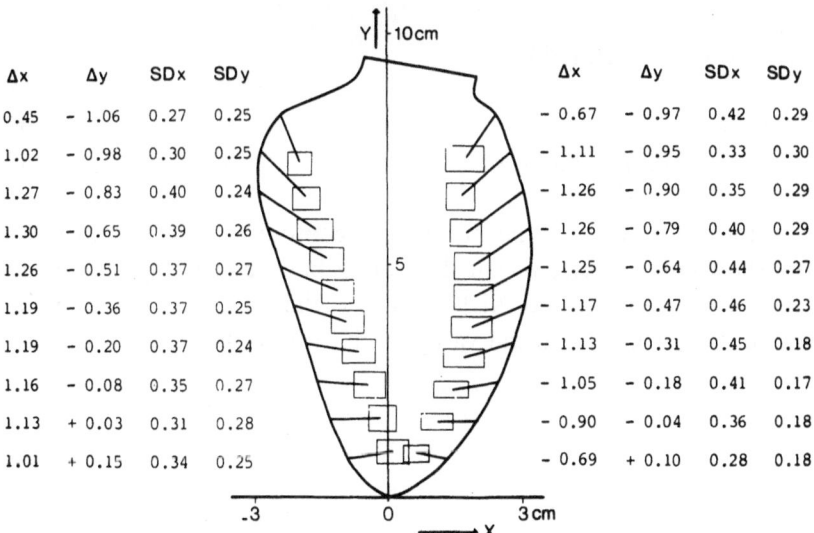

Δx	Δy	SDx	SDy		Δx	Δy	SDx	SDy
0.45	− 1.06	0.27	0.25		− 0.67	− 0.97	0.42	0.29
1.02	− 0.98	0.30	0.25		− 1.11	− 0.95	0.33	0.30
1.27	− 0.83	0.40	0.24		− 1.26	− 0.90	0.35	0.29
1.30	− 0.65	0.39	0.26		− 1.26	− 0.79	0.40	0.29
1.26	− 0.51	0.37	0.27		− 1.25	− 0.64	0.44	0.27
1.19	− 0.36	0.37	0.25		− 1.17	− 0.47	0.46	0.23
1.19	− 0.20	0.37	0.24		− 1.13	− 0.31	0.45	0.18
1.16	− 0.08	0.35	0.27		− 1.05	− 0.18	0.41	0.17
1.13	+ 0.03	0.31	0.28		− 0.90	− 0.04	0.36	0.18
1.01	+ 0.15	0.34	0.25		− 0.69	+ 0.10	0.28	0.18

Fig. XI.9. Mean systolic left ventricular endocardial landmark pathways in normal human individuals. The x- and ȳ-components of each pathway are expressed as △x and △y. The rectangles represent the standard deviations of △x and △y.

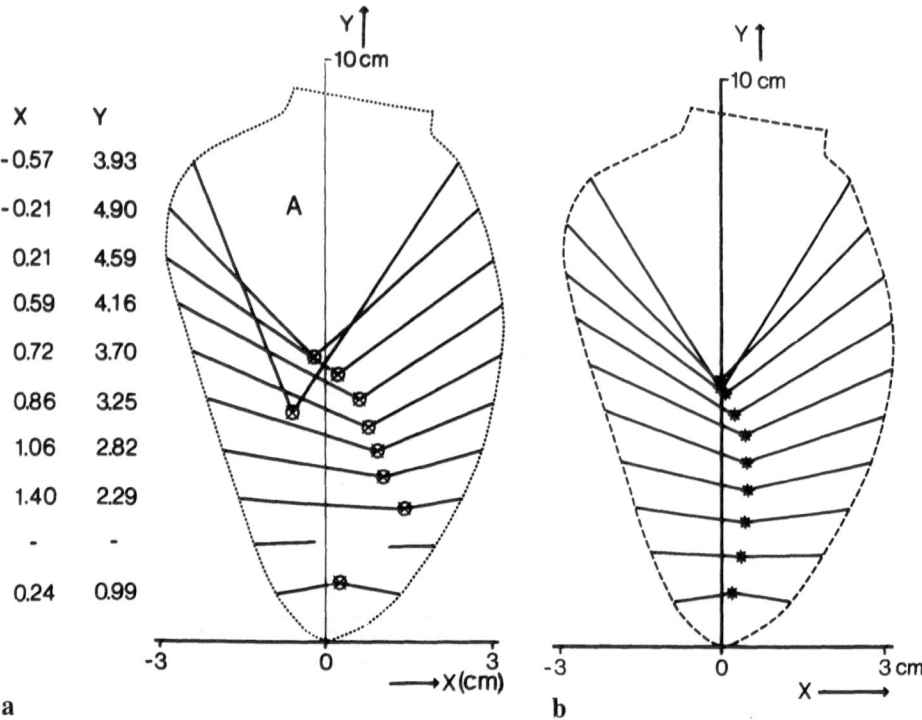

Fig. XI.10a. Points of intersection of the pathways extending from the 10 pairs of opposing starting points.

Fig. XI.10b. Points of intersection of the pathways and direction of regional wall motion using the mathematical expression described in the text.

points will move are defined by:

$$x_p = (x_a + x_i)/2 \qquad \text{(XI.5)}$$
$$y_p = L \cdot (0.57 - 0.53|1 - 1.1 \, y/L|^{1.4}) \qquad \text{(XI.6)}$$

Applying these formulas to the normalized contour of figure XI.8 yields the positions shown in Fig. XI.10b. The differences between corresponding pathway directions in Fig. XI.10a and XI.10b are less than 4 degrees, except for the pathway starting from the mitral valve fornix, where the difference equals 9.7 degrees.

Discussion

Quantitative analysis of left ventricular endocardial wall motion from angiocardiograms in humans has been hampered by the lack of an accurate and widely accepted procedure to define the direction of systolic motion of the endocardial border. Early experience with our automated endocardial outlining system suggested the recognition of endocardial landmarks, which reappeared so regularly in consecutive analyzed frames of the cineangiograms, that they could be followed over substantial parts of the cardiac cycle [13]. Although in general, one particular landmark cannot be followed over the complete systolic period because there may be some rotation of the ventricle along its long axis and because of the squeezing of contrast out of the intertrabecular spaces, it is possible to interpolate between neighboring landmark pathways in order to obtain well-defined systolic landmark pathways. This interpolation may be justified on the basis that neighboring landmarks belong to closely connected endocardial structures and as such follow the same direction of motion as observed in a particular projection. Evidently, from the observed landmark trajectories no conclusions may be drawn about wall motion in another plane than the one shown on the cineangiogram. The aim of this study was to test the hypothesis that the motion pattern of the landmarks in fact reflects the motion pattern of actual anatomical structures at the endocardial border and that these therefore can be used as natural markers.

It is obvious, that in humans no direct proof of this hypothesis can be obtained as this would require endocardial marker insertion, being the only accurate method to assess local endocardial wall motion. As an alternative, the described animal experiment was designed to compare the motion patterns of the endocardial landmarks with those from metal markers. The metal markers were inserted via a percutaneous retrograde transvascular approach, in order to minimize the damage afflicted to the myocardium. Analysis of the hemodynamic variables and the ECG, before and after marker insertion, indeed showed no sign of significant cardiac damage resulting from the procedure. In one pig a minor change in the T-wave was observed. In no case did visual inspection of the myocardium at autopsy reveal any significant damage at the positions of marker insertion. In all cases, the depth of insertion of the markers into the myocardium was found to be the same, i.e. up to the level of the interface between the body of the marker and the actual harpoon. As illustrated in Fig. XI.2 the choice of the lateral projection for the pig left ventricles is evident, as this view results in a projection of the heart similar to the RAO-view in humans. Linear regression analysis of the endocardial landmark and metal marker pathways in pigs, showed an acceptable correlation coefficient for the y-components ($r = 0.86$), but a lower correlation coefficient for the x-components ($r = 0.74$). A significant difference was also found between the slopes of the two regression equations, being 1.0 and 1.2 for the y- and x-directions, respectively. This discrepancy can be explained by the apparent and exaggerated endocardial inward motion, in a direction perpendicular to the endocardial wall, as observed on the contrast angiogram. For nearly all measured endocardial locations, this increased motion has a much larger x- than y-component and thus influences primarily the observed x-components of the landmark pathways. Especially the papillary muscle area of the pig left ventricles appears to be very sensitive for this phenomenon (Fig. XI.7). This overestimation of true systolic wall motion is caused by the squeezing of contrast media out of the intertrabecular spaces and from the papillary muscle area; this phenomenon has also been observed by other groups [6, 14–16]. The discrepancies in percent overall wall thickening between the contrast media methods [17–19], the bead and clip methods [2] and the ultrasonic crystal methods [20, 21] also point in this direction. Comparison of the direction of motion of the endocardial landmarks and the marker pathways, shows a rather high correlation ($r = 0.86$) with a small standard-error-of-the-estimate of 10.3°. In this comparison, the data from the apical pathways were excluded because of the fact that small deviations in the determination of the x- or y-components will result in large errors in the determination of the angle α. The slight underestimation of α by the landmark pathways is also partly influenced by the exaggerated wall motion in the x-direction. In addition, if the positions of the harpoons do not remain in exactly the same plane as defined by the angiographic silhouette over the systolic period, shortening of the motion of the metal markers in the x-direction will occur. Finally, it should be realized that a small, though definite intra-observer variability in the drawing of the landmark pathways exists, which further explains the uncertainty in the estimation of α and $\triangle y$. Earlier measurements showed that the observer variability in the y-direction of the landmarks equals 1.4 mm (s.d.) [11]. From all the data presented, it may be concluded that the landmark trajectories indeed represent the motion of actual anatomical landmarks and thus may serve as a noninvasive marker method. As illustrated in Fig. XI.8, the variations in shape of the analyzed human ventricles, are distributed in a regular manner over the entire wall and show a narrow range. Variations in the valvular anatomy and variations in their spatial orientation with respect to the X-ray system have almost no influence on the normalization procedure applied in this study. Other ways of normalization usually lead to greater variations: if, for example, the junction of the mitral valve and aortic valve is chosen to define the y-axis, the deviations at the basal ventricular sites will be twice as large.

In the human as well as in the animal studies, the y-components of the endocardial landmark trajectories show a gradually decreasing magnitude from base to apex. This agrees with the systolic descent of the base of the heart, as observed by many authors in animal experiments [1, 22–24] as well as in human studies [6, 25]. The apical landmark motion in the y-direction is very small, although in many cases visual inspection of the contrast angiogram would suggest a considerable apical upward motion towards the base. The apical motion of the pig and human left ventricles is shown in more detail in Fig. XI.11.

Note the apparent systolic upward motion of the apex resulting from the X-ray contrast angiographic imaging procedure, which simply follows the moving contrast border. This seeming contradiction is caused by complete extrusion of contrast media from the apex in late systole. From the analysis of contrast angiograms, many authors came to the erroneous conclusion, that the apex moves considerably towards the base during systole, which led to an overestimation of long axis shortening [25–27]. In addition, contrast angiograms, par-

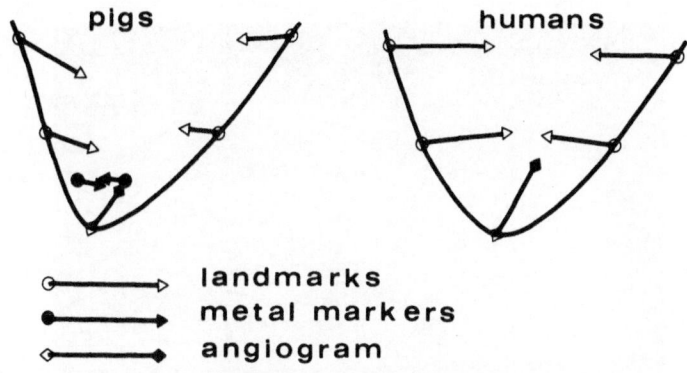

Fig. XI.11. Mean systolic wall motion of human and pig left ventricles near the apex on the basis of the metal markers, anatomical landmarks and the apical angiographic contrast border.

ticularly those in the RAO-view, suggest a substantial rotation of the apex along the left ventricular long axis, a phenomenon which is partially due to extrusion of dye by the posterior papillary muscle. However, earlier studies with epicardial and endocardial markers unmistakably showed that the apex is remarkably stationary during systole [1, 6, 22]. In accordance with these observations, the systolic motion of the apical metal markers, as shown in Fig. XI.11, is very small, although the contrast angiogram would often suggest considerable apical upward motion and rotation. These apparent changes are evident from inspection of Fig. XI.12, which depicts the end-systolic situation of the same ventricle of Fig. XI.2. Finally, a human study with implanted mid-wall metal markers showed very similar results with one minor difference, explained by the fact that mid-wall markers will always show less motion in the x-direction than endocardial structures due to wall thickening [28].

The discrepancies between metal marker motion and the angiographic observations do not suggest that the clinical value of the angiogram is low. The angiogram, by its nature, primarily shows the resulting motion of blood induced by the contracting ventricular walls. For that reason, angiographic measurements on wall motion must be interpreted with caution. In fact, as a result of the squeezing behavior of the ventricular walls the angiogram may even be more sensitive in the assessment of minor changes in regional wall function than implanted markers. It is clear, that models for the quantitative analysis of the angiogram, particularly those proposed for the assessment of endocardial wall motion, should take the above mentioned observations into account. It must be clear from the above, that one should not use the apparent end-systolic apex position to correct for the suggested apical lift and rotation. Although the desire to correct for extra cardiac motion is certainly very logical, the methods commonly used probably cause larger errors than they intend to avoid. In general, suspended respiration during angiography will eliminate the major source of extracardiac motion in the majority of patients.

256

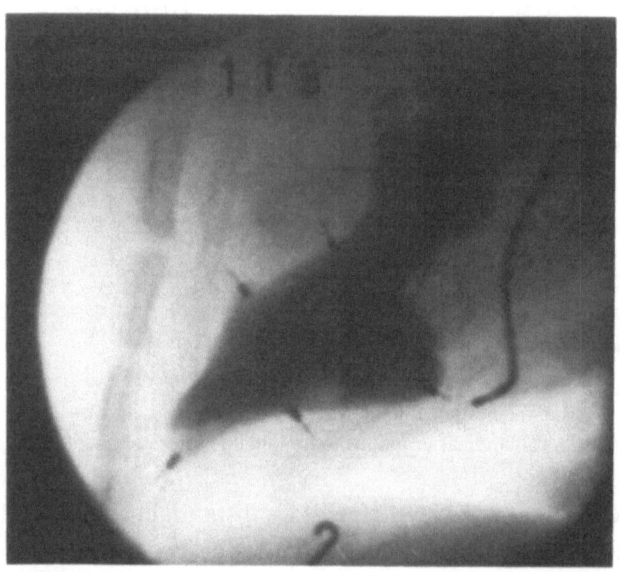

Fig. XI.12. End-systolic frame of left ventricular cineangiocardiogram after marker insertion. The corresponding end-diastolic frame is shown in Fig. XI.2. Squeezing of contrast from the apex may result in an apparent rotation and ascent of the apex as observed on the contrast angiogram, while the end-diastolic and end-systolic metal marker positions remain at a nearly identical position (see Fig. XI.6: 6b).

The mathematical description of the landmark pathway directions in humans can be used advantageously for the study of wall motion in general. The process of manually indicating the mitral valve fornix can be automated by means of the following algorithm. At first, the algorithm searches for an isosceles triangle as indicated in Fig. XI.4 with a maximal base length. Next, it determines an isosceles triangle at the ventricular base with a base length equal to 78% of the earlier determined maximal value. This latter triangle is then used to define the required rectangular coordinate system with respect to which all subsequent calculations are performed.

In conclusion, the motion patterns of landmarks appearing at the endocardial border, as detected with an automated technique for the analysis of cineangiograms, reflect the motion patterns of actual anatomical structures. From this technique, a model for normal endocardial wall motion has been derived, which provides the basis for further developments of methods to quantify regional left ventricular function in clinical practice [29].

References

1. Rushmer RF, Crystal DK, Wagner C: The functional anatomy of ventricular contraction. Circ Res 1: 162–170, 1953.
2. Mitchell JH, Wildenthal K, Mullins CB: Geometrical studies of the left ventricle utilizing biplane cinefluorography. Fed Proc 28: 1334–1343, 1969.
3. Carlsson E, Milne ENC: Permanent implantation of endocardial tantalum screws: A new technique for functional studies of the heart in the experimental animal. J Assoc Can Radiol 19: 304–309, 1967.
4. Ingels NB, Daughters GT, Stinson EB, Alderman EL: Measurement of midwall myocardial dynamics in intact man by radiography of surgically implanted markers. Circulation 52: 859–867, 1975.
5. Harrison DC, Goldblatt A, Braunwald E, Glick G, Mason DT: Studies on cardiac dimensions in intact, unanesthetized man. I. Description of techniques and their validation. Circ Res 13: 448–467, 1963.
6. McDonald IG: The shape and movements of the human left ventricle during systole. Am J Cardiol 26: 221–229, 1970.
7. Brower RW, ten Katen HJ, Meester GT: Direct method for determining regional myocardial shortening after bypass surgery from radiopaque markers in man. Am J Cardiol 41: 1222–1229, 1978.
8. Wildenthal K, Mitchell JH: Dimensional analysis of the left ventricle in unanesthetised dogs. J. Appl Physiol 27: 115–119, 1969.
9. Chapman CB, Baker O, Reynolds J, Bonte FJ: Use of biplane cinefluorography for measurement of ventricular volume. Circulation 18: 1105–1117, 1958.
10. Chaitman BR, Bristow JB, Rahimtoola SH: Left ventricular wall motion assessed by using fixed external reference systems. Circulation 48: 1043–1054, 1973.
11. Slager CJ, Hooghoudt TEH, Reiber JHC, Schuurbiers JCH, Booman F, Meester GT: Left ventricular contour segmentation from anatomical landmark trajectories and its application to wall motion analysis. Comp in Cardiol: 347–350, 1979.
12. Brower RW: Evaluation of pattern recognition rules for the apex of the heart. Cathet and Cardiov Diagn 6: 145–157, 1980.
13. Slager CJ, Reiber JHC, Schuurbiers JCH, Meester GT: Automated detection of left ventricular contour. Concept and application. In: Roentgen-Video-Techniques for Dynamic Studies of Structure and Function of the Heart and Circulation. PH Heintzen, JH Bürsch, (Eds.). Georg Thieme Publishers, Stuttgart: 158–167, 1978.
14. Herman MV, Heinle RA, Klein MD, Gorlin R: Localized disorders in myocardial contraction. Asynergy and its role in congestive heart failure. New Eng J Med 277: 222–232, 1967.
15. Chapman CB, Baker O, Mitchell JH, Collier RG: Experiences with a cinefluorographic method for measuring ventricular volume. Am J Cardiol 18: 25–30, 1966.
16. Hugenholtz PG, Kaplan E, Hull E: Determination of left ventricular wall thickness by angiocardiography. Amer Heart J 78: 513–522, 1969.
17. Sandler H, Dodge, HT: Left ventricular tension and stress in man. Circ Res 13: 91–104, 1963.
18. Eber LM, Greenberg HM, Cooke JM and Gorlin R: Dynamic changes in left ventricular free wall thickness in the human heart. Circulation 39: 455–464, 1969.
19. Dumesnil JG, Ritman EL, Frye RL, Gau GT, Rutherford BD, Davies GD: Quantitative determination of regional left ventricular wall dynamics by Roentgen Videometry. Circulation 50: 700–708, 1974.
20. Sasayama S, Franklin D, Ross J Jr, Kemper WS, McKown D: Dynamic changes in left ventricular wall thickness and their use in analyzing cardiac function in the conscious dog. Am J Cardiol 38: 870–879, 1976.
21. Osakada G, Sasayama S, Kawai C, Hirakawa A, Kemper WS, Franklin D and Ross J Jr: The

analysis of left ventricular wall thickness and shear by an ultrasonic triangulation technique in the dog. Circ Res 47: 173–181, 1980.

22. Hamilton WF, Rompf JH: Movements of the base of the ventricle and the relative constancy of the cardiac volume. Amer J Physiol 102: 559–565, 1932.

23. Tsakiris AG, von Bernuth G, Rastelli GC, Bourgeois MJ, Titus JL, Wood EH: Size and motion of the mitral valve annulus in anesthetized intact dogs. J Appl Physiol 30: 611–618, 1971.

24. Hinds JE, Hawthorne EW, Mullins CB, Mitchell JH: Instantaneous changes in the left ventricular lengths occurring in dogs during the cardiac cycle. Fed Proc 28: 1351–1357, 1969.

25. Brower RW, Meester GT: Computer based methods for quantifying regional left ventricular wall motion from cine ventriculograms. Comp in Cardiol: 55–62, 1976.

26. Leighton RF, Wilt SM, Lewis RP: Detection of hypokinesis by a quantitative analysis of left ventricular cineangiograms. Circulation 50: 121–127, 1974.

27. Rickards A, Seabra-Gomes R, Thurstone P: The assessment of regional abnormalities of the left ventricle by angiography. Eur. J Cardiol 5: 167–182, 1977.

28. Ingels NB, Mead CW, Daughters GT, Stinson EB, Alderman EL: A new method for assessment of left ventricular wall motion. Comp in Cardiol: 57–61, 1978.

29. Slager CJ, Hooghoudt TEH, Serruys PW, Schuurbiers JCH, Reiber JHC, Verdouw PD, Hugenholtz PG: Quantitative assessment of regional left ventricular motion. J Amer Coll Cardiol 7, No. 2, 1986.

XII. The cardiovascular database and the coronary reporting system

Introduction

As soon as coronary and left ventricular cineangiograms are analyzed quantitatively on a more or less routine basis for clinical diagnostic or research studies, the need arises very quickly to store all the quantitative results in a database. The advantages of such approach are evident: (1) structurized storage of these quantitative data; (2) readily accessibility of the data and results presented in a convenient manner; and (3) possibility of statistical analysis of the results of studies using standardly available statistical packages.

Because of the large amounts of data involved in the quantitative analyses by CAAS, the database should be filled automatically by the computer following the analyses; both from a standpoint of efficiency and the elimination of possibly occurring errors by manual procedures, these quantitative data should not be entered individually by a data-typist. For our purposes, it was most convenient to store the data in a hierarchical manner, i.e. per patient. The majority of the databases in use in cardiological centers are filled by data-typists or cardiologists and these data are usually organized in a nonhierarchical manner, i.e. per investigation (not per patient) [1, 2]. In this context, investigation is defined as one of many possible angiographic procedures, such as pre-PTCA, post-PTCA, diagnostic angiographic procedure, etc. Various databases have been designed for large computer systems [3, 4], but not for a minicomputer such as the PDP 11/44 or PDP 11/73. Since a practically useful database did not exist for our minicomputer systems, we decided to develop our own database system.

Our goal was to store the quantitative data of every patient in a hierarchical manner, which requires a hierarchical approach. A disadvantage of this type of database due to the structure in which the data are stored is that all levels need to be assessed before a complete overview of the analysis data of a specific coronary or left ventricular intervention becomes available. To partially overcome this slight inconvenience, a coronary reporting program has been developed that allows a summary of the quantitative data from a particular intervestigation to be presented in a schematic diagram of the coronary tree on the video monitor. This reporting program extracts all required information from the database.

At this point in time the following situation exists in our laboratory: cinefilms of patients are analyzed with the CAAS program and the quantitative data are stored automatically in the CAAS database. To obtain a readily interpretable overview of the analysis data of a specific investigation the reporting program is used. In the near future a retrieval program will be available allowing statistical analysis of the data. In the remainder of this chapter a more detailed description of the CAAS database and the reporting program will be given; the nomenclature as used by Date will be followed [5].

CAAS database

The hierarchial structure of the CAAS database is given in figure XII.1. Every rectangle represents a segment of the database containing one or more parameters (fields). The field descriptions for each segment are given in the Appendix; for each field the following information is provided:
– Field description
– Field unit
– Field range (minimum and maximum values).
The first or root segment is PATIENT. This segment contains fields providing general information about the patient, e.g. his/her name, date of birth, patient identification, etc. Segment PATIENT is the so-called parent of segments CATH and FREETEXT. In segment CATH information about the catheterization procedure, such as the cinefilm number, catheterization time and date, fluorescense duration, etc., plus other relevant patient data are stored. In segment FREETEXT a field 'text' has been defined, which may contain a comment line for this patient.

Segment CATH is the parent of segments FREETEXT and STUDY. This segment FREETEXT is similar to the one described above, while segment STUDY contains the name of the clinical or research study and the patient's study number (or identification). Segment STUDY is the parent of segment INVESTIGATION. In this segment the type of angiographic investigation performed as defined in the introduction, is stored. This segment INVESTIGATION is the parent of segments (coronary) SEGMENT, SEGMENT BYPASS and LVRAO. (Note: there is a segment named 'SEGMENT' and a segment named 'SEGMENT BYPASS'). The segment SEGMENT contains the name of the segment (of the coronary tree) that was analyzed, while segment SEGMENT BYPASS contains the identification (name) of a possibly analyzed bypass graft. In segment LVRAO information about the X-ray system settings used during left ventriculography in the RAO projection, such as the geometry of the X-ray gantry, size image intensifier, film speed, etc. are stored. As the RAO-view is the preferred and

261

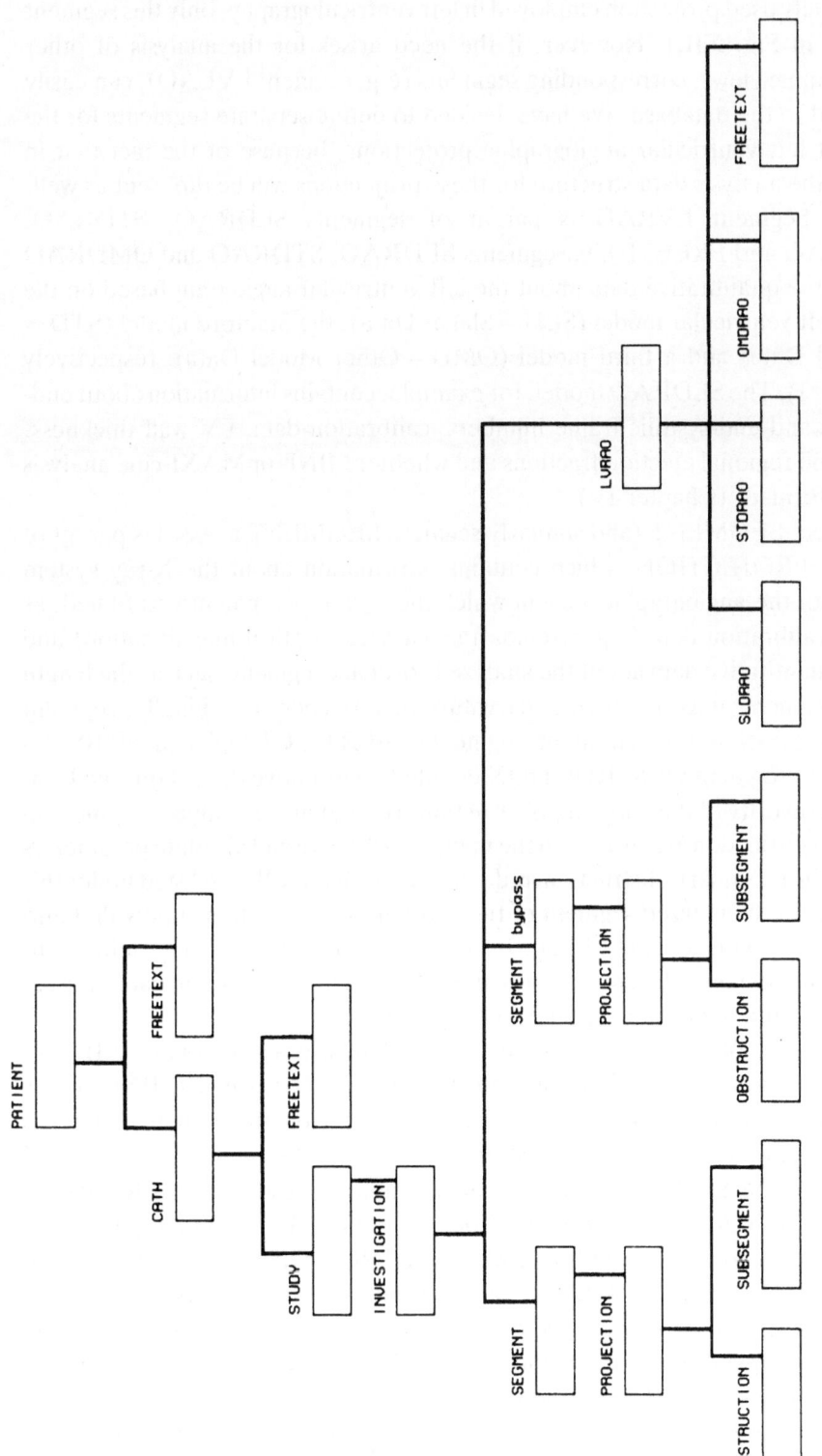

Fig. XII.1. Hierarchial structure of CAAS database.

most widely used projection employed in left ventriculography, only this segment is given in Fig. XII.1. However, if the need arises for the analysis of other angiographic views, corresponding segments (e.g. segment LVLAO), can easily be added to the database. We have decided to define separate segments for the different left ventricular angiographic projections, because of the fact that in general the analysis data structure for these projections will be different as well. Finally, Segment LVRAO is parent of segments SLDRAO, STDRAO, OMDRAO and FREETEXT; segments SLDRAO, STDRAO and OMDRAO contain the quantitative data about the left ventricular angiogram based on the Slager left ventricular model (SLD = Slager Data), the Stanford model (STD = Stanford Data) and a third model (OMD = Other Model Data), respectively (Chapter I). The SLDRAO model, for example, contains information about end-diastolic and end-systolic frame numbers, calibration data, LV wall thickness, global and regional ejection fractions and whether MINI- or MAXI-cine analysis was performed. (Chapter IV).

Segment SEGMENT (and similarly segment SEGMENT BYPASS) is parent of segment PROJECTION, which contains information about the X-ray system settings of the angiographic view in which the coronary segment was filmed, as well as calibration data (e.g. size contrast catheter, optical magnification) and global quantitative data about the analyzed coronary segment, such as the length of the segment, edge roughness, curvature quality code, etc. Finally, segment PROJECTION is the parent of segments OBSTRUCTION and SUBSEGMENT. In segment OBSTRUCTION detailed quantitative data about the location and severity of the coronary obstructions (if any) in the analyzed segment in the given projection are stored; all the measured relative and absolute parameters describing a coronary obstruction as described in Chapter III are listed under this segment. Each analyzed segment of the coronary tree is further subdivided into subsegments with lengths of approximately 0.5 cm (Ch. III). The minimum, maximum and mean diameter values and the standard deviation in each subsegment are listed under the segment SUBSEGMENT.

An example of an occurrence in the CAAS database is given in Fig. XII.2. In this particular example patient Johnson was catheterized twice. The ID-numbers of the catheterization films are + 84-12 and + 84-86. Note that film nr. + 84-86 is of poor quality. Film nr. + 84-86 has been used for two clinical studies, PTCA and DRUG A. For the PTCA study two angiographic investigations, PRE-PTCA and POST-PTCA, were performed. From the POST-PTCA angiographic investigation two coronary segments (the MAIN and RCA-DIST) were analyzed with the CAAS. Segment RCA-DIST was analyzed in two views, the RAO- and LAO-view. In the LAO-view two obstructions were found at locations 304 and 307 (for an explanation of these numbers, see Ch. III). The RCA-DIST segment was divided into 8 subsegments in the LAO-view.

Similar information as for the RCA-DIST segment is available for the analyzed bypass segment; however, no obstruction was found in this segment. From the

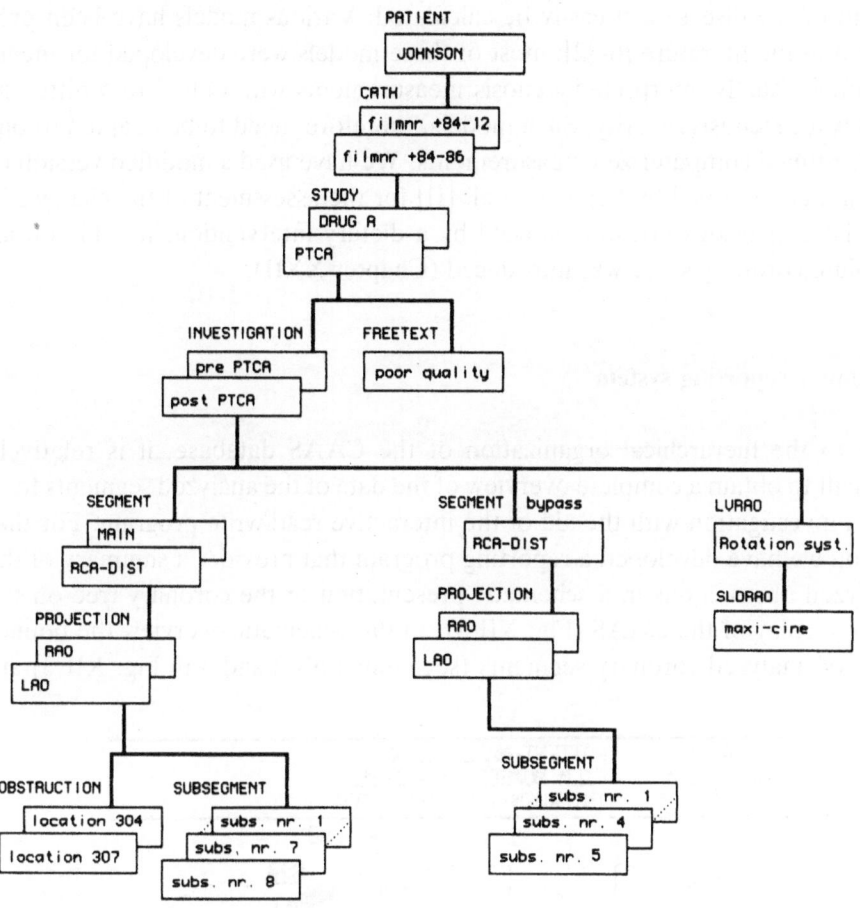

Fig. XII.2. Example of an occurrence in the CAAS database.

post-PTCA investigation left ventricular function was analyzed in the RAO-view according to the Slager model with the MINI-cine program.

N.B.: Cath. segments with filmnr + 84-12 and filmnr. + 84-86 are both connected to the segment with patient Johnson; for reasons of clarity, only one of these segments has been followed further down.

The database is filled automatically with data as provided by CAAS. In addition to this automated mode, an interactive program has been written that allows the user to read from or write to the database. Some changes in the structure of the database (such as adding new fields or segments and deleting fields) are possible, without destroying old data.

Access to the database is only possible by entering a password. Every password has a privileged number assigned to it, indicating the type of access to the database (read only, read/write, read/write/delete).

Once all the obstructions in a patient's coronary angiogram have been analyzed and stored in the database, a coronary score or index being a measure for the

extent of the disease can easily be calculated. Various models have been presented in the literature [6–12]; most of these models were developed for incorporating visually interpreted stenosis measurements with only 4 to 5 different
classes for stenosis severity. Such models, therefore, need to be adapted to our
more refined computerized measurements. We have used a modified version of
the model described by Leaman et al. [11] for the assessment of the changes in
arterial dimensions possibly induced by a dietary intervention; in addition an
absolute coronary score was introduced (Chapter XXII).

Coronary reporting system

Due to the hierarchical organization of the CAAS database, it is relatively
difficult to obtain a complete overview of the data of the analyzed segments for a
given investigation with the aid of the interactive read/write program. For that
reason we have developed a reporting program that provides a summary of the
analyzed obstructions in a schematic presentation of the coronary tree on the
video display of the CAAS (Fig. XII.3). In this schematic overview the boundaries of analyzed coronary segments (segments no's 2 and 6 in Fig. XII.3) are

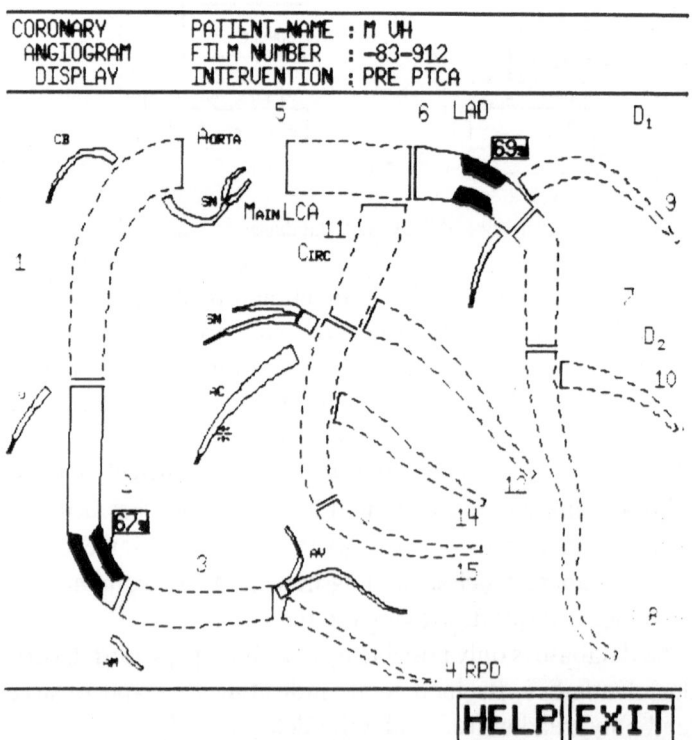

Fig. XII.3. Schematic diagram of coronary tree with analyzed obstructions displayed to scale.

displayed with continuous lines, those of nonanalyzed segments with interrupted lines. If an obstruction was found in a coronary segment, this obstruction is displayed to scale in the segment with the interpolated percentage diameter stenosis measurement presented next to it. If the obstruction was analyzed in different views, only the most severe percentage diameter stenosis measurement is displayed. In the schematic presentation of Fig. XII.3 the analyzed segments 2 and 6 each contained an obstruction. The percentages diameter stenosis were 67% and 69%, respectively. At the top of the overview, the name of the patient (M VH), the film number (-83-912) and the type of the angiographic investigation (PRE-PTCA) are presented. At the bottom of the overview two command fields, HELP and EXIT, are available. Command fields can be selected with the aid of the writing tablet. If the field HELP is selected, a help page is shown containing information about the usage of the program. Exiting from the program is achieved by selecting the field EXIT.

Such coronary reporting system provides the clinician with a readily understandable picture about the extent of the patient's coronary artery disease and is therefore an extremely helpful tool in clinical decision making and as a research tool. A hardcopy of this page can be filed in the patient's status.

Besides this overview page, all the other detailed quantitative data about analyzed coronary segments can also be made available to the clinician on the video monitor by selecting a particular coronary segment with the writing tablet

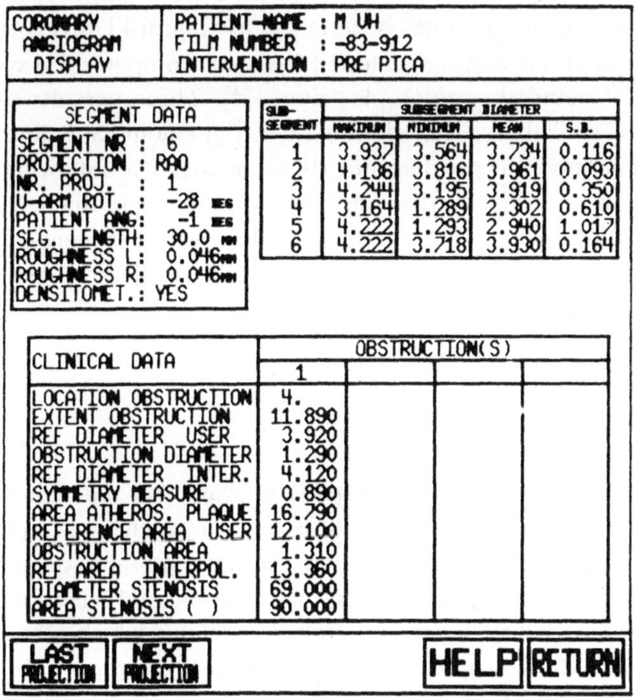

CORONARY ANGIOGRAM DISPLAY	PATIENT-NAME : M VH FILM NUMBER : -83-912 INTERVENTION : PRE PTCA				

SEGMENT DATA	SUB-SEGMENT	SUBSEGMENT DIAMETER			
		MAXIMUM	MINIMUM	MEAN	S.D.
SEGMENT NR : 6	1	3.937	3.564	3.734	0.116
PROJECTION : RAO	2	4.136	3.816	3.961	0.093
NR. PROJ. : 1	3	4.244	3.195	3.919	0.350
U-ARM ROT. : -28 DEG	4	3.164	1.289	2.302	0.610
PATIENT ANG. : -1 DEG	5	4.222	1.293	2.940	1.017
SEG. LENGTH: 30.0 MM	6	4.222	3.718	3.930	0.164
ROUGHNESS L: 0.046mm					
ROUGHNESS R: 0.046mm					
DENSITOMET.: YES					

CLINICAL DATA	OBSTRUCTION(S)			
	1			
LOCATION OBSTRUCTION	4.			
EXTENT OBSTRUCTION	11.890			
REF DIAMETER USER	3.920			
OBSTRUCTION DIAMETER	1.290			
REF DIAMETER INTER.	4.120			
SYMMETRY MEASURE	0.890			
AREA ATHEROS. PLAQUE	16.790			
REFERENCE AREA USER	12.100			
OBSTRUCTION AREA	1.310			
REF AREA INTERPOL.	13.360			
DIAMETER STENOSIS	69.000			
AREA STENOSIS ( )	90.000			

LAST PROJECTION	NEXT PROJECTION		HELP	RETURN

Fig. XII.4. Presentation of quantitative data about the LAD-lesion from Fig. XII.3.

cursor. An example of such a video page is given in Fig. XII.4; in this case the results for coronary segment 6 from Fig. XII.3 were selected. This page contains information about the angiographic view, the length of the analyzed segment, the roughness data of the contours and whether densitometric analysis was performed (left upper block), the maximum, minimum, mean and standard deviations of the diameter values in the various coronary subsegments (right upper block), and the detailed data about the analyzed coronary obstruction(s) (lower block). If this obstruction was filmed and analyzed in more than one view, similar data can be retrieved for another view by selecting NEXT PROJECTION with the writing tablet cursor. By selecting field LAST PROJECTION the preceding page is displayed again. By selecting field EXIT the program returns to the schematic overview as in Fig. XII.3.

The display program is very user-friendly. All the interactions between the user and the program take place by means of the writing tablet; under certain conditions error messages are displayed on the video-screen. For example: if the nonanalyzed segment 9 is selected in Fig. XII.3 the following message will appear on the screen: 'SELECTED SEGMENT WAS NOT ANALYZED'. By pointing at the CONTINUE-field, the message will disappear and the user may continue. In the near future the coronary reporting package will be extended such that it can be applied in routine clinical practice. In these situations the cinefilm is not analyzed by the CAAS and the cardiologist may enter the visually interpreted data about the location and severity of coronary obstructions in such a schematic overview. A similar program has been in use at Stanford University [13].

Sapoznikov et al. have also developed a graphic computerized system for the presentation of detailed angiographic data [14]. Three variants of the model circulation are available: a left dominant, a right dominant, and a balanced circulation. The model is divided into 116 segments. The following parameters can be assessed and displayed in the model: percentage diameter narrowing (from the view in which the lesion appears most severe), the length of the lesion and diameter of the distal coronary vessel, as well as collateral vessels, coronary artery bypass grafts, and coronary artery spasm.

Summary

A database system has been developed, in which all the demographic and quantitative data from the computer processing of a patient film can be stored and retrieved. By applying statistical software packages on these quantitative data, the results from clinical research studies can be evaluated scientifically.

In addition, a coronary display program is available which provides an overview of the localization, extent and severity of analyzed coronary obstructions for a given patient's angiographic investigation.

References

1. Willems JL, Piessens J: Implementation and experiences with a computer based coronary artery reporting and information system. Comp Cardiol: 465–470, 1977.
2. Miller MR: Development of a customized database management system for the cardiac catheterization laboratory.
3. Bolson EL, Brown BG, Dodge HT: Quantitative coronary arteriography – use of a general DBMS for reporting results of a lesion progression study. Comp Cardiol: 141–144, 1980.
4. Covvey HD, McAlister NH, Cass W, Wigle ED: CRSS – A clinical database system in a datacenter environment. Comp Cardiol: 175–178, 1982.
5. Date CJ: An introduction to database systems. I. Addison-Wesley Publishing Company, Reading, 1982.
6. Humphries JO'N, Kuller L, Ross RS, Friesinger GC, Page EE: Natural history of ischemic heart disease in relation to arteriographic findings. A twelve year study of 224 patients. Circulation 49: 489–497, 1974.
7. Gensini GG: Coronary Arteriography. Futura Publishing Co, Mount Kisco, N.Y., 1975.
8. Feuerlicht J, Stone DL, Cattell MR, Donaldson RM, Balcon R: A computer aided assessment of an index for scoring coronary angiograms. Comp Cardiol: 461–464, 1977.
9. Brandt PWT, Partridge JB, Wattie WJ: Coronary Arteriography; method of presentation of the arteriogram report and a scoring system. Clin Radiol 28: 361–365, 1977.
10. Balcon R, Cattell MR, Stone DL, Feuerlicht G: A computer generated index for the assessment of coronary angiography. Acta Med Scand S 615: 25–31, 1978.
11. Leaman DM, Brower RW, Meester GT, Serruys PW, Brand M van den: Coronary artery atherosclerosis: severity of the disease, severity of angina pectoris and compromised left ventricular function. Circulation 63: 285–292, 1981.
12. Moise A, Théroux P, Taeymans Y, Waters DD, Lespérance J, Fines P, Descoings B, Robert P: Clinical and angiographic factors associated with progression of coronary artery disease. J Amer Coll Cardiol 3: 659–667, 1984.
13. Hamilton KK, Alderman EL, Silverman JF, Sanders WJ: Computer reporting of coronary arteriograms using interactive graphics. Comp Cardiol: 111–116, 1979.
14. Sapoznikov D, Halon DA, Lewis BS, Gotsman MS: A graphic computerized system for reporting and analysis of coronary angiograms. Comp Biom Res 16: 334–339, 1983.

Appendix. Definitions of the fields in the individual segments of the CAAS-database.

Fields of segment: PATIENT

Description		range	
	Unit	Minimum	Maximum
Patient name			
Patient initials			
Maiden name			
Patient identification			
Date of birth			
Date of death			
Blood group			
Male or female			

Fields of segment: CATH

Description	Unit	Range Minimum	Maximum
Film number			
Hospital of catheterization			
Number cath. lab.		1.	10.
Date of catheterization			
Time of catheterization			
Name angiographist			
Fluorescence duration	min	1.	60.
Age of patient	year	0.	99.
Height of patient	cm	20.00	220.00
Weight of patient	kg	1.00	120.00
Body surface area	m²	1.00	5.00
Left or right dominant			
Diagnostic index AHA			

Fields of segment: FREETEXT

Description	Unit	Range Minimum	Maximum
Text			

Fields of segment: STUDY

Description	Unit	Range Minimum	Maximum
Type of study			
Patient study identification			

Fields of segment: INVESTIGATION

Description		Range	
	Unit	Minimum	Maximum
Angiographic investigation			
Therapy (code)		1.	500.

Fields of segment: SEGMENT

Description		Range	
	Unit	Minimum	Maximum
Segment name			

Fields of segment: LVRAO

Description		Range	
	Unit	Minimum	Maximum
Type of X-ray gantry			
X-ray unit			
U-arm rotation	deg	− 180.	180.
Patient angle (SKEW)	deg	− 90.	90.
Distance focus-isocenter	cm	0.	100.
Distance isocenter-object	cm	− 100.	100.
Distance image intens.-isocenter	cm	0.	100.
Size image intensifier	inch	0.	20.
Film speed	frms/s	0.	200.
ED quality code		0.00	10.00
ES quality code		0.00	10.00
Heart rate	bmp	20.	250.
Analyst			
File name			

Fields of segment: SLDRAO

Description	Unit	Range	
		Minimum	Maximum
Analysis method			
End-diastolic frame 1		1.	10000.
End-diastolic frame 2		1.	10000.
End-systolic frame		1.	10000.
Frame, aortic valve opening		1.	10000.
Optical magnification		0.70	4.00
Calibration object			
Size calibration object	cm	0.00	20.00
Calibration factor	mm/pel	0.00	10.00
LV Long axis	cm	6.00	20.00
ED volume index	ml/m^2	40.00	400.00
Ejection fraction	%	0.00	100.00
Wall thickness	cm	0.00	10.00
Regional contribution EF, sgm 1	%	−5.00	30.00
Regional contribution EF, sgm 2	%	−5.00	30.00
Regional contribution EF, sgm 3	%	−5.00	30.00
Regional contribution EF, sgm 4	%	−5.00	30.00
Regional contribution EF, sgm 5	%	−5.00	30.00
Regional ejection fraction 1	%	−100.00	100.00
Regional ejection fraction 2	%	−100.00	100.00
Regional ejection fraction 3	%	−100.00	100.00
Regional ejection fraction 4	%	−100.00	100.00
Regional ejection fraction 5	%	−100.00	100.00
Regional ejection fraction 6	%	−100.00	100.00
Regional ejection fraction 7	%	−100.00	100.00
Regional ejection fraction 8	%	−100.00	100.00
Regional ejection fraction 9	%	−100.00	100.00
Regional ejection fraction 10	%	−100.00	100.00
Regional ejection fraction 11	%	−100.00	100.00
Regional ejection fraction 12	%	−100.00	100.00
Regional ejection fraction 13	%	−100.00	100.00
Regional ejection fraction 14	%	−100.00	100.00
Regional ejection fraction 15	%	−100.00	100.00
Regional ejection fraction 16	%	−100.00	100.00
Regional ejection fraction 17	%	−100.00	100.00
Regional ejection fraction 18	%	−100.00	100.00
Regional ejection fraction 19	%	−100.00	100.00
Regional ejection fraction 20	%	−100.00	100.00
End-diastolic diameter 1	cm	0.50	12.00
End-diastolic diameter 2	cm	0.50	12.00
End-diastolic diameter 3	cm	0.50	12.00
End-diastolic diameter 4	cm	0.50	12.00
End-diastolic diameter 5	cm	0.50	12.00
End-diastolic diameter 6	cm	0.50	12.00

	Unit	Minimum	Maximum
End-diastolic diameter 7	cm	0.50	12.00
End-diastolic diameter 8	cm	0.50	12.00
End-diastolic diameter 9	cm	0.50	12.00
End-diastolic diameter 10	cm	0.50	12.00
Date of insertion in database			

Fields of segment: PROJECTION

Description		Range	
	Unit	Minimum	Maximum
Projection name			
Type of X-ray gantry			
X-ray unit			
U-arm rotation	deg	− 180.	180.
Patient angle (SKEW)	deg	− 90.	90.
Distance focus-isocenter	cm	0.	100.
Distance isocenter-object	cm	− 100.	100.
Distance image intens.-isocenter	cm	0.	100.
Size image intensifier	inch	0.	20.
Film frame number		1.	10000.
Size contrast catheter	fren	0.00	10.00
Calibration factor	mm/pel	0.00	1.00
Optical magnification		0.70	4.00
Segment length	mm	0.00	100.00
Roughness left	mm	0.00	10.00
Roughness right	mm	0.00	10.00
Mean edge roughness	mm	0.00	10.00
Curvature segment		0.00	1000.00
Quality code		0.00	10.00
Number of subsegments		0.	20.
Densitometry			
Analyst			
File name			
Date of insertion in database			

272

Fields of segment: OBSTRUCTION

Description	Unit	Range Minimum	Maximum
Segmental location obstruction		0.	32000.
Extent obstruction	mm	0.00	100.00
Obstruction diameter	mm	0.00	10.00
Obstruction area	mm²	0.00	100.00
Symmetry measure obstruction		0.00	1.00
Area atherosclerotic plaque	mm²	0.00	100.00
Reference diameter; user-def.	mm	0.00	10.00
Reference diameter; comp.-def.	mm	0.00	10.00
Reference area; user-def.	mm²	0.00	100.00
Reference area; comp.-def.	mm²	0.00	100.00
Perc. diam. stenosis; comp.-def.	%	0.00	100.00
Perc. area stenosis; comp.-def.	%	0.00	100.00
Poisseuille resistance	mmHg·s/ml	0.00	10000.00
Turbulent resistance	mmHg·s/ml	0.00	10000.00
Inflow angle	deg	−360.00	360.00
Outflow angle	deg	−360.00	360.00

Fields of segment: SUBSEGMENT

Description	Unit	Range Minimum	Maximum
Subsegment number		1.	20.
Maximum diameter	mm	0.00	10.00
Minimum diameter	mm	0.00	10.00
Mean diameter	mm	0.00	10.00
Standard deviation	mm	0.00	10.00

Part Two
Clinical Applications

XIII. Influence of intracoronary nifedipine on left ventricular function, coronary vasomotility, and myocardial oxygen consumption

Summary

The effect of intracoronary nifedipine on regional and global left ventricular performance, coronary vasomotility, and myocardial oxygen consumption is reported. Left ventricular pressures and volume indices of contractility and relaxation were simultaneously recorded in five patients without coronary artery disease. In these patients, nifedipine in the left main coronary artery not only delayed (+115 ms) anterior wall contracton, but also slowed (3.5 vs 1.9 cm/s) and depressed it (−26%), resulting in a depression of global left ventricular ejection. This asynchrony and depression of regional contraction is considered to be responsible for the slowed isovolumic contraction and relaxation of the whole ventricle.

In 10 other patients with coronary artery disease, coronary sinus blood flow and myocardial oxygen consumption were measured before and after intracoronary nifedipine. The observed decrease in myocardial oxygen consumption (−28%) depended primarily on a decrease in contractility and left ventricular performance.

In a third study group of 12 patients with coronary artery disease, the effects of intracoronary nifedipine on the coronary vasomotility of 40 coronary segments (normal, prestenotic, stenotic, poststenotic) were quantitatively determined. Left ventricular hemodynamics and coronary sinus saturation were monitored while the cineangiograms were recorded before and after nifedipine. Nifedipine provoked vasodilatation of the normal (+10.3%), prestenotic, stenotic (+4 to 30%), and poststenotic (+16.4%) coronary segments, which persisted after the disappearance of its direct effects on the myocardium. This transient regional 'cardioplegic' effect of nifedipine, associated with an increase in coronary blood flow, a reduction in myocardial oxygen consumption, and a vasodilatation of the epicardial vessels is likely to be beneficial during temporary coronary occlusion such as occurs in spasm or transluminal angioplasty.

Introduction

Direct intracoronary injection of nifedipine is used increasingly in an effort to reverse spontaneously occurring or induced spasm [1, 2] and to restore coronary blood flow. Recently introduced techniques, such as transluminal angioplasty and fibrinolytic recanalization of coronary artery thrombosis have also become indications [3, 4] for injecting nifedipine directly into the affected coronary artery, since it is argued that the specific inhibitory action of nifedipine on contractile energy expenditure may favorably influence the oxygen supply/demand ratio for ischemic or potentially ischemic cardiac cells in the affected region.

Because of the potential value of this drug, it is necessary to determine to what extent selective intracoronary bolus injection depresses left ventricular performance in man and/or reduces the myocardial oxygen consumption while at the same time dilating the coronary artery system.

Patients and methods

Patients and design of the study

For the first part of the study, five patients (32 to 55 years) were catheterized because of suspected coronary artery disease. Four had atypical chest pain and one had exertional angina, but all proved to have normal coronary arteries, with ejection fractions well within the normal range. One patient, however, had asymmetrical septal hypertrophy without outflow obstruction and one had electrocardiographic evidence of left ventricular hypertrophy without strain.

Pressures were recorded with a tip-manometer mounted on an 8 F catheter*. Derived variables were calculated on line by a computer system [5]. A 30° right anterior oblique ventriculogram (50 frames per second) was obtained by injection of 0.75 ml/kg 76% Urografin**. When diagnostic coronary arteriography showed normal coronary arteries, informed consent was obtained for the remainder of the study. This included an additional left ventricular cineangiogram 30 seconds after a bolus injection of 0.075 to 0.175 mg nifedipine into the left main coronary artery. The injection was made no sooner than 20 minutes and only after left ventricular end-diastolic pressure and the contractility variables were identical with those recorded before the initial angiogram.

The patient's position was kept unchanged in relation to the X-ray equipment during both angiograms. Movement of the diaphragm was excluded by shallow inspiration, taking care to prevent the Valsalva manoeuvre.

---

* Millar Instruments, Inc., Houston, Texas, USA.
** Schering AG, Berlin, Bergkammen, GFR.

Analysis of isovolumic indices during ventriculography

The on-line computer system provides the following data: peak left ventricular pressure (mmHg), left ventricular end-diastolic pressure (mmHg), and peak positive rate of change of pressure (pk + dP/dt in mmHg/s). In addition, isovolumic relaxation phase variables were calculated: peak negative rate of change of pressure (pk −dP/dt) and the time constant of relaxation (T) by the least squares fit of $P = e^{At+B}$ (T = −1/A) from the moment of pk −dP/dt to the opening of the mitral valve [6]. The opening of the mitral valve was defined from the angiographic frame preceding that in which nonopacified blood first entered the left ventricle. In all cases mitral valve opening was identified in the same frame by two independent observers [6].

Analysis of global and regional left ventricular function during systole and diastole

From all cineangiograms one complete cardiac cycle was analyzed frame-by-frame with the Contouromat. End diastole was defined as the moment when the derivative of left ventricular pressure first exceeded 200 mmHg/s. In all cases this point coincided with the maximal measured volume. End systole was defined at the occurrence of the incisura of the central aortic pressure, recorded with a tip-manometer of a 5 F catheter*. Early diastole was defined as the interval between the opening of the mitral valve and minimal ventricular diastolic pressure. Early diastolic left ventricular inflow volume was measured as an absolute value (ml), and early diastolic mean inflow rate was calculated as the ratio between the difference of ventricular volumes at minimal pressure and opening of the mitral valve and the time interval corresponding to the number of frames between them.

Regional left ventricular displacement was determined frame by frame for the 20 segments as described in Chapter IV (Fig. XIII.1). Regional wall velocity was computed as the first-derivative of the instantaneous displacement function. Mean wall velocity ($\overline{V}$) was calculated from end diastole to end systole (Fig. XIII.1). For each of the 20 segments the CREF-value was computed as described in Chapter IV.

Diastolic pressure-volume relations were determined from the minimal diastolic pressure to the beginning of the 'a' wave. The natural logarithm of pressure was used in a linear regression analysis of pressure and volume from which a slope k was derived. Changes in k were taken as changes in volume stiffness [7].

---

* Millar Instruments Inc, Houston, Texas, USA.

278

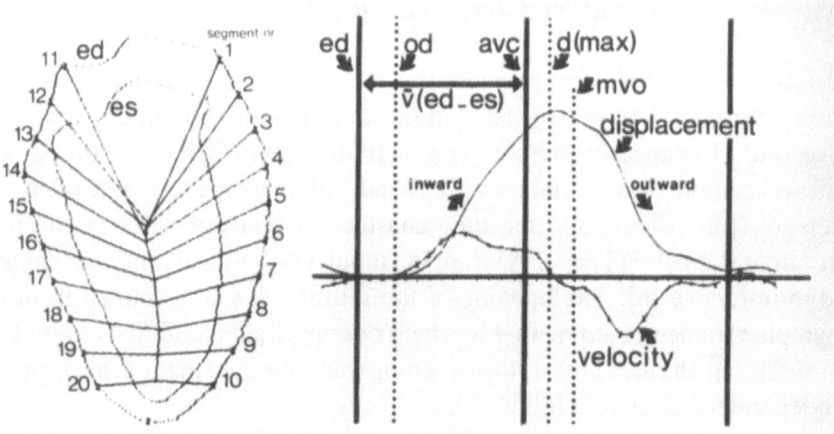

Fig. XIII.1. End-diastolic and end-systolic left ventricular contours, as detected with the automated analysis system. On these silhouettes is superimposed a system of coordinates along which segmental left ventricular wall displacement is detected. Left ventricular wall velocity – first-derivative of wall displacement – is derived from these data. ED, end diastole; ES, end systole; OD, onset of displacement; $\overline{V}$(ED-ES), mean systolic wall velocity; D(max), maximal inward wall displacement; MVO, mitral valve opening; AVC, aortic valve closure.

Coronary sinus blood flow measurement and myocardial oxygen consumption

In the second part of this study, the effect of intracoronary injection of nifedipine on coronary sinus blood flow and myocardial oxygen consumption was determined in 10 other patients (54 to 68 years), who all had significant coronary heart disease.

Blood flow was measured via the continuous thermodilution method of Ganz et al. [8]. The position of the external thermistor was assessed by injection of 3 ml contrast material before the intracoronary injection of 0.1 mg nifedipine.

Before injecting nifedipine, the blood oxygen content in the aorta and the coronary sinus was determined* and baseline data for flow and aortic pressures were obtained during 60 seconds. Thirty seconds and three minutes after the intracoronary administration of nifedipine these measurements were repeated and changes in myocardial oxygen consumption computed.

Quantitative coronary angiography

For the third part of the study, coronary artery dimensions were quantified in 12 patients (33 to 59 years), again catheterized for suspected coronary artery disease. Two patients had completely normal coronary arteries, one had single

---

* Lex-O_2-CON, Lexington Instruments Corporation, Waltham, Massachusetts, USA.

vessel disease, six had double vessel disease, and three had triple vessel disease, all with obstructions of 70% diameter narrowing or more. The effects of intra-coronary injection of nifedipine on coronary vasomotility were studied in four consecutive coronary cineangiograms. Before the angiographic study, a fiberoptic catheter* was inserted into the coronary sinus and the O_2 saturation was continuously measured [9]. The left ventricular pressure was also recorded continuously with a dual tip-manometer and analyzed for changes in left ventricular contractility, reflected by peak dP/dt, peak V_{CE}, and V_{max} [5]. A total of 40 coronary segments was selected for quantitative angiographic analysis. Eight were stenotic in nature, five were prestenotic, 17 were poststenotic, and 10 were normal. Before injecting the nifedipine, two baseline coronary angiograms (C1, C2) were performed five minutes apart. The second control angiogram (C2) was carried out to study the effect of the contrast agent itself on the artery. Five minutes later, 0.15 mg nifedipine was injected within 20 seconds into the left main coronary artery.

A third angiogram (N1) was then obtained as soon as the coronary sinus saturation reached its maximum value, usually within 30 seconds. The final coronary angiogram (N2) was recorded when the coronary sinus saturation had returned to its control values, usually within five minutes. All arteriograms were obtained via the Sones technique and recorded on Kodak 35 mm cinefilm at the rate of 50 frames per second with the biplane Cardioskope U**. The contrast medium, 76% Urografin was injected at a flow rate of 3 ml/s with a Medrad injector. Coronary arterial dimensions were quantitated with the CAAS system. It is emphasized that the X-ray system settings were not changed during consecutive filming after drug injection. Calibration of the diameter values in mm is, therefore, not necessary for comparative changes. The results after nifedipine administration are then expressed as relative changes in diameters, with respect to the control situation.

Results

Global systolic and diastolic left ventricular function

Left ventricular pressure and volume measurements before and 30 seconds after intracoronary nifedipine are shown in Tables XIII.1a and XIII.1b. The heart rates remained essentially unchanged, while peak systolic pressure, peak positive dP/dt, peak negative dP/dt, and peak V_{CE} and V_{max} decreased significantly. In addition, the end-diastolic pressure became raised and the time constant of relaxation increased. End-diastolic volumes did not change significantly, but there was an increase in the end-systolic volume, with a consistent decrease in

---

* Siemens AG, Henkestrasse, Erlangen, GBR.
** American Optical Company, Southbridge, Massachusetts, USA.

Table XIII.1a. Left ventricular volume measurements and derived indices.

Case No.	Dose IC nifedipine (mg)	Heart rate/min		EDVI (ml/m²)		ESVI (ml/m²)		SI (ml/m²)		EF (%)	
		C	N	C	N	C	N	C	N	C	N
1	0.075	75	74	75.1	79.1	21.4	29.9	53.6	49.2	71.4	62.1
2	0.15	67	72	92.0	89.1	26.4	43.6	65.6	45.5	71.3	51.0
3	0.175	66	66	80.4	88.4	27.3	47.2	53.1	41.1	65.9	46.5
4	0.125	70	86	122.6	101.5	34.4	51.5	88.1	50.0	71.9	49.2
5	0.1	66	71	69.2	60.6	11.7	26.1	57.5	34.4	83.0	56.8
	Mean	69	74	88	84	24	40	64	44	73	53
	s.d.	±4	±7	±21	±15	±8	±11	±15	±6	±6	±6
	p-value	n.s.		n.s.		<0.002		<0.03		<0.005	

IC, intracoronary; EDVI, End-diastolic volume index; ESVI, end-systolic volume index; SI, stroke index; EF, ejection fraction; C, control; N, nifedipine.

stroke index and thus ejection fraction. Because of this decrease in cardiac output, and in spite of the transient reduction in blood pressure, the total systemic resistance remained unchanged. In four of five patients, the mean rate of flow, measured during the early diastolic filling period, between the mitral valve opening and the point of minimal pressure declined.

The relation between left ventricular diastolic pressure and volume after

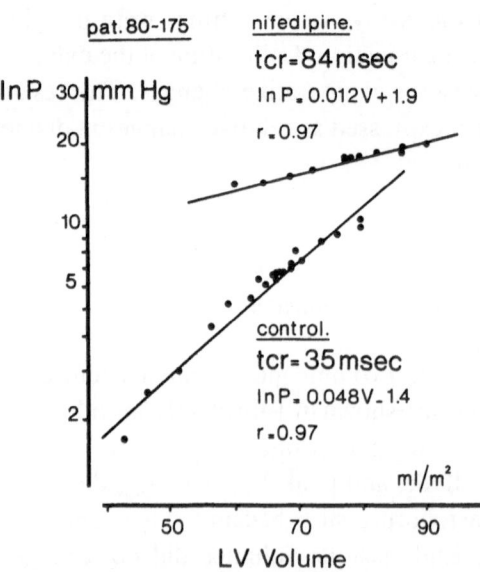

Fig. XIII.2. Pressure-volume relation during diastole before and after nifedipine. Linear regression equation of the relation between the natural logarithm of left ventricular pressure (ln P) and left ventricular volume is shown. Intracoronary nifedipine results in a reduction in the slope (k) of the regression line. TCR, time constant of relaxation.

Table XIII.1b. Left ventricular pressure measurements and derived indices.

Case No.	P_{min} (mmHg) C	N	k_p/ml C	N	EDP (mmHg) C	N	peak(+) dP/dt (mmHg/s) C	N	peak V_{CE}/s C	N
1	0.3	6.5	0.125 r=0.88	0.045 r=0.96	8.7	17.4	1830	1460	47	39
2	6	13.1	0.029 r=0.97	0.007 r=0.72	20.8	23	1440	1110	29	24
3	1.4	14	0.048 r=0.97	0.012 r=0.97	9.9	21	1410	1020	36	20
4	0	13	0.061 r=0.96	0.031 r=0.97	12.1	22.8	1470	1130	38	25
5	0.3	8.1	0.158 r=0.89	0.049 r=0.98	10.4	21.6	1730	1020	54	22
Mean	1.6	11	0.084	0.029	12	21	1576	1148	41	26
s.d.	±2.5	±3	±0.054	±0.019	±5	±2	±191	±182	±10	±8
p-value	0.005		0.03		0.01		0.005		0.05	

P_{min}, left ventricular minimal diastolic pressure; k_p, slope of diastolic logarithmic pressure volume relation; EDP, end-diastolic pressure; dP/dt, rate of change of pressure. Values expressed as means ± s.d.

Case No.	V_{max}/s C	N	Peak LVP (mmHg) C	N	ESP (mmHg) C	N	TSR (dyne·s/cm⁵) C	N	Peak(−) dP/dt (mmHg/s) C	N	TCR (ms) C	N
1	59	50	138	132	71	70	1054	1137	2081	1454	35.4	60.8
2	41	31	98	91	79	59	879	962	1367	1073	51.5	70.3
3	41	26	101	95	81	59	1114	1180	1792	825	35.1	84.2
4	48	30	120	113	94	82	763	974	1520	1248	43.2	68.2
5	58	34	135	91	102	58	1364	1233	2164	1310	21.0	47.5
Mean	50	34	118	105	86	66	1035	1097	1785	1182	37	66
s.d.	±9	±9	±19	±18	±12	±10	±231	±123	±345	±242	±11	±13
p-value	0.005		n.s.		0.05		n.s.		0.02		0.01	

TSR, total systemic resistance; V_{CE}, velocity of contractile elements (dP/dt/P); V_{max}, VCE linearly extrapolated to P = 0 mmHg; LVP, left ventricular pressure; ESP, pressure at aortic valve closure; TCR, time constant of relaxation; C, control; N, nifedipine.

nifedipine is illustrated by one example (Fig. XIII.2). It is evident that the entire diastolic pressure-volume relation is shifted so that, at any given volume, pressure is higher. This effect was consistently seen after each administration of nifedipine. The slope (k) of the ln P vs volume line, – an index of volume stiffness – however, was considerably reduced in all patients.

282

Regional left ventricular function

The profound effect of intracoronary nifedipine on left ventricular wall motion and its time sequence is shown in Fig. XIII.3. Before administration of nifedipine, displacement of the anterior and inferior wall was seen, 29 and 28 ms, respectively, after end diastole (Table XIII.2). After injection of nifedipine into the main stem of the left coronary artery, the onset of displacement of the anterior wall was delayed an additional 115 ms (p<0.001), while the inferior wall was delayed by 44 ms (p<0.001). For each segment the timing relation between aortic valve closure and the occurrence of the maximal wall displacement is shown in Fig. XIII.4. Before nifedipine, the maximal displacement of the anterior wall

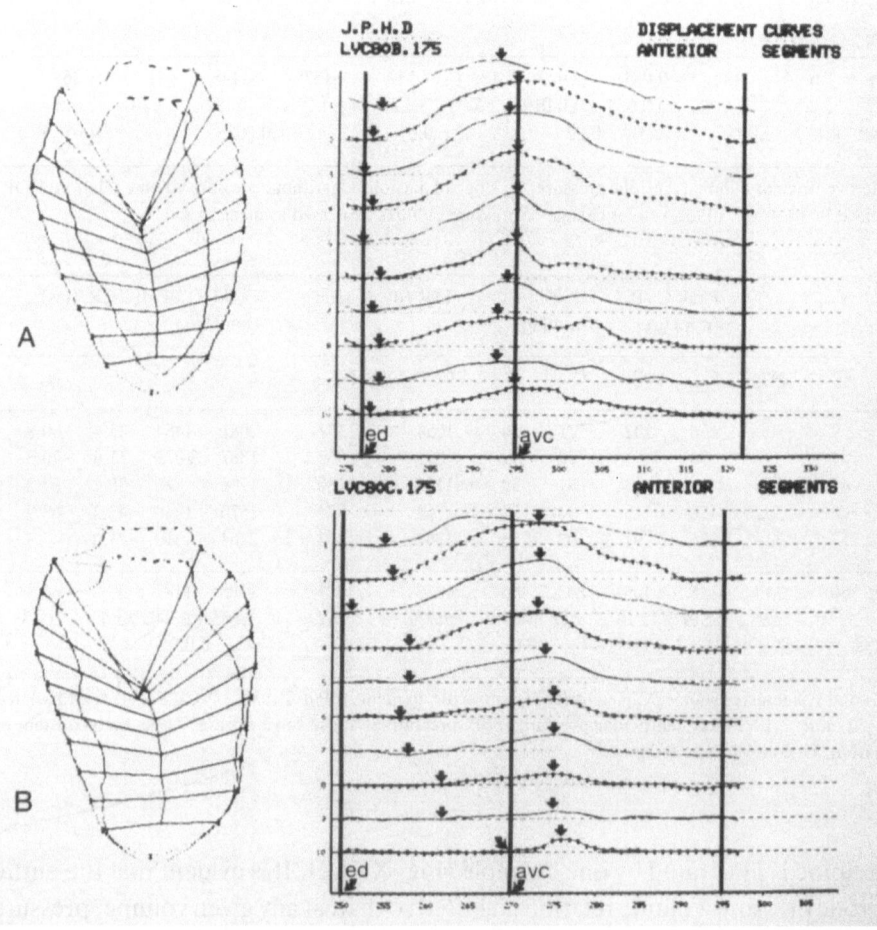

Fig. XIII.3. Effect of nifedipine into the left main coronary artery on left ventricular anterior wall motion and its time sequence. Arrows indicate onset and the moment of maximal segmental wall displacement. Nifedipine induces a delay in onset of displacement, a decrease in the extent of segmental wall motion, and a delay in the maximal wall displacement. (A) Control left ventriculogram. (B) Left ventriculogram after nifedipine. ED, end diastole; AVC, aortic valve closure.

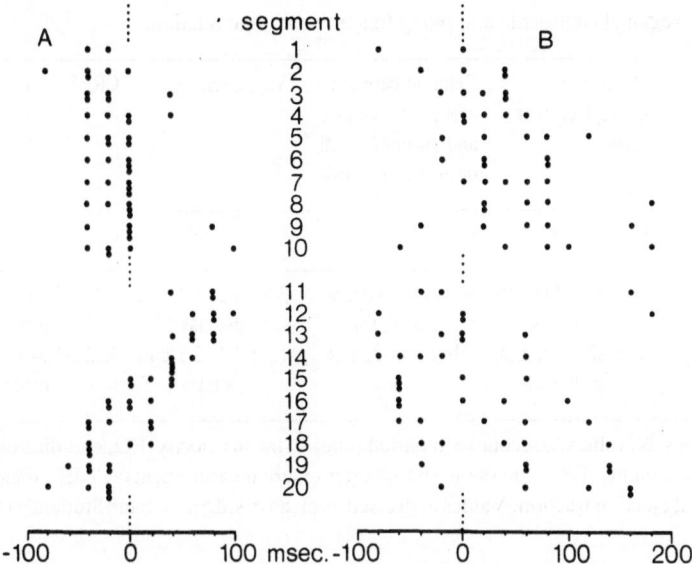

Fig. XIII.4. Time relation between aortic valve closure (time zero) and the occurrence of maximal wall displacement before (A) and after (B) intracoronary nifedipine. In 13 of 200 segments the moment of maximal wall displacement could not be determined accurately. These data are omitted in the figure.

occurred 11 ms before aortic valve closure. In contrast, with the anterior wall segments, the infero-posterior wall segments did not reach their maximal wall displacement synchronously. The maximal displacement of the five postero-basal segments (no. 11–15) occurred between 20 and 100 ms after aortic valve closure so that the maximal wall displacement of the entire inferior wall fell, on average, 10 ms after aortic valve closure. After nifedipine, the moment of maximal wall displacement for the anterior wall shifted from end systole (11 ms before aortic valve closure) to early diastole (60 ms after aortic valve closure). The antero-lateral and the apical segment of the anterior wall, as well as the apical segment of the inferior wall appear to be the most affected. On the contrary, the postero-basal wall segments reach their maximum in end systole, instead of early diastole.

The measurement of mean systolic wall velocity after nifedipine showed a decrease which was again more pronounced in the anterior wall (Table XIII.2) than in the inferior wall. The individual regional pump function data for all 20 segments before and after the intracoronary administration of nifedipine are given in Fig. XIII.5. Though these data demonstrated a myocardial depression affecting the whole ventricle, the antero-lateral and apical segments were most severely affected. Two patients with a dominant left coronary artery showed an impressive reduction of the pump function of their postero-basal wall segments as well. Under the influence of nifedipine, the mean values of regional contribution to global ejection fraction decreased from 3.33 to 2.46% (p<0.0001) for the anterior wall and from 3.32 to 2.85% (p<0.0001) for the inferior wall.

Table XIII.2. Regional contractile and pump function and time relation.

	Delay of onset of displacement (ms)		Relation between aortic valce closure and maximum wall displacement (ms)		V_{ED-ES} (cm/s)		CREF (%)	
	C	N	C	N	C	N	C	N
Anterior wall segments	29 ± 27	144 ± 95	-11 ± 31	60 ± 56	3.5 ± 1.2	1.9 ± 1.2	3.33 ± 1.46	2.46 ± 1.29
	p<0.0001		p<0.0001		p<0.0001		p<0.0001	
Inferior wall segments	28 ± 27	72 ± 70	10 ± 44	22 ± 76	3.5 ± 1.1	2.3 ± 1.0	3.32 ± 1.34	2.85 ± 1.29
	p<0.0001		n.s.		p<0.0001		p<0.0001	

C, control values; N, values 30 seconds after nifedipine; V, mean velocity; ED, end-diastole (based on pressure measurement); ES, end-systole (based on pressure measurement); CREF, regional contribution to global ejection fraction. Values expressed as mean ± s.d.; p, p-value Student's t test (paired data).

Coronary sinus blood flow and myocardial oxygen consumption

Thirty seconds after intracoronary administration of nifedipine, coronary sinus blood flow increased significantly (p<0.005) from 103 ml/min to 155 ml/min, but returned to the pre-administration values within three minutes (Table XIII.3). Simultaneously, mean aortic blood pressure dropped from 111 mmHg, to 98 mmHg, then returned to control values. Despite this transient decrease in perfusion pressure, coronary vascular resistance was significantly reduced (1.15 versus 0.66 mmHg/ml per min; p<0.0002). Thirty seconds after nifedipine, the coronary sinus oxygen content almost doubled (from 6.0 to 11.9 ml/100 ml; p<0.0001), and this was reflected in a considerable narrowing of the aortic-coronary sinus oxygen difference (from 12.7 to 6.3 ml/100 ml; p<0.0001). In this group of patients, the net increase in myocardial blood flow was smaller than expected from the narrowing of the aortic-coronary sinus oxygen difference, reflecting a reduced myocardial oxygen consumption (from 13.4 to 9.6 ml/min; p<0.01).

Quantitative coronary cineangiography

Hemodynamic data assessing the effects of nifedipine on the epicardial coronary arteries are shown in Table XIII.4. Peak systolic pressure remained constant during both control cineangiograms, but decreased by 14 mmHg immediately after the intracoronary injection of nifedipine (p<0.05). This acute change was transient so that by the time the fourth coronary angiogram was recorded, the left ventricular pressure had already returned to its control value of 135 mmHg. End-diastolic pressure showed a significant increase from 19 to 25 mmHg (p<0.001) 30

Table XIII.3. Effect of intracoronary nifedipine (0.15 mg) on coronary sinus blood flow and myocardial oxygen consumption in 10 patients with coronary artery disease.

	HR (min^{-1})			Mean aortic pressure (mmHg)			CSBF (ml/min)		
	C	N1	N2	C	N1	N2	C	N1	N2
Mean	65	74	65	111	98	112	103	155	109
s.d.	±8	±8	±9	±13	±13	±10	±30	±40	±36
C vs N1	p<0.002			p<0.0005			p<0.0005		
C vs N2	n.s.			n.s.			n.s.		
C vs N2	p<0.0005			P<0.0005			P<0.001		

CVR (mmHg/ml per min)			(Ao-Cs) O$_2$ (ml/100 ml)			CS O$_2$ content (ml/100 ml)			MVO$_2$ (ml/min)		
C	N1	N2	C	N1	N2	C	N1	N2	C	N1	N2
1.15	0.66	1.12	12.7	6.3	11.9	6.0	11.9	6.6	13.4	9.6	13.7
±0.31	±0.15	±0.35	±1.5	±1.6	±1.1	±1.1	±1.4	±0.7	±4.9	±3.1	±6.1
	p<0.0002			p<0.0001			p<0.0001			p<0.01	
	n.s.			p<0.005			p<0.02			n.s.	
	p<0.0005			p<0.0001			p<0.0001			p<0.01	

C, control values; N1, values 30 seconds after nifedipine; N2, values 3 minutes after nifedipine; HR, heart rate; CSBF, coronary sinus blood flow; CVR, coronary vascular resistance; (Ao–Cs) O$_2$, aortic/coronary sinus O$_2$ difference; MVO$_2$ myocardial oxygen consumption; p, p-value Student's test (paired data). Values expressed as mean ± s.d.

Table XIII.4. Pressure derived variables and coronary sinus saturation during the two control (C1, C2) and the two post-nifedipine cineangiograms (N1, N2) (Mean ± SEM).

	Peak LVSP (mmHg)	LVEDP (mmHg)	V$_{max}$ (s^{-1})	Peak dP/dt (mmHg/s)	Peak V$_{CE}$ (s^{-1})	CS$_{O2}$ sat (%)
C1	135 ± 11.5	18 ± 2.6	47.8 ± 2.3	1722 ± 191	35.5 ± 3.8	36.0 ± 3.0
C2	137 ± 11.6	19 ± 2.6	45.0 ± 2.1	1607 ± 120	32.0 ± 2.5	36.0 ± 3.2
N1	123 ± 8.4	25 ± 3.1	36.7 ± 2.8	1333 ± 139	24.3 ± 2.4	63.0 ± 4.7
N2	135 ± 11.0	22 ± 2.6	47.5 ± 1.9	1629 ± 139	31.3 ± 2.6	35.3 ± 1.1
C1 vs N1	p<0.05	p<0.002	p<0.005	p<0.02	p<0.02	p<0.01
C1 vs N2	n.s.	n.s.	n.s.	n.s.	n.s.	n.s.
C2 vs N1	p<0.005	p<0.001	p<0.002	p<0.05	p<0.01	p<0.005
C2 vs N2	n.s.	n.s.	n.s.	n.s.	n.s.	n.s.
N1 vs N2	P<0.03	n.s.	p<0.002	p<0.02	p<0.01	p<0.005

Abbreviations: Peak LVSP, peak left ventricular systolic pressure; LVEDP, left ventricular end-diastolic pressure; V$_{max}$, maximal velocity of contractile element; dP/dt, first-derivative LV pressure; peak V$_{CE}$, peak velocity of contractile element; CS$_{O2}$ sat, coronary sinus oxygen saturation; p, p-value Student's t test (paired); n.s., not significant.

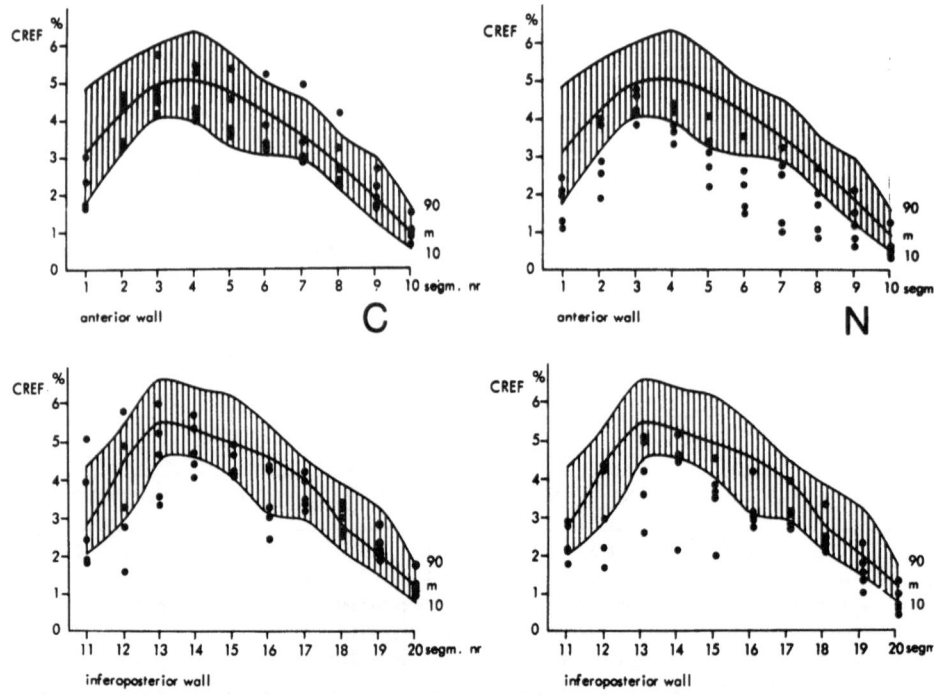

Fig. XIII.5. Effect of nifedipine into the left main coronary artery on regional contribution to global ejection fraction (CREF). Left side of the Figure: individual CREF values (five patients) in the anterior and infero-posterior wall segments before nifedipine injection. Shaded areas represent the normal range of CREF values. Right side of the Figure: after nifedipine an overall depression of regional pump function is observed which is more pronounced in the anterior (segments 1–8) and apical (9, 10, 19, 20) areas.

seconds after nifedipine had been administered. During the fourth cinefilm, the end-diastolic pressure was still slightly, but not significantly, raised. After the intracoronary injection of nifedipine, peak dP/dt and V_{max} decreased simultaneously by 17 and 18% and both variables returned to their control values by the time of the fourth coronary cineangiogram. As for the coronary sinus saturation, 30 seconds after the intracoronary administration of nifedipine there was a pronounced increase from 36% to 63% occurring simultaneously with the drop in V_{max}. It must be emphasized that five minutes after the intracoronary injection of nifedipine, there remained no detectable effect of nifedipine on the coronary sinus O_2 saturation or on contractility. The effects of nifedipine on the mean diameter of 10 normal, five prestenotic, and 16 poststenotic segments are given in Table XIII.5 and shown in Fig. XIII.6. One of the 17 poststenotic segments was excluded from the statistical analysis because it showed a paradoxical reduction of 60% in diameter after nifedipine. There is no significant difference in the mean diameter between the first and the second control cinefilm. After administration of nifedipine (film N2), all segments ($N = 29$) showed an increase of 12%

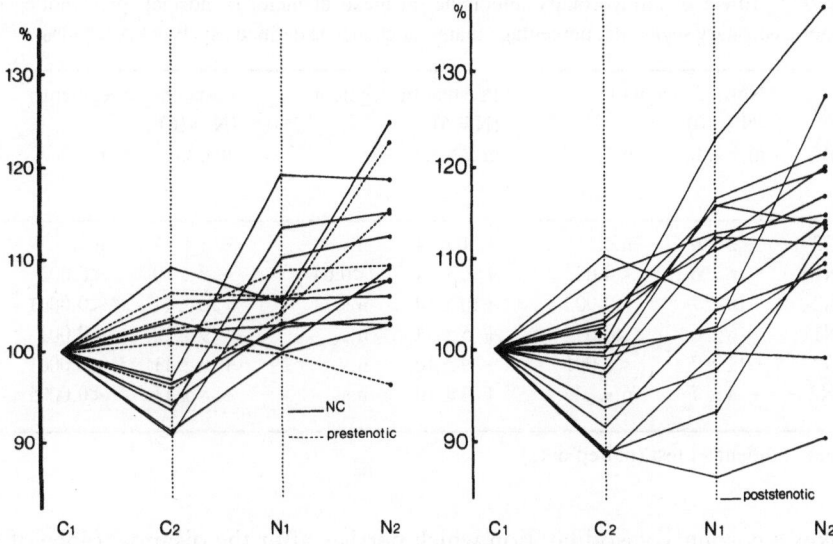

Fig. XIII.6. Effect of intracoronary nifedipine on the mean diameter of 10 normal (NC), five prestenotic, 17 poststenotic coronary segments during two control cineangiograms (C1, C2), and two cineangiograms after nifedipine (N1, N2). The individual diameter measurements are expressed as percentages with respect to C1 = 100%. Arrow indicates a segment which shows paradoxical reduction of 60% after nifedipine injection (see text).

(p<0.0001) in mean diameter, except for three coronary segments (one prestenotic, two poststenotic in series in the same artery).

These changes in detail were as follows. Thirty seconds after the intracoronary injection of nifedipine there was already a small, but significant vasodilatation (C1 vs N1, 6.2%, p<0.02; C2 vs N1, 7.9%, p<0.05) of the normal coronary segments. Five minutes later, on the last film (N2), there was an additional increase in mean diameter so that an overall increase of 10.3% (p<0.002) in mean diameter was observed between C1 and N2 and a 12.0% increase (p<0.001) between films C2 and N2. Similar changes were seen in the prestenotic coronary segments (Table XIII.5).

Thirty seconds after nifedipine there was also a significant increase in the luminal diameter of the poststenotic segments (C1 vs N1, 8.3%, p<0.002 and C2 vs N1, 9%, p<0.001). This vasodilatation persisted and increased further: all 16 segments showed an increase in mean diameter with an average of 15.7% (p <0.0001) between films C1 and N2 and an average increase of 16.4% (p <0.0001) between films C2 and N2. Seven of the eight stenotic areas also dilated with nifedipine and their luminal diameters increased in absolute terms over a range of 4 to 30% (Table XIII.6). There was a slight reduction in diameter in one segment.

It is clear that the normal, prestenotic, stenotic, and poststenotic segments remained in a state of vasodilatation even when V_{max} and the coronary sinus saturation had returned to their control values. In other words, nifedipine

Table XIII.5. Effect of intracoronary nifedipine on mean diameter of normal, prestenotic, and poststenotic coronary segments; percentage diameter change is defined as: $(B-A)/A \times 100\%$.

A	B	Normal segment (N = 10)		Prestenotic segment (N = 5)		Poststenotic segment (N = 16)	
		m ± s.d. %	p	m ± s.d. %	p	m ± s.d. %	p
C1 vs C2		− 2 ± 6	n.s.	+ 1 ± 4	n.s.	− 1 ± 7	n.s.
C1 vs N1		+ 6 ± 6	<0.02	+ 6 ± 4	<0.04	+ 8 ± 10	<0.002
C1 vs N2		+10 ± 7	<0.002	+10 ± 10	n.s.	+16 ± 11	<0.0001
C2 vs N1		+ 8 ± 6	<0.05	+ 5 ± 4	n.s.	+ 9 ± 10	<0.001
C2 vs N2		+12 ± 7	<0.001	+ 9 ± 10	n.s.	+16 ± 11	<0.0001
N1 vs N2		+ 4 ± 7	n.s.	+ 4 ± 10	n.s.	+ 8 ± 11	<0.0005

p, p-value, Student's t test (paired data).

provokes a coronary vasodilatation which persists after the disappearance of its direct effects on the myocardium.

Discussion

Global and regional left ventricular function

Earlier studies of the direct effect of nifedipine on the myocardium were carried out in this laboratory in patients in whom radiopaque markers had been implanted on the epicardium at the time of bypass surgery [10].

The question remained, however, to what extent regional endocardial movement was affected. In order to investigate this aspect, frame by frame analysis of

Table XIII.6. Luminal diameters of eight stenotic lesions during control cineangiogram (C1) and after (N2) intracoronary administration of nifedipine; luminal diameters are expressed in pixels.

Control C1	Nifedipine N2	Luminal diameter change (%)
4.73	6.18	31
9.92	12.59	27
10.93	13.67	25
10.31	12.63	22.5
13.75	16.10	17
13.97	15.29	9.4
8.32	8.68	4.3
9.84	8.90	− 9.5

Luminal diameter change is defined as: $(N-C)/C \times 100$, and expressed as a percentage.

the left ventricular cavity outline provided the opportunity to investigate the relation between changes in regional endocardial wall motion and alterations in left ventricular isovolumic contraction and relaxation, which have been described after intracoronary administration of nifedipine [11]

Asynchrony in regional wall motion in itself could explain the disturbance in isovolumic contraction, the depressed systolic function, and the abnormalities in relaxation [12, 13]. In other words, the teamwork which must exist between the different parts of a ventricle to provide maximal mechanical efficiency during ejection might be simply disrupted by the regional administration of nifedipine, without implying a true reduction in regional myocardial performance. It has been suggested that the primary abnormality induced by intracoronary nifedipine could be a delayed onset of contraction without abnormal function. If this theory was correct, all disturbances described above could be the result of an electrophysiological delay in the activation of the Purkinje fibres, but recent work of Dangman and Hoffman [14] showing that has all but excluded this possibility. It is more likely that the changes in isovolumic contraction and relaxation reflect either globally altered myocardial contractility or asynchrony of the electromechanical coupling within the sarcomere population. The data obtained from the analysis of endocardial wall motion favor the former hypothesis. A delay in the onset of wall displacement (Table XIII.2) and a profound change in the timing relation between aortic valve closure and peak inward displacement of the individual wall segments were clearly shown. Normally, contraction ends in a synchronous manner, except for some physiological late contraction of the inferobasal area (Fig. XIII.4). After nifedipine a considerable delay (Table XIII.2) of the anterior segments (4–8) and apical segments (8–10, 18–20) was seen, while contraction of the infero-basal segments (11–15) ended earlier. The mean velocity of systolic wall displacement ($\overline{V}_{ED-ES}$) was significantly reduced (Table XIII.2). Furthermore, after intracoronary administration of nifedipine, regional contribution to ejection fraction of the anterior and inferior wall segments decreased, respectively, by 26 and 14%.

Intracoronary nifedipine not only slows and depresses the segmental contraction, but also delays and prolongs it.

This latter observation led us to analyze another phenomenon. Since the volume of the ventricle is, by definition, constant during the relaxation period – defined in terms of valve movement – inward movement in one area must be compensated for by outward movement elsewhere. This is illustrated and shown quantitatively in Fig. XIII.7. Displacement 1 (D_1) expresses for the individual segments the systolic inward wall displacement from end diastole to aortic valve closure. Between aortic valve closure and mitral valve opening the majority of the anterior and infero-apical segments show a persisting inward wall motion, in contrast with the infero-basal segments which move outward. Column D_2 (displacement 2) expresses the net effect of inward and outward wall displacement as computed just before mitral valve opening.

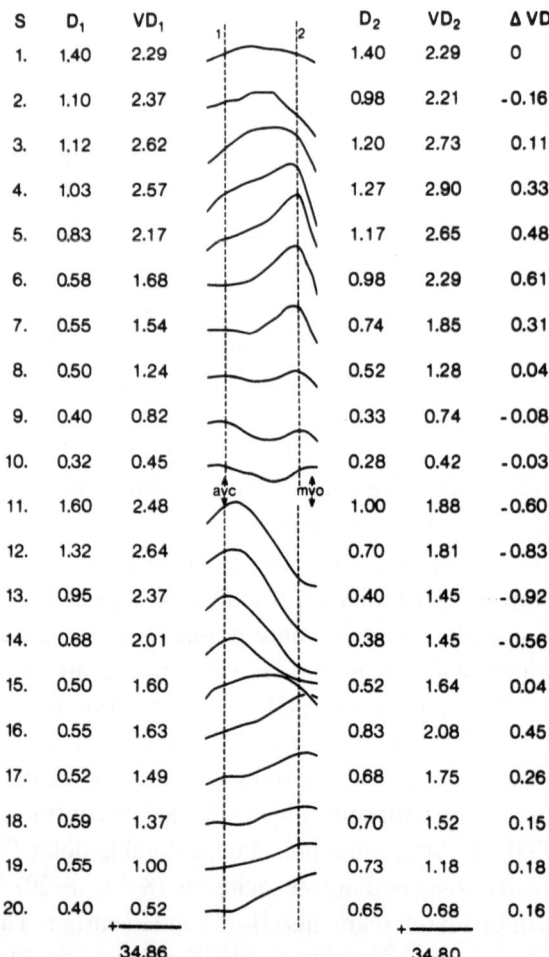

S	D$_1$	VD$_1$			D$_2$	VD$_2$	Δ VD
1.	1.40	2.29			1.40	2.29	0
2.	1.10	2.37			0.98	2.21	-0.16
3.	1.12	2.62			1.20	2.73	0.11
4.	1.03	2.57			1.27	2.90	0.33
5.	0.83	2.17			1.17	2.65	0.48
6.	0.58	1.68			0.98	2.29	0.61
7.	0.55	1.54			0.74	1.85	0.31
8.	0.50	1.24			0.52	1.28	0.04
9.	0.40	0.82			0.33	0.74	-0.08
10.	0.32	0.45			0.28	0.42	-0.03
11.	1.60	2.48	avc	mvo	1.00	1.88	-0.60
12.	1.32	2.64			0.70	1.81	-0.83
13.	0.95	2.37			0.40	1.45	-0.92
14.	0.68	2.01			0.38	1.45	-0.56
15.	0.50	1.60			0.52	1.64	0.04
16.	0.55	1.63			0.83	2.08	0.45
17.	0.52	1.49			0.68	1.75	0.26
18.	0.59	1.37			0.70	1.52	0.15
19.	0.55	1.00			0.73	1.18	0.18
20.	0.40	0.52			0.65	0.68	0.16
		34.86				34.80	

Fig. XIII.7. Segmental wall motion after intracoronary nifedipine during the isovolumic relaxation phase, between the closure of the aortic valve (AVC) and the opening of the mitral valve (MVO). See also Fig. XIII.1. S: segment number; D$_1$: segmental wall displacement (cm) between end diastole (ED) and AVC; D$_2$: segmental wall displacement (cm) between ED and MVO; VD$_1$: segmental volume displacement (ml) between ED and AVC; VD$_2$: segmental volume displacement (ml) between ED and MVO; ΔVD: changes in segmental volume between AVC and MVO, expressed in ml.

From the displacement D$_1$ and D$_2$ the segmental volume displacements are computed. The total volume displaced between end diastole and aortic valve opening equals that displaced between end diastole and mitral valve opening. Thus, the ventricular volume remains constant while a variety of segmental wall motion changes takes place. In studying this illustration it becomes obvious that changes in the rate of pressure relaxation may not only reflect a globally altered myocardial relaxation, but also heterogeneity in activation and performance within the sarcomere population, with continuation of contraction and tension development extending into the isovolumic period. In other words, impaired relaxation of the ventricle as a whole must not automatically be equated with impaired relaxation at a cellular level.

Fleckenstein et al. [15] have indicated that electromechanical decoupling occurs after nifedipine which leads to decrease in actin-myosin interaction. The negative inotropic effect on the heart which was recorded and the upward shift in left ventricular diastolic pressure volume curves observed in this study are probably an expression of that fundamental biochemical effect: nifedipine interrupts the normal process by which calcium is transported to the cell, lowers the cytosolic calcium and inhibits and delays contraction of the myocardial wall so that there is delay in diastolic interaction of contractile elements. This could be a reasonable explanation for the upward shift in left ventricular diastolic pressure volume curves. On the other hand, residual diastolic interaction between contractile elements – caused by an increased cytosolic calcium [16] – has also been proposed as a possible explanation for the upward shift in diastolic pressure volume relations seen during angina [17, 18].

Cultures of dissociated beating ventricular cells from chick embryos manifested a negative inotropic response to calcium antagonism [19]. That is, amplitude and velocity of contraction of the individual cells decreased in the presence of the drug, while there was no effect on velocity of cell wall motion during relaxation. Higher calcium concentrations, however, did cause a slowing in the rate of relaxation and a decrease in the amplitude of contraction as though the cells were in a constant state of partial contracture. Thus, the apparently conflicting observations are reconciled since the changes induced in cultured cells by high calcium concentrations are reversed by calcium antagonists, indicating 'that calcium antagonist can dramatically improve systolic and diastolic function of a calcium-overloaded myocardial cell'.

Coronary blood flow and myocardial oxygen consumption

In our patients the myocardial oxygen consumption decreased by 28% after intracoronary injection of nifedipine. From our hemodynamic and angiographic data we assume that the decrease in myocardial oxygen consumption depended primarily on a decrease in contractility and left ventricular performance. This interpretation, however, is open to question, since despite an increase in global coronary blood flow, a decrease in endocardial flow and oxygen supply could make the endocardium ischemic and consequently alter its mechanical performance. Others have pointed to the fact that after administration of a coronary vasodilator endocardial capillary blood flow may actually decrease because of an epicardial coronary 'steal' phenomenon [20].

This difference in regional blood flow response is seen particularly when coronary blood flow is increased in the presence of a critical stenosis of a large coronary artery [21, 22]. In these circumstances, when flow is increased as a result of arteriolar dilatation distal to the stenosis, transmural perfusion becomes heterogeneous because of the greater increase in epicardial flow [23]. In the present study we do not have any experimental evidence which would allow us to rule out this possibility, but Henry et al. [24] have shown that, in dogs subjected to coronary occlusion, nifedipine increases collateral flow to the ischemic myocardium. This increase was accompanied by a relative increase in endocardial perfusion, a phenomenon that was particularly prominent in the ischemic zone [24].

Quantitative coronary angiography

Although it has been proved that nifedipine dilates the coronary arteries, particularly in patients with variant angina, there have been few reports showing whether this drug actually dilates the coronary artery at the point of the stenotic lesions or at points distal to fixed obstructions [25].

The present study provides quantitative measurements of the effects of nifedipine on the epicardial coronary artery after direct intracoronary administration. This route of administration was used in order to dissociate its coronary vasodilator action from its direct myocardial effect and afterload reduction [10, 26]. When nifedipine (0.1 mg) was intravenously injected, it had no detectable hemodynamic effects. When nifedipine was regionally administered, it had a transient negative inotropic effect, associated with a transient increase in coronary blood flow and decrease in myocardial oxygen consumption. The vasodilatation of all three, the prestenotic, stenotic, and poststenotic coronary segments, persisted, however, much longer than the hemodynamic effects, at least during the period of observation in this study. This observation raises the possibility that there are distinct differences in the response to nifedipine between the myocardial cells and the smooth muscle cells in the coronary vascular wall.

Another essential question is: what effect do large vessel vasomotor tone and distal arteriolar resistance have on a proximal lesion? In isolated perfused human coronary arteries, a decrease in perfusion pressure can lead to a 'dynamic' increase in resistance to flow across an elastic and eccentric stenosis [27].

The study has even shown experimentally that the administration of a coronary vasodilator could induce a fall into distending pressure of the poststenotic coronary segment, resulting in a passive collapse of the wall of the stenotic segment and an increase in resistance to flow [28–30].

An explanation for these conflicting possibilities may be that in the experimental studies the vasodilators affected primarily the distal arteriolar coronary bed leading to a reduction in poststenotic intraluminal pressure, whereas in the clinical studies the epicardial large coronary arteries were primarily affected in their prestenotic as well as in their poststenotic segments [31].

Conclusion

Intracoronary nifedipine not only delays and prolongs the segmental contraction, but also slows and depresses it. It is suggested that a decreased cytosolic calcium might induce delayed diastolic interaction between contractile elements which could be a reasonable explanation for alteration of the isovolumic relaxation and for the upward shift in the left ventricular pressure volume curve after intracoronary administration of nifedipine. We presume that the decrease in myocardial oxygen consumption depends primarily on a decrease in contractility and left ventricular performance. Finally, we showed that the vasodilatation of the epicardial vessels after intracoronary nifedipine persists longer than its direct effects on the myocardium. In conclusion, the transient regional 'cardioplegic' effect of nifedipine, associated with an increase in coronary blood flow, a reduction in MVO_2, and a vasodilatation of the epicardial vessels, is likely to be beneficial during temporary coronary occlusion.

References

1. Hugenholtz PG, Michels HR, Serruys PW, Brower RW: Nifedipine in the treatment of unstable angina, coronary spasm and myocardial ischemia. Am J Cardiol 47: 163–173, 1981.
2. Bertrand ME, Lablanche JM, Tilmant PY: Treatment of Prinzmetal's variant angina. Role of medical treatment with nifedipine and surgical coronary revascularization combined with plexectomy. Am J Cardiol 47: 174–178, 1981.
3. Serruys PW, van den Brand M, Brower RW, Hugenholtz PG: Regional cardioplegia and cardioprotection during transluminal angioplasty, which role for nifedipine? Eur Heart J 4 (Suppl C): 115–121, 1983.
4. Serruys PW, van den Brand M, Hooghoudt TEH, Simoons ML, Fioretti P, Ruiter J, Fels PW, Hugenholtz PG: Coronary recanalization in acute myocardial infarction: immediate results and potential risks. Eur Heart J 3: 404–415, 1982.
5. Meester GT, Bernard N, Zeelenberg C, Brower RW, Hugenholtz PG: A computer system for real time analysis of cardiac catheterization data. Cathet Cardiovasc Diagn 1: 113–132, 1975.
6. Fioretti P, Brower RW, Meester GT, Serruys PW: Interaction of left ventricular relaxation and filling during early diastole in human subjects. Am J Cardiol 46: 197–203, 1980.
7. Gaasch WH, Levine HJ, Quinones MA, Alexander JK: Left ventricular compliance: mechanisms and clinical implications. Am J Cardiol 38: 645–653, 1976.
8. Ganz W, Tamura K, Marcus HS, Donoso R, Yoshido S, Swan HJC: Measurement of coronary sinus blood flow by continuous thermodilution in man. Circulation 44: 181–195, 1971.
9. Hugenholtz PG, Verdouw PD, Meester GT: Fiberoptics in cardiac catheterization. II. Practical applications. In: Dye Curves: The Theory and Practice of Indicator Dilution. DA Bloomfield (Ed.). University Park Press, Baltimore/London/Tokyo: 285–311, 1974.
10. Serruys PW, Brower RW, ten Katen HJ, Bom AH, Hugenholtz PG: Regional wall motion from radiopaque markers after intravenous and intracoronary injections of nifedipine. Circulation 63: 584–591, 1981.
11. Rousseau MF, Veriter C, Detry JMR, Brasseur L, Pouleur H: Impaired early left ventricular relaxation in coronary artery disease: effects of intracoronary nifedipine. Circulation 62: 764–772, 1980.

294

12. Altieri PI, Wilt SM, Leighton RF: Left ventricular wall motion during the isovolumic relaxation period. Circulation 48: 499–505, 1973.
13. Gibson DG, Doran JH, Traill TA, Brown DJ: Regional abnormalities of left ventricular wall movement during isovolumic relaxation in patients with ischemic heart disease. Eur J Cardiol 7, Suppl: 251–264, 1978.
14. Dangman KH, Hoffman BF: Effects of nifedipine on electrical activity of cardiac cells. Am J Cardiol 46: 1059–1067, 1980.
15. Fleckenstein A von, Tritthart H, Döring HJ, Byon KY: BAY a 1040-ein hochaktiver Ca^{++}-antagonistischer Inhibitor der elektro-mechanischen Koppelungsprozesse im Warmblüter-Myokard. Arzneim Forsch 22: 22–33, 1972.
16. Lewis MJ, Grey AC, Henderson AH: Determinants of hypoxic contracture in isolated heart muscle preparations. Cardiovasc Res 13: 86–94, 1979.
17. Grossman W, Serizawa T, Carabello BA: Studies on the mechanism of altered left ventricular diastolic pressure-volume relations during ischaemia. Eur Heart J 1 (Suppl A) 141–147, 1980.
18. Grossman W, Barry WH: Diastolic pressure-volume relations in the diseased heart. Fed Proc 39: 148–155, 1980.
19. Lorell BH, Barry WH: Effects of verapamil on myocardial systolic and diastolic function during calcium overload. Circulation 62 (Supp III): 293 (Abstract), 1980.
20. Lipscomb K, Gould KL: Mechanism of the effect of coronary artery stenosis on coronary flow in the dog. Am Heart J 89: 60–67, 1975.
21. Gould KL, Lipscomb K, Calvert C: Compensatory changes of the distal coronary vascular bed during progressive coronary constriction. Circulation 51: 1085–1094, 1975.
22. Nakamura M, Matsuguchi H, Mitsutake A, Kikuchi Y, Takeshita A, Nakagaki O, Kuroiwa A: The effect of graded coronary stenosis on myocardial blood flow and left ventricular wall motion. Basic Res Cardiol 72: 479–491, 1977.
23. Weintraub WS, Hattori S, Agarwal J, Bodenheimer MM, Banka VS, Helfant RH: Variable effect of nifedipine on myocardial blood flow at three grades of coronary occlusion in the dog. Circ Res 48: 937–942, 1981.
24. Henry PD, Shuchleib R, Clark RE, Perez JE: Effect of nifedipine on myocardial ischemia: analysis of collateral flow, pulsatile heat and regional muscle shortening. Am J Cardiol 44: 817–824, 1979.
25. Schulz W, Kober G, Krauss G, Kaltenbach M: Influence of intracoronary and intravenous nifedipine on diameters of coronary vessels and stenoses. In: Unstable Angina Pectoris. W Rafflenbeul, PR Lichtlen, R Balcon (Eds.). Georg Thieme Verlag, Stuttgart/New York: 259–265, 1981.
26. Kaltenbach M, Schulz W, Kober G: Effects of nifedipine after intravenous and intracoronary administration. Am J Cardiol 44: 832–838, 1979.
27. Logan SE: On the fluid mechanics of human coronary artery stenosis. IEEE Trans Biomed Eng 22: 327–334, 1975.
28. Walinsky P, Santamore WP, Wiener L, Brest AN: Dynamic changes in the haemodynamic severity of coronary artery stenosis in a canine model. Cardiovasc Res 13: 113–118, 1979.
29. Santamore WP, Walinsky P: Altered coronary flow responses to vasoactive drugs in the presence of coronary arterial stenosis in the dog. Am J Cardiol 45: 276–285, 1980.
30. Schwartz JS, Carlyle PF, Cohn JN: Effect of dilation of the distal coronary bed on flow and resistance in severely stenotic coronary arteries in the dog. Am J Cardiol 43: 219–224, 1979.
31. Gould KL: Dynamic coronary stenosis. Am J Cardiol 45: 286–292, 1980.

XIV. Effect of intracoronary thrombolytic therapy on global and regional left ventricular function. A three years experience with randomization

Summary

The effect of myocardial reperfusion on regional left ventricular function has been quantitated by analysis of segmental wall motion in 185 patients enrolled in a randomized trial comparing thrombolysis with conventional treatment in patients with acute myocardial infarction. When analyzing the hemodynamic data on an 'intention to treat' basis, we found a significant preservation of left ventricular function after thrombolytic therapy when compared to conventional treatment. In addition, the wall motion analysis showed that a significant improvement of regional function in the 'infarct zone' was observed in inferior infarction as well as in anterior infarction, although significant changes in regional function of the remote 'noninfarct zone' were observed at the acute as well as the chronic stage.

However, our follow-up data indicate that as yet it has not been resolved whether this method of treatment does indeed improve prognosis in patients with acute myocardial infarction. Accordingly, we maintain the view that such invasive treatment should not be generally applied until more follow-up data become available from larger randomized trials.

Introduction

Since the initial publication by Rentrop et al., it has been confirmed that acutely occluded coronary arteries can be recanalized by intracoronary infusion of a fibrinolytic agent [1]. Reestablishment of antegrade flow might prevent myocardium, made temporarily ischemic by coronary occlusion, from progressing to complete necrosis or alternatively might support marginally viable cells [2]. Animal experiments have shown that restoration of coronary blood flow may save myocardium [3, 4, 5] and improve survival [3], if the reperfusion is instituted within a few hours after coronary occlusion. However, it is still uncertain whether these results are applicable in humans. The risk of angiography in the first hours of myocardial infarction is not negligible [6] and may outweigh the potential benefit of the recanalization; reperfusion of ischemic myocardium might be harmful because of the occurrence of serious arrhythmias [7], intramyocardial hemorrhage [8, 9] and calcium overload of myocardial cells with subsequent death as a result of too rapid reperfusion – the oxygen paradox [10].

To answer the question as to whether this approach to the treatment of patients with acute myocardial infarction will be ultimately beneficial to most patients with acute myocardial infarction, a carefully designed randomized trial was started in June 1981 at the Thoraxcenter. This study includes detailed analysis of the influence of myocardial reperfusion on left ventricular (LV) function two weeks after attempted recanalization, as well as identical studies on those patients assigned to conventional treatment (CT) in addition to a long-term follow-up with end points such as mortality and reinfarction rate. In the randomized trials, published thus far, the assessment of global ejection fraction has mainly been employed for this purpose [11–14].

However, any improvement of global left ventricular function after successful recanalization of a coronary artery might be caused by several factors: salvage of jeopardized myocardium, compensatory hyperactivity of other wall segments [15, 16] or changes in pre- and afterload.

In an effort to solve this problem, the effect of myocardial reperfusion on regional left ventricular function has been quantitated by analysis of segmental wall motion.

Patient selection and methods

The randomized trial of thrombolysis in acute myocardial infarction is a multicenter study supported by the Interuniversity Cardiology Institute in the Netherlands. The study was initiated at the Thoraxcenter in June 1981. The Free University in Amsterdam and the Zuiderziekenhuis in Rotterdam have participated in the trial since January 1983, and the St. Annadal Hospital in Maastricht since August 1983. The present analysis is limited to the first 185 patients enrolled at the Thoraxcenter between June 1981 and June 1984.

Patient selection

Patients were eligible for the trial if they had been admitted within 4 hours after the onset of chest pain with a duration of 20 minutes or more and with ECG-signs compatible with myocardial infarction. ST-segment elevation of 0.2 mV or greater should be present in one of the precordial leads and/or 0.1 mV in a limb lead, despite of treatment with oral or intravenous nitroglycerine and/or nifedipine. In addition, patients were included with 0.2 mV ST-segment depression in

precordial leads, compatible with posterior wall infarction. The following exclusion criteria were used:
– Age over 70 years
– Previous treatment with streptokinase
– Bypass surgery of the vessels corresponding to the infarct location
– Recent trauma including traumatic resuscitation
– Gastro-intestinal bleeding or ulcer within 3 months
– Hematuria within 3 months
– Cerebrovascular accident within 3 months
– Pregnant or menstruating women
– Mental confusion precluding informed consent
– Anticipation of follow up problems.

Study protocol

A flow chart of the protocol is presented in figure XIV.1. Eligible patients who did not meet the exclusion criteria were entered in the trial. These patients were registered by a central telephone answering service. The physician at the CCU called the answering service and provided administrative data including patient's initials, sex, date of birth and clinical state. The answering service then opened the randomization envelope and provided treatment allocation. Informed con-

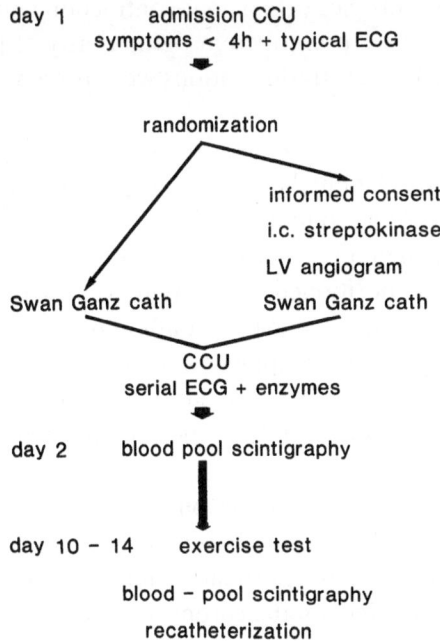

Fig. XIV.1. Flow chart of the procedures in the current randomized trial at the Thoraxcenter.

sent was asked from patients allocated to thrombolytic treatment only [17]. Seven patients refused the intervention, while informed consent was obtained in 86 patients; 92 were assigned to conventional treatment (CT). Patients who refused consent were treated according to the conventional treatment protocol. Data analysis was based on the 'intention to treat' principle. Thus patients who refused acute angiography were analyzed as part of the thrombolysis group, following original treatment allocation.

Conventional treatment was guided by hemodynamic monitoring. Both in the control group and in patients allocated to thrombolysis it was attempted to achieve an 'optimal' hemodynamic state characterized by light sedation, a heart rate between 60 and 90 beats per minute, systolic blood pressure between 100 and 140 mmHg and absence of left ventricular failure with the pulmonary capillary wedge pressure below 12 mmHg. Guidelines for treatment have been described in detail [18] and include the use of beta blockers when heart rate was greater than 90 bpm with systolic blood pressure over 100 mmHg in the absence of heart failure; nitroprusside when systolic blood pressure was greater than 150 mmHg; nitroglycerine and furosemide in the presence of heart failure; atropine and/or temporary ventricular pacing in the case of bradycardia and dobutamine in patients with systolic blood pressure lower than 100 mmHg. In addition intra-aortic balloon counter pulsation was used for the treatment of cardiogenic shock.

All patients were treated with heparine followed by acenocoumarol (Sintrom®) until hospital discharge. After discharge anticoagulants were continued only in patients with ventricular aneurysm, intraventricular thrombus, mitral incompetence or large ventricles with a poor contraction pattern. Beta blockers, metoprolol 2×100 mg, were prescribed in the majority of patients starting between 7 and 14 days unless contra-indications were present. Other therapy was prescribed as needed.

In patients assigned to streptokinase treatment, a nitroglycerine infusion ($100\,\mu g/kg/min$) was started immediately and the patients were transferred to the catheterization laboratory as soon as possible. Lidocaine was also given intravenously in a dose of 2 mg/min. After puncturing the femoral vein and artery a pacemaker catheter was positioned in the right ventricle. Next, coronary arteriography of the artery suspected to be thrombosed was performed. A nonionic contrast agent (Amipaque®) was employed as contrast medium. After identification of the thrombosed coronary branch, 50 mg heparin was administered intravenously together with 250 mg acetylsalicylic acid and 100 mg diadresone F^R, a corticosteroid.

Before starting the intracoronary perfusion with streptokinase, 3 mg isosorbide dinitrate was injected into the thrombosed coronary artery over 1 min, with monitoring of the aortic pressure. Coronary arteriography was then repeated to evaluate any spasmolytic effect on the coronary occlusion. Intracoronary perfusion with streptokinase was carried out at a rate of 4000 units/min to a maximum of 250,000 units of streptokinase, diluted in 500 ml of physiological solution, at a flow rate of 8 ml/min. Coronary angiograms were repeated every 15 minutes until the chest pain disappeared. The appearance of ventricular extrasystoles or any other conduction disturbance was also an indication to reangiogram the artery. If there were no signs of recanalization, an attempt was made to administer strep-tokinase locally in a higher concentration by passing a thin catheter (French 2) with a radiopaque tip through the Judkins catheter (French 8). After completion of the streptokinase infusion, nitroglycerine and lidocaine infusions were ceased and complete left and right coronary arteriography was performed. If the clinical condition was stable with left ventricular end-diastolic pressure below 35 mmHg, left ventriculography in the RAO projection was done. In 31 patients, per-cutaneous transluminal coronary angioplasty was performed in the same session, 20 to 60 minutes after the end of streptokinase infusion, in order to prevent early and late reocclusion [19]. The day before discharge from the intermediate care area, coronary arteriography and left ventricular angiography were obtained both in the control group (CT) and the trombolysis-treated (TR) group.

In 125 patients, left ventriculograms of sufficient quality were obtained to permit automated analysis with the Contouromat. The small number of late angiograms was due to the following factors. In the thrombolysis group, 7 patients refused the thrombolytic therapy after randomization, three of them died within 10 days; 3 other patients died during attempted fibrinolysis; one patient sustained a fatal reinfarction shortly after successful fibrinolysis; two were transferred to another hospital; eight underwent coronary artery bypass-grafting after thrombolysis because of symptoms and 12 refused to cooperate with the follow-up study. In the conventionally treated group, six patients died in the hospital before catheterization could be performed; eighteen refused the cathe-terization and there were three LV angiograms of insufficient quality to permit automated analysis. Thus, at the chronic stage, 65 left ventricular angiograms were available for analysis in the control group and 60 angiograms in the throm-bolysis group.

Both groups are similar with regard to the infarct localization on the electrocar-diogram and the involved vessel. The CT-group includes 20 patients with pre-vious infarction compared with 13 in the thrombolysis group (ns). Their data provide the essence of this study (Table XIV.1).

Analysis of global and regional LV function

Global and regional left ventricular function was studied from the 30° right anterior oblique left ventricular cineangiogram and analyzed with the Con-touromat with the MAXI-cine program. The segmental CREF-values in the antero-basal (segments 1–5), antero-lateral (segments 5–9), apical (segments 9, 10, 19 and 20), inferior (segments 15–19) and postero-basal (segments 11–15) wall regions were compared in the CT-group and in the TR-group.

Table XIV.1. Clinical and angiographic data in 125 patients with LV angiogram at two weeks

	Conventional treatment (CT)	p-value	i.c. Thrombolysis (TR)
Number of patients	65	n.s.	60
Infarct localization			
Anterior/lateral	33 (51%)	n.s.	34 (57%)
Inferior/posterior	32 (49%)	n.s.	26 (43%)
Previous infarction	20 (31%)	n.s.	13 (22%)
Infarct related vessel			
LAD	26 (40%)	n.s.	29 (48%)
LCX	11 (17%)	n.s.	8 (13%)
RCA	28 (43%)	n.s.	23 (38%)
Infarct related vessel patency	30 (46%)	= 0.003	48 (80%)

Abbreviations: i.c. = intracoronary; LAD = left anterior descending coronary artery; LCX = left circumflex; RCA = right coronary artery; n.s. = nonsignificant.

Statistical analysis

Data are expressed as mean ± s.d.; paired or unpaired t-tests of Student were applied to the hemodynamic data whenever appropriate. Differences in baseline characteristics between groups were tested by the Fisher's exact test.

Results

The effect of the thrombolytic therapy is shown by 80% patency of the infarct related vessel in the intervention group versus 46% patency in the control group (p = 0.003) at two weeks (Table XIV.1).

In Table XIV.2 the hemodynamic data of the control group are compared to those of the thrombolysis group. Almost all the parameters listed in this table are significantly different in both groups. The global left ventricular ejection fraction in the thrombolysis group was 10% (p-value 10^{-3}) higher than in the control group and this was mainly due to a smaller end-systolic volume in the thrombolysis group, (38 ml/m² versus 55 ml/m² in the control group, p-value<.0001). Most prominent is the smaller percentage of abnormally contracting segments in the thrombolysis group: 7.8% versus 15.5% [20]. In addition, the end-diastolic pressure and volume were significantly higher in the control group than in the thrombolysis group, whereas the mean aortic pressure and heart rate were not different at the time of the hemodynamic investigation. Table XIV.3 shows the hemodynamic data of both groups after exclusion of the patients with the pre-

Table XIV.2. Left ventricular hemodynamics prior to discharge.

	CT (N = 65)		TR (N = 60)		p-value
HR [bpm]	79	± 16	75	± 13	n.s.
mean AoP [mmHg]	92	± 14	94	± 14	n.s.
EDP [mmHg]	22	± 8	18	± 8	<.003
EDV [ml/m²]	99	± 27	81	± 20	<.001
ESV [ml/m²]	55	± 27	38	± 15	<.0001
EF [%]	45	± 14	55	± 11	<.001
SV [ml/m²]	42	± 13	44	± 12	n.s.
CI [1/min/m²]	3.2± 0.9		3.3± 0.9		n.s.
ACS [%]	15.5 ± 15		7.8 ± 10		<.002

Values are expressed as mean ± s.d.; Student test for unpaired data.
Abbreviations: HR = heart rate; AoP = aortic pressure; EDP = end-diastolic pressure; EDV = end-diastolic volume; ESV = end-systolic volume; EF = ejection fraction; SV = stroke volume; CI = cardiac index; ACS = abnormally contracting segments [24]. CT = conventional treatment; TR = thrombolysis.

vious infarction (20 in the control group and 13 in the thrombolysis group). It appears that the differences observed in the entire group (n = 125 patients) after conventional treatment or thrombolytic therapy are still present and significant, although less marked, when corrected for the uneven incidence of patients with previous infarction. In the thrombolysis group, the ejection fraction is 6% (p<0.02) higher than in the control group, while the end-systolic volume is 11 ml/m² (p<0.02) smaller than in the control group. From these results we may conclude, that attempted treatment with intracoronary streptokinase leads to preservation of global left ventricular function even when the results are pre-

Table XIV.3. Left ventricular hemodynamics prior to discharge in patients without previous myocardial infarction.

	CT (N = 45)		TR (N = 47)		p-value
HR [bpm]	79	± 17	74	± 12	n.s.
mean AoP [mmHg]	94	± 15	94	± 16	n.s.
EDP [mmHg]	21	± 8	18	± 8	<.05
EDV [ml/m²]	94	± 25	82	± 20	<.02
ESV [ml/m²]	48	± 23	37	± 15	<.02
EF [%]	50	± 14	56	± 11	<.02
SV [ml/m²]	45	± 14	46	± 11	n.s.
CI [1/min/m²]	3.3± 0.9		3.4± 0.8		n.s.
ACS [%]	11.7 ± 14		7.3 ± 10		n.s.

Abbreviations as in Table XIV.2.

302

sented on an 'intention to treat' basis. However, the crucial question remains as to whether we can ascribe these differences in global LV function to the salvage of previously jeopardized myocardium in the area supplied by recanalized vessel.

In an effort to answer this question, segmental wall motion was analyzed in patients with anterior and inferior infarction. In Table XIV.4 and Fig. XIV.2 the global and regional LV functions of patients with inferior infarction are presented. The global LVEF shows a 11% difference ($p < 0.01$) in favor of the thrombolysis group and this difference in EF is due to a significantly ($p < 0.005$) smaller end-systolic volume ($35 \, ml/m^2$) as compared to the end-systolic volume ($56 \, ml/m^2$) of the control group. Also the end-diastolic pressure, the end-diastolic volume and the percentage of the abnormally contracting segments are smaller in the thrombolysis group. In Fig. XIV.2, the CREF values of the patients with inferior infarction assigned to thrombolysis are compared with those assigned to conventional treatment. Subnormal CREF values were observed in the infero-posterior wall (segments 11–18) as expected, but a significantly less marked depression in regional pump function was observed in patients assigned to thrombolysis. No difference in regional function of the anterior wall was observed. In Table XIV.7 and Fig. XIV.2C the changes in global and regional LV function from the acute stage (immediately after recanalization) to the chronic stage (two weeks later) in the patients with inferior infarction are presented. When the recanalization is successful and the infarct related vessel remains patent at two weeks, no significant change in the global hemodynamics is observed. This contrasts with a significant improvement within two weeks of the inferior wall associated with the subsidence of the compensatory functioning of the anterior wall (Fig. XIV.2C). This latter phenomenon is particularly prominent in the patients who underwent at the acute phase a combined procedure of recanalization and angioplasty (Fig. XIV.2D).

In Table XIV.5 and Fig. XIV.3, the global and regional LV functions of patients with anterior myocardial infarction are shown. A significant ($p < 0.02$)

Table XIV.4. LV hemodynamics in inferior infarction prior to discharge.

	CT (N = 32)		TR (N = 26)		p-value
HR [bpm]	80	± 17	72	± 12	n.s.
mean AoP [mmHg]	92	± 15	98	± 17	n.s.
EDP [mmHg]	21	± 8	18	± 7	n.s.
EDV [ml/m²]	100	± 26	75	± 23	<.001
ESV [ml/m²]	56	± 26	35	± 16	<.005
EF [%]	45	± 13	56	± 11	<.01
SV [ml/m²]	43	± 12	42	± 11	n.s.
CI [1/min/m²]	3.3 ± 0.9		3.0 ± 0.8		n.s.
ACS [%]	13.9 ± 15		2.5 ± 4		<.001

Abbreviations as in Table XIV.2; CT = conventional treatment; TR = thrombolysis.

8% difference in ejection fraction is shown between both groups due to a smaller end-systolic volume in the thrombolysis group, 40 ml/m² versus 55 ml/m² in the control group (p < .02). Fig. XIV.3 clearly indicates that this 8% difference in LVEF in favor of the thrombolysis group is essentially due to a better regional pump function of the inferior wall and, to a smaller extent, better regional pump function of the basal segment of the anterior wall (Fig. XIV.3A).

Moreover, it must be pointed out that these results have been analyzed on 'an intention to treat basis' and that the thrombolysis group can be subdivided in three subsets of patients: (a) patients with either unsuccessful recanalization or late occlusion; (b) patients with successful recanalization and late patency of the IRV (Infarct Related Vessel); (c) patients who underwent a successful recanalization, immediately followed by angioplasty.

In the patient who could not be successfully recanalized the segmental function of the anterior wall was the worst, while the greatest preservation of regional function of the anterior wall was observed in the patients who underwent a combined procedure of recanalization and angioplasty.

In Table XIV.6 and Fig. XIV.3C, the serial (acute, and after two weeks) changes in global and regional LV function of the patients with anterior infarction are shown. Following successful recanalization, no significant change in global hemodynamics could be demonstrated. In these patients the small but significant improvement of the anterior wall observed between the acute and chronic stage was partially masked by the disappearance of the compensatory functioning of the inferior wall (Table XIV.6). Conversely, when recanalization was unsuccessful this resulted in a significant deterioration of the global parameters: decrease of 5% in ejection fraction (p < .05), increase in ESV from 34 to 46 ml/m² (p < .01), in EDV from 75 to 89 ml (p < .05).

These changes in global function corresponded with deterioration of the regional function in the anterior, apical and apico-inferior segments.

Table XIV.5. LV hemodynamics in anterior infarction prior to discharge.

	CT (N = 33)	TR (N = 34)	p-value
HR [bpm]	77 ± 14	78 ± 13	n.s.
mean AoP [mmHg]	92 ± 14	91 ± 14	n.s.
EDP [mmHg]	23 ± 7	18 ± 8	< .02
EDV [ml/m²]	97 ± 27	86 ± 17	= .05
ESV [ml/m²]	55 ± 29	40 ± 14	< .02
EF [%]	46 ± 14	54 ± 11	< .01
SV [ml/m²]	42 ± 14	46 ± 11	n.s.
CI [l/min/m²]	3.1 ± 0.9	3.5 ± 0.9	n.s.
ACS [%]	16.9 ± 16	11.2 ± 12	n.s.

Abbreviations as in Table XIV.2.

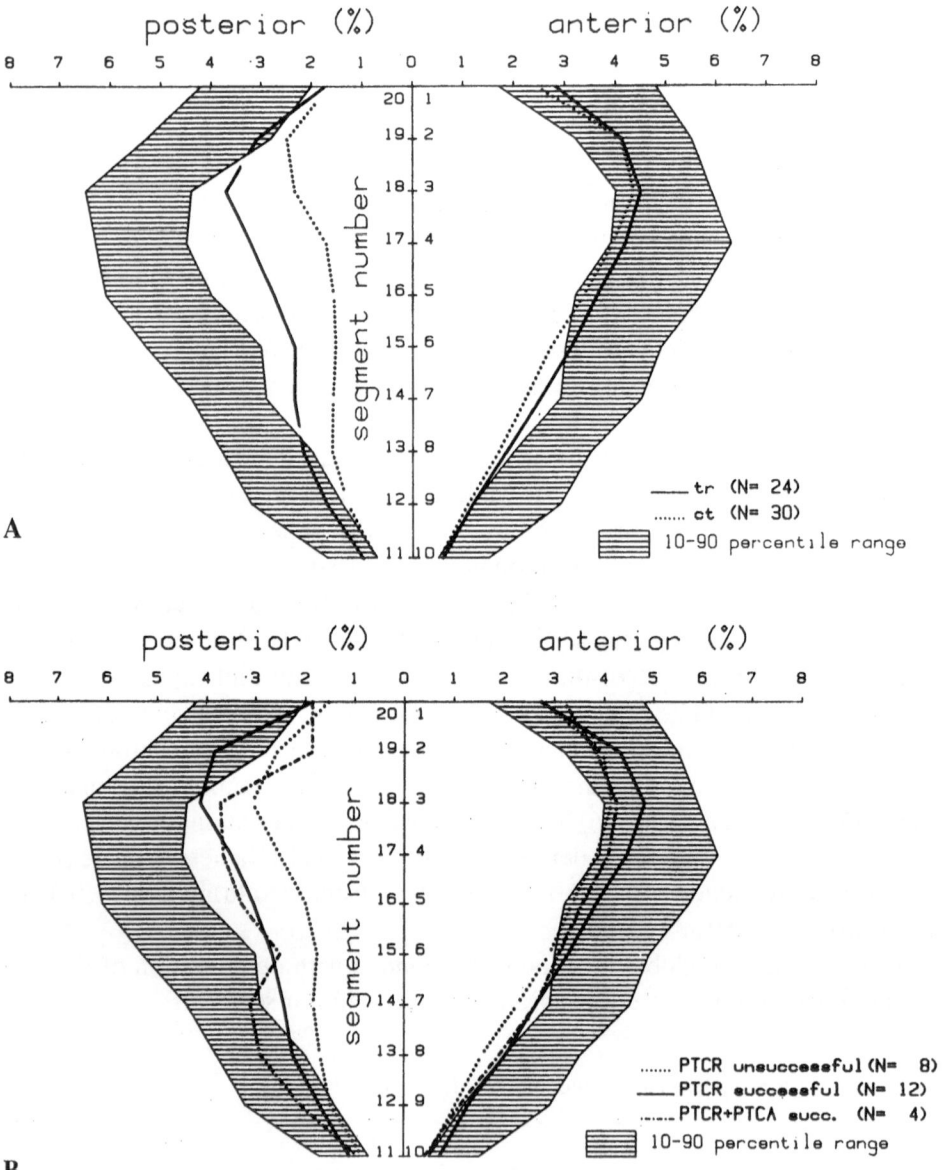

Fig. XIV.2. A. Regional contribution to global ejection fraction (CREF) in 20 segments of the left ventriculogram in patients with inferior infarction. Shaded areas represent the normal range. The regional pump function of the inferior wall (segments 11 to 20) in the thrombolysis treated group (solid line) is markedly less depressed than in the conventionally treated group (dotted lines).

B. Regional contribution of the inferior wall to global ejection fraction at the chronic stage in the

305

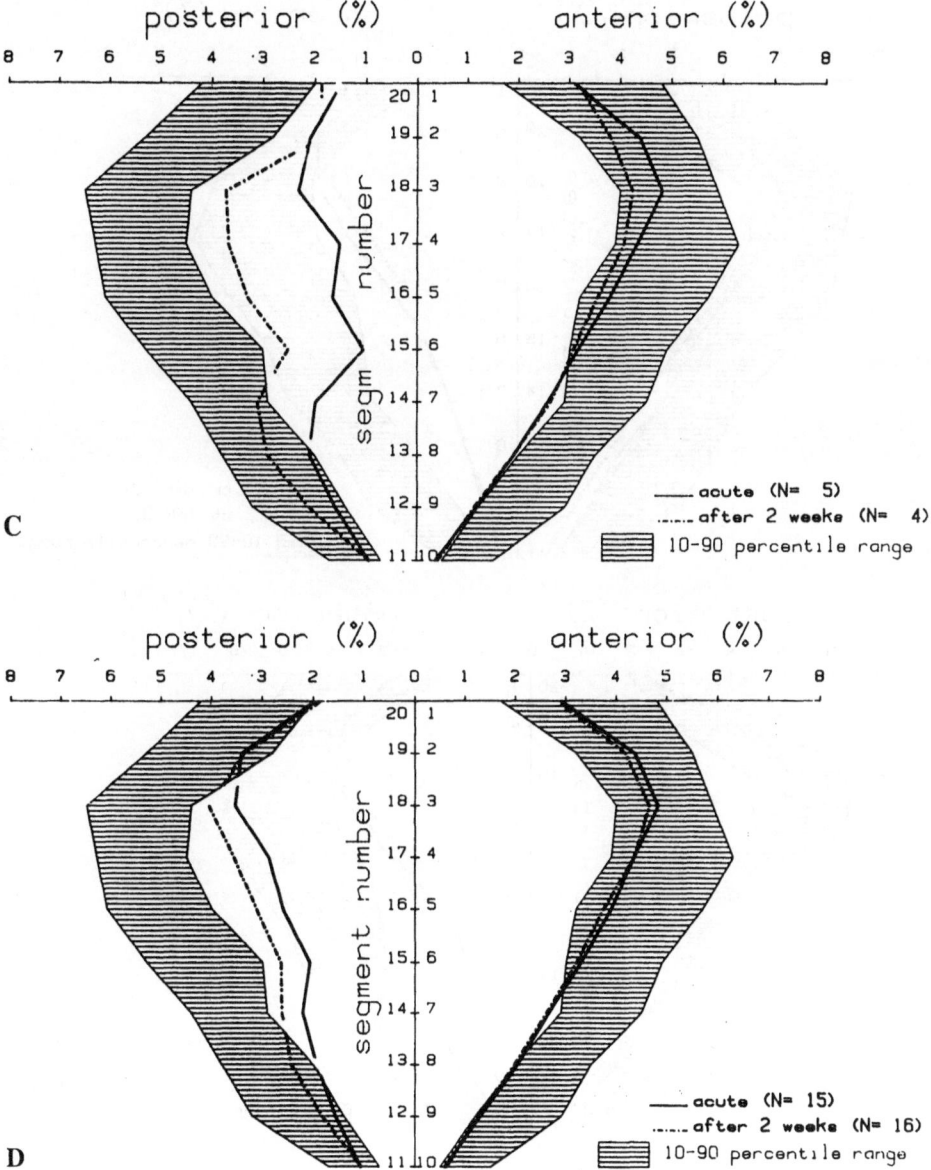

thrombolysis group, according to the success of the recanalization at the acute stage.

C. Change in CREF from the acute (solid line) to the chronic stage (dotted line) in patients (N = 16) with an inferior infarction, who underwent a successful recanalization.

D. Change in CREF from the acute (solid line) to the chronic stage (dotted line) in patients (N = 5) with an inferior infarction who underwent a combined procedure of recanalization and angioplasty.

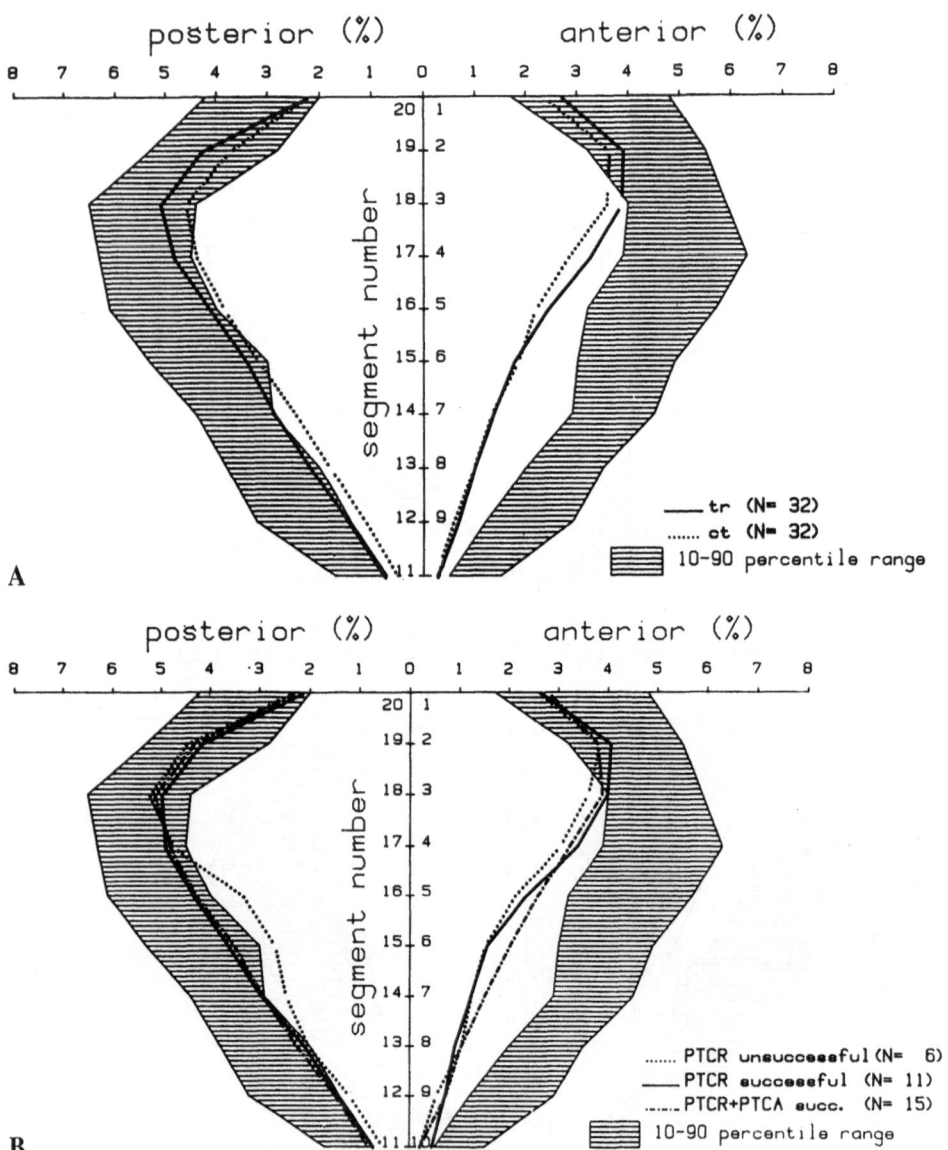

A

B

Table XIV.6. Thrombolysis group: serial LV hemodynamics in anterior infarction.

	Successful (N = 26)			Unsuccessful (N = 6)		
	Acute	p-value	Chronic	Acute	p-value	Chronic
HR [bpm]	81 ± 12	n.s.	76 ± 13	87 ± 16	n.s.	77 ± 15
AoP [mmHg]	89 ± 12	n.s.	92 ± 8	87 ± 16	n.s.	95 ± 21
EDP [mmHg]	23 ± 9	n.s.	19 ± 8	18 ± 7	n.s.	18 ± 11
EDV [ml/m²]	84 ± 21	n.s.	88 ± 20	75 ± 18	<.05	89 ± 18
ESV [ml/m²]	40 ± 15	n.s.	41 ± 15	34 ± 10	<.01	46 ± 16
EF [%]	52 ± 10	n.s.	55 ± 11	54 ± 7	<.05	49 ± 13
SV [ml/m²]	42 ± 11	<.03	48 ± 14	39 ± 10	n.s.	43 ± 12

Abbreviations as previously. Values are expressed as mean ± sd; Student t-test for paired data.

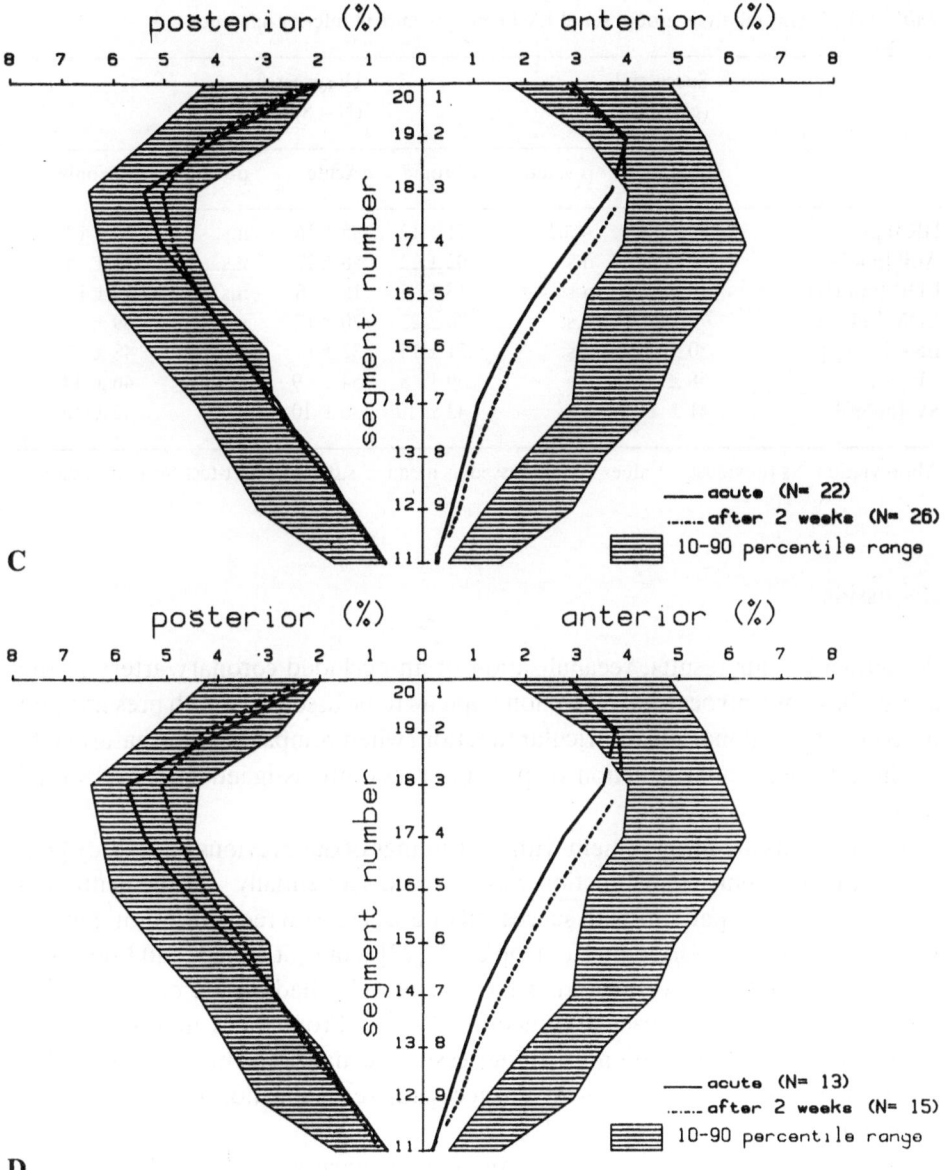

Figure XIV.3. A. The mean CREF values in patients with anterior infarction are shown as in Fig. XIV.2. The regional pump function of the antero-basal segment (segments 1 to 5) is slightly better in the thrombolysis group, while the function of the entire opposite inferior wall is better after thrombolysis as compared to conventional treatment.

B. Regional contribution of the anterior wall to global ejection fraction at the chronic stage in the thrombolysis group, according to the success of the recanalization at the acute stage.

C. Change in CREF from the acute (solid line) to the chronic stage (dotted line) in patients (N = 26) with an anterior infarction who underwent a successful recanalization.

D. Change in CREF from the acute (solid line) to the chronic stage (dotted line) in patients (N = 15) with an anterior infarction who underwent a combined procedure of recanalization and angioplasty.

Table XIV.7. Thrombolysis group: serial LV hemodynamics in inferior infarction.

	Successful (N = 16)			Unsuccessful (N = 8)		
	Acute	p-value	Chronic	Acute	p-value	Chronic
HR [bpm]	82 ± 15	<.02	71 ± 12	85 ± 16	n.s.	75 ± 12
AoP [mmHg]	97 ± 10	n.s.	102 ± 12	88 ± 17	n.s.	91 ± 5
EDP [mmHg]	19 ± 7	n.s.	18 ± 5	18 ± 8	n.s.	19 ± 12
EDV [ml/m2]	70 ± 14	n.s.	70 ± 22	70 ± 17	<.02	89 ± 21
ESV [ml/m²]	30 ± 9	n.s.	31 ± 13	32 ± 10	<.01	48 ± 17
EF [%]	58 ± 10	n.s.	59 ± 8	54 ± 9	< .02	46 ± 14
SV [ml/m²]	41 ± 11	n.s.	43 ± 10	36 ± 10	n.s.	42 ± 16

Abbreviations as previously. Values are expressed as mean ± s.d.; Student t-test for paired data.

Discussion

As shown by our results, recanalization of an occluded coronary artery in the acute phase of a myocardial infarction appears to be associated with preservation of global and regional left ventricular function, when compared to the natural fate of the left ventricular function of patients randomly assigned to conventional treatment.

These results are in agreement with the findings of our previous pilot study [21], where the left ventricular function was assessed sequentially – at the acute and chronic stages – in patients with successful or unsuccessful recanalization. Similar results have been reported by Rentrop et al. [22], Ganz et al. [23] and Mathey et al. [24]. Thereafter, several studies have been published on the effect of early reperfusion on left ventricular function [25–28]. From these nonrandomized studies it appeared that patients with successful recanalization had a higher global ejection fraction than those with unsuccessful recanalization or conventional treatment.

Also, it appeared that the left ventricular damage was less in patients with spontaneous recanalization demonstrated by the existence of an open infarct vessel at 4–6 weeks after the acute event than in those with an occluded infarct vessel [25]. Schwartz et al. demonstrated improvement of left ventricular function only when recanalization was achieved within four hours [26]. According to Rentrop et al., only some subgroups showed an improved left ventricular function after thrombolysis: those with collaterals, those with incomplete obstruction before intervention and those in whom complete obstruction was permanently recanalized [27].

Although these studies have aroused great interest, their results have been mainly based on series in which patients with successful thrombolysis were compared with patients in whom the procedure failed. Such analysis carries considerable bias, since patients in whom thrombolysis succeeded are not necessarily similar to those in whom the intervention failed.

This bias can be ruled out only by means of a properly conducted randomized trial and the analysis of the data on an 'intention to treat' basis. However, in such a trial it is difficult to follow the sequence: determination of patient eligibility, coronary arteriography, randomization and attempted reperfusion of patients randomized to special therapy. In this sequence, patients with evolving infarcts who are randomized to conventional therapy would be obliged to undergo emergency coronary arteriography without sufficient potential benefit to outweigh the attendant risk. To overcome this difficulty, we randomized all patients who were eligible on clinical grounds but obtained consent for performing coronary arteriography only from those assigned to reperfusion therapy. This procedure has been proposed by Zelen for the comparison of a new method of treatment with an accepted mode of therapy [17].

When analyzing the hemodynamic data on an 'intention to treat' basis, we found a significant preservation of left ventricular function after thrombolytic therapy when compared to conventional treatment. The results of the four completed randomized trials [11–14] and the still ongoing trial conducted at the Thoraxcenter Rotterdam, are conflicting. Khaja et al. [11] found that i.c. streptokinase was more effective than placebo (i.c. infusion of dextrose) in achieving reperfusion. However, they detected no improvement of left ventricular function as a result of reestablished coronary flow measured at treatment, at 12 days and at five months. Kennedy et al. [13] and Leiboff et al. [14] demonstrated no difference in the radionuclide determined ejection fraction at discharge in patients with anterior or inferior myocardial infarction treated with intracoronary streptokinase or controls. However, it may be argued that the intervention in these studies was instituted rather late. In the study of Khaja et al. [11], the time period between chest pain and infusion of streptokinase was 5.4 hours, and in the study of Kennedy et al. [13] this time period was between 3 and 12 hours in the majority of the patients.

Schwartz et al. [30] clearly demonstrated benefit only in early reperfusion (within four hours) but not in late reperfusion (later than 4 hours), which is in agreement with animal experiments. These 3 studies are counter-balanced by the results of the study by Anderson et al. [12] and the preliminary results from our study. Both studies show that i.c. streptokinase appears to have a beneficial effect on the left ventricular function.

However, it should be appreciated that measurement of the global ejection fraction is a rather crude method which may not detect improvement of left ventricular function. More sophisticated techniques are required for analysis of left ventricular function. Since only the infarction area is at risk and can potentially benefit from reperfusion, mixing data from areas of the ventricle which may benefit from reperfusion with data from areas which cannot benefit from reperfusion will make it harder to detect any real effect of reperfusion. Determination of changes in regional rather than global ventricular function is now recognized as the proper way to study patients before and after reperfusion [16, 29, 30].

Stack et al. [29] determined regional and global ventricular performance before, 24 hours after, and 16 days after intracoronary streptokinase. All reperfused patients showed improvement of regional shortening in the jeopardized region (p = 0.01), but the global ejection fraction showed no improvement or a decrease in half of these patients. The global ejection fraction before streptokinase was increased by compensatory increases of wall motion in the noninfarction regions of the heart, while the global ejection fraction 16 days later was decreased by subsidence of the compensatory increases of wall motion of the noninfarcted regions of the heart. However, when appropriate regional techniques for evaluation of the jeopardized myocardium were utilized, significant salvage of myocardium was indicated by recovery of contractile function in patients who were reperfused during the first 6 hours of myocardial infarction.

Very similar results were shown by Sheehan et al. [16], who utilized computerized measurements of motion along 100 chords around the left ventricle. Regional hypokinesia improved in 41% of patients with reperfusion by streptokinase and subsequent coronary bypass grafting and in 30% of patients with reperfusion by streptokinase alone.

No improvement was seen in patients who did attain reperfusion. However, the ejection fraction did not discriminate between reperfused and nonreperfused patients. Due to increased motion of the noninfarction regions of the heart, the global ejection fraction often was normal in acute myocardial infarction despite severe regional hypokinesia in the infarction area. Late after infarction, the subsidence of increased motion in the noninfarction regions of the heart often masked significant improvement in regional hypokinesia. These authors concluded that early thrombolysis in acute myocardial infarction results in improved left ventricular function, and regional wall motion must be measured to adequately assess this effect.

Our results show that a significant improvement of regional function in the 'infarct zone' is observed in inferior infarction as well as in anterior infarction, although significant changes in regional function of the remote 'noninfarct zone' were observed at the acute as well as at the chronic stage [31–34].

The results of the four published reports on randomized trials of SK i.c. in acute myocardial infarction, strengthen our opinion that the ultimate benefits of this invasive treatment are yet to be established. The clinical benefits of thrombolytic therapy could not easily be demonstrated. Although dramatic improvements have been reported in a few patients in cardiogenic shock [35], or in patients with complete occlusion of the left main coronary artery [36], the clinical course at the coronary care unit (CCU) of patients with and without thrombolysis was similar [37].

Earlier we reported no differences in early and late mortality, reinfarction, angina or exercise test data between patients assigned to streptokinase treatment and controls [38]. At present, 302 patients have been enrolled in the ongoing trial supported by the Interuniversity Cardiology Institute and the conclusions remain similar [39]. Actuallly, this finding is not surprising. If indeed the major effect of early recanalization is preservation of left ventricular function and a greater LVEF, then the beneficial effects on mortality will become evident only when large series of patients are studied.

Sanz et al. [40] and de Feyter et al. [41] reported better one year survival after myocardial infarction in patients with higher LVEF, independent of the extent of coronary disease. Similar data were found in a follow-up study of 214 hospital survivors at the Thoraxcenter [42]. Pooling the results of these studies, a relationship between the one year mortality rate and the LVEF could be constructed (Fig. XIV.4).

If these data were applied to the observed improvement of left ventricular ejection fraction from 45% in controls versus 55% in patients allocated to thrombolysis, the one year mortality would be reduced from approximately 16% to 10% after thrombolysis, which corresponds to our observations and the data from the Western Washington trial. In order to demonstrate this difference in mortality with p = 0.05 and a power of 80%, approximately 1800 patients should be enrolled in the study.

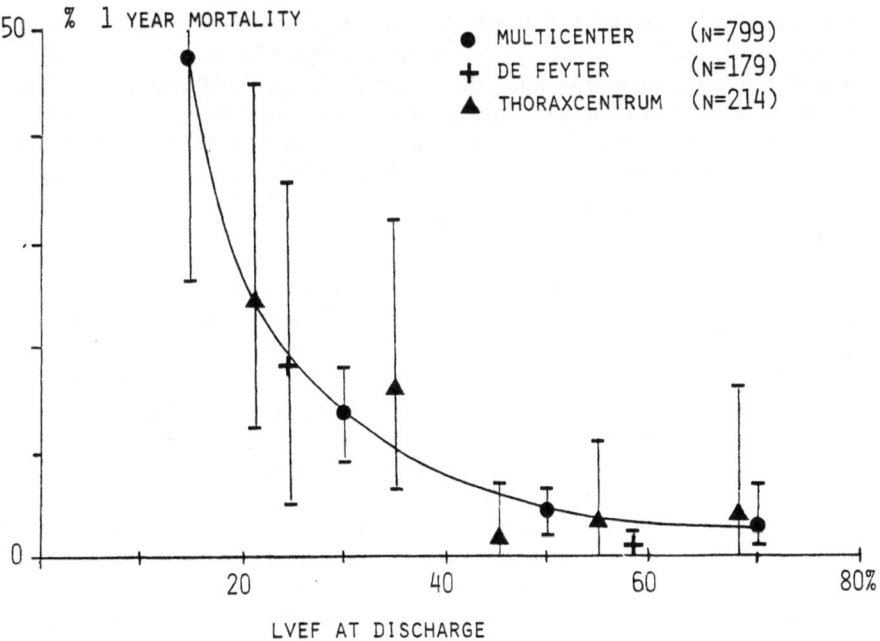

Figure XIV.4. Relationship between one year mortality and left ventricular ejection fraction at discharge. Data from three different studies [40–42] were pooled. Vertical bars represent 95% confidence limits.

312

The combined analysis of all randomized trials on intracoronary thrombolysis [43] indicates that as yet it has not been resolved whether this method of treatment does indeed improve prognosis in patients with acute myocardial infarction. Accordingly, we maintain the view that such invasive treatment should not be generally applied until more follow-up data become available. On the other hand, the accumulated experience indicates that some patients do benefit from early recanalization. Analysis of subgroups may be used to select those patients who are most likely to benefit from thrombolysis.

Finally, the development of tissue plasminogen activator is likely to reduce the risk of bleeding after thrombolysis [44, 45], which would render this intervention more applicable in clinical practice.

References

1. Rentrop P, Blanke H, Karsch KR, Kreutzer H: Initial experience with transluminal recanalization of the recently occluded infarct-related coronary artery in acute myocardial infarction. Comparison with conventionally treated patients. Clin Cardiol 2: 92–105, 1979.
2. Reimer KA, Lowe JE, Rasmussen MM, Jennings RB: The wavefront phenomenon of ischemic cell death. 1. Myocardial infarct size vs. duration of coronary occlusion in dogs. Circulation 56: 786–794, 1977.
3. Baughman KL, Maroko PR, Vatner SF: Effects of coronary artery reperfusion on myocardial infarct size and survival in conscious dogs. Circulation 63: 317–323, 1981.
4. Lavallee M, Cox D, Patrick TA, Vatner SF: Salvage of myocardial function by coronary artery reperfusion 1, 2, and 3 hours after occlusion in conscious dogs. Circ Res 53: 235–247, 1983.
5. Bush LR, Buja LM, Samowitz W, Rude RE, Wathen M, Tilton GD, Willerson JT: Recovery of left ventricular segmental function after long-term reperfusion following temporary coronary occlusion in conscious dogs. Comparison of 2- and 4-hour occlusions. Circ Res 53: 248–263, 1983.
6. Serruys PW, Brand M van den, Hooghoudt TEH, Simoons ML, Fioretti P, Ruiter J, Fels PW, Hugenholtz PG: Coronary recanalization in acute myocardial infarction: immediate results and potential risks. Eur Heart J 3: 404–415, 1982.
7. Corr PB, Witkowski FX: Potential electrophysiologic mechanisms responsible for dysrhythmias associated with reperfusion of ischemic myocardium. Circulation 68 (Supp. I): 16–24, 1983.
8. Bresnahan GF, Roberts R, Shell WE, Ross J Jr, Sobel BE: Deleterious effects due to hemorrhage after myocardial reperfusion. Am J Cardiol 33: 82–86, 1974.
9. Mathey DG, Schofer J, Kuck K-H, Beil V, Klöppel G: Transmural, haemorrhagic myocardial infarction after intracoronary streptokinase. Clinical, angiographic, and necropsy findings. Br Heart J 48: 546–551, 1982.
10. Hearse J, Humphry SM, Bullock GR: The oxygen paradox and the calcium paradox: two facets of the same problem? J Mol Cell Cardiol 10: 641–668, 1978.
11. Khaja F, Walton JA, Brymer JF, Lo E, Osterberger L, O'Neill WW, Colfer HT, Weiss R, Lee T, Kurian T, Goldberg AD, Pitt B, Goldstein S: Intracoronary fibrinolytic therapy in acute myocardial infarction. Report of a prospective randomized trial. N Engl J Med 308: 1305–1311, 1983.
12. Anderson JL, Marshall HW, Bray BE, Lutz JR, Frederick PR, Yanowitz FG, Datz FL, Klausner SC, Hagan AD: A randomized trial of intracoronary streptokinase in the treatment of acute myocardial infarction. N Engl J Med 308: 1312–1318, 1983.
13. Kennedy JW, Ritchie JL, Davis KB, Fritz JK: Western Washington randomized trial of intracoronary streptokinase in acute myocardial infarction. N Engl J Med 309: 1477–1482, 1983.

14. Leiboff RH, Katz RJ, Wasserman AG, Bren GB, Schwartz H, Varghese J, Ross AM: A randomized, angiographically controlled trial of intracoronary streptokinase in acute myocardial infarction. Am J Cardiol 53: 404–407, 1984.

15. Rigaud M, Rocha P, Boschat J, Farcot JC, Bardet J, Bourdarias JP: Regional left ventricular function assessed by contrast angiography in acute myocardial infarction. Circulation 60: 130–139, 1979.

16. Sheehan FH, Mathey DG, Schofer J, Krebber H-J, Dodge HT: Effect of interventions in salvaging left ventricular function in acute myocardial infarction: a study of intracoronary streptokinase. Am J Cardiol 52: 431–438, 1983.

17. Zelen M: A new design for randomized clinical trials. N Engl J Med 300: 1242–1245, 1979.

18. Simoons ML, Serruys PW, Fioretti P, Brand M van den, Hugenholtz PG: Practical guidelines for treatment with beta-blockers and nitrates in patients with acute myocardial infarction. Eur Heart J 4 (Suppl. D): 129–135, 1983.

19. Serruys PW, Wijns W, Brand M van den, Ribeiro V, Fioretti P, Simoons ML, Kooijman CJ, Reiber JHC, Hugenholtz PG: Is transluminal coronary angioplasty mandatory after successful thrombolysis? Quantitative coronary angiographic study. Br Heart J 50: 257–265, 1983.

20. Feild BJ, Russell RO, Dowling JT, Rackley CE: Regional left ventricular performance in the year following myocardial infarction. Circulation 46: 679–689, 1972.

21. Hooghoudt TEH, Serruys PW, Reiber JHC, Slager CJ, Brand M van den, Hugenholtz PG: The effect of recanalization of the occluded coronary artery in acute myocardial infarction on left ventricular function. Eur Heart J 3: 416–421, 1982.

22. Rentrop KP, Blanke H, Karsch KR: Effects of nonsurgical coronary reperfusion on the left ventricle in human subjects compared with conventional treatment. Am J Cardiol 49: 1–8, 1982.

23. Ganz W, Buchbinder N, Marcus H, Mondkar A, Maddahi J, Charuzi Y, O'Connor L, Shell W, Fischbein MC, Kass R, Miyamoto A, Swan HJC: Intracoronary thrombolysis in evolving myocardial infarction. Am Heart J 101: 4–13, 1981.

24. Mathey DG, Kuck K-H, Tilsner V, Krebber H-J, Bleifeld W: Nonsurgical coronary artery recanalization in acute transmural myocardial infarction. Circulation 63: 489–497, 1981.

25. Feyter PJ de, Eenige MJ van, Wall EE van der, Bezemer PD, Engelen CL van, Funke-Kupper AJ, Kerkkamp HJ, Visser FC, Roos JP: Effects of spontaneous and streptokinase-induced recanalization on left ventricular function after myocardial infarction. Circulation 67: 1039–1044, 1983.

26. Schwartz F, Schuler G, Katus H, Hofmann M, Manthey J, Tillmanns H, Mehmel HC, Kübler W: Intracoronary thrombolysis in acute myocardial infarction: duration of ischemia as a major determinant of late results after recanalization. Am J Cardiol 50: 933–937, 1982.

27. Rentrop P, Smith H, Painter L, Holt J: Changes in left ventricular ejection fraction after intracoronary thrombolytic therapy. Results of the Registry of the European Society of Cardiology. Circulation 68 (Supp. I): 55–66, 1983.

28. Smalling RW, Fuentes F, Matthews MW, Freund GC, Hicks CH, Reduto LA, Walker WE, Sterling RP, Gould KL: Sustained improvement in left ventricular function and mortality by intracoronary streptokinase administration during evolving myocardial infarction. Circulation 68: 131–138, 1983.

29. Stack RS, Phillips HR III, Grierson DS, Behar VS, Kong Y, Peter RH, Swain JL, Greenfield JC Jr: Functional improvement of jeopardized myocardium following intracoronary streptokinase infusion in acute myocardial infarction. J Clin Invest 72: 84–95, 1983.

30. Cribier A, Berland J, Champoud O, Moore N, Behar P, Letac B: Intracoronary thrombolysis in evolving myocardial infarction. Sequential angiographic analysis of left ventricular performance. Br Heart J 50: 401–410, 1983.

31. Corday E, Kaplan L, Meerbaum S, Brasch J, Constantini C, Lang T-W, Gold H, Rubins S, Osher J: Consequences of coronary arterial occlusion on remote myocardium: effects of occlusion and reperfusion. Am J Cardiol 36: 385–394, 1975.

314

32. Wyatt HL, Forrester JS, da Luz PL, Diamond GA, Chagrasulis R, Swan HJC: Functional abnormalities in nonoccluded regions of myocardium after experimental coronary occlusion. Am J Cardiol 37: 366–372, 1976.

33. Mathes P, Romig D, Sack D, Erhardt W: Experimental myocardial infarction in the cat. I. Reversible decline in contractility of noninfarcted muscle. Circ Res 38: 540–546, 1976.

34. Naccarella FF, Weintraub WS, Agarwal JB, Helfant RH: Evaluation of 'Ischemia at a distance': effects of coronary occlusion on a remote area of left ventricle. Am J Cardiol 54: 869–874, 1984.

35. Mathey D, Kuck KH, Remmecke J, Tilsner V, Bleifeld W: Transluminal recanalization of coronary artery thrombosis: a preliminary report of its application in cardiogenic shock. Eur Heart J 1: 207–212, 1980.

36. Feyter PJ de, Serruys PW: Thrombolysis of acute total occlusion of the left main coronary artery in evolving myocardial infarction. Am J Cardiol 53: 1727–1729, 1984.

37. Fioretti P, Simoons ML, Serruys PW, Brand M van den, Fels PW, Hugenholtz PG: Clinical course after attempted thrombolysis in myocardial infarction. Results of pilot studies and preliminary data from a randomized trial. Eur Heart J 3: 422–432, 1982.

38. Serruys PW, Wijns W, Simoons ML, Suryapranata H, Planellas J, Domburg R van, Fioretti P, Feyter PJ de, Brand M van den, Hugenholtz PG: Effects of intracoronary thrombolytic therapy on left ventricular function and mortality in patients with acute myocardial infarction. Preliminary results of the Thoraxcenter randomized trial. Eur Heart J 1985 (in press).

39. Simoons ML, Brand M van den, Zwaan C de, Verheugt FWA, Remme WJ, Serruys PW, Bär F, Res J, Krauss XH, Vermeer F, Lubsen J: Improved survival after early thrombolysis in acute myocardial infarction. A randomised trial by the Interuniversity Cardiology Institute in The Netherlands. Lancet 2: 578–582, 1985.

40. Sanz G, Castañer A, Betriu A, Magriña J, Roig E, Coll S, Paré JC, Navarro-López F: Determinants of prognosis in survivors of myocardial infarction: a prospective clinical angiographic study. N Engl J Med 306: 1065–1070, 1982.

41. Feyter PJ de, Eenige MJ van, Dighton DH, Visser FC, Jong J de, Roos JP: Prognostic value of exercise testing, coronary angiography and left ventriculography 6–8 weeks after myocardial infarction. Circulation 66: 527–536, 1982.

42. Fioretti P, Brower RW, Simoons ML, Das SK, Bos RJ, Wijns W, Reiber JHC, Lubsen J, Hugenholtz PG: Prediction of mortality in hospital survivors of myocardial infarction. Comparison of predischarge exercise testing and radionuclide ventriculography at rest. Br Heart J 52: 292–298, 1984.

43. Yusuf S, Collins R, Peto R, Furberg C, Stampfer MJ, Goldhaber SZ, Hennekens CH: Intravenous and intracoronary fibrinolytic therapy in acute myocardial infarction: overview of results on mortality, reinfarction and side-effects from 33 randomized controlled trials. Eur Heart J 6: 556–585, 1985.

44. Collen D, Verstraete M: Systemic thrombolytic therapy of acute myocardial infarction? Circulation 68: 462–465, 1983.

45. Werf F van de, Ludbrook PA, Bergmann SR, Tiefenbrunn AJ, Fox KAA, Geest H de, Verstraete M, Collen D, Sobel BE: Coronary thrombolysis with tissue-type plasminogen activator in patients with evolving myocardial infarction. N Engl J Med 310: 609–613, 1984.

XV. Effect of coronary occlusion during percutaneous transluminal angioplasty in man on left ventricular chamber stiffness and regional diastolic pressure-radius relations.

Summary

The effect of repeated (3 to 10) and transient (15 to 75 sec) abrupt coronary occlusions on the global and regional chamber stiffness was studied in 9 patients undergoing angioplasty (PTCA) of a single proximal left anterior descending coronary artery stenosis. The left ventricular high fidelity pressure and volume relation was obtained prior to and after the procedure, as well as during coronary occlusion, after 20 seconds (N = 9) and after 50 seconds (N = 5). During ischemia, there was an upward shift of the pressure-volume relation. The nonlinear simple elastic constant of chamber stiffness increased from 0.0273 ± 0.017 (mean $\pm$ s.d.) pre-PTCA to 0.0621 ± 0.026 after 20 sec of occlusion (p<0.05) and to 0.0605 ± 0.015 after 50 sec of occlusion (p<0.01). In 6 patients, the post-PTCA value remained higher than the control value, but at the group level the mean value (0.0529 ± 0.037) was not statistically different. The regional stiffness was determined from the changes in the length of 6 segmental radii during diastole, from the lowest diastolic to the end-diastolic pressure. The regional constant of elastic stiffness was unaffected in the nonischemic zone. In the adjacent and ischemic zones, the regional stiffness was increased during occlusion (p<0.05). These regional abnormalities in diastolic function persisted at the time of post-PTCA measurements, 12 minutes after the end of the procedure. This suggests that recovery of a normal diastolic function after repeated ischemic injuries is delayed after restoration of a normal blood flow and systolic function.

Introduction

An increase in left ventricular diastolic pressure relative to volume has been described in patients during pacing and exercise-induced ischemia [1, 2] as well as during spontaneous angina at rest [3]. The observed upward shift of the entire pressure-volume relation reflects an increased chamber stiffness. From these data it could not be inferred that the intrinsic diastolic properties of the myocardium were altered, since many other factors, such as delayed and incomplete left ventricular relaxation or extrinsic compression by the right ventricle and the pericardium, may be involved [4, 5].

Studies in man [6] using a combined echocardiographic and hemodynamic technique during pacing induced ischemia related the shift in the left ventricular pressure-volume relation to a regional increase in myocardial stiffness of the ischemic zone. Similar data were obtained in open-chest anesthetized dogs during high demand ischemia induced by pacing tachycardia in an angina physiology model [7]. When low flow ischemia was induced by acute coronary occlusion in closed-chest anesthetized [8] and conscious [9] dogs, an increase in myocardial wall stiffness with upward shift of the diastolic pressure-volume curve was observed as well. The latter was prevented by inferior vena cava occlusion evidencing the modulating role of the right ventricular loading conditions. In patients with coronary disease, interruption of blood flow induced by transient balloon inflation during percutaneous transluminal coronary angioplasty (PTCA) is a situation which mimics the experimental abrupt coronary occlusion in the animal laboratory. This provides a unique opportunity to study the mechanical and metabolic effects of low flow ischemia in man. Earlier, we reported the dynamic changes in the left ventricular hemodynamics and geometry during PTCA [10 and Ch. XVIII] and demonstrated the perfect reversibility after the procedure of the abnormalities in global and regional systolic functions induced by repeated transluminal occlusions.

The aim of the present study was to analyze the changes in diastolic function induced by coronary occlusion. We determined whether an upward shift in the diastolic pressure-volume relation was actually observed, whether this increase in chamber stiffness, if any, was reversible and could be ascribed to an increased regional stiffness of the ischemic zone.

Patients and methods

Patients

The present study includes 9 patients (1 female and 8 males) with normal resting left ventricular function and wall motion who underwent a percutaneous transluminal coronary angioplasty of a proximal and isolated left anterior descending (LAD) coronary artery stenosis. No patient had had previous infarction. The distal vessel was not filled by collaterals, as shown by diagnostic angiography. One of the 10 previously reported [10] patients was excluded because the small number of available data points due to a higher heart rate precluded valuable analysis of the diastolic function. All patients gave their informed consent and there were no complications related to the research procedure. Medications (beta-blocker, calcium antagonist and long acting nitrates) were not discontinued on the day of the PTCA procedure, but no particular premedication was administered to the patient prior to the angioplasty procedure.

Prior to the approval of the protocol by the Thoraxcenter ethics committee, a feasibility study was performed including an analysis of the effect of nonionic contrast media on the left ventricular function. Details regarding the angioplasty procedure used in our laboratory have been published elsewhere [11 and Ch. XVI].

Study protocol

Simultaneous left ventricular pressure and volume were obtained by contrast ventriculography before the angioplasty procedure was started (N = 9), after a median occlusion period of 20 seconds (range 15–27) during the second dilatation (N = 9), after a median occlusion period of 48 seconds (range 46–59) during the fourth dilatation (N = 5) and a median time of 12 min after the end of the angioplasty procedure (N = 9). A total of 3 to 10 occlusions were performed; the duration of each balloon inflation ranged from 15 to 75 seconds. According to the recommendation by the ethics committee, no investigational occlusions were carried out after completion of a technically successful dilatation. In four patients, this result was achieved after three dilatations so that angiographic data after 48 seconds (fourth occlusion) are only available in 5 out of 9 patients.

These sequential angiograms were made only after the return to baseline of the end-diastolic pressure and of the left ventricular pressure-derived isovolumic parameters of contractility and relaxation, which were available on line during the procedure. The interval between two angiograms was at least 10 minutes. Care was taken to maintain the patient's position unchanged with respect to the X-ray equipment and to reduce diaphragm movement by shallow inspiration. The left ventricular pressure was measured with a Millar micro-manometer on an 8F pigtail catheter. The contrast ventriculograms (30 degrees right anterior oblique at 50 frames/second) were obtained by injection of 0.75 ml/kg of a nonionic contrast medium (Metrizamide, Amipaque®).

Data analysis

Frame-by-frame left ventricular volumes and the corresponding pressures were simultaneously obtained from a complete cardiac cycle as previously described [12]. The ventricular contours were automatically detected with the Contouromat and the volumes calculated according to Simpson's rule. The end-diastolic pressure was defined at that point on the pressure trace at which the derivative of the pressure first exceeded 200 mmHg/sec [12] and in all cases coincided with the largest left ventricular volume. End systole was defined with reference to the pressure tracing, at the occurrence of the dicrotic notch of the central aortic pressure. The left ventricular pressure decay during the isovolumic relaxation was quantified as previously described [10] using a bi-exponential model, where Tau 1 represents the time constant of early relaxation (during the first 40 msec after the peak negative dP/dt).

In the present study, the length of the 20 segmental radii defined by the endocardial landmark model was measured frame-by-frame. Among these, we selected 3 pairs of segments located in the core of the ischemic zone (antero-lateral and apical segments), in the nonischemic zone (antero-basal and postero-basal segments) and immediately adjacent to the ischemic zone (inferior and anterior segments), as shown in Fig. XV.1. The linear correlation coefficients between repeated measurements in 20 patients ranged from 0.96 to 0.99 (SEE = 0.4 to 1.4%) for the same operator and from 0.91 to 0.99 (SEE = 0.4 to 2.3%) for two different operators.

Calculations

For the evaluation of the global chamber stiffness, the left ventricular pressure (P) and volume (V) data obtained every 20 msec starting at the lowest diastolic pressure and ending at the end-diastolic pressure were fitted by a simple elastic

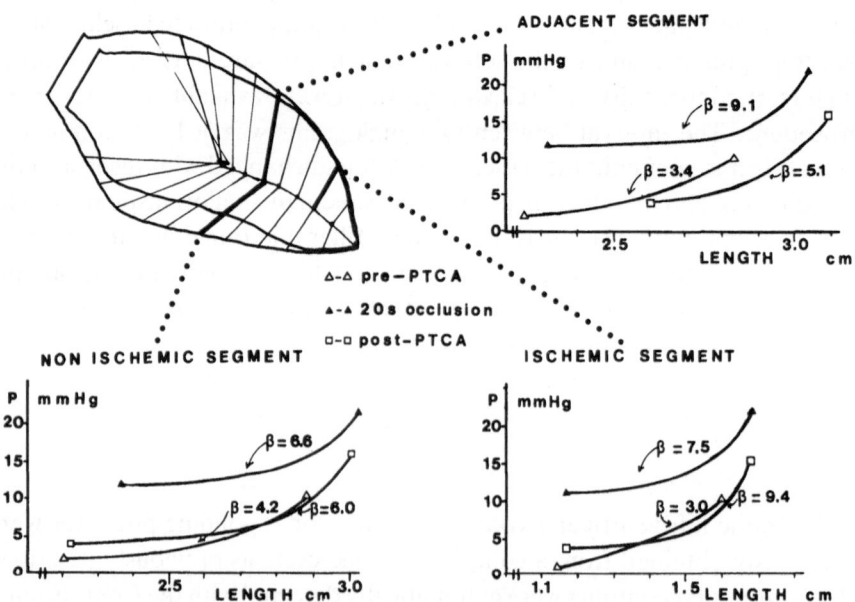

Fig. XV.1. Pressure-length relation in the core of the ischemic zone (antero-apical segment), in the nonischemic zone (postero-basal segment) and in the segment immediately adjacent to the ischemic zone.

model: $P = \alpha e^{\beta V} + C$, where α = intercept (mmHg), β = constant of elastic chamber stiffness and C = baseline pressure (mmHg). The three constants of this equation (α, β, C) were determined using an iteration procedure until the best nonlinear curve fit was obtained [13].

For the evaluation of the regional chamber stiffness, the left ventricular pressure and the segment radius length (L) data were fitted in a similar way for each of the six (1, 2, ... n) analyzed segmental radii: $P = \alpha_1 \cdot e^{\beta_1 \cdot L} + C_1$, where β_1 represents the regional elastic stiffness constant for a given segment 1. The same approach was applied previously by others to pressure-length relations obtained by ultrasonic subendocardial crystals [14], as well as to pressure- circumference relations obtained by contrast ventriculography [8].

Statistical analysis

Results are given for all patients (N = 9) and the subgroup analyzed after 50 sec of occlusion (N = 5), either as mean ± standard deviation or as median values using analysis of variance for repeated measurements. Comparisons between pre-PTCA, post-PTCA and 20 sec occlusion conditions were performed in 9 patients. The pre-, post-PTCA and 50 sec occlusion data were compared in the subgroup of 5 patients. When overall significance was found, multiple comparisons were used to delineate which paired comparisons were significantly different at the 0.05 level.

Results

The left ventricular volumes at the lowest diastolic pressure as well as at end-diastole did not change significantly during and after angioplasty, while the end-systolic volume and Tau 1, the time constant of early relaxation, increased markedly ($p<0.01$) already after 20 seconds of occlusion (Table XV.1). The lowest diastolic ($p<0.05$) and the end-diastolic ($p<0.01$) pressures were significantly increased in the subgroup of patients studied after 50 seconds of LAD occlusion.

After completion of the procedure, all the parameters returned towards control values. This increase in pressure relative to volume during transluminal occlusion resulted in an upward shift of the entire pressure-volume relation as shown for a representative patient in Fig. XV.2. The calculated parameters of global chamber stiffness showed a similarly increased constant of elastic stiffness (β) after 20 seconds as well as after 50 seconds of LAD occlusion. The baseline pressure increased significantly ($p<0.01$) only after 50 seconds of coronary occlusion.

No change in the intercept (α) was observed (Table XV.2). All but one patients

Table XV.1. Hemodynamic variables before PTCA, at 20 and 50 sec after LAD occlusion and after the PTCA procedure.

| | pre-PTCA | | 20 sec occl | 50 sec occl | post-PTCA | |
	all (N=9)	subgroup (N=5)	all (N=9)	subgroup (N=5)	all (N=9)	subgroup (N=5)
Pmin [mmHG]	8	8	12	15*	8	6
V at Pmin [ml/m²]	50	50	55	59	53	53
EDP [mmHg]	20	16	22	30°	19	18
EDV [ml/m²]	78	78	82	87	84	86
ESV [ml/m²]	28	28	36°	44"	27	27
Tau 1 [msec]	58	56	77"	74*	56	57

Abbreviations: PTCA = percutaneous transluminal coronary angioplasty; P = pressure, V = volume; ED = end-diastolic; ES = end-systolic; Tau 1 = time constant of early relaxation; median values are shown; p versus pre- and post-PTCA: * = p<0.05; ° = p<0.01; " = p<0.001.

showed an increase in chamber stiffness during coronary occlusion which, after the procedure, returned to values not significantly different from the pre-PTCA value. However, in 6 patients, the post-PTCA value remained higher than the control value. The changes in the constant of regional chamber stiffness (β_1) showed a marked and persistent increased stiffness in the ischemic zone as well as in the adjacent inferior segment (Table XV.3 and Fig. XV.1). The regional stiffness in the nonischemic zone and in the adjacent anterior segment was not affected by the coronary occlusions. No significant changes in the nonlinear

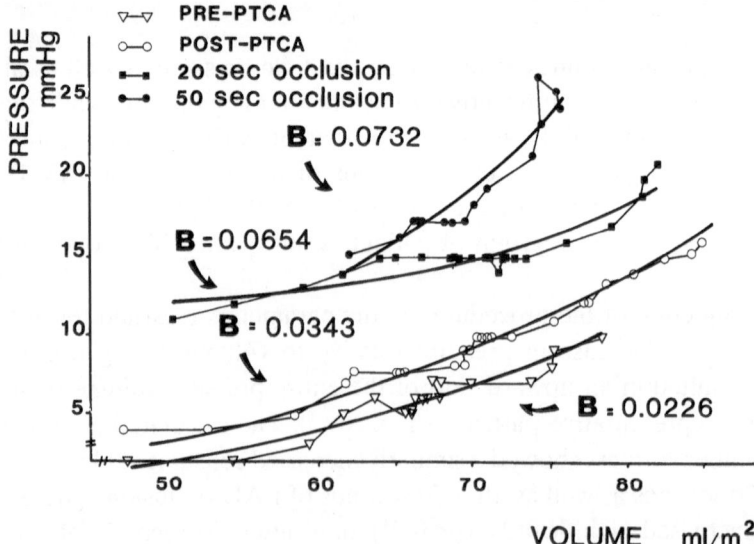

Fig. XV.2. Diastolic pressure-volume relation in a respresentative patient, showing an increased constant of elastic chamber stiffness after 20 seconds, as well as after 50 seconds of LAD occlusion.

Table XV.2. Global left ventricular chamber stiffness.

	Intercept (mmHg)	Constant of elastic stiffness	Baseline pressure (mmHg) C
All Patients (N=9)	n.s.	*	n.s.
Pre-PTCA	4.6 ± 4.9	0.0273 ± 0.017	−1.4 ± 9.5
20 sec occlusion	1.2 ± 3.3	0.0621 ± 0.026*	5.2 ± 8.3
Post-PTCA	1.2 ± 1.5	0.0529 ± 0.037	2.8 ± 4.7
Subgroup (N=5)	n.s.	°	°
Pre-PTCA	5.3 ± 5.9	0.0214 ± 0.007	−5.8 ± 7.4
50 sec occlusion	0.2 ± 0.3	0.0605 ± 0.015*	9.4 ± 2.7°
Post-PTCA	1.9 ± 1.8	0.0396 ± 0.027	0.8 ± 5.6

Values are mean ± s.d.; * = $p<0.05$; ° = $p<0.01$; n.s. = nonsignificant; abbreviations as previously; overall and paired (versus pre-PTCA) significance values are given.

elastic constant (α_1) were observed for the regional pressure-radius relations. Similar shifts in the baseline pressure as for the global diastolic function were measured, since the same left ventricular pressure data were used for both calculations of global and regional stiffness.

Discussion

The major finding of the present study was that ischemia induced by complete occlusion of the left anterior descending coronary artery increased the regional

Table XV.3. Regional left ventricular chamber stiffness β_1 = constant of regional elastic stiffness.

Zone Segment	Nonischemic antero-basal	Adjacent anterior	Ischemic antero-lateral	apical	Adjacent inferior	Nonischemic postero-basal
All patients (N=9)	n.s.	n.s.	*	n.s.	n.s.	n.s.
Pre-PTCA	1.59	3.92	3.11	2.93	2.76	4.03
20 sec occl.	3.03	4.03	5.63	4.97	6.59	5.01
Post-PTCA	2.73	2.59	6.45*	7.16	5.98	3.64
Subgroup (N=5)	n.s.	n.s.	0.05+	0.05+	°	n.s.
Pre-PTCA	1.59	3.45	2.81	1.09	1.52	2.59
50 sec occl.	4.13	4.81	5.39	6.16	7.56*	5.54
Post-PTCA	1.98	3.71	5.59	7.16	6.93	4.35

Given are median values; + the statistical significance was borderline at the 0.05 level; * = $p<0.05$; ° = $p<0.01$;overall and paired (versus pre-PTCA) significance values are given; abbreviations as previously.

chamber stiffness of the ischemic anterior wall, even during an occlusion as short as 20 seconds. Parallel to this increase in regional stiffness, the global stiffness of the left ventricle increased significantly (Table XV.2). In experimental studies [8, 9], an increase in global chamber stiffness was only seen when the area rendered ischemic was large, such as during acute occlusion of the left anterior descending coronary artery.

The baseline pressure (constant C) increased slightly from -1.4 to 5.2 mmHg 20 sec and from -5.8 to 9.4 mmHg 50 sec after acute coronary occlusion (Table XV.2). This increase in baseline pressure reflects the upward shift of the diastolic pressure-volume relation during coronary occlusion, which was 6.6 mmHg after 20 sec and 15.2 mmHg after 50 sec.

Twelve minutes after the end of the procedure including repeated (3 to 10) and brief (15 to 75 sec) occlusions, angiocardiography was repeated. The parameters of global and regional systolic function were back to normal, as shown from the indices of isovolumic contraction, relaxation and segmental wall motion [10]. In contrast, the parameters of regional diastolic function were still abnormal (Table XV.3), while the constant of global chamber stiffness and the baseline pressure remained slightly elevated. How can these persisting diastolic abnormalities be explained, when complete recovery of systolic function and relaxation has occurred?

The significance of the upward shift in the pressure-volume and pressure-radius relations is still the subject of controversy. In most studies, this was attributed to changes in diastolic myocardial stiffness, delayed left ventricular relaxation and/ or loss of elastic recoil due to left ventricular asynergy [5–9]. Ventricular interaction with changes in right ventricular loading conditions were also considered to be responsible for the upward shift of the diastolic pressure-volume curve during acute myocardial ischemia [9, 15].

However, the upward shift was observed with and without pericardium [16], suggesting no constrictive effect of the pericardium on the diastolic filling of the left ventricle. A limitation of the present study is that diastolic function was assessed from pressure-volume and pressure-radius relations using the slope of these relations, fitted by a simple elastic model, as a measure of global and regional chamber stiffness. Using these measurements, it cannot be inferred that the intrinsic diastolic properties of the myocardium are affected by acute coronary occlusion, since this requires analysis of left ventricular wall stress and strain [4]. Heretofore, regional wall thickness measurements are needed which cannot be obtained accurately at 20 msec intervals from the left ventricular angiocardiograms. The strain data should be normalized for a reference unloaded muscle length, i.e. at a transmural pressure of 0 mmHg, and this cannot be obtained easily during cardiac catheterization in man. Thus, at least theoretically, coronary and other extrinsic factors such as the right ventricular loading conditions [4, 5] may have contributed to the apparent increase in chamber stiffness. The coronary perfusion, or the so-called 'erectile effect' [4] is not likely to account for the increased stiffness in the core of the ischemic zone.

During coronary occlusion, inflation of the dilatation balloon results on average in a 44% decrease in regional blood flow [17], hereby reducing the myocardial wall blood volume. Likewise, the post-PTCA measurements were obtained at a time where an increased myocardial turgor due to reactive hyperemia is no more expected. The increase in regional stiffness observed in the adjacent inferior segment could, however, be related to an increased turgor as the collateral flow to that area might increase during left anterior descending occlusion [18].

The role of the ventricular loading conditions is controversial. In an angina physiology model [7], where ischemia was induced by pacing in the presence of high-grade coronary stenoses, upward shifts in the pressure-volume and pressure-length relations were found, even when the influence of right ventricular distension was removed by vena caval occlusion. However, such high demand, high flow situation does not necessarily compare to the low flow ischemia induced during PTCA. This situation rather mimicks the experimental coronary occlusion in the animal laboratory. In such a model, Hess et al. [9] showed that the 'myocardial wall stiffness is increased during complete coronary occlusion when there is systolic thinning of the ischemic wall'. In these conscious chronically instrumented dogs with opened pericardium, this alteration in the intrinsic diastolic properties of the muscle resulted in the expected upward shift of the pressure-volume curve. However, this upward shift was prevented by inferior vena cava obstruction, emphasizing that the right ventricular loading conditions and the ventricular interaction have a modulating role and can offset the increase in pressure. Thus, despite the limitations of the present study, the observed changes in global and regional diastolic chamber stiffness are in accordance with previous experimental work [8, 9, 14], showing an increase in the myocardial stiffness during coronary occlusion. The mechanism by which ischemia increases the myocardial stiffness remains speculative and may depend on the pathophysiology of a given ischemic condition. In the acute coronary occlusion model [8, 9], systolic overstretch of the ischemic muscle fibers was thought to be responsible for the diastolic thinning of the ischemic wall and the increase in resting muscle length. This 'creep' effect causes the ischemic myocardium to operate at a higher point on the sarcomere pressure-length relation, and thus at an increased stiffness level. Although no significant change in end-diastolic volume was observed throughout the procedure, it cannot be excluded that 'creep' actually occurred. Echocardiographic studies from our and other laboratories [20] have shown evidence of wall thinning during balloon occlusion of the proximal left anterior descending coronary artery and during attacks of variant angina.

Another possible mechanism refers to the concept of residual diastolic myosin-actin interaction [21], which may lead to increased stiffness of the ischemic wall as well. Interestingly, we found similar increases in the constant of elastic chamber stiffness after 20 and after 50 seconds of occlusion, while left ventricular asynchrony and late shortening of the ischemic wall were observed only at 20 seconds

[10]. This increased chamber stiffness observed at 20 seconds may only be apparent and related more to an increase in viscous resistance than to early filling.

Although experimental data [22] showed that viscous forces are negligible in the intact ventricle at low filling velocity and in the absence of hypertrophy, this probably does not hold during ischemia. Asynchrony and late shortening affect the stiffness of rat heart trabeculae [23] and it was shown recently in humans, that early diastolic filling can be kept normal during ischemia despite delayed relaxation and loss of elastic recoil (increase in end-systolic volume) by increasing the left atrial driving pressure [24]. It is well known that diastolic properties are better characterized by a viscoelastic rather than a simple elastic stress-strain relation [25]. However, the present angiocardiographic data did not allow to quantitate properly strain rates which are essential for determining diastolic viscous effects. Due to the use of the simple elastic model, the stiffness constant that we calculated includes both elastic and viscous forces. Finally, the abnormalities of the regional diastolic function were still present 12 minutes after the procedure, despite normalization of the rate of relaxation. The latter does not exclude the presence of abnormal myocardial 'tone'. As recently emphasized [7], such failure of complete myofilament inactivation implies a reduced extent of relaxation, which is not necessarily synonymous to a reduced rate of relaxation as measured from the time constant of isovolumic left ventricular pressure decay.

In summary, we can conclude that complete coronary occlusion of the left anterior descending coronary artery in man is associated with profound alterations in diastolic chamber stiffness, which persist well after restoration of myocardial blood flow and of a normal systolic function. The analysis of diastolic function may prove a sensitive tool in assessing the possibly deleterious effects of repeated coronary occlusions during PTCA. The need to detect any persisting dysfunction becomes an even greater concern as the number of dilated vessels and the duration of balloon inflation tend to increase, hereby enhancing both the extent and the severity of ischemia. Further work is needed to document the time course of the recovery of a normal regional diastolic function, and to address the responsible derangements of subcellular metabolism, as the mechanisms of the observed abnormalities are not yet fully understood.

References

1. Mann T, Brodie BR, Grossman W, McLaurin LP: Effect of angina on the left ventricular diastolic pressure-volume relationship. Circulation 55: 761–766, 1977.
2. Carroll JD, Hess OM, Hirzel HO, Krayenbuehl HP: Exercise-induced ischemia: the influence of altered relaxation on early diastolic pressures. Circulation 67: 521– 528, 1983.
3. Sharma B, Behrens TW, Erlein D, Hodges M, Asinger RW, Francis GS: Left ventricular diastolic properties and filling characteristics during spontaneous angina pectoris at rest. Am J Cardiol 52: 704–709, 1983.
4. Glantz SA, Parmley WW: Factors which affect the diastolic pressure-volume curve. Circ Res 42: 171–180, 1978.
5. Grossman W, Serizawa T, Carabello BA: Studies on the mechanism of altered left ventricular

diastolic pressure-volume relations during ischemia. Eur Heart J 1 (Suppl. A): 141–147, 1980.

6. Bourdillon PD, Lorell BH, Mirsky I, Paulus WJ, Wynne J, Grossman W: Increased regional myocardial stiffness of the left ventricle during pacing-induced angina in man. Circulation 67: 316–323, 1983.

7. Momomura S-i, Bradley AB, Grossman W: Left ventricular diastolic pressure-segment length relations and end-diastolic distensibility in dogs with coronary stenoses. An angina physiology model. Circ. Res 55: 203–214, 1984.

8. Hess OM, Koch R, Bamert C, Krayenbuehl HP: Regional wall stiffness during acute myocardial ischaemia in the canine left ventricle. Eur Heart J 1: 435–443, 1980.

9. Hess OM, Osakada G, Lavelle JF, Gallagher KP, Kemper WS, Ross J Jr: Diastolic myocardial wall stiffness and ventricular relaxation during partial and complete coronary occlusions in the conscious dog. Circ Res 52: 387–400, 1983.

10. Serruys PW, Wijns W, Brand M van den, Meij S, Slager CJ, Schuurbiers JCH, Hugenholtz PG, Brower RW: Left ventricular performance, regional blood flow, wall motion, and lactate metabolism during transluminal angioplasty. Circulation 70: 25–36, 1984.

11. Serruys PW, Wijns W, van den Brand M, Ribeiro V, Fioretti P, Simoons ML, Kooijman CJ, Reiber JHC, Hugenholtz PG: Is transluminal coronary angioplasty mandatory after successful thrombolysis? Br Heart J 50: 257–265, 1983.

12. Meester GT, Bernard N, Zeelenberg C, Brower RW, Hugenholtz PG: A computer system for real time analysis of cardiac catheterization data. Cath and Cardiov Diagn 1: 113–123, 1975.

13. Hess OM, Grimm J, Krayenbuehl HP: Diastolic simple elastic and viscoelastic properties of the left ventricle in man. Circulation 59: 1178–1187, 1979.

14. Theroux P, Franklin D, Ross J Jr, Kemper WS: Regional myocardial function during acute coronary artery occlusion and its modification by pharmacologic agents in the dog. Circ Res 35: 896–908, 1974.

15. Shirato K, Shabetai R, Bhargava V, Franklin D, Ross J Jr: Alteration of the left ventricular diastolic pressure segment length relation produced by the pericardium: effects of cardiac distension and afterload reduction in conscious dogs. Circulation 57: 1191–1198, 1978.

16. Serizawa T, Carabello BA, Grossman W: Effect of pacing-induced ischemia on left ventricular diastolic pressure-volume relations in dogs with coronary stenoses. Circ Res 46: 430–439, 1980.

17. Serruys PW, Brand M van den, Brower RW, Hugenholtz PG: Regional cardioplegia and cardioprotection during transluminal angioplasty, which role for nifedipine? Eur Heart J 4 (Suppl. C): 115–121, 1983.

18. Wahr DW, Ports TA, Botvinick EH, Dae M, Schechtmann N, Hattner RS, Turley K: The effects of coronary angioplasty and reperfusion on myocardial flow distribution. Circulation 70 (Pt. II): II–299 (Abstract), 1984.

19. Das SK, Serruys PW, Brand M van den, Domenicucci S, Vletter WB, Roelandt J: Acute echocardiographic changes during percutaneous coronary angioplasty and their relationship to coronary blood flow. J Cardiovasc Ultrason 2: 269–271, 1983.

20. Distante A, Rovai D, Picano E, Moscarelli E, Palombo C, Morales MA, Michelassi C, L'Abbate A: Transient changes in left ventricular mechanics during attacks of Prinzmetal's angina: An M-mode echocardiographic study. Am Heart J 107: 465–472, 1984.

21. Nayler WG, Williams A: Relaxation in heart muscle: Some morphological and biochemical considerations. Eur J Cardiol 7 (Suppl.): 35–50, 1978.

22. Pouleur H, Karliner JS, Le Winter MM, Covell JW: Diastolic viscous properties of the intact canine left ventricle. Circ Res 45: 410–419, 1979.

23. Wiegner AW, Allen GJ, Bing OHL: Weak and strong myocardium in series: implications for segmental dysfunction. Am J Physiol 235 (6): H776–H783, 1978.

24. Carroll JD, Hess OM, Hirzel HO, Krayenbuehl HP: Dynamics of left ventricular filling at rest and during exercise. Circulation 68: 59–67, 1983.

25. Rankin JS, Arentzen CE, McHale PA, Ling D, Anderson RW: Viscoelastic properties of the diastolic left ventricle in the conscious dog. Circ Res 41: 37–45, 1977.

XVI. Is transluminal coronary angioplasty mandatory after successful thrombolysis? A quantitative coronary angiographic study

Summary

Percutaneous transluminal coronary angioplasty has been advocated as a mandatory procedure to prevent reocclusion after successful thrombolysis in acute myocardial infarction. This study describes our experience with both procedures over a 12 month period. Out of 105 patients catheterized in the acute phase of myocardial infarction, 64 were recanalized with 250.000 units of streptokinase, while in 25 patients recanalization could not be achieved. In the remaining sixteen, the infarct related vessel was patent at the time of the procedure. Eighteen of the 78 patients who had a patent infarct related vessel at the end of the recanalization procedure underwent transluminal angioplasty immediately afterwards.

Postlysis angiograms were analyzed quantitatively with a computerized measurement system. The contours of the relevant arterial segments were detected automatically. Reference diameter, minimal obstruction diameter, length of the lesions, and percentage diameter stenosis were averaged from multiple views. In 31% of our patients a diameter stenosis of less than 50% was found, whereas one of 70% or more was seen only in 19% of the patients. Eleven stenotic lesions, recanalized at the acute stage, reoccluded in the short term, and in the long term eight other patients sustained a reinfarction in the same myocardial territory. Seventeen of these 19 recanalized lesions had a diameter stenosis of 58% or more.

In view of these results, we felt justified in combining recanalization and angioplasty in 18 patients selected from the most recent admissions. In these patients, the mean diameter stenosis decreased from 59% to 30% and mean pressure gradient from 41 to 8 mmHg. Late follow-up showed reocclusion in one case.

Although percutaneous transluminal coronary angioplasty does not seem to be mandatory at the acute stage in the majority of patients, it is feasible to undertake in one sitting and seems to prevent reocclusion in patients selected on the basis of quantitative angiographic criteria.

Introduction

Salvage of ischemic but still viable myocardium around areas of myocardial infarction is currently a topic of much clinical interest. The removal of obstruction of the nutrient artery by intracoronary thrombolysis in the first hours after the onset of myocardial infarction [1–3] has provided a new approach which is undergoing randomized trials in our own and other institutions [4–6]. Since there is often residual stenosis, additional transluminal angioplasty and/or coronary artery bypass grafting have been advocated as a mandatory procedure after successful recanalization. It has been argued that a severe residual stenosis in the area of the previous occlusion might cause reocclusion over the ensuing days [7–11]. In order to elucidate this question, quantitative angiographic analysis was applied to recanalized vessels of 78 patients who had an open infarct related vessel at the end of the procedure. Tentative answers were formulated on three questions: How severe are the residual lesions after 'successful' thrombolysis? Is it possible to identify those lesions that are liable to reocclude in the short term? In order to prevent reocclusion after initial successful recanalization, is transluminal angioplasty a mandatory procedure?

Patients and methods

Between September 1980 and December 1982, coronary recanalization was attempted in 105 patients. Different procedures were used since our first experience with intracoronary thrombolysis in September 1980. They have been described elsewhere [4]. In the current randomized trial, patients below 65 years of age were selected, without a history of haemorrhagic diathesis of previous cerebrovascular accident. On admission all patients suffered from chest pain lasting less than four hours. The electrocardiogram showed typical myocardial infarction with ST elevation. The combination of hypotension (systolic pressure below 90 mmHg) and sinus tachycardia (heart rate over 100 beats/minute) led to temporary exclusion, but if the hemodynamic condition of the patient returned to normal quickly, he could still be included in the study. Informed consent was obtained from all patients assigned to thrombolytic treatment. Immediately after admission, an infusion of glyceryl trinitrate was started and as soon as possible the patient was transferred to the catheterization laboratory. Prophylactic lidocaine was given intravenously in a dose of 2 mg/min.

Technique of intracoronary streptolysis

After puncturing the femoral vein and artery a pacemaker catheter was positioned in the right ventricle. Heparin 50 mg, was administered intravenously as well as 250 mg acetosalicylic acid and 100 mg diadresone F®. A nonionic contrast agent (Amipaque®) was used as a contrast medium for coronary angiography of the artery suspected to be thrombosed; subsequently 0.2 mg nifedipine was injected into the occluded artery over a period of three minutes, while the aortic pressure was monitored.

Coronary angiography was then repeated to evaluate the spasmolytic effect on the coronary occlusion. Intracoronary perfusion with streptokinase was carried out at a rate of 4000 units per minute to a maximum of 250.000 units of streptokinase, diluted in 500 ml physiological solution at a flow rate of 8 ml per minute. Coronary angiograms were repeated every 15 minutes until the chest pain disappeared. The appearance of ventricular extrasystoles or any conduction disturbance was an additional reason to revisualize the artery. If there were no signs of recanalization, an attempt was made to administer streptokinase locally in a higher concentration by passing a thin catheter (French 2 or 3) with a radiopaque tip through the Judkins catheter (French 8). After the procedure, selective coronary angiography in multiple projections was performed with an ionic contrast medium (Urografin® 76%).

All arteriograms were recorded on Kodak 35 mm cinefilm at the rate of 25 frames/s. The stenotic areas were filmed in two different projections in stenoses of the right coronary artery and of the left circumflex coronary artery, and in at least three projections, including one cranio-caudal, in stenoses of the left anterior descending artery.

Technique of percutaneous transluminal coronary angioplasty

In 18 patients an attempt was made to dilate the residual stenosis. In 16 patients, PTCA was performed in the same session, 20 to 60 min after the end of streptokinase infusion. In two other patients, PTCA was performed in a second session, respectively 8 hours and 12 days later. Via a 9F, 16 cm long introducing sheath, a guiding catheter was directed into the stenotic area under fluoroscopic and pressure control. In four of the 18 successfully treated cases, we used a balloon catheter with an outer diameter of 3.7 mm, in the 14 other patients its outer diameter was 3 mm. The mean pressure gradient across the stenotic lesion was computed on line after 20 seconds of data acquisition. Two to 9 (mean 4.5; s.d. 2.3) balloon inflations were performed for a period of 10 to 70 s (mean 49; s.d. 12) at a pressure of 4 to 8 bar (mean 6; s.d. 1). After the dilatation procedure the sheath was left in place for the next 24 hours, while the patients were monitored in the coronary care unit.

All patients received heparin (20.000 U/24h) followed by oral coumarin until discharge from the hospital. Anticoagulants were continued after discharge in patients with left ventricular aneurysm or recognized mural thrombus in the left ventricle. In addition, nifedipine was given, 10 mg every four hours, for two days in patients treated with streptokinase [12].

Quantitative angiographic analysis

The quantitative analysis of selected coronary segments was carried out with the Cardiovascular Angiography Analysis System (CAAS). The severity of a coronary obstruction was determined in terms of the interpolated percentage diameter stenosis measurement.

Results

Patency of the infarct related vessel, acute and chronic stage

The angiographic findings at the beginning and at the end of the recanalization procedure are given in Fig. XVI.1. In 64 patients, thrombolysis was successful and after recanalization, transluminal angioplasty was performed in 20 of these 64 patients. In 16 other patients the infarct related vessel was found to be patent at the first coronary angiogram. In two of the 16 cases, occlusion of an initially patent artery occurred during the procedure. Thus, 78 infarct related vessels were patent at the end of the catheterization procedure. In 25 patients we did not succeed in recanalizing the thrombosed arteries.

Fifty-seven patients, excluding those who had undergone PTCA in the acute phase, agreed to be restudied angiographically two weeks later (Fig. XVI.2). In forty-one patients, the infarct related vessel was still patent at the chronic stage. Five lesions, which had remained occluded at the acute stage, were found recanalized at this point; in seven other patients the coronary arteries which had been successfully recanalized at the acute stage were now found to be reoccluded. This observation suggests a reocclusion rate of 17% two weeks after recanalization.

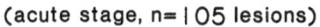

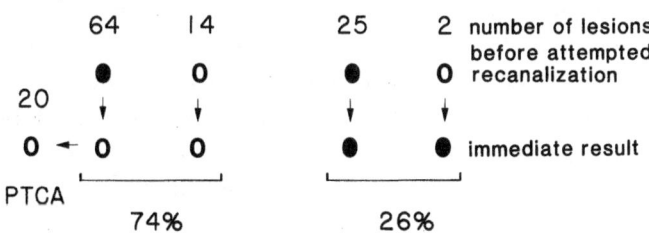

(acute stage, n=105 lesions)

December 82

Fig. XVI.1. Results of attempts at intracoronary thrombolysis in 105 patients. The upper line represents the initial angiographic findings, the lower line the state of the infarct related vessel at the end of the procedure. ● = occluded vessel; ○ = patent vessel.

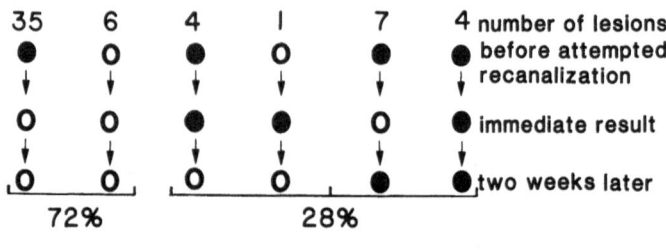

| 35 | 6 | 4 | 1 | 7 | 4 number of lesions |

occlusion rate at 2 weeks = 7/42 = 17%

Fig. XVI.2. Infarct related vessel patency at the chronic stage (two weeks after attempted throm-bolysis) in 57 patients. ● = occluded vessel; ○ = patent vessel.

Moreover, in the long term follow-up (mean 8.3 months) eight other patients sustained a reinfarction in the same myocardial territory, which was documented with the electrocardiogram and cardiac enzymes: two of them were restudied angiographically and in one patient the infarct related vessel had reoccluded. Finally, four lesions which had remained occluded at the acute stage were still occluded at the chronic stage.

Quantitative angiographic analysis

The individual data of the quantitative analysis of 75 stenotic lesions are given in Fig. XVI.3. Three lesions could not be analyzed because of the poor quality of the angiograms. Each depicted value represents the average value of measurements obtained in different angiographic projections. The median value for the refer-ence diameter is 2.98 mm, whereas the 10th and 90th percentiles are 2.22 mm and 4.20 mm, respectively; the median value for the minimal obstruction diameter is 1.32 mm, and the values of the 10th and 90th percentiles are 0.78 mm and 1.88 mm, respectively. As for the length of the lesion, the median value is 9 mm, while values of the 10th and 90th percentiles are 5 and 16 mm, respectively. Figure XVI.4 is a histogram of the percentage diameter stenosis measured on 75 stenotic lesions after the successful thrombolysis. At the acute stage, the median value for the percentage diameter stenosis is 58% in this group of 75 patients; the values of the 10th and 90th percentiles are 37% and 74%, respectively. A percentage diameter stenosis less than 50% is measured in 31% of the patients, whereas a diameter stenosis greater or equal to 70% is seen only in 19%. When comparing the percentage diameter stenosis in a subgroup of 26 individual lesions, analyzed in identical projections in the acute and chronic stage, no significant improvement or deterioration of the recanalized lesions at the chronic stage could be demon-strated (Fig. XVI.5).

There are, of course spectacular individual changes in diameter stenosis, but for the whole group the percentage diameter stenosis does not change signifi-

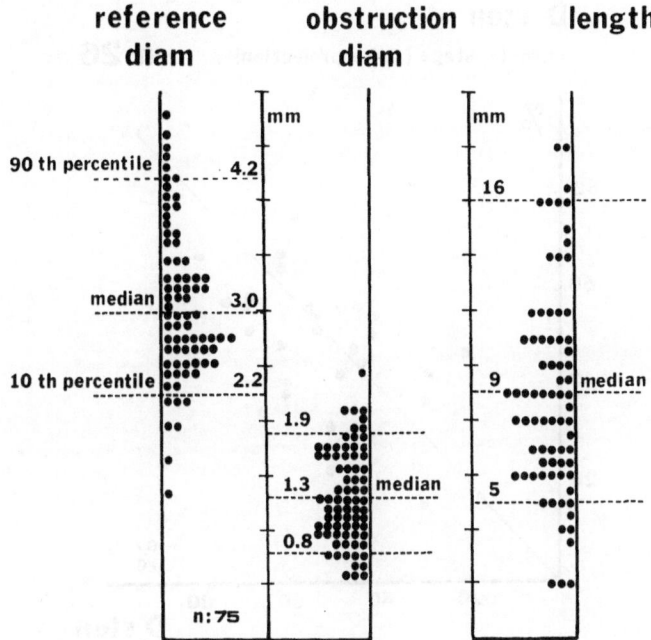

Fig. XVI.3. Individual data for the reference and obstruction diameters as well as the length of the obstructions of 75 lesions. The dotted lines represent the 10th and 90th percentiles and the median values.

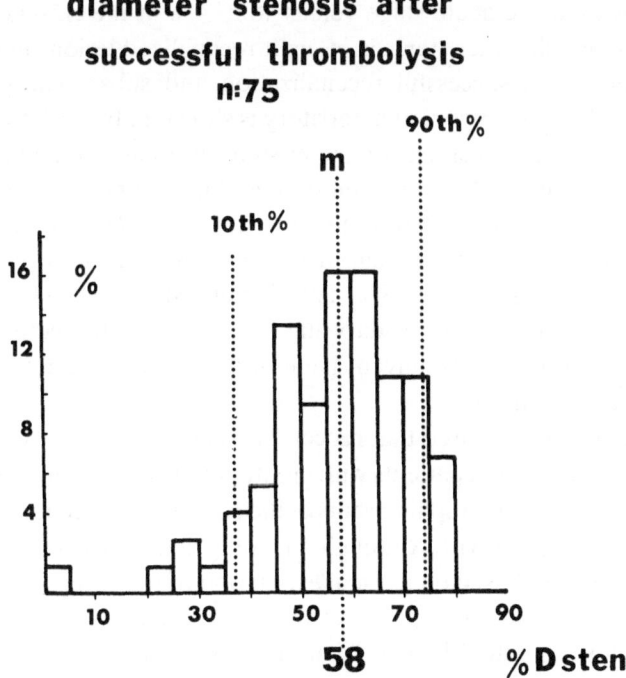

Fig. XVI.4. Histogram (in percentage distribution) of the percentage diameter stenosis measured on 75 lesions after successful thrombolysis. The median value and the 10th and 90th percentiles are given.

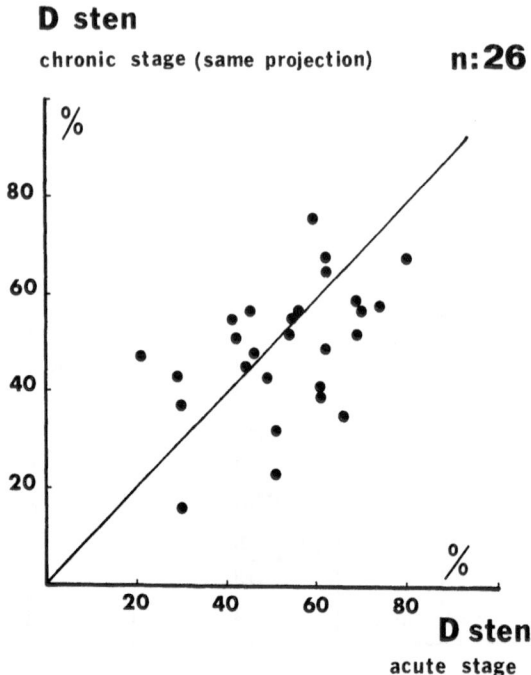

D sten

chronic stage (same projection)   **n:26**

%

D sten

acute stage

Fig. XVI.5. Percentage diameter stenosis of 26 stenotic lesions analyzed in the same projection at the acute and chronic stage.

cantly: $54 \pm 16\%$ at the acute stage versus $48 \pm 14\%$ at the chronic stage.

The percentage diameter stenosis of eight recanalized lesions in patients who initially underwent a successful recanalization and subsequently sustained a reinfarction in the same myocardial territory is shown in Fig. XVI.6. Six of eight stenotic lesions had a percentage diameter stenosis greater or equal to 58% (the median value) immediately after thrombolysis. The second column represents 11 stenotic lesions which reoccluded at the acute stage (N = 4) or at the chronic stage (N = 7) after they had been recanalized. All of them had a percentage diameter stenosis greater than or equal to 58%. The diameter stenoses of 14 stenotic lesions found to be patent at the first coronary angiogram during the acute phase of their myocardial infarction are also given. Nine of them had a diameter stenosis less than 58% (median value).

From these data it appeared that reocclusion and recurrent myocardial infarction were more frequent in patients with greater than 58% diameter stenosis after recanalization. The angiographic results of the combined procedure performed in 18 patients are also shown. Although the selection and decision to perform angioplasty had been based on a visual evaluation of the severity of the lesion at the time of the procedure, it appears retrospectively that 13 of the 18 lesions had a diameter stenosis greater than 58% after thrombolysis. In these 18 patients angioplasty decreased the average percentage diameter stenosis from 59% (s.d.: 9.9%) to 30% (s.d.: 9.9%) and the minimal obstruction diameter increased from

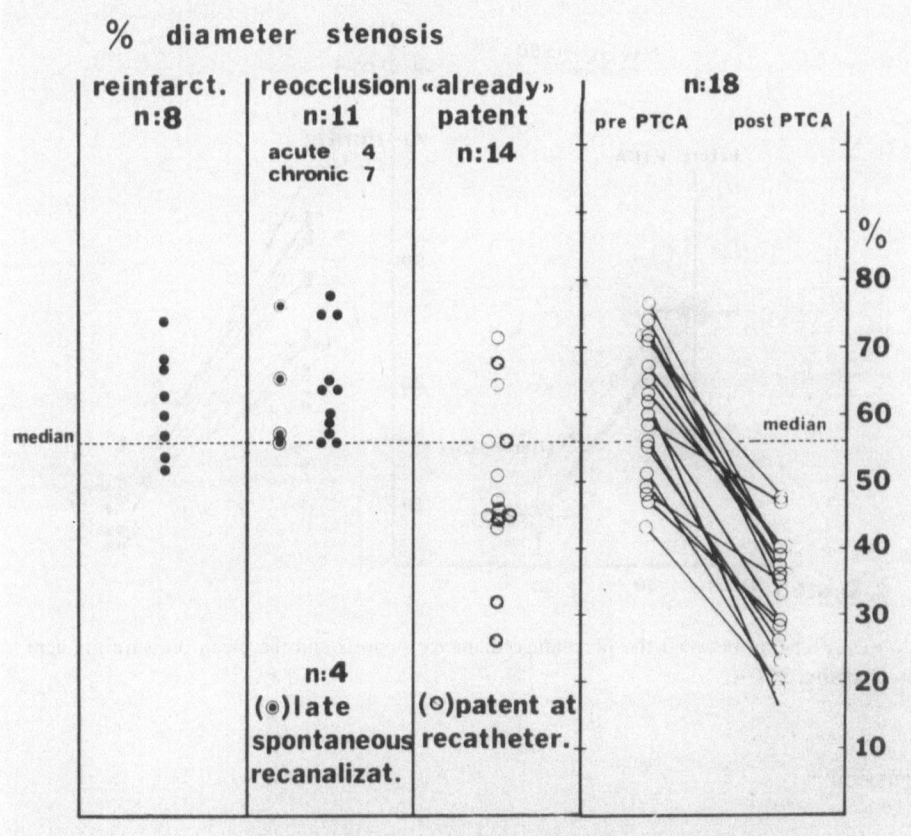

Fig. XVI.6. Percentage diameter stenosis of coronary lesions in a subset of patients with reinfarction, reocclusion, late 'spontaneous recanalization' or with 'already' patent infarct related vessels. In the last column the changes in percentage diameter stenosis after PTCA are given.

1.3 mm (s.d.: 0.4 mm) to 2.2 mm (s.d.: 0.3 mm). This reduction in diameter stenosis was highly significant (p<0.0001) and was associated with a significant decrease in mean pressure gradient from 41 mmHg (s.d.: 17 mmHg) to 8 mmHg (s.d.: 5 mmHg) (Fig. XVI.7). On the basis of the changes in pressure gradient, dilatation had not been necessary in two of these patients.

Fifteen out of the 18 patients who underwent PTCA were restudied angiographically after a mean follow-up of four months (range from 10 days to 11 months). In all but one, the dilated vessel was patent. One patient developed exertional angina three months later. A restenosis at the site of the previous occlusion was successfully dilated a second time.

334

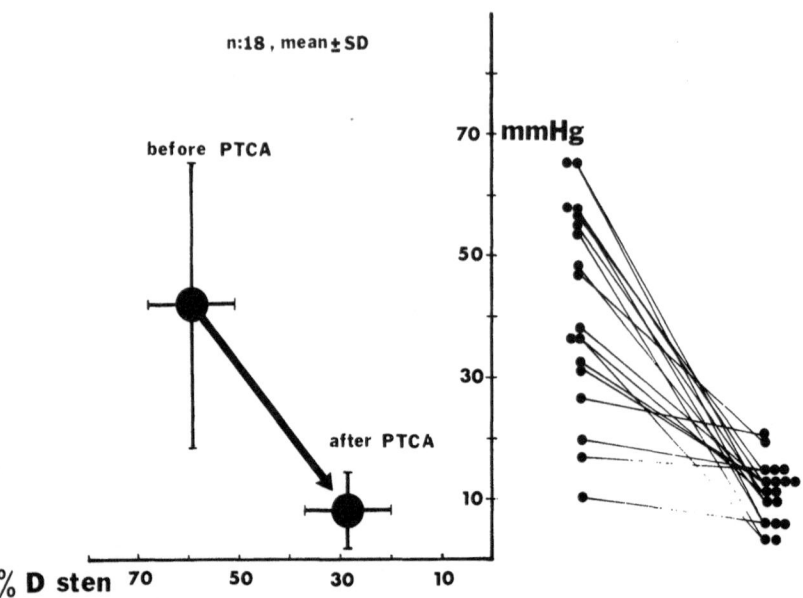

Fig. XVI.7. Relation between the percentage diameter stenosis and the mean pressure gradient before and after PTCA.

Discussion

In this chapter it is shown that intracoronary streptokinase infusion and percutaneous transluminal coronary angioplasty can be carried out in the same session in an effort to enhance reperfusion. The issue, however, is not whether these combined interventions can be performed safely in the setting of acute infarction, but rather whether one is justified in doing so. The present work is a tentative answer to this question and its conclusions are based on the results of quantitative angiographic analysis of recanalized vessels.

Since at the end of the procedure, 31% of our patients had a recanalized vessel with a percentage diameter stenosis below 50%, whereas a diameter stenosis greater than 50% was seen in the remainder, we had no evidence of a major residual thrombus at the site of the stenosis. No retention of contrast medium or staining of a distal thrombus was seen, so residual clot, reported by others [13–15] appears unlikely as well. Furthermore, it has been the custom to continue the streptokinase treatment for about 30 minutes after patency has already been established.

On the other hand, severe residual stenosis of the recanalized vessel has been reported by other groups [10,16]. Their reports are based on visual and therefore subjective interpretation of the stenotic lesions. Overestimation and excessive variations by intra- or interobserver error have been reported [17, 18]. These discrepancies led us to evaluate the exact condition of the stenotic lesions after successful lysis by an objective, computer aided, interpretation.

In 14 cases with clear clinical, electrocardiographic, and enzymatic signs of an acute infarction, the diseased vessel was patent at the time of coronary angiography. In these patients long lasting vasospasm superimposed on organic lesions may have led to transient occlusion and myocardial infarction [19, 20]. Another possibility is that the clot had already lysed in the meantime. In nine out of these 14 patients, the infarct related vessel had a mild stenotic lesion, a factor that might have facilitated the reopening of the vessel. This is the more likely as these patients were started on an intravenous perfusion of glyceryl trinitrate before intracoronary lysis was attempted. In patients with transmural acute myocardial infarction and coronary arterial thrombi, histologic sections of coronary arteries have been shown to be narrowed by the atherosclerotic plaque alone to 33 to 98% (mean 81%), at the site of the thrombus [21]. When histological cross-sectional areas are compared to cross-sectional areas derived from diameter measurements, our quantitative angiographic results *in vivo* are consistent with the histologic findings. Furthermore, it is remarkable how closely the obstruction diameters after successful thrombolysis correspond with the postmortem findings reported by Fulton [22] as shown in Fig. XVI.8.

In one third of our patients the myocardial infarction had occurred when the relevant artery showed a stenosis of less than 50%. Gertz et al. have shown experimentally that endothelial damage and thrombus formation may occur at the site of focal arterial constriction even when the reduction in luminal diameter by itself is insufficient to alter significantly the rate of flow [23].

As shown by Fulton in his elegant study on the morphology of coronary thrombotic occlusions, atherosclerotic lesions are usually of a complex nature [22]. In two thirds of his cases, a break or a tear in the luminal lining exposed blood flowing to the material composing the underlying lesion. He postulated that this was the probable cause of platelet aggregation and fibrin deposition [24, 25]. In half of his cases, a haemorrhagic dissection was found which resulted in an apparent reduction of the lumen. Successful thrombolysis could again expose the material of the atheromatous lesion to flowing blood.

Whether the thrombogenic activity of this material would be as active as it was in the first instance remains speculative, but secondary thrombotic occlusion may occur. Accordingly, there are strong theoretical reasons for adopting antithrombotic measures after successful thrombolysis. On the other hand, instrumental dilatation of the coronary artery stenosis underlying the occlusive thrombus might produce desquamation of endothelium and shearing of the superficial portion of endothelial plaque, possibly altering its thrombogenic propensity. Subsequent fibrosis and healing appear to cause further enlargement of the lumen and thereby may improve local rheology [26]. Thus, arguably, it might be advisable to perform angioplasty even in patients with a stenosis of less than 50%.

Reported rates of reocclusion vary between less than 10% [27] to 25% [28]. In this study two weeks after thrombolysis, the reocclusion rate was 17%. Moreover,

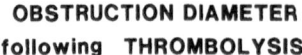

OBSTRUCTION DIAMETER
following **THROMBOLYSIS**

LUMEN DIAMETER
before **THROMBOTIC OCCLUSION**

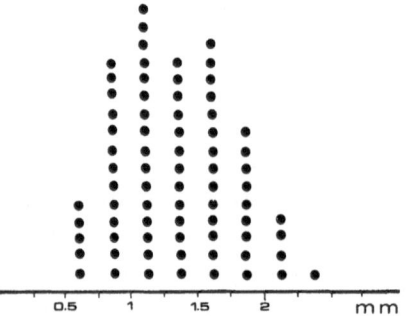

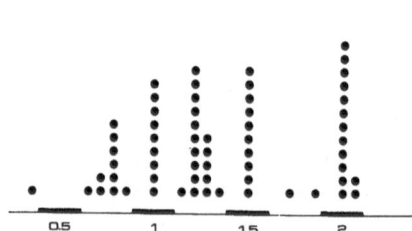

Fig. XVI.8. Lumen diameter 'before thrombotic occlusion' in 63 patients with fatal infarct (modified with permission from Fulton [22]) compared with our *in vivo* angiographic measurement of obstruction diameter after thrombolysis.

during follow-up, eight patients sustained reinfarction in the same myocardial region, so that reocclusion and/or reinfarction might affect 25% of our patients who had undergone a successful recanalization. Thus it seems rational at the acute stage to dilate recanalized arteries with a residual stenosis greater than 58% since these stenotic lesions are liable to early reocclusion. This concept was supported by our observations that during streptokinase infusion, reocclusion occurred in four patients (Fig. XVI.6) despite intravenous or intracoronary administration of glyceryl trinitrate or nifedipine. Here PTCA might have been the only way to restore blood flow adequately and to prevent immediate reocclusion. As emphasized by Meyer et al., the advantages of the combined procedure are savings in time and money [11]. The same introducing sheath can be used, the catheterization laboratory equipment and the personnel have to be used only once, and it appears to be less strenuous for the patient. To date no reocclusions have occurred during such immediate dilation of the critical stenosis. Fifteen out of the 18 patients who underwent PTCA were restudied angiographically after a median follow-up of four months (range from 10 days to 11 months). In all but one patient, the dilated vessel has remained patent. All 17 patients have been followed at the outpatient clinic at three months intervals. The mean period of follow-up has been seven months and the longest one year. None of these patients has sustained a reinfarction thus far.

These observations indicate that PTCA immediately after thrombolysis is a safe and reasonable procedure when after lysis of the obstruction a 58% stenosis is still present. This combined approach seems to result in a lower rate of reocclusion or reinfarction than thrombolysis alone. As further randomized trials are necessary to show the ultimate benefit of thrombolysis in acute myocardial infarction, it is recommended that during them the additional value of immediate PTCA is investigated.

References

1. Boucek RJ, Murphy WP Jr: Segmental perfusion of the coronary arteries with fibrinolysin in man following a myocardial infarction. Am J Cardiol 6: 525–533, 1960.
2. Chazov EI, Matveeva LS, Mazaev AV, Sargin KE, Sadovshaya BK, Ruda Y: Intracoronary administration of fibrinolysin in acute myocardial infarct. Ter Arkh 48: 8–19, 1976.
3. Rentrop P, Blanke H, Köstering K, Karsch KR: Acute myocardial infarction: intracoronary application of nitroglycerin and streptokinase in combination with transluminal recanalization. Clin Cardiol 5: 354–361, 1979.
4. Serruys PW, Brand M van den, Hooghoudt TEH, Simoons ML, Fioretti P, Ruiter J, Fels PW, Hugenholtz PG: Coronary recanalization in acute myocardial infarction: immediate results and potential risks. Eur Heart J 3: 404–415, 1982.
5. Hooghoudt TEH, Serruys PW, Reiber JHC, Slager CJ, Brand M van den, Hugenholtz PG: The effect of recanalization of the occluded coronary artery in acute myocardial infarction on left ventricular function. Eur Heart J 3: 416–421, 1982.
6. Khaja F, Lo E, Osterberger L, Walton JA Jr, Brymer JF, O'Neill WW, Goldstein S, Pitt B, Lee TG, Goldberg AD: Intracoronary fibrinolytic therapy in acute myocardial infarction: preliminary report of a randomized trial. Am J Cardiol 49: 961 (Abstract), 1982.
7. Meltzer RS, Brand M van den, Serruys PW, Fioretti P, Hugenholtz PG: Sequential intracoronary streptokinase and transluminal angioplasty in unstable angina with evolving myocardial infarction. Am Heart J 104: 1109–1111, 1982.
8. Goldberg S, Urban P, Greenspon A, Berger BC, Walinsky P, Maroko P: Reperfusion in acute myocardial infarction. Am J Cardiol 49: 1033 (Abstract), 1982.
9. Hartzler GO, Rutherford BD, McConahay DR: Percutaneous coronary angioplasty with and without prior streptokinase infusion for treatment of acute myocardial infarction. Am J Cardiol 49: 1033 (Abstract), 1982.
10. Gold HK, Leinbach RC, Palacios IF, Block PC, Buckley MJ, Akins CW, Daggett WM, Austen WG: Effects of immediate angioplasty on coronary patency following infarct therapy with streptokinase. Am J Cardiol 49: 1033 (Abstract), 1982.
11. Meyer J, Merx W, Schmitz H, Erbel R, Kiesslich T, Dörr R, Lambertz H, Bethge C, Krebs W, Bardos P, Minale C, Messmer BJ, Effert S: Percutaneous transluminal coronary angioplasty immediately after intracoronary streptolysis of transmural myocardial infarction. Circulation 66: 905–913, 1982.
12. Fioretti P, Simoons ML, Serruys PW, Brand M van den, Fels PW, Hugenholtz PG: Clinical course after attempted thrombolysis in myocardial infarction. Results of pilot studies and preliminary data from a randomized trial. Eur Heart J 3: 422–432, 1982.
13. Hugenholtz PG, Rentrop P: Thrombolytic therapy for acute myocardial infarction: quo vadis? A review of the recent literature. Eur Heart J 3: 395–403, 1982.
14. Rentrop KP, Blanke H, Karsch KR, Rahlf G, Leitz K: Infarktgrössenbegrenzung durch nichtchirurgische Rekanalisation der Koronararterien. Dtsch Med Wschr 106: 765–770, 1981.
15. Gangadharan V, Ramos RG, Hauser AM, Westveer DC, Timmis GC, Gordon S: Intracoronary streptokinase: evidence for continued iatrogenic or spontaneous thrombolysis after termination of infusion. Am J Cardiol 49: 973 (Abstract), 1982.
16. Rutsch W, Schartl M, Mathey D, Kuck K, Merx W, Dörr R, Rentrop P, Blanke H: Percutaneous transluminal coronary recanalization: Procedure, results and acute complications. Am Heart J 102: 1178–1181, 1981.
17. Zir LM, Miller SW, Dinsmore RE, Gilbert JP, Hartborne JW: Interobserver variability in coronary angiography. Circulation 53: 627–632, 1976.
18. Detre KM, Wright E, Murphy ML, Takaro T: Observer agreement in evaluating coronary angiograms. Circulation 52: 979–986, 1975.
19. Oliva PB, Breckinridge JC: Arteriographic evidence of coronary arterial spasm in acute myocardial infarction. Circulation 56: 366–374, 1977.

338

20. Maseri A, L'Abbate A, Baroldi G, Chierchia S, Marzilli M, Ballestra AM, Severi S, Parodi O, Biagini A, Distante A. Pesola A: Coronary vasospasm as a possible cause of myocardial infarction. A conclusion derived from the study of 'preinfarction' angina. New Eng J Med 299: 1271–1277, 1978.
21. Brosius III FC, Roberts WC: Significance of coronary arterial thrombus in transmural acute myocardial infarction. A study of 54 necropsy patients. Circulation 63: 810–816, 1981.
22. Fulton WFM: The morphology of coronary thrombotic occlusions relevant to thrombolytic intervention. In: Transluminal Coronary Angioplasty and Intracoronary Thrombolysis, Coronary Heart Disease IV. M Kaltenbach, A Grüntzig, K Rentrop, WD Bussman (Eds.). Springer-Verlag, Berlin/Heidelberg/New York: 244–252, 1982.
23. Gertz SD, Uretsky G, Wajnberg RS, Navot N, Gotsman MS: Endothelial cell damage and thrombus formation after partial arterial constriction: relevance to the role of coronary artery spasm in the pathogenesis of myocardial infarction. Circulation 63: 476–486, 1981.
24. Friedman M, Bovenkamp GJ van den: The pathogenesis of a coronary thrombus. Am J Pathol 48: 19–44, 1966.
25. Harland WA, Holburn AM: Coronary thrombosis and myocardial infarction. Lancet 2: 1158–1160, 1966.
26. Block PC, Baughman KL, Pasternak RC, Fallon JT: Transluminal angioplasty: correlation of morphologic and angiographic findings in an experimental model. Circulation 61: 778–785, 1980.
27. Rentrop P, Blanke H, Karsch KR, Kaiser H, Köstering H, Leitz K: Selective intracoronary thrombolysis in acute myocardial infarction and unstable angina pectoris. Circulation 63: 307–317, 1981.
28. Merx W, Dörr R, Rentrop P, Blanke H, Karsch KR, Mathey DG, Kremer P, Rutsch W, Schmutzler H: Evaluation of the effectiveness of intracoronary streptokinase infusion in acute myocardial infarction: Postprocedure management and hospital course in 204 patients. Am Heart J 102: 1181–1187, 1981.

XVII. Assessment of percutaneous transluminal coronary angioplasty by quantitative coronary angiography: diameter versus densitometric area measurements

Summary

Cineangiograms of 138 patients who underwent percutaneous transluminal coronary angioplasty (PTCA) were analyzed quantitatively. In a first study group (120 patients) the severity of the obstructive lesions derived from the automatically detected contours was evaluated in absolute terms as well as in percentage diameter reduction. In a second group of patients, 18 coronary lesions were selected for their extreme severity and symmetric aspect prior to angioplasty as assessed from multiple views. In the second group, the densitometric percentage area stenosis was used to assess the changes in cross-sectional area after PTCA and compared to the circular percentage area stenosis computed from the diameter measurements. Before PTCA, there existed a good agreement between the densitometric percentage area stenosis and the circular percentage area stenosis measurements. After PTCA, important discrepancies between these two types of measurements were observed. It is suggested that these discrepancies in results after PTCA can be accounted for by asymmetric morphological changes in luminal cross section, which cannot be assessed accurately from diameter measurements in a single plane view.

Introduction

When comparing percentage luminal narrowing of obstructions in coronary angiograms only the discrete dimensions at the site of the obstruction and at the so-called normal caliber of the vessel are incorporated. However, the prestenotic and poststenotic segments of a coronary vessel consist of subtle combinations of stenotic and ectatic areas and this fact alone creates a major problem in the quantification of the degree of luminal narrowing [1].

Previous studies on the hemodynamic effects of a stenosis in an artery have demonstrated that the most critical determinant of the severity is the minimal luminal cross-sectional area [2–5]. Assessment of the percentage area reduction in a stenotic area from diameter measurements obtained from a single projection assumes a symmetrical circular cross section, an assumption which will not always be true. In fact, Freudenberg and Lichtlen estimate that 70% of coronary artery stenoses are eccentric rather than concentric [6]. Even a technique of quantitating area stenosis from two orthogonal measurements and computing the area based on an elliptical model would fail to describe an asymmetrical lesion accurately [7]. However, some clue to the presence of this asymmetry will exist, since the observed density is markedly reduced in that area, even though the caliber of the vessel seems normal. It has been demonstrated in Chapter VII, that the true luminal cross sections of a contrast-filled coronary artery can be computed from a single X-ray projection by densitometric analysis.

From the above, it is clear that an objective and reproducible technique of quantitating cross-sectional area stenosis and normal luminal area both in absolute terms and in relative percentage changes is needed, if one is to evaluate the efficacy of transluminal coronary angioplasty in a quantitative sense.

Cineangiograms of 138 patients who underwent percutaneous transluminal coronary angioplasty (PTCA) were analyzed with the CAAS and the results before and after dilation are presented. In a first study group (120 patients), the severity of the obstructive lesions derived from the automatically detected contours was evaluated in absolute terms as well as in percentage diameter reduction. In the second group (18 patients), the severity of the lesion was derived from the densitometric measurements and expressed in percentage area stenosis.

Methods

Quantitative analysis of coronary obstructions

The quantitative analysis of selected coronary segments was carried out with the CAAS. The reference diameters and the percentages diameter reduction of the obstructions were computed according to the interpolated technique. The densitometric analysis was carried out according to the technique described in Chapter VII. The densitometric percentage area reduction of an obstruction was obtained by comparing the minimal area value at the obstruction with the reference area value computed following an interpolative approach similar to the method for diameter measurements (Chapter III).

An illustrative example of the results of this technique applied to an aortacoronary bypass graft, successfully dilated and filmed in two orthogonal views, is presented in Fig. XVII.1. The percentage diameter stenosis from the LAO-view is only 19%; if circular cross sections were assumed, this would result in a circular percentage area stenosis of 34%. However, the image shows a much greater decrease in density level at the obstruction than one would expect from

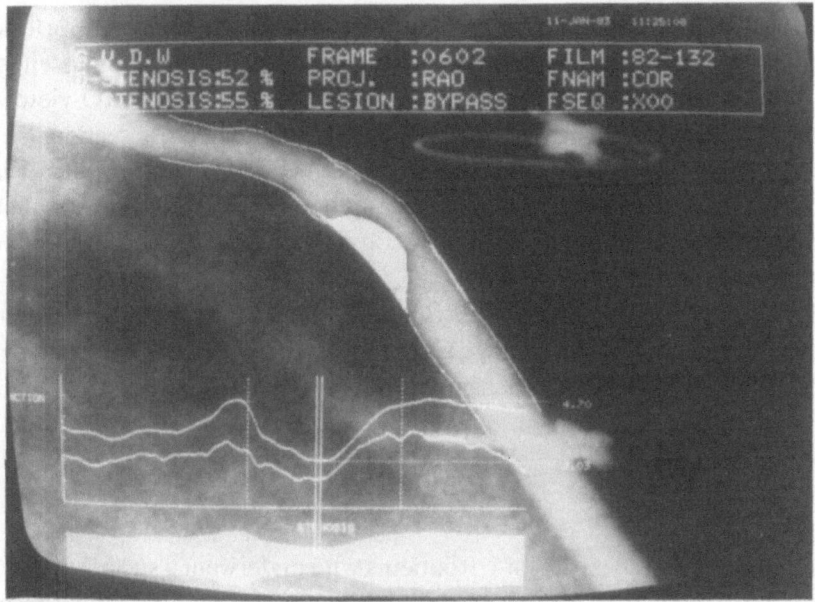

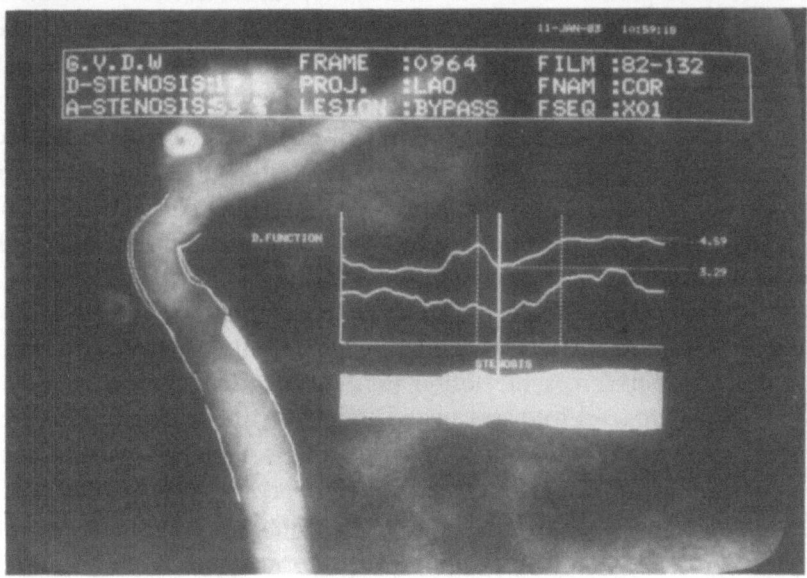

Fig. XVII.1. Contours and densitometric analyses of the severity of an obstruction in the same aortacoronary bypass graft, filmed in right (RAO, upper photograph) and left (LAO, lower photograph) anterior oblique projections. In each illustration, the diagnostic diameter function (upper curve) and the densitometric area function (lower curve) are displayed on the video image. The white areas are a measure for the 'atherosclerotic' plaque and are defined by the difference between the actual luminal contours, detected by the computer and the reconstructed (original) reference contours. The densitometric area stenosis (A-STENOSIS) measured in the orthogonal projections were found to be 53% and 55%, respectively, whereas the diameter stenosis (D-STENOSIS) based on the detected contours was equal to 19% in the LAO-projection and 52% in the RAO-projection.

the apparent decrease in diameter, suggesting the presence of an eccentric lesion. Indeed, the densitometric analysis provides a 53% densitometric area stenosis.

The RAO-view gives a 52% diameter stenosis. If only this RAO-view was available without densitometric analysis, then a circular cross-sectional area stenosis of 77% would be our best approximation of cross-sectional narrowing, thus overestimating the severity of the disease; in this view a 55% densitometric area stenosis was measured, which is very consistent with the 53% densitometric area stenosis from the LAO-view.

If only the diameter measurements from the two views were available, then by elliptical approximation a percentage area stenosis of 61% would be found, being an overestimation of the 'true' densitometric area stenosis.

Study population

The first study group consisted of 120 patients who underwent a successful PTCA between September 1981 and December 1982; within 6 months after the procedure 50 of these patients agreed to undergo repeat cardiac catheterization.

The second study group consisted of 18 patients in whom the densitometric percentage area stenosis technique was used to assess the changes in percentage cross-sectional area before and after PTCA. All data were obtained from single projections. The lesions were selected for their extreme severity and symmetric aspect before angioplasty as assessed from multiple views. PTCA was performed according to the technique of Grüntzig, using the equipment of Schneider (20–3.0 or 20–3.7 mm balloon), via a femoral route. In all cases, the pressure gradient across the obstructive lesion was recorded before and after dilatation. The inflation pressure ranged from 4 to 10 atm, while the duration of the inflation was usually 30 to 60 seconds. Attempts at dilating the stenotic lesion were repeated as long as the gradient across the lesion persisted (4 to 10 times). Before the procedure all patients received aspirin and nifedipine; β-blocking drugs were not discontinued. During the procedure heparin and low-molecular-weight dextran were administered intravenously; direct intracoronary injection of nifedipine and isosorbide dinitrate was performed before the dilatation. To visualize the effect of the procedure, coronary angiography was performed immediately before and after transluminal angioplasty. Lateral, antero-posterior, oblique, and hemiaxial views were usually obtained.

Results

In the first study group the quantitative analysis was limited to computation of the diameter values, derived from the detected contours. The severity of the obstructive lesion was expressed in relative percentage narrowing and in absolute values (mm). For statistical analysis the average value of the measurements obtained in multiple angiographic projections (2 to 6 views) were determined for each individual. The results for the 138 lesions of the first study group are summarized in Table XVII.1. On the average, the interpolated reference diameter remained unchanged after PTCA; the obstruction diameter increased from 1.28 ± 0.40 mm (mean $\pm$ s.d.) to 2.24 ± 0.57 mm (p<0.001); the interpolated percentage diameter stenosis was thus reduced from $62 \pm 12\%$ to $34 \pm 15\%$ (p<0.001).

Three groups of individual data are shown in Fig. XVII.2 according to the severity of the interpolated percentage diameter stenosis before PTCA. Prior to PTCA, 26% of the lesions had a percentage diameter stenosis ranging from 71 to 100%, while 58% of the lesions ranged between 51 and 70%. In the remaining 16% of the lesions that were dilated, the percentage diameter stenosis was less then 51%. In 4 of these patients, PTCA was performed immediately after intracoronary fibrinolysis [8]; in 18 other instances, we felt justified to dilate a second, less critical lesion during the same session.

The quantitative angiographic follow-up of the minimal obstruction diameters in 50 successfully dilated lesions is shown in Fig. XVII.3. A change superior to the total measurement variability of repeated coronary cineangiography and quantitative analysis (0.44 mm for obstruction diameter, i.e. 2 standard deviations (s.d.) of the difference of duplicate measurements) was considered as significant [9].

In 22 of these lesions, the residual obstruction diameter, measured immediately after PTCA, remained unchanged over a period of 6 months. In 16 other patients, some degree of restenosis occurred, while late further improvement was observed in the remaining twelve.

In the second group, the densitometric percentage area stenosis was used to assess the changes in cross-sectional area after PTCA and compared with the circular percentage area stenosis computed from the diameter measurements. The comparative data are shown in Table XVII.2 and Fig. XVII.4. Before PTCA, there exists a good agreement between the densitometric percentage area stenosis and the circular percentage area stenosis (standard deviation of the difference = 5.0 %-area stenosis). After PTCA, important discrepancies between these two types of measurements are observed (s.d. of the difference = 18% area stenosis). It is suggested that these discrepancies in results after PTCA can be accounted for by asymmetric morphological changes in luminal cross

Table XVII.1. Effect of PTCA on 138 obstructive lesions in the first study group.

	Before PTCA	After PTCA	p-value
Reference diameter (mm)	3.40 ± 0.68	3.34 ± 0.70	n.s.
Obstruction diameter (mm)	1.28 ± 0.40	2.24 ± 0.57	0.001
Diameter stenosis (%)	62 ± 12	34 ± 15	0.001

n.s. = not significant; PTCA = percutaneous transluminal coronary angioplasty

344

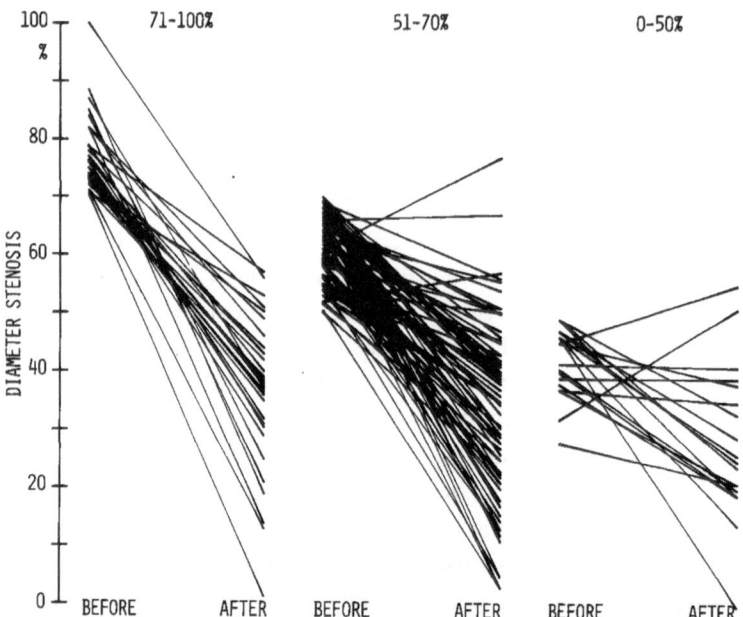

Fig. XVII.2. Individual data of change in percentage diameter stenosis for three subsets of coronary stenoses according to the initial severity. In the group with a stenosis ⩾71%, the diameter stenosis decreased on the average from 76% ± 7 to 33% ± 15. In the intermediate group (51–70%), the diameter stenosis decreased from 63% ± 6 to 33% ± 15, while in the last group (0–50%) it decreased from 42% ± 6 to 25% ± 6.

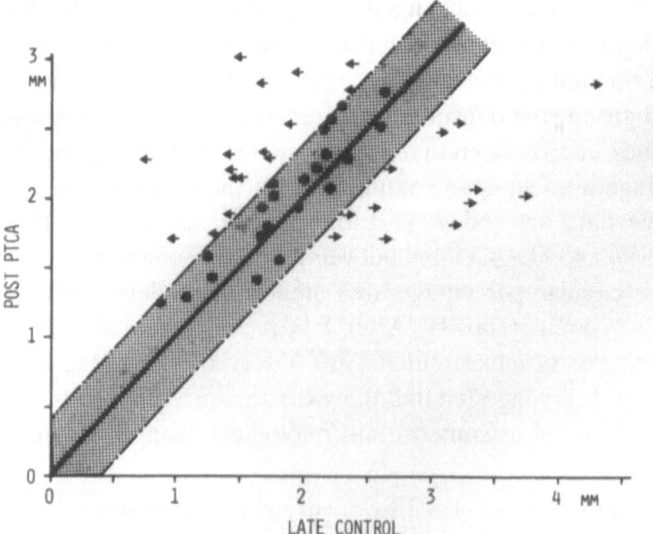

Fig. XVII.3. Quantitative angiographic follow-up after 6 months (late control) of the minimal obstruction diameter (mm) in 50 successfully dilated lesions with comparison to the same parameter immediately after the dilatation. The shaded area represents the total measurement variability (±2 standard deviations) of repeated coronary cineangiography and quantitative analysis. Symbols: ← = late deterioration of the initial angiographic results; ● = unchanged minimal obstruction diameter; → = late improvement.

Table XVII.2. Percentage area stenosis derived from detected contours versus densitometric area measurement, before and after angioplasty (PTCA).

Pt. No.	Before PTCA			After PTCA		
	% Circular A-sten	% Densito- metric A-sten	Difference	% Circular A-sten	% Densito- metric A-sten	Difference
1	69	69	0	24	9	− 15
2	93	93	0	57	71	14
3	94	97	4	33	44	11
4	73	85	12	36	64	28
5	85	89	4	73	75	2
6	88	92	4	42	47	5
7	85	90	5	19	44	25
8	70	71	1	21	36	15
9	85	90	5	52	35	− 17
10	93	93	0	23	47	24
11	57	61	4	54	58	4
12	96	99	3	46	17	− 29
13	95	94	− 1	83	82	− 1
14	84	82	− 2	60	46	− 14
15	89	93	4	66	71	5
16	84	89	5	51	66	15
17	88	94	6	28	36	12
18	90	77	− 13	44	10	− 34
mean	84%	87%	2.3%	45%	48%	2.8%
Corr Coeff:	0.89		s.d. 5%	0.62		s.d. 18%

A-sten = area stenosis; Corr Coeff = correlation coefficient; PTCA = percutaneous transluminal coronary angioplasty; s.d. = standard deviation.

section, which cannot be assessed accurately from diameter measurements in a single-plane view.

Discussion

Whenever a lesion appears to be of different severity when viewed from multiple projections, asymmetry should be suspected. In this study, asymmetry is considered present when the percentage diameter stenosis measured in one angiographic view exceeded that measured in another view by more than 2 standard deviations of the method used. As shown in Chapter V, the total measurement variability of repeated coronary cineangiography and quantitative analysis was 7.2% for the interpolated percentage diameter stenosis. In a study reported previously [10] , when 120 lesions were analyzed in several orthogonal projections, asymmetric lesions were seen in more than half of the cases (Fig. XVII.5).

346

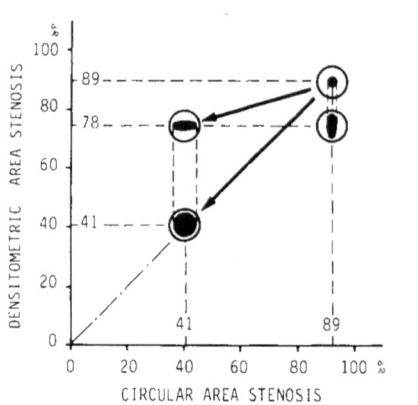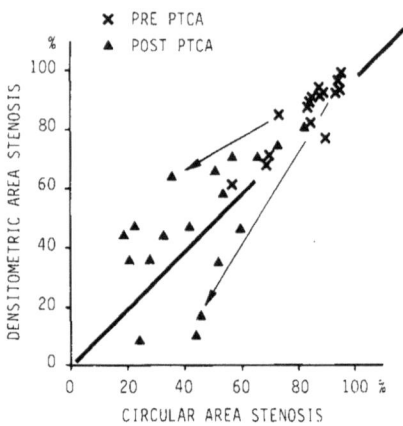

Fig. XVII.4. Left, schematic representation of the potential asymmetric morphologic changes in luminal cross section during angioplasty. Let us assume before PTCA a circular cross section (area stenosis: 89%) at the site of the stenosis. After angioplasty, three hypothetical situations are observed: (1) an elliptical cross section with the long axis perpendicular to the image intensifier; (2) an elliptical cross section with the long axis parallel to the image intensifier; and (3) an enlarged cross section. From the figure, it is clear that for the 2 asymmetric dilatations, the %-area stenosis (41% and 89%) derived from diameter measurements assuming a circular cross-sectional model differs from the densitometric %-area stenosis (78%). Right, before and after (PRE and POST) PTCA comparison between densitometric area stenosis and area stenosis derived from the diameter measurements.

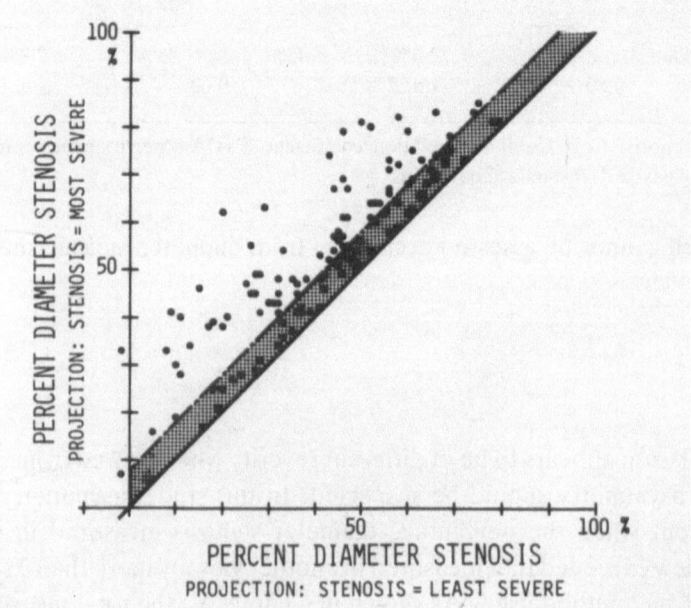

Fig. XVII.5. Asymmetry of 120 obstructive lesions analyzed in more than one projection. On the horizontal axis, percentage diameter stenosis measured in the less severe angiographic projection; on the vertical axis, percentage diameter stenosis of the same lesion measured in the most severe projection.

This shows that an atheromatous lesion may not always involve the entire circumference of the vessel but frequently results in an asymmetric or eccentric lesion. From postmortem data, it has been proven that a diseased vessel often looks like an exaggerated ellipse in which, ultimately, a slit-like lumen with a crescent shape represents the 'artery' [11]. It has been argued that this latter aspect is a product of postmortem arterial fixation with sectioning in the unpressurized state [12, 13]; yet the present data indicate that this is not an artifact. The corollary of these considerations is that the severity of the lesion to be dilated should be quantitated in as many angiographic views as possible when its efficacy is to be assessed by diameter measurements.

For the entire group the mean diameter stenosis before PTCA was 62%, as an average of multiple views. For the subset of lesions exceeding 50%, it was 69%. This value is almost 10% lower than that commonly reported when values are based on subjective reading of angiograms [14–16]. Such visual interpretation of diameter reductions is subject to systematic overestimation of the severity of the stenosis, as has been shown by several investigators [17, 18]. Luminal reductions greater than 90% with minimal obstruction diameter of 0.35 mm are unlikely to be crossed even by a low-profile deflated balloon catheter, which has a mean diameter of 0.8 mm. One must further keep in mind that a value of 80% of mean diameter stenosis commonly reported before PTCA corresponds to a 96% reduction of the luminal area. Again, this is unlikely to occur in patients with chronic stable angina because this would have limited the resting coronary blood flow at rest to a minimum. In fact, such restrictions are incompatible with adequate blood supply, unless collaterals are present [19].

On the other hand, a diameter stenosis of 69% measured in a single projection could be consistent with a cross-sectional area stenosis between 80 and 97% as shown in Fig. XVII.6. The latter also illustrates the varying results in percentage

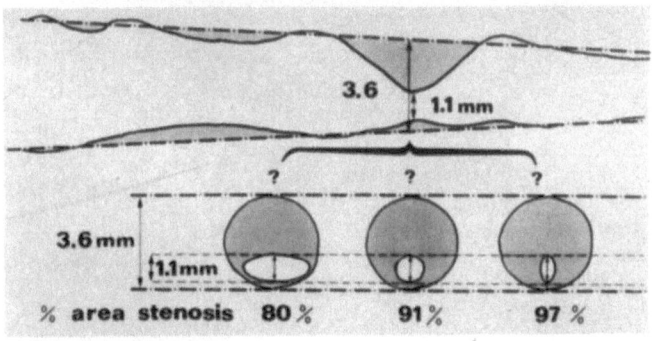

Fig. XVII.6. Schematic representation of a coronary obstruction with an interpolated diameter stenosis of 69% measured in a single projection. The percentage area stenosis, computed from diameter measurements, varied between 80% and 97% depending on the circular or elliptical model applied for the computation.

area stenosis, assessed from diameter measurements in a single view, depending on whether a circular or an elliptical model is applied.

The results of cross-sectional area measurements obtained in the second study group suggest the creation of asymmetric lesions after angioplasty. As demonstrated elegantly by Block et al. in rabbit arteries after experimentally induced atherosclerotic lesions, transluminal angioplasty leads to the breaking of the intimal surface of the atherosclerotic lesion [20]. This split may extend to the internal elastic membrane. Angiography performed after such procedures in the rabbit frequently shows an irregular column of contrast in this area. As suggested

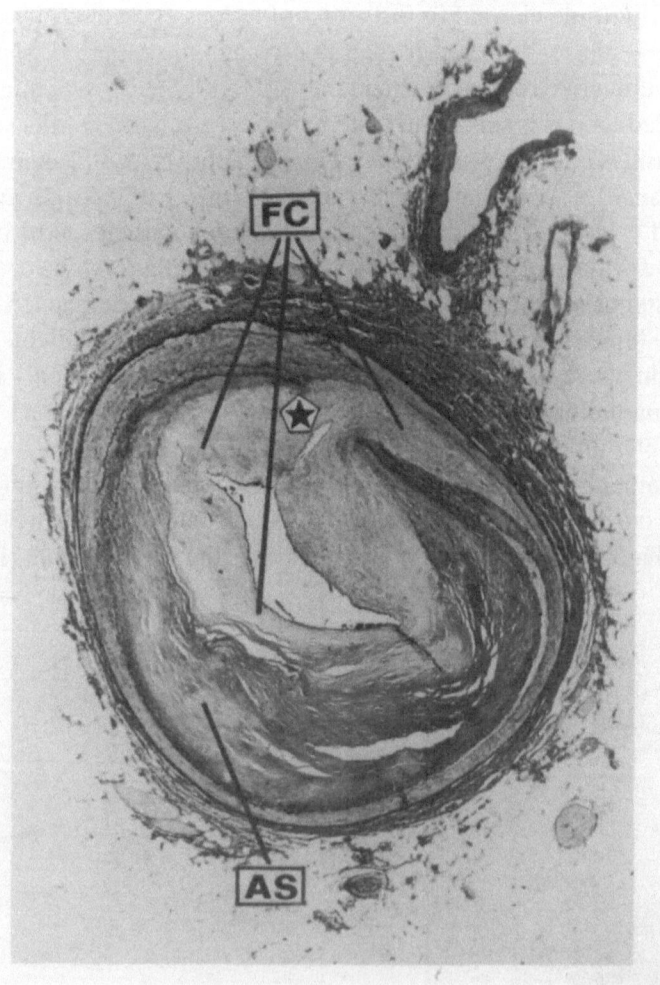

Fig. XVII.7. Histologic section through a stenotic lesion successfully dilated five months before the death of the patient. A disruption of the medial layer (star) is present, which had led to medial dissection. The false channel and the major part of the lumen are filled with fibrocellular tissue (FC). The pre-existent atherosclerotic plaque (AS) is readily identified.

by the investigators, these irregularities must certainly represent contrast material within the remains of the atherosclerotic plaque. Recently, human coronary arteries that had undergone angioplasty were analyzed. They have shown changes identical to those seen in animal models [21–23]. Such a disruption of the medial layer creating a slit-like appendix to the original lumen is shown in Fig. XVII.7. Because this tear in the wall is filled by fibrocellular tissue, it must be inferred that the asymmetric morphological aspect is not a postmortem artefact.

In conclusion, our angiographic study suggests that changes in the luminal area of an artery, produced by the mechanical disruption of its internal wall, cannot be assessed accurately from the detected contours of the vessel from a single plane angiographic view. Therefore, the diagnostic value of this type of measurement is restricted by the fact that the angioplastic changes are eccentric in nature. To obviate this limitation, the use of densitometry to compute cross-sectional areas from single views is advocated.

References

1. Roberts WC: The coronary arteries and left ventricle in clinically isolated angina pectoris. Circulation 54: 388–390, 1976.
2. Mates RE, Gupta RL, Bell AC, Klocke FJ: Fluid dynamics of coronary artery stenosis. Circ Res 42: 152–162, 1978.
3. Lipscomb K, Hooten S: Effect of stenotic dimensions and blood flow on the hemodynamic significance of model coronary arterial stenoses. Am J Cardiol 42: 781–792, 1978.
4. Harrison DG, White CW, Hiratzka LF, Wright CB, Doty CB, Miller MR, Eastham CL, Marcus ML: Can the significance of a coronary stenosis be predicted by quantitative coronary angiography? Circulation 64 (Supp IV): 160 (Abstract), 1981.
5. Collins SM, Skorton DJ, Harrison DG, White CW, Eastham CL, Hiratzka LF, Doty DB, Marcus ML: Quantitative computer-based videodensitometry and the physiological significance of a coronary stenosis. Comp in Cardiol: 219–222, 1982.
6. Freudenberg H, Lichtlen P: Postmortale Koronarangiographie. In: Koronarangiographie. PR Lichtlen (Ed) Verlag Dr Med D. Straube, Erlangen: 341–357, 1979.
7. Brown BG, Bolson EL, Dodge HT: Arteriographic assessment of coronary atherosclerosis. Review of current methods, their limitations and clinical application. Arteriosclerosis 2: 2–15, 1982.
8. Serruys PW, Wijns W, Brand M van den, Ribeiro V, Fioretti P, Simoons ML, Kooijman CJ, Reiber JHC, Hugenholtz PG: Is transluminal coronary angioplasty mandatory after successful thrombolysis? Quantitative coronary angiographic study. Br Heart J 50: 257–265, 1983.
9. Serruys PW, Hooghoudt TEH, Reiber JHC, Slager C, Brower RW, Hugenholtz PG: Influence of intracoronary nifedipine on left ventricular function, coronary vasomotility, and myocardial oxygen consumption. Br Heart J 49: 427–441, 1983.
10. Wijns W, Serruys PW, Brand M van den, Reiber JHC, Suryapranata H, Hugenholtz PG: Progression to complete coronary obstruction without myocardial infarction in patients who are candidates for Percutaneous Transluminal Angioplasty: a 90-Day Angiographic Follow-Up. In: Prognosis of Coronary Heart Disease – Progression of Coronary Arteriosclerosis. H Roskamm, (Ed). Springer-Verlag, Berlin: 190–195, 1983.
11. Roberts WC, Buja LM: The frequency and significance of coronary arterial thrombi and other observations in fatal acute myocardial infarction. A study of 107 necropsy patients. Am J Med 52: 425–433, 1972.

12. Arnett EN, Isner JM, Redwood DR, Kent KM, Baker WP, Ackerstein H, Roberts WC: Coronary artery narrowing in coronary heart disease: comparison of cineangiographic and necropsy findings. Ann Int Med 91: 350–356, 1979.
13. Brown BG, Petersen R: Computer-assisted measurements of coronary artery stenosis. Reply to letter to the editor. Circulation 60: 1196, 1979.
14. Cowley MJ, Vetrovec GW, Wolfgang TC: Efficacy of percutaneous transluminal coronary angioplasty: technique, patient selection, salutary results, limitations and complications. Am Heart J 101: 272–280, 1981.
15. Meier B, Gruentzig AR, Goebel N, Pyle R, Gosslar W von, Schlumpf M: Assessment of stenoses in coronary angioplasty. Inter- and intraobserver variability. Int J Cardiol 3: 159–169, 1983.
16. Kent KM, Bentivoglio LG, Block PC, Cowley MJ, Dorros G, Gosselin AJ, Grüntzig A, Myler RK, Simpson J, Stertzer SH, Williams DO, Fisher L, Gillespie MJ, Detre K, Kelsey S, Mullin SM, Mock MB: Percutaneous Transluminal Coronary Angioplasty: Report from the Registry of the National Heart, Lung and Blood Institute. Am J Cardiol 49: 2011–2020, 1982.
17. Cherrier F, Booman F, Serruys PW, Cuillière M, Danchin N, Reiber JHC: L'angiographie coronaire quantitative. Application à l'évaluation des angioplasties transluminales coronaires. Arch Mal Coeur 74: 1377–1387, 1981.
18. Gerbrands JJ, Reiber JHC, Booman F: Computer processing and classification of coronary occlusions. In: Pattern Recognition in Practice. ES Gelsema, LN Kanal (Eds.). North Holland Publishing Company: 223–233, 1980.
19. McMahon MM, Brown BG, Cukingnan R, Rolett EL, Bolson E, Frimer M, Dodge HT: Quantitative Coronary Angiography: measurement of the 'critical' stenosis in patients with unstable angina and single-vessel disease without collaterals. Circulation 60: 106–113, 1979.
20. Block PC, Baughman KL, Pasternak RC, Fallon JT: Transluminal Angioplasty: correlation of morphologic and angiographic findings in an experimental model. Circulation 61: 778–785, 1980.
21. Holmes DR, Vlietstra RE, Mock MB, Reeder GS, Smith HC, Bove AA, Bresnahan JF, Piehler JM, Schaff HV, Orszulak TA: Angiographic changes produced by Percutaneous Transluminal Coronary Angioplasty. Am J Cardiol 51: 676–683, 1983.
22. Block PC, Myler RK, Stertzer S, Fallon JT: Morphology after transluminal angioplasty in human beings. New Engl J Med 305: 382–385, 1981.
23. Essed CE, Brand M van den, Becker AE: Transluminal coronary angioplasty and early re-stenosis. Fibrocellular occlusion after wall laceration. Br Heart J 49: 393–396, 1983.

XVIII. Left ventricular performance, regional blood flow, wall motion and lactate metabolism during transluminal angioplasty

Summary

The response of left ventricular function, coronary blood flow, and myocardial lactate metabolism during percutaneous transluminal coronary angioplasty (PTCA) was studied in a series of patients undergoing the procedure. From four to six balloon inflation procedures per patient were performed with an average duration per occlusion of 51 ± 12 sec (mean $\pm$ s.d.) and a total occlusion time of 252 ± 140 sec. Analysis of left ventricular hemodynamics in 19 patients showed that the relaxation parameters, peak negative rate of change in pressure, and early time constants of relaxation, responded earliest to short-term coronary occlusion (peak effect at 17 ± 7 sec), while other parameters, such as peak pressure, left ventricular end-diastolic pressure, and peak positive rate of change in pressure, responded more gradually, suggesting a progressive depression of myocardial mechanics throughout the procedure. Left ventricular angiograms, available from 14 patients, indicated an early onset of asynchronous relaxation concurrent with the early response in peak negative dP/dt and the time constant of early relaxation. All hemodynamic functions fully recovered within minutes after the end of PTCA. Mean blood flow in the great cardiac vein and proximal coronary sinus and the hyperemic response were measured in 20 patients. Before PTCA mean flow in the great cardiac vein was 69 ± 17 ml/min and in the coronary sinus it was 129 ± 34 ml/min. Reactive hyperemia (great cardiac vein) was 55% after the first PTCA and 91% after the third. A more pronounced reaction was observed when the residual functional coronary stenosis was reduced in subsequent dilatations. Arteriovenous lactate difference appeared constant during the first two occlusions (control $+ 0.11$ mmol/liter, first PTCA -0.87 mmol/liter, and second PTCA -0.82 mmol/liter) and did not increase during subsequent occlusions. Within minutes after the procedure lactate balance was again positive, demonstrating the reversibility of the metabolic disturbances after repeated ischemia. The results of this study indicate that there is no permanent dysfunction of global or regional myocardial mechanics, myocardial blood flow, or lactate metabolism after PTCA with four to six coronary occlusions of 40 to 60 seconds.

Introduction

Until recently the measurement in man of left ventricular geometry and hemo-dynamics early after an abrupt occlusion of a major coronary artery has not been feasible. Percutaneous transluminal coronary angioplasty (PTCA), however, now provides a unique opportunity to study the time course of changes during the transient interruption of coronary flow by the balloon occlusion sequence in patients with single-vessel disease and without angiographically demonstrable collateral circulation [1, 2]. We report the dynamic changes in left ventricular hemodynamics in 19 patients and the concurrent left ventricular geometric changes assessed by angiography in another group of 14 patients during PTCA. In a third group of patients regional blood flow and lactate metabolism were analyzed during reactive hyperemia after repeated occlusions of the left anterior descending coronary artery. These different studies were undertaken to investig-ate the sequence of events during transient ischemia induced by PTCA and to determine whether or not the effects of ischemia after repeated occlusions were reversible.

Materials and methods

Study population and protocol

After a feasibility study of the effect of nonionic contrast media on left ventricular function, permission from the Thoraxcenter Ethics Committee was granted to obtain left ventricular angiograms during transluminal occlusions. All patients in this study gave their informed consent and there were no complications directly related to the research procedure.

For the first part of the study data were collected from 19 adult patients undergoing temporary coronary occlusion of a diseased left coronary artery during PTCA. Four of these patients had had a previous myocardial infarction. Records were analyzed during the first successful PTCA procedure for each patient.

For the second part of the study, 14 patients were selected from 356 consecutive patients in whom angioplasty was attempted. These patients met the inclusion criteria by having isolated obstructive lesions of one coronary vessel (left anterior descending artery in 10 patients, right coronary in four, left circumflex in one) and normal resting left ventricular function and wall motion. Four patients had mild essential hypertension and elevated left ventricular filling pressures (end-dia-stolic pressure ≥ 25 mmHg). During the PTCA procedure the number of transluminal occlusions performed per patient was 4.9 ± 2.2 (mean $\pm$ s.d.). The average duration of each occlusion was 51 ± 12 sec (mean $\pm$ s.d.) and the total occlusion time during the whole procedure was 252 ± 140 sec (mean $\pm$ s.d.). With a tipmanometer on a No. 8F pigtail catheter, pressures were recorded and derived indices were calculated off-line by a computer system [3, 4]. Three to four ventriculograms (30 degrees right anterior oblique at 50 frames/sec) were obtained by injection of 0.75 ml/kg of a nonionic contrast medium (metrizamide, Amipaque). The hemodynamic and angiographic investigations were performed before the PTCA procedure was begun, after 20 sec of occlusion during the second dilatation, after 50 sec of occlusion during the fourth dilatation, and again 5 minutes after completion of the PTCA procedure. These sequential left ventricular angiograms were made only after the values for left ventricular end-diastolic pressure and the various isovolumetric parameters had returned to those recorded before the initial angiogram. In all cases the interval between two angiograms was at least 10 minutes. Care was taken to maintain the patient's position unchanged in relation to the X-ray equipment during the consecutive angiograms. Diaphragm movement was kept to a minimum by instructing patients to keep inspiration shallow and to avoid the Valsalva manoeuvre.

For the third part of the study, data were collected from 20 other patients with proximal lesions in the left anterior descending artery. Coronary sinus and great cardiac vein blood flow were measured by the continuous thermodilution method with a Baim catheter [5, 6]. The main objective of this measurement was to detect changes in the global and regional blood flows, as well as in the regional lactate metabolism, during the reactive hyperemia after consecutive episodes of transluminal occlusion. In the beginning of the investigation the position of the distal thermistor in the great cardiac vein was determined by injection of 3 ml of contrast medium. After each balloon deflation coronary sinus and great cardiac vein flows were measured for 10 sec. The continuous infusion for thermodilution was then interrupted to allow blood withdrawal from the great cardiac vein. Lactate was assayed enzymatically according to Apstein et al. [7] with the AutoAnalyzer II (Technicon, Tarrytown, NY). Blood (4 ml) for lactate measurements was rapidly deproteinized with an equal volume of cold 8% perchloric acid ($HClO_4$) and centrifuged. The supernatant was analyzed on the AutoAnalyzer and compared with standard curves made with lithium lactate in 4% $HClO_4$.

Analysis of pressure-derived indices during systole and diastole

Left ventricular pressure was measured with a Millar micromanometer catheter and digitized at 250 samples/sec. Combined analog and digital filtering resulted in an effective time constant of less than 10 msec. We used an updated version of the beat-to-beat program described previously [3, 4] that also incorporates the capability of acquiring a calibrated pressure signal and storing it on disk or tape for

354

subsequent off-line analysis. The latter procedure was followed for all PTCA procedures. For off-line analysis of pressure relaxation the following definitions were used: (1) pressure at the beginning of isovolumetric relaxation (P_b) is the pressure at the point at which dP/dt is minimal (maximum negative dP/dt), and (2) pressure at end of isovolumetric relaxation (P_e) is the pressure less than or equal to the previous end-diastolic pressure, but not less than 1 mmHg.

Although it is possible that the latter definition may result in P_e being measured just after mitral valve opening, estimation of the time constants using more stringent criteria, such as end-diastolic pressure + 10 mmHg, did not result in a significantly better estimation, and on the contrary failed to measure the time constants during high heart rates.

Peak left ventricular pressure, left ventricular end-diastolic pressure, peak negative dP/dt, peak positive dP/dt, and the relationship between dP/dt/pressure and pressure linearly extrapolated to pressure = 0 (V_{max}), where V_{max} is maximal velocity, were computed on-line after a data acquisition of 20 seconds.

Determination of relaxation parameters

Three techniques have been implemented for the off-line beat-to-beat calculation of the relaxation parameters [8–10]. All require a minimum of eight samples (over 32 msec) between P_b and P_e.

Semilogarithmic model
The semilogarithmic model used was: $P(t) = P_o e^{-t/T}$, where P is pressure; t is time; P_o is equivalent to P_b when a true exponential decay is present starting from the time of peak negative dP/dt; the fit for the first 40 msec ($n \geq 8$), T_1, is biexponential [10]; the fit after 40 msec ($n \geq 3$), T_2, is biexponential [10]; and the fit for all points ($n \geq 8$), T, is monoexponential. The P_o and T parameters are estimated from a linear least squares fit of $Ln\ P = -t/T + Ln\ P_o$.

Exponential model
The exponential model used was: $P(t) = P_o e^{-t/T} + P_1$, with nonlinear least squares fit of P, for P_o, P_1, and T. P_1 represents the offset pressure the system relaxes to for $t \geq T$. The isovolumetric relaxation period is modeled only monoexponentially.

Derivative model
The derivative model used was: $P(t) = P_o e^{-t/T} + P_1$ or $dP/dt = -1/T \cdot (P(t)-P_1)$, with linear least squares fit of dP/dt vs P for T and P, starting at 16 msec after P_b until P_e.

Analysis of global and regional left ventricular function during systole and diastole

A complete cardiac cycle was analyzed frame-by-frame with the Contouromat for all cineangiograms. End-diastolic pressure was defined as that point on the pressure trace at which the derivative of the pressure first exceeded 200 mmHg/ sec and in all cases coincided with the maximal measured left ventricular volume [3]. End systole was defined, with reference to the pressure tracing, at the occurrence of the dicrotic notch of the central aortic pressure. To analyze the regional left ventricular function, the computer generated a system of coordinates along which the left ventricular displacement was determined frame-by-frame in 20 segments (Fig. XVIII.1) (Chapter IV).

Segmental wall velocity was computed as the first-derivative of the instantaneous displacement function. Mean ejection phase wall velocity for each segment was calculated from end diastole to end systole (Fig. XVIII.1). Segmental volume was computed from the local radius (R) and the height of each segment (1/10 of left ventricular long-axis length L) according to the formula $\pi R^2 L/20$. When normalized for end-diastolic volume, the systolic segmental volume change can be considered as a parameter of regional pump function (Fig. XVIII.2). During systole this parameter expresses quantitatively the contribution of a particular segment to global ejection fraction, termed regional contribution to global ejection fraction (Chapter IV). The sum of the values for all 20 segments equals the global ejection fraction. Diastolic function was analyzed in terms of volume stiffness. Pressure-volume relationships were determined from the lowest diastolic pressure to the beginning of the 'a' wave. The natural logarithm of pressure was used in a linear regression analysis of pressure and volume from which a slope (K) was derived. Changes in K were taken as changes in volume stiffness [11].

Results

Analysis of pressure-derived indices during systole and diastole

Hemodynamic parameter values for a control beat just before occlusion, at peak effect in terms of the change in negative dP/dt and T_1 (occurring, on average, at 17 ± 7 sec), and at the end of the occlusion (occurring, on average, at 53 ± 12 sec) are summarized in Table XVIII.1. No attempt was made to average consecutive beats or to select beats with respect to the respiratory cycle. An example of a continuous recording of V_{max} positive and negative dP/dt, T_1, T_2, T, end-diastolic pressure and peak pressure is illustrated in Fig. XVIII.3.

There was no important change in heart rate during the PTCA procedure. The pattern of change in peak left ventricular pressure, left ventricular end-diastolic pressure, peak positive dP/dt, and V_{max}, however, suggest a progressive depres-

356

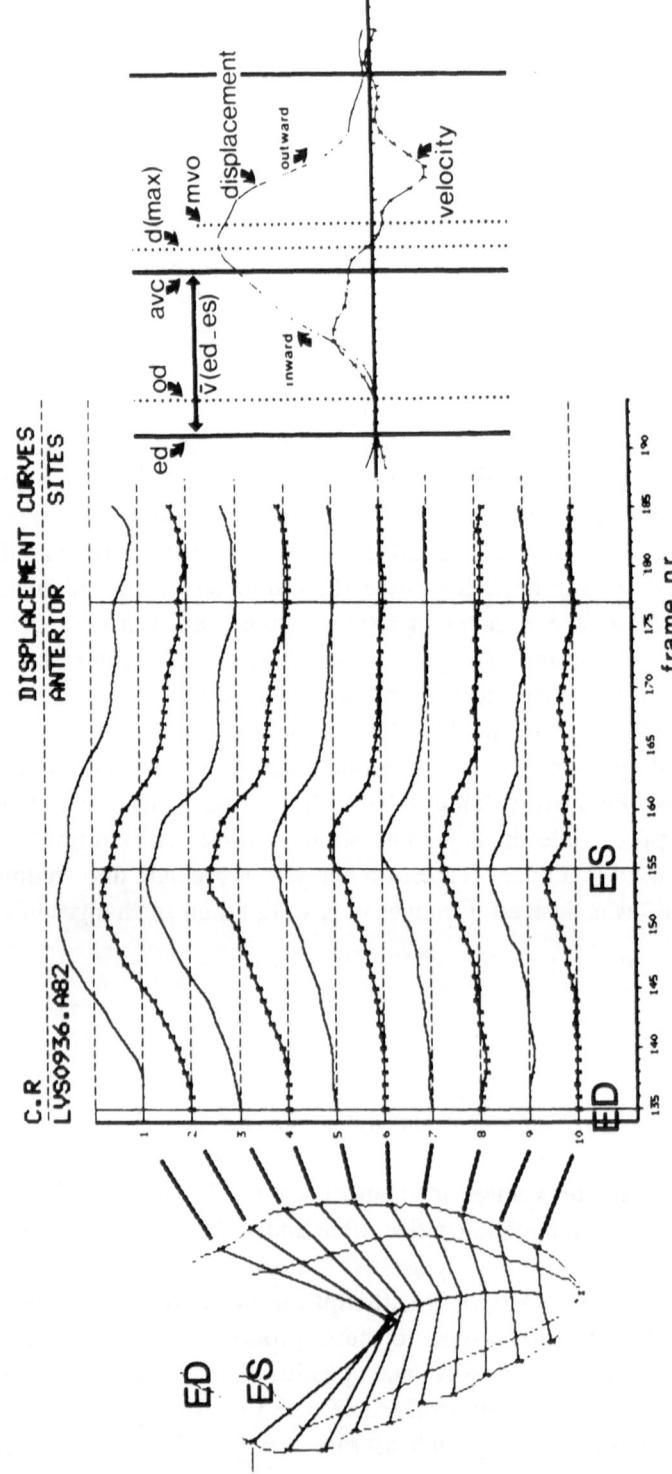

Fig. XVIII.1. End-diastolic and end-systolic left ventricular contours, as detected by the automated analysis system. Superimposed on these silhouettes is a system of coordinates along which segmental left ventricular wall displacement is detected. Left ventricular wall velocity, the first derivative of wall displacement, is derived from these data. ed = end diastole; es = end systole; od = onset of displacement; v̄(ed−es) = mean ejection phase wall velocity; d(max) = maximal inward wall displacement; mvo = nitral valve opening.

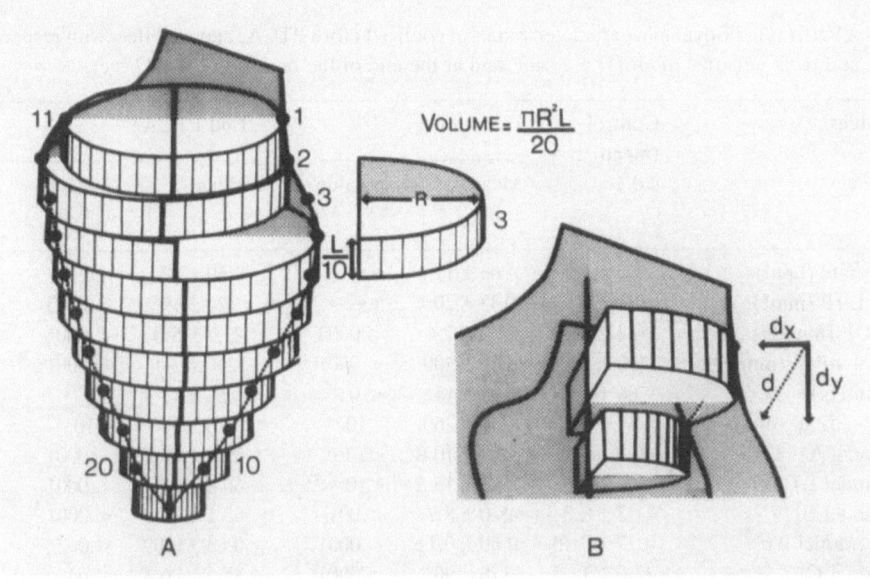

Fig. XVIII.2. Method for computing regional contribution to ejection fraction (CREF): The volume of each segment (slice volume) is computed according to the formula shown in the figure. The change in systolic volume is derived from the regional displacement and is mainly a consequence of the decrease in radius (R) of a half slice, which is expressed by the x-component (dx) of the displacement vector (d). L = left ventricular long-axis length extending from base to apex.

$$\text{CREF (\%)} = \frac{\text{(ED-ES) slice volume}}{\text{Global ED volume}} \times 100.$$

sion in myocardial mechanics without any indication of an early peak. The pressure at which the isovolumetric relaxation phase was considered to begin (P_b) was not altered appreciably during PTCA in spite of the drop in peak left ventricular pressure and peak negative dP/dt.

Within 4 or 5 beats after occlusion, a deformation appeared in the ascending limb of the negative dP/dt curve (Fig. XVIII.4) and in the next 10 seconds this deformation gradually increased so that the irregularity in the curve reached the same height as peak negative dP/dt, which had progressively decreased to its nadir. In the next 20 to 50 sec, peak negative dP/dt began to return towards control levels with a resolution of the irregularity in the ascending limb of its curve. At 50 sec, this parameter recovered to 77% of the preocclusion value and the deformity was no longer present.

This deformation of the negative dP/dt signal at the early phase of the occlusion indicates that the time course of left ventricular pressure decay deviates substantially from the monoexponential model usually proposed and also that asynchronous contraction or relaxation may be involved at the very beginning of the transluminal occlusion. Therefore, biexponential fitting of the pressure curve was computed during the isovolumetric relaxation, primarily because the pressure curve, when plotted on semilogarithmic paper, was observed to follow two straight lines rather than the one predicted by the monoexponential mode.

Table XVIII.1. Hemodynamic parameter values at control before PTCA, at peak effect with respect to T_1, and peak negative dP/dt (17 ± 7 sec), and at the end of the occlusion (52 ± 12 sec).

Variables	Control (mean ± s.d.)	Peak effect Mean ± s.d.	p-value	End PTCA Mean ± s.d.	p-value
Heart rate (bpm)	67 ± 12	66 ± 11	n.s.	69 ± 12	n.s.
Peak LVP (mmHg)	137 ± 21	133 ± 20	n.s.	124 ± 19	<.0003
LVEDP (mmHg)	16.4 ± 6.4	19.3 ± 7.4	<.0003	23.7 ± 5.0	<.0001
Peak + dP/dt (mmHg/s)	1490 ± 330	1300 ± 200	<.0001	1260 ± 250	<.0001
P_b (mmHg)	86 ± 14	90 ± 15	<.04	84 ± 13	n.s.
Peak − dP/dt (mmHg/s)	1710 ± 320	1240 ± 260	$<10^{-6}$	1320 ± 380	$<10^{-5}$
T (model A)	46.4 ± 8.1	58.4 ± 10.8	$<10^{-6}$	59.4 ± 10.2	<.0001
T_1 (model B)	53.0 ± 7.6	81.7 ± 15.3	$<10^{-6}$	66.2 ± 13.0	<.0001
T_2 (model B)	41.3 ± 8.8	48.0 ± 8.7	<.001	55.1 ± 10.8	<.0001
T_2/T_1 (model B)	0.77 ± 0.10	0.60 ± 0.11	<.0001	0.83 ± 0.09	<.002
T (model C)	72.6 ± 18.5	178 ± 96	<.0001	85.5 ± 26.4	<.04
T (model D)	63.2 ± 11.8	120 ± 57	<.0001	76.3 ± 24.3	<.01

All time constant values are in milliseconds. LVP = left ventricular pressure; LVEDP = left ventricular end-diastolic pressure. Computation models: A = single constant without offset; B = double time constant without offset; C = time constant from dP/dt; D = single time constant with offset P_1.

The second half of Table XVIII.1 summarizes the results with the different techniques for computing the relaxation parameters. While major differences are apparent in the magnitude of the time constants, however computed, they all showed a highly significant slowing of relaxation early during PTCA and recovery and return to near-control levels by the end of the procedure. The behavior of the two time constants (T_1, T_2) during PTCA is illustrated in Fig. XVIII.3.

Generally the time constants computed from the logarithm of pressure were smaller and showed less variation than those computed from the other two models. The major discrepancies are apparent at the peak effect of PTCA. This is also reflected in the p (significance)-value. The ratio T_2/T_1, an index of asynchrony [10], showed a drop of 0.17 from 0.77 (control) to 0.60 (peak effect), but within 53 sec not only returned to the control level but exceeded it slightly. After 53 sec of occlusion, the region perfused by the occluded coronary artery could no longer be considered to be asynchronous, but was probably akinetic and not actively contributing to either contraction or relaxation.

Global left ventricular function during systole and diastole

The left ventricular pressures and volumes measured before, during, and after angioplasty are listed in Table XVIII.2. During the four sequential cine-an-

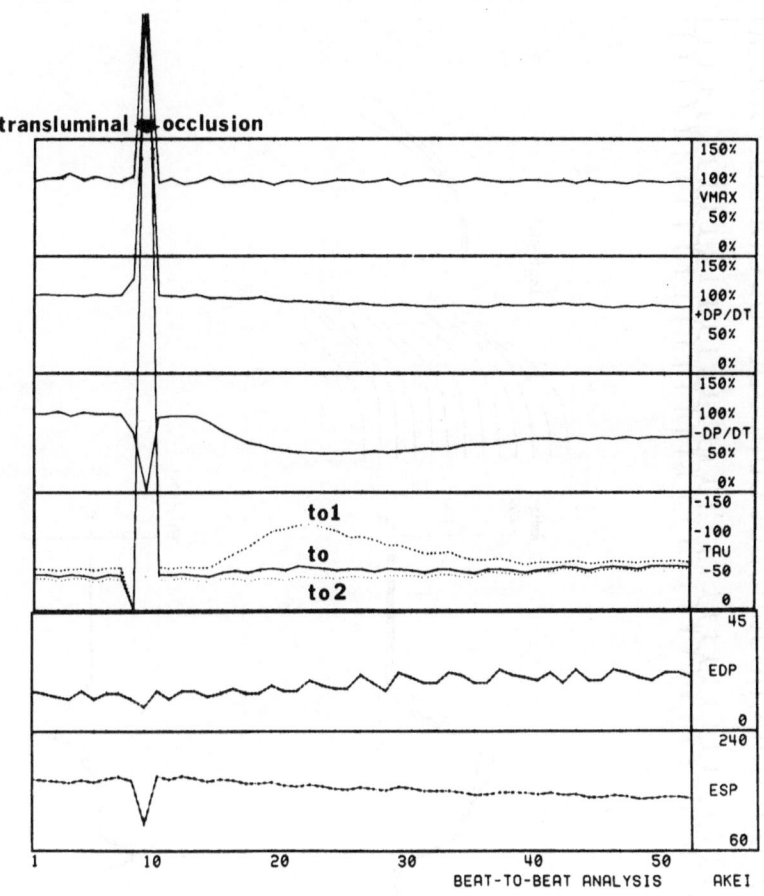

Fig. XVIII.3. Hemodynamic measurements in a patient during PTCA. From top to bottom, maximal velocity of the contractile elements (V_{max}), peak negative and positive dP/dt expressed as percentages of control values; the time constants of relaxation to_1 (dashed line), to (solid line), and to_2 (dotted line) (scale 50 msec); end-diastolic pressure (EDP, scale 15 mmHg); and peak systolic pressure (ESP, scale 60 mmHg, with 60 mmHg offset). The break in the data at beat 10 corresponds to inflation of the PTCA balloon.

giographic investigations the heart rates were almost identical, whereas the isovolumetric indices of contraction and relaxation recorded during the second (20 sec occlusion) or the third (50 sec occlusion) left ventricular angiograms showed changes very similar to those described in the first group of results (Table XVIII.1). Occlusion of a major coronary artery for only 20 sec resulted in a significant ($p < 0.005$) increase in end-systolic volume (from 31 ± 9 to 37 ± 9 ml/ m^2), while the end-diastolic volume remained unchanged after 20 sec and even after 50 sec of transluminal occlusion. At 50 sec the ejection fraction decreased from 62% to 48% ($p < 0.005$) and this decrease was essentially due to an increase in end-systolic volume from 29 ± 7 to 41 ± 9 ml/m^2 ($p < 0.005$).

An example of the relationship between left ventricular diastolic pressure and

360

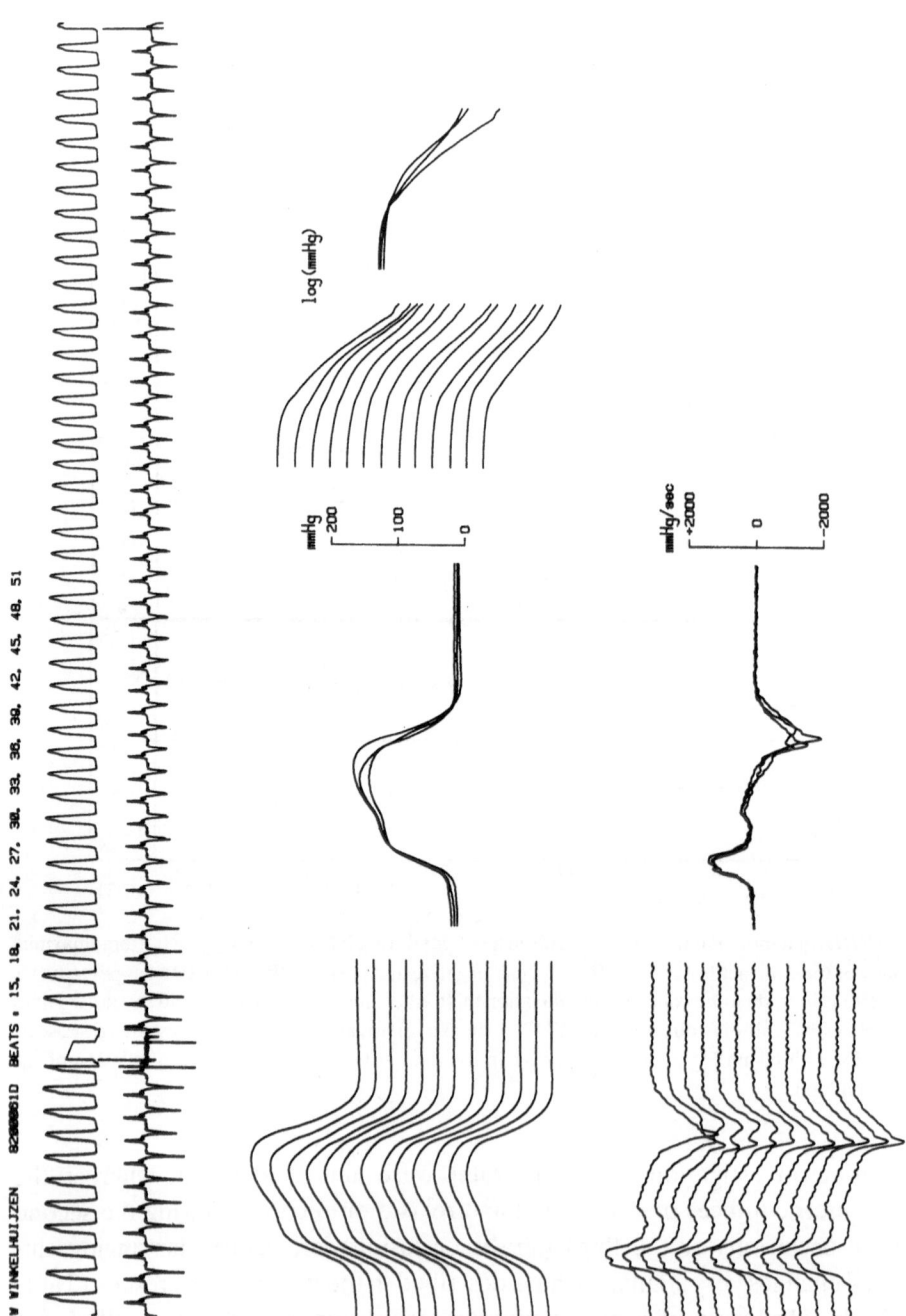

Fig. XVIII.4. Effects of coronary artery occlusion on left ventricular pressure (mmHg) and positive and negative dP/dt (mmHg/sec). The break in the recording at beat 15 corresponds with the inflation of the balloon. On the left are displayed the left ventricular pressures and positive and negative dP/dt's of individual beats (15, 18, 21, and so forth) while the natural logarithm of the pressure is shown on the right. The decrease in negative dP/dt is associated with an irregularity in the upstroke of the negative dP/dt curve. After 30 sec (beat 42) peak negative dP/dt starts to return toward a more normal shape of the signal.

Table XVIII.2. Hemodynamic parameter values before PTCA, at 20 and 50 sec after occlusion, and after the PTCA procedure.

Variables	Before PTCA		20 sec occlusion (total group; N = 14)	50 sec occlusion (subgroup; N = 9)	After PTCA	
	Total group (N = 14)	Subgroup (N = 9)			Subgroup (N = 9)	Total group (N = 14)
HR (bpm)	62 ± 16	59 ± 18	61 ± 13	62 ± 14	63 ± 11	64 ± 11
EDV (ml/m²)	81 ± 15	79 ± 14	81 ± 15	81 ± 16	78 ± 11	77 ± 11
SV (ml/m₂)	31 ± 9	29 ± 7	37 ± 9+	41 ± 9+	26 ± 15	27 ± 7*
SV (ml/m²)	50 ± 11	49 ± 11	44 ± 12*	39 ± 14*	52 ± 10	50 ± 9
EF (%)	61 ± 8	62 ± 6	54 ± 8+	48 ± 12+	66 ± 6	64 ± 7
Peak LVP (mmHg)	154 ± 30	151 ± 35	142 ± 29	145 ± 37	148 ± 25	147 ± 21
Peak + dP/dt (mmHg.sec⁻¹)	1403 ± 304	1356 ± 257	1312 ± 320	1278 ± 317	1442 ± 384	1412 ± 333
V_{max} (sec⁻¹)	39 ± 9	40 ± 8	39 ± 9	34 ± 10*	43 ± 12	42 ± 11
ESP (mmHg)	95 ± 18	92 ± 22	90 ± 19	98 ± 24	91 ± 15	90 ± 14
Peak – dP/dt (mmHg.sec⁻¹)	1727 ± 322	1614 ± 267	1268 ± 355+	1404 ± 370*	1665 ± 296	1664 ± 243
T_1 (msec)	55 ± 8	55 ± 6	79 ± 17+	68 ± 16+	56 ± 7.5	54 ± 7
T_2 (msec)	44 ± 7	43 ± 7	51 ± 8*	59 ± 8+	45 ± 8	45 ± 9
Pmin (mmHg)	10 ± 5	8 ± 3	11 ± 4	16 ± 6+	8 ± 5	8 ± 4
EDP (mmHg)	22 ± 8	18 ± 6	22 ± 7	29 ± 5*	21 ± 5	20 ± 6
K ln P/V (ml⁻¹)	0.0244 ± 0.009	0.0239 ± 0.008	0.0314 ± 0.016	0.0431 ± 0.018	0.0349 ± 0.016	0.0339 ± 0.013

HR, heart rate; EDV, end-diastolic volume; ESV, end-systolic volume; SV, stroke volume; EDV, ESV and SV have been normalized for body surface area; EF, ejection fraction; LVP, left ventricular pressure; ESP, end-systolic pressure; Pmin, left ventricular minimal diastolic pressure; EDP, left ventricular end-diastolic pressure; K ln P/V, natural logarithmic slope of diastolic pressure-volume relationship. * $p < .05$ compared with before PTCA, paired Student t test; + $p < .005$, compared with before PTCA, paired Student t test.

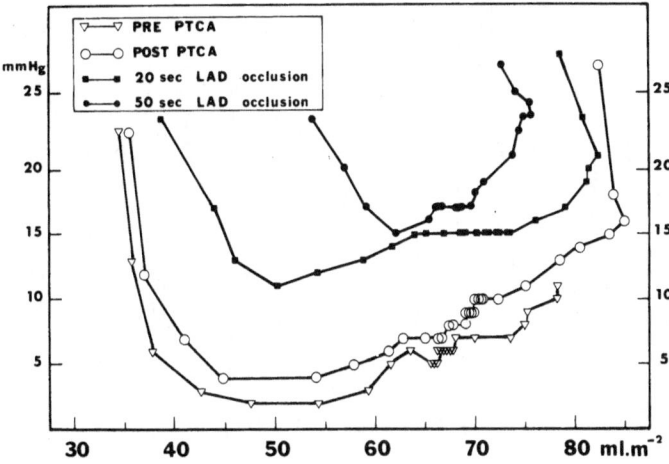

Fig. XVIII.5. Diastolic pressure-volume relationships during PTCA. During occlusion there is a gradual shift upward and to the right in the diastolic pressure-volume relationship. LAD = left anterior descending artery.

362

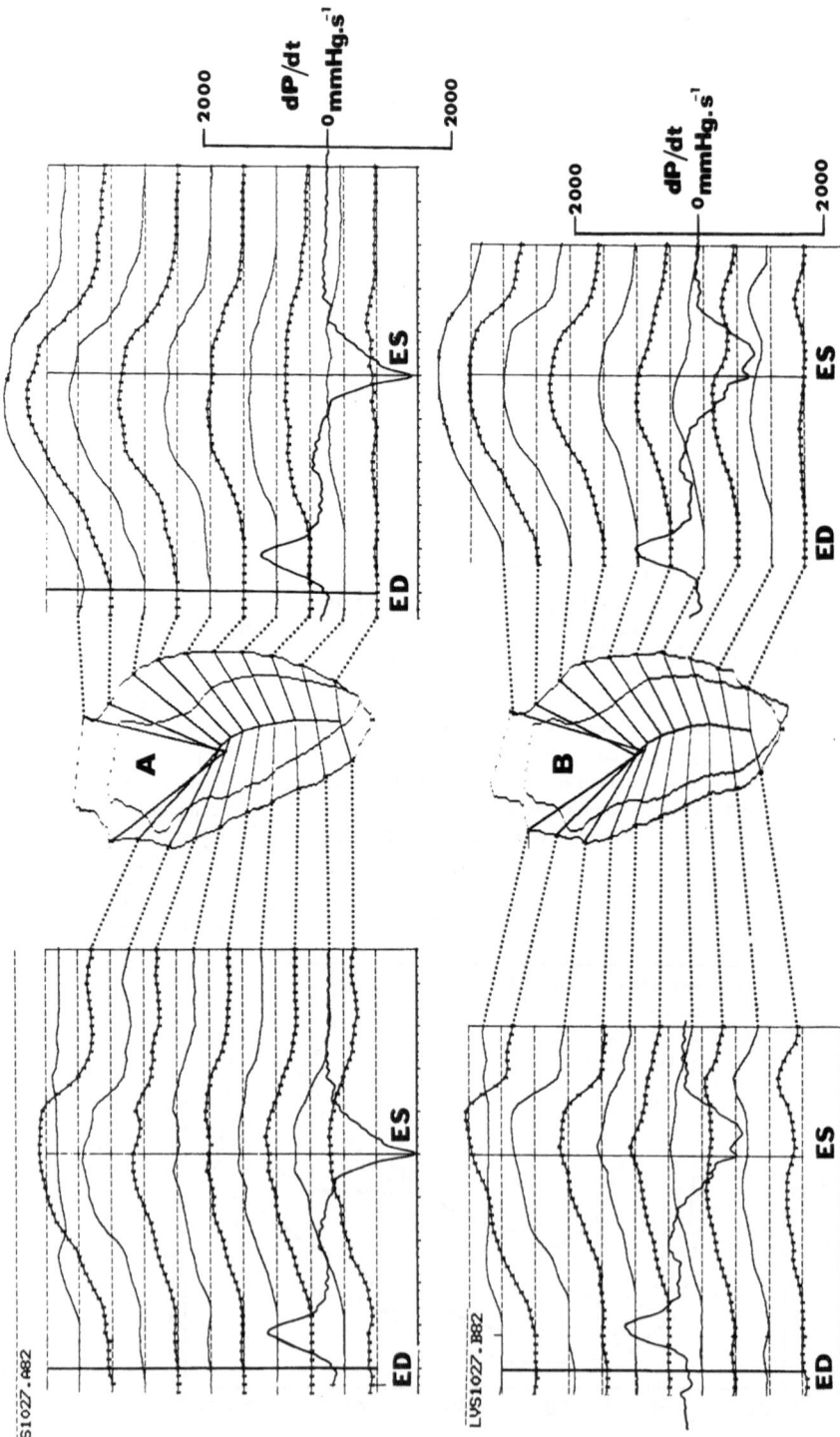

Fig. XVIII.6. Left ventricular wall displacement studied in 20 separate segments, 10 in the anterior (right) and 10 in the infero-posterior (left) wall. A typical example of the relationship between segmental wall displacement and dP/dt curve is observed before PTCA (A) and after 20 sec (B) of occlusion of the left anterior descending artery. After 20 sec of occlusion, the notch in the dP/dt curve corresponds to a second wave of inward wall displacement in the antero-apical and infero-apical segments.

volume during transluminal occlusion is illustrated in Fig. XVIII.5. It is evident that the entire diastolic pressure-volume relationship during transluminal occlusion was gradually shifted upward and to the right so that at any given volume, the diastolic pressures were higher. This effect was consistently observed after 50 sec of occlusion. Furthermore, the K constant, considered to be an index of volume stiffness, was significantly increased after 50 sec of transluminal occlusion (Table XVIII.2). Nevertheless, the hemodynamic and cineangiographic investigations performed after completion of the PTCA procedure demonstrated the perfect reversibility of these changes in volume as well as the normalization of the different pressure-derived indices.

Regional left ventricular function

The profound effect of a 20 sec occlusion of the left anterior descending artery on left ventricular wall motion and its time sequence is shown in Fig. XVIII.6. The delay in onset of displacement with respect to end-diastole as well as the time relationship between the aortic valve closure and the occurrence of the maximal wall displacement is illustrated in Fig. XVIII.7. The onset of displacement of the

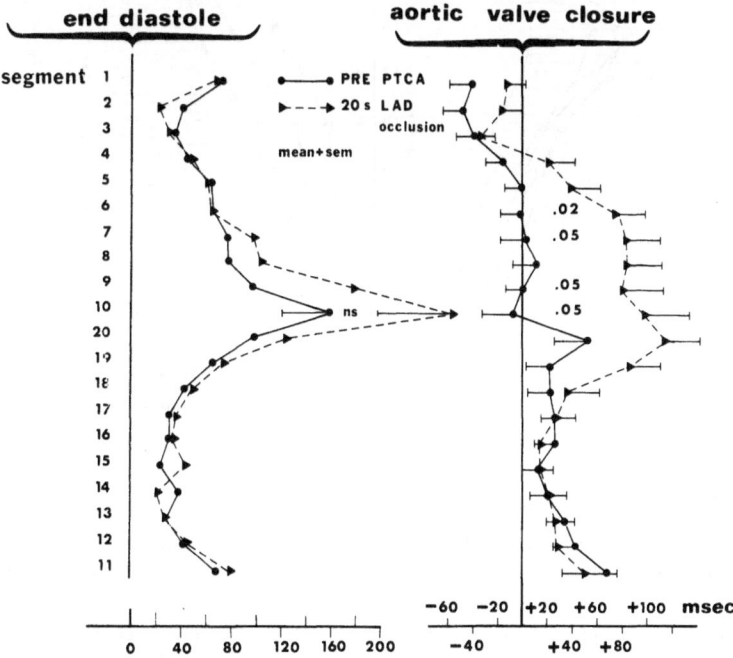

Fig. XVIII.7. Delay (msec) in onset of displacement for the 20 individual wall segments with respect to end diastole (time zero) before and after 20 sec of occlusion of the left anterior descending artery. Time relationship between aortic valve closure (time zero) and the occurrence of maximal wall displacement before and after 20 sec of occlusion of the left anterior descending artery.

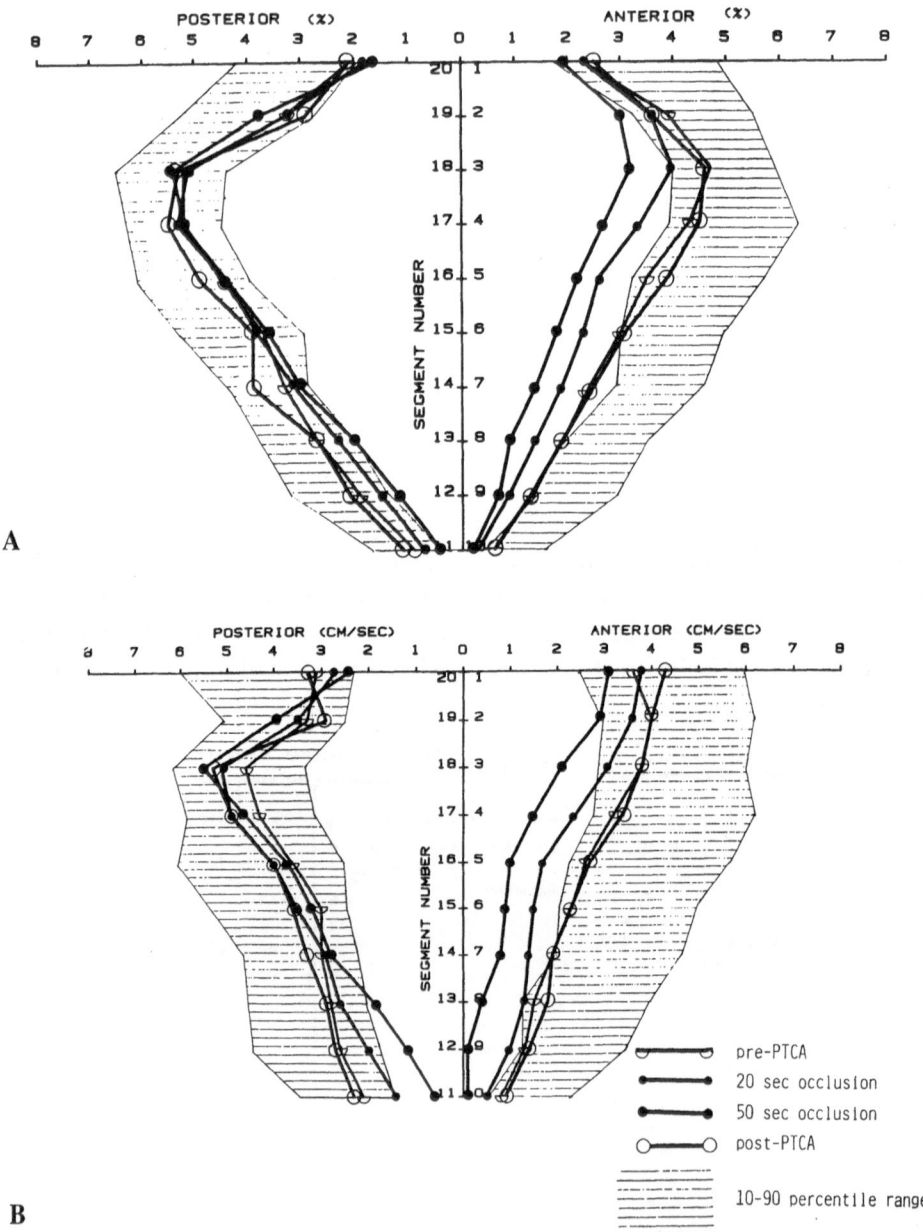

Fig. XVIII.8. (A) Display of the computed CREF's (regional contributions to ejection fraction) after a 20 or 50 sec occlusion of the left anterior descending artery. On the x-axis the CREF's of the anterior and infero-posterior wall areas are displayed (%), while on the y-axis the segment numbers of the anterior wall (1 to 10) and of the infero-posterior wall (11 to 20) are depicted. The shaded zones represent the 10th to 90th percentile area of CREF's in normal individuals. (B) Mean ejection phase velocity before PTCA and after 20 and 50 sec occlusions of the left anterior descending artery. On the x-axis the velocity values of the anterior and infero-posterior wall areas are displayed (cm/sec), while on the y-axis the segment numbers of the anterior wall (1–10) and of the infero-posterior wall (11–20) are depicted. The shaded zones represent the 10th to 90th percentile areas in normal individuals.

anterior and inferior walls was not significantly affected after 20 sec occlusion of the left anterior descending artery. On the contrary, the moment of maximal wall displacement for the anterior wall shifted from end systole to early diastole. The antero-lateral segment (Nos. 6 and 7 on Fig. XVIII.7), the apical segment (Nos. 9 and 10) of the anterior wall, and the apical segment (Nos. 20 and 19) of the inferior wall appeared to be most affected.

The measurement of mean ejection phase velocity after 20 and 50 sec occlusion of the left anterior descending artery showed a decrease which was again more pronounced in the anterior wall segments (Fig. XVIII.8). The regional wall motion and wall velocity (Fig. XVIII.8) showed a similar response to occlusion of this coronary artery. These data clearly demonstrate a progressive myocardial depression that affected specifically the antero-lateral and apical segments (Table XVIII.3).

It must be emphasized that all these ischemic changes were transient and perfectly reversible, as demonstrated by the regional analysis of the last cine-angiogram performed after completion of the whole procedure.

Table XVIII.3. Ejection phase velocity and regional contribution to ejection fraction (CREF).

Segment No.	Mean ejection phase velocity (cm/sec)				CREF (%)			
	Before PTCA (N = 10)	15 sec occl. (N = 10)	45 sec occl. (N = 7)	After PTCA (N = 10)	Before PTCA (N = 10)	15 sec occl. (N = 10)	45 sec occl. (N = 7)	After PTCA (N = 10)
1	3.6 ± 1.0	3.8 ± 1.5	3.1 ± 1.5	$4.3 \pm 1.5^*$	2.3 ± 0.4	2.3 ± 0.5	1.9 ± 0.7	$2.5 \pm 0.5°$
2	4.0 ± 1.3	$3.6 \pm 1.2^*$	$2.9 \pm 1.5°$	4.0 ± 1.8	3.9 ± 0.9	3.6 ± 0.8	$3.0 \pm 1.0^*$	3.6 ± 0.8
3	3.8 ± 1.2	$3.1 \pm 1.3^*$	$2.1 \pm 1.4^+$	3.8 ± 1.6	4.7 ± 0.9	$4.0 \pm 0.8^+$	$3.2 \pm 1.0^+$	4.6 ± 0.8
4	3.2 ± 1.0	$2.4 \pm 1.3^*$	$1.5 \pm 1.5^+$	3.4 ± 1.4	4.3 ± 1.0	$3.4 \pm 1.0°$	$2.7 \pm 1.4^+$	4.5 ± 0.7
5	2.6 ± 0.9	$1.7 \pm 1.1^*$	$1.0 \pm 1.4^+$	2.7 ± 1.1	3.5 ± 1.0	$2.6 \pm 1.0^*$	$2.2 \pm 1.6^+$	3.9 ± 0.6
6	2.3 ± 0.8	$1.5 \pm 0.9°$	$0.9 \pm 1.3^+$	2.3 ± 0.8	3.0 ± 0.8	$2.3 \pm 0.9°$	$1.8 \pm 1.5°$	3.1 ± 0.4
7	1.9 ± 0.8	1.4 ± 1.0	$0.8 \pm 1.3^*$	1.9 ± 0.7	2.4 ± 0.7	$1.9 \pm 0.1^*$	$1.4 \pm 1.2°$	2.5 ± 0.5
8	1.5 ± 0.6	1.3 ± 0.9	$0.4 \pm 1.2^*$	1.8 ± 1.0	1.9 ± 0.5	$1.4 \pm 0.7^*$	$0.9 \pm 0.8^+$	1.9 ± 0.7
9	1.3 ± 0.5	1.0 ± 1.0	0.1 ± 1.0	1.4 ± 0.9	1.3 ± 0.4	$0.9 \pm 0.6^*$	$0.7 \pm 0.8^*$	1.3 ± 0.6
10	0.8 ± 0.7	0.5 ± 1.3	0.1 ± 0.9	0.9 ± 0.9	0.6 ± 0.3	0.3 ± 0.5	0.2 ± 0.6	0.6 ± 0.5
11	3.1 ± 1.0	2.7 ± 0.7	$2.4 \pm 0.7^*$	3.3 ± 0.9	2.1 ± 0.4	1.8 ± 0.3	$1.6 \pm 0.3^+$	2.1 ± 0.4
12	3.3 ± 2.0	3.5 ± 2.1	4.0 ± 2.3	2.9 ± 1.5	3.3 ± 1.2	3.3 ± 1.4	3.8 ± 1.5	2.9 ± 1.3
13	4.6 ± 1.3	5.1 ± 1.0	$5.5 \pm 1.2^*$	5.3 ± 1.7	5.2 ± 0.7	5.1 ± 0.7	5.4 ± 1.0	5.3 ± 1.1
14	4.3 ± 1.0	$4.9 \pm 0.8^*$	4.6 ± 1.0	4.9 ± 1.4	5.2 ± 0.5	5.3 ± 0.3	5.2 ± 0.4	5.5 ± 0.8
15	3.6 ± 0.6	$4.0 \pm 0.7^*$	3.7 ± 1.0	4.0 ± 1.1	4.5 ± 0.4	4.4 ± 0.5	4.4 ± 0.4	$4.9 \pm 0.6^*$
16	3.0 ± 0.5	3.5 ± 0.9	3.2 ± 1.1	3.6 ± 1.3	3.7 ± 0.4	3.8 ± 0.4	3.6 ± 0.3	3.9 ± 0.5
17	3.0 ± 0.6	2.9 ± 1.0	2.8 ± 1.2	3.3 ± 1.3	3.3 ± 0.5	3.1 ± 0.5	3.0 ± 0.7	3.9 ± 0.5
18	2.8 ± 0.7	2.6 ± 0.9	$1.9 \pm 1.1^+$	2.9 ± 1.2	2.7 ± 0.5	$2.3 \pm 0.3^*$	$2.0 \pm 0.5^+$	2.7 ± 0.5
19	2.6 ± 0.5	$2.0 \pm 0.7^*$	$1.2 \pm 1.0^+$	2.7 ± 1.1	1.9 ± 0.5	$1.5 \pm 0.3^*$	$1.2 \pm 0.4^+$	2.1 ± 0.5
20	2.1 ± 0.9	1.4 ± 1.1	$0.6 \pm 1.0^+$	2.3 ± 1.2	0.9 ± 0.4	0.7 ± 0.3	$0.4 \pm 0.5^+$	1.1 ± 0.4

Values are mean $\pm$ s.d. * p <0.05; $°$ p <0.01; $^+$ p <0.005 vs before PTCA

Coronary blood flow and lactate metabolism

During the initial dilatation, the mean duration of angioplasty balloon inflation was 41 ± 13 sec and during the subsequent dilatations the duration of inflation was gradually increased up to 54 ± 12 sec in a subset of four patients who underwent six consecutive dilatations (Table XVIII.4).

The mean blood flow in the great cardiac vein in 20 patients before the first inflation was 69 ± 17 ml/min, falling to 49 ± 23 ml/min (p $<10^{-5}$) during the first inflation and rising to 107 ± 31 ml/min (p $<10^{-5}$) after the first balloon deflation.

The mean hyperemic increase in great cardiac vein flow was 38 ml/min above the control flow value after the first inflation compared with 63 ml after the third inflation (p $<.01$; Fig. XVIII.9).

Proximal coronary sinus blood flow before the first dilation was 129 ± 34 ml/min, falling to 92 ± 27 ml/min (p $<10^{-5}$) during transluminal occlusion and rising to 152 ± 44 ml/min (p $<10^{-4}$) after the first balloon deflation.

During the peak reactive hyperemia that followed the third dilatation, the coronary sinus blood flow was 161 ± 31 ml/min. There was no difference in resting pre-PTCA and post-PTCA levels of great cardiac vein or coronary sinus blood flow.

The arteriovenous lactate measurements are also listed in Table XVIII.4. The control measurements showed a difference of $+0.11 \pm 0.2$ mmol/liter, which decreased to -0.87 ± 0.70 and -0.82 ± 0.57 mmol/liter after the first and the second dilatations, respectively. After the third dilatation the lactate difference was -0.44 ± 0.34 mmol/liter, which was not significantly different from the values recorded after the first and the second dilatation; after the fourth, the fifth and the sixth dilatations the number of measurements was too small to demonstrate a significant increase or decrease in lactate production.

Discussion

Global and regional left ventricular performance

The earliest (1 to 15 sec after occlusion) and most sensitive hemodynamic indicator of regional perfusion deficit proved to be an impairment in early relaxation, with extreme prolongation of T_1, the time constant of the early relaxation phase. If the premise of the two time constant models previously described [10] is correct, then the early change in T_1 with constant T_2 represents an exacerbation in the asynchrony of relaxation. This is illustrated by the change in negative dP/dt and wall displacement induced by a 20 sec coronary occlusion (Fig. XVIII.6, B). Within 4 or 5 beats after occlusion, a distinct deformation appears in the ascending limb of the negative dP/dt curve and in the next 10 seconds this deformation reaches the same height as peak negative dP/dt, which in the meantime has

Table XVIII.4. Reactive hyperemia and arteriovenous lactate difference after sequential transluminal occlusions.

	Before PTCA (range)	First occl. (range)	Second occl. (range)	Third occl. (range)	Fourth occl. (range)	Fifth occl. (range)	Sixth occl. (range)	After PTCA (range)
No. of patients	20	20	20	19	9	7	4	20
Average duration of transluminal occlusion per patient (sec)	–	41 ± 13* (10,60)	44 ± 14 (20,70)	51 ± 15 (25,90)	52 ± 11 (30,70)	54 ± 11 (30,65)	54 ± 12 (40,75)	–
p-value (vs first occlusion)			<.005	<.005	<.02	<.02	n.s.	
Coronary sinus blood flow (ml/min)	129 ± 34 (101,152)	152 ± 44 (97,203)	155 ± 37 (101,203)	161 ± 31 (110,210)	167 ± 40 (116,200)	161 ± 44 (95,187)	–	144 ± 35 (110,189)
p-value (vs before PTCA)		<.001	<.001	<.0005	<.01	<.01		n.s.
GCV flow (ml/min)	69 ± 17 (40,99)	107 ± 31 (66,152)	127 ± 39 (81,210)	132 ± 22 (109,167)	112 ± 33 (66,160)	109 ± 33 (67,167)	110 ± 33 (99,152)	82 ± 9 (63,87)
p-value (vs before PTCA)		<.001	<.0005	<.0005	<.002	<.02	n.s.	n.s.
Aorto-GCV difference in lactate (mmol/l)	+0.11 ± 0.2 (−0.45,0.4)	−0.87 ± 0.70 (−2.10,0.17)	−0.82 ± 0.57 (−2.10,0.02)	−0.44 ± 0.34 (−0.89,0.0)	−0.62 ± 0.42 (−1.50,0.18)	−0.64 ± 0.37 (−1.30,0.13)	–	+0.18 ± 0.09 (0.06,0.31)
p-value (vs before PTCA)		$<10^{-4}$	$<10^{-6}$	$<10^{-4}$	$<10^{-5}$	<.01		n.s.

GCV = great cardiac vein.

* Mean ± s.d.

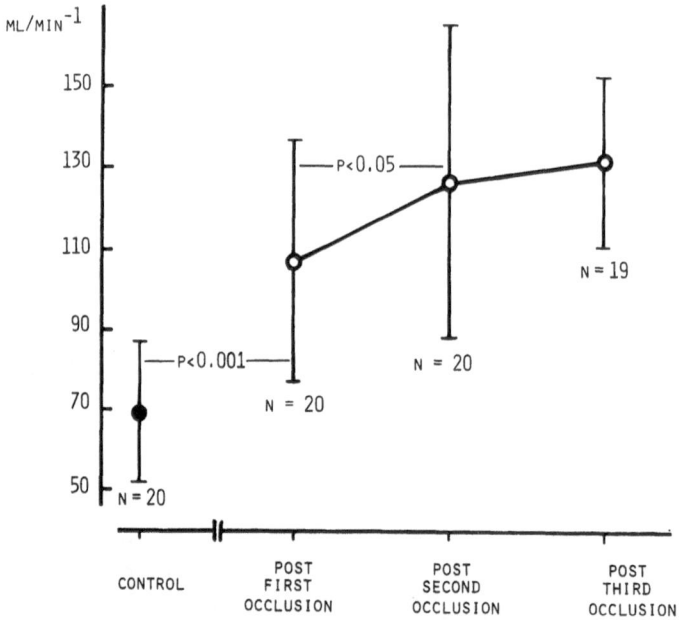

Fig. XVIII.9. Great cardiac vein flow during control measurements and after three sequential episodes of reactive hyperemia.

progressively decreased to its nadir. Accompanying this change in negative dP/dt, the ischemic segments exhibit a biphasic inward-outward wall displacement that occurs after valve closure and peak negative dP/dt. During the remainder of relaxation and rapid filling the ischemic segments display a second wave of inward wall displacement. The beginning of this second wave of wall displacement in early diastole corresponds closely in time to the irregularity in dP/dt. In the same way, the peak inward displacement of the control segment is consistently observed near the notching in the dP/dt. Shortly after this point, the pressure ceases to have a relaxation time constant T_1 and abruptly switches to T_2. On the other hand, after 50 sec of occlusion the majority of the ischemic segments are akinetic and exhibit an increased regional stiffness, whereas T_1 tends to return toward less abnormal values. In our study, at 50 sec the deformity in negative dP/dt was no longer present.

The connection between transient asynergy, myocardial ischemia, and alteration in the time course of relaxation was pointed out as early as 1969 by Tyberg et al., [12] who designed an experimental preparation consisting of two papillary muscles in series. They demonstrated that when one muscle of the pair is hypoxic but still contracting it disturbs the time course of the total fall in tension generated by the two muscles much more than when one of the muscles in series is not contracting at all and infinitely stiff [12]. More recent studies in conscious animals after experimental coronary occlusion have indicated that ventricular dyssynchrony due to late systolic contraction and relaxation in different regions can produce marked effects on the linearity and maximal rate of fall in pressure in the left ventricle [13–15].

Our results suggest that a similar phenomenon may occur in the intact human heart during acute ischemia. At 20 sec the late systolic outward displacement of the ischemic segment is probably passive and due to a simultaneously increased and active inward displacement of the nonischemic segments. Conversely the early diastolic inward displacement of the ischemic segments must correspond to an accelerated outward displacement of the normal segment. Ultimately after 20 sec of ischemia the ischemic zone acts as an additional elastic element in series with the actively contracting and relaxing nonischemic segment. This mechanism is consistent with the model of left ventricular pressure relaxation recently proposed by our group [10] in which it is assumed that the observed time constant T_l results from the combined action of that fraction of the myocardium in the process of relaxing and the remaining fraction in which relaxation has not yet been initiated.

Coronary hemodynamics

The mean great cardiac vein flow of 69 ml/min reported here is well within the range previously reported [5, 6, 16]. This is in agreement with Rothman et al., [17] who reported a flow of 76 ml/min before angioplasty. In their study the mean hyperemic increase in great cardiac vein flow was 29.9% above control flow after the first inflation, compared with 59.3% above control after the final inflation.

In our patients the mean hyperemic increase in great cardiac vein flow was 55% after the first dilatation and 91% after the third dilatation (Fig. XVIII.9). In a subset of nine patients who needed more than three dilatations to satisfactorily reduce the transstenotic gradient, the values of reactive hyperemia were less elevated, ranging between 58% and 63%. As observed by Rothman et al., [17] more pronounced reactive hyperemia developed when the residual functional coronary stenosis associated with the deflated PTCA balloon was reduced by subsequent dilatations.

In general, our values for reactive hyperemia are higher than those found by Rothman et al. [17]. This difference might be explained by the difference in the mean duration of balloon inflation which was 9.8 ± 3.7 sec in their patients compared to 41 ± 13 sec in our patients. These prolonged occlusion times (41 to 54 sec) are due to the fact that we kept the balloon inflated as long as the patient did not manifest any clinical signs of ischemia. In fact, we have noticed that the duration of balloon inflation could be gradually prolonged during subsequent dilatations, as if the anginal threshold had increased following these repeated occlusions.

Metabolic disturbances

Recently, coronary sinus K^+ concentration was measured continuously in two patients undergoing angioplasty of significant stenoses of their left anterior descending coronary arteries [18]. The recordings obtained from these patients show that, although coronary sinus K^+ levels did not change significantly during coronary occlusion, a transient rise occurred when the occlusion was removed. After reducing pressure in the balloon, the coronary sinus K^+ levels began to rise within 8 sec. This fits exactly with the timing of peak reactive hyperemia observed in our study and by Rothman et al. [17]. In our patients, blood samples were obtained 10 to 15 seconds after the start of deflation. Since we could not record the great cardiac vein flow during the sampling period, we did not express our results in terms of lactate efflux. The less elevated concentration (-0.44 mmol/liter) in the great cardiac vein after the third sequential occlusion does not necessarily reflect a reduction in lactate production since the reactive hyperemia measured before the sampling was significantly ($p < .05$) greater (132 ml/min) than that measured during the first and second occlusions.

As a first approximation, the amount of lactate lost from the ischemic tissue during the first two occlusions seems to be constant and at least does not increase with subsequent occlusions. The crucial conclusion to be drawn from the observation that a few minutes after termination of this procedure the lactate balance again becomes positive is that the metabolic disturbances induced by repeated ischemia are reversible.

Clinical implications

Experimental data on atherosclerotic vessel segments have shown that volume reduction of atherosclerotic tissue is related to the duration of pressure application. These findings have led many clinicians to use longer inflation durations (30 to 60 sec) during PTCA [19, 20]. On the other hand, Braunwald and Kloner [21] have recently addressed the question of whether the myocardium can become chronically, even permanently, 'stunned' as a consequence of repeated episodes of myocardial ischemia. Although most episodes of transient ischemia produced in our patients during PTCA were not as severe as those produced in animal studies [13, 14, 22], the total duration of episodes during PTCA has increased considerably since our initial experience; the median is now 4 min and in a few cases it has exceeded ten minutes in our laboratory [2]. This total occlusion time of 4 min might be excessive since it has been demonstrated in conscious dogs that the return of myocardial function is delayed after periods of coronary occlusion as brief as 100 sec. In this case, however, hyperemia that occurs normally during reperfusion is prevented by a residual subtotal occlusion [23] and there is no such occlusion after successful PTCA. In this respect, the results of the present study seem to be reassuring since there is no evidence of global or regional myocardial dysfunction even after four to six coronary occlusions of 40 to 60 sec each.

References

1. Das SK, Serruys PW, Brand M van den, Domenicucci S, Vletter WB, Roelandt J: Acute echocardiographic changes during percutaneous coronary angioplasty and their relationship to coronary blood flow. J Cardiovasc Ultrasonogr 2: 269–271, 1983.
2. Serruys PW, Brand M van den, Brower RW, Hugenholtz PG: Regional cardioplegia and cardioprotection during transluminal angioplasty, which role for nifedipine? Eur Heart J 4 (Suppl C): 115–121, 1983.
3. Meester GT, Bernard N, Zeelenberg C, Brower RW, Hugenholtz PG: A computer system for real time analysis of cardiac catheterization data. Cath Cardiovasc Diagn 1: 113–132, 1975.
4. Meester GT, Zeelenberg C, Bernard N, Gorter S: Beat to beat analysis of cardiac catheterization data. Comp in Cardiol: 63–65, 1974.
5. Baim DS, Rothman MT, Harrison DC: Improved catheter for regional coronary sinus flow and metabolic studies. Am J Cardiol 46: 997–1000, 1980.
6. Baim DS, Rothman MT, Harrison DC: Simultaneous measurement of coronary venous blood flow and oxygen saturation during transient alterations in myocardial oxygen supply and demand. Am J Cardiol 49: 743–752, 1982.
7. Apstein CS, Puchner E, Brachfeld N: Improved automated lactate determination. Anal Biochem 38: 20–34, 1970.
8. Rousseau MF, Veriter C, Detry JM, Brasseur L, Pouleur H: Impaired early left ventricular relaxation in coronary artery disease: effects of intracoronary nifedipine. Circulation 62: 764–772, 1980.
9. Thompson DS, Waldron CB, Juul SM, Naqvi N, Swanton RH, Coltart DJ, Jenkins BS, Webb-Peploe MM: Analysis of left ventricular pressure during isovolumic relaxation in coronary artery disease. Circulation 65: 690–697, 1982.
10. Brower RW, Meij S, Serruys PW: A model of asynchronous left ventricular relaxation predicting the bi-exponential pressure decay. Cardiovasc Res 17: 482–488, 1983.
11. Gaasch WH, Levine HJ, Quinones MA, Alexander JK: Left ventricular compliance: Mechanisms and clinical implications. Am J Cardiol 38: 645–653, 1976.
12. Tyberg JV, Parmley MW, Sonnenblick EH: In-vitro studies of myocardial asynchrony and regional hypoxia. Circulation 25: 569–579, 1969.
13. Theroux P, Ross J Jr, Franklin D, Covell JW, Bloor CM, Sasayama S: Regional myocardial function and dimensions early and late after myocardial infarction in the unanesthetized dog. Circ Res 40: 158–165, 1977.
14. Theroux P, Ross J Jr, Franklin D, Kemper WS, Sasayama S: Regional myocardial function in the conscious dog during acute coronary occlusion and responses to morphine, propranolol, nitroglycerine and lidocaine. Circulation 53: 302–314, 1976.
15. Kumada T, Karliner JS, Pouleur H, Gallagher KP, Shirato K, Ross J Jr: Effects of coronary occlusion on early ventricular diastolic events in conscious dogs. Am J Physiol 237: H542–H549, 1979.
16. Feldman RL, Conti CR, Pepine CJ: Regional coronary venous flow responses to transient coronary artery occlusion in human beings. J Am Coll Cardiol 2: 1–10, 1983.
17. Rothman MT, Baim DS, Simpson JB, Harrison DC: Coronary hemodynamics during percutaneous transluminal coronary angioplasty. Am J Cardiol 49: 1615–1622, 1982.
18. Webb SC, Rickards AF, Poole-Wilson PA: Coronary sinus potassium concentration recorded during coronary angioplasty. Br Heart J 50: 146–148, 1983.

372

19. Schmitz HJ, Meyer J, Kiesslich T, Effert S: Greater initial dilatation gives better late an-giographic results in percutaneous coronary angioplasty (PTCA). Circulation 66 (Supp. II): II-123 (Abstract), 1982.
20. Kaltenbach M, Kober G: Can prolonged application of pressure improve the results of coronary angioplasty (TCA)? Circulation 66 (Supp. II): II-123 (Abstract), 1982.
21. Braunwald E, Kloner RA: The stunned myocardium: prolonged, postischemic, ventricular dysfunction. Circulation 66: 1146–1149, 1982.
22. Heijndrickx GR, Millard RW, McRitchie RJ, Maroko PR, Vatner SF: Regional myocardial function and electrophysiological alterations after brief coronary artery occlusion in conscious dogs. J Clin Invest 56: 978–985, 1975.
23. Pagani M, Vatner SF, Baig H, Braunwald E: Initial myocardial adjustments to brief periods of ischemia and reperfusion in the conscious dog. Circ Res 43: 83–92, 1978.

XIX. The role of vascular wall thickening during changes in coronary artery tone

Summary

In eighteen patients with resting as well as exertional angina, maximal changes in coronary artery diameter were measured after administration of ergometrine, followed by intracoronary isosorbide dinitrate. Analysis of angiograms was carried out with the CAAS system. Mean minimal obstruction diameters of twenty stenotic lesions decreased from 2.2 mm to 1.0 mm ($p<10^{-7}$) five minutes after 0.4 mg ergometrine, and increased to 2.7 mm ($p<10^{-8}$) after 3 mg isosorbide dinitrate. Using geometric principles, diameter changes occurring at the adjacent nonstenotic segments after drug administration were used to predict minimal and maximal dimensions of the stenotic lesions. This geometric concept could only predict the observed reactivity after ergometrine in four out of twenty stenotic segments: six lesions proved hyporeactive, while unexpected spasm occurred in six segments. The extent of vasodilation by isosorbide dinitrate could be predicted by this theory in half of the cases.

We conclude that geometric principles cannot adequately explain the reactivity of the coronary arteries to ergometrine in patients with resting as well as exertional angina: this concept seems more applicable to vasodilation.

Introduction

In human coronary artery disease with exertional angina pectoris, it is generally assumed that a 'fixed' stenosis exists, i.e. a permanent obstruction, so that ischemia results only when flow requirements of the myocardium exceed the flow capacity of the diseased vessel. Recently, the hypothesis has been developed that increased coronary arterial vasomotor tone superimposed on a pre-existing obstruction, which by itself is not impeding coronary flow in rest, is another pathophysiologic mechanism leading to angina pectoris during exercise [1, 2]. Furthermore, it has been clearly established that the arteries of patients with inappropriate vasomotor tone like those with spontaneous spasm are hypersensitive to a variety of stimuli, one of which is ergometrine, at the site of atherosclerotic lesions [3–10]. MacAlpin [11] has proposed that this hypersensitivity is due to enhanced vasoconstriction at the point where the atheromatous lesion enchroaches upon the lumen, the degree of vasoconstriction being related to the severity of the encroachment i.e. a mechanism determined by geometric considerations.

The present study was undertaken in order to determine whether this geometric concept also could explain the hyperreactivity of arteries in patients with proven vasospastic angina. In 18 patients with exertional as well as resting angina, the maximal changes in coronary arterial diameter were measured both after a vasoconstrictive test with ergometrine and after a coronary dilating agent, isosorbide dinitrate.

Using geometric principles, diameter changes occurring at the adjacent non-stenotic segments after drug administration were used to predict minimal and maximal dimensions of the stenotic lesions.

Methods

Patients selection and test procedure

After informed consent, eighteen patients, all with exertional as well as resting angina, underwent coronary angiography using the femoral technique. Medication was discontinued 24 hours before catheterization. Patients with left main disease were not eligible for the study, and patients with spontaneous angina during catheterization were also excluded. Five minutes after a baseline coronary angiogram (control), 0.4 mg ergometrine (Methergin® = methylergometrine) was injected intravenously, and a second arteriogram was obtained 5 minutes after the control film, or as soon as the patient developed chest pain or/and electrocardiographic ST-segment changes. Subsequently, 3 mg isosorbide dinitrate (Risordan®) was administered in the coronary artery and a third coronary angiogram obtained 2 minutes hereafter.

The X-ray system was maintained in exactly the same position during the sequential angiographic studies so that no differences in projection occurred.

Quantitative angiographic analysis

For each individual patient arterial dimensions were measured at specific distances from identifiable branch points in diastolic frames with the CAAS-system. An example of the computer output of an analyzed lesion in a right coronary artery at different states of vasomotion is given in Fig. XIX.1, a-c.

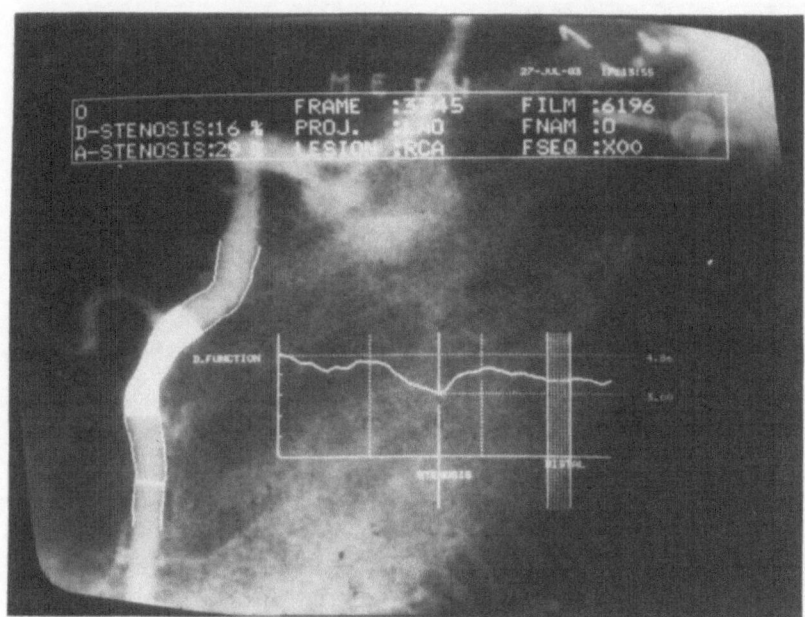

a

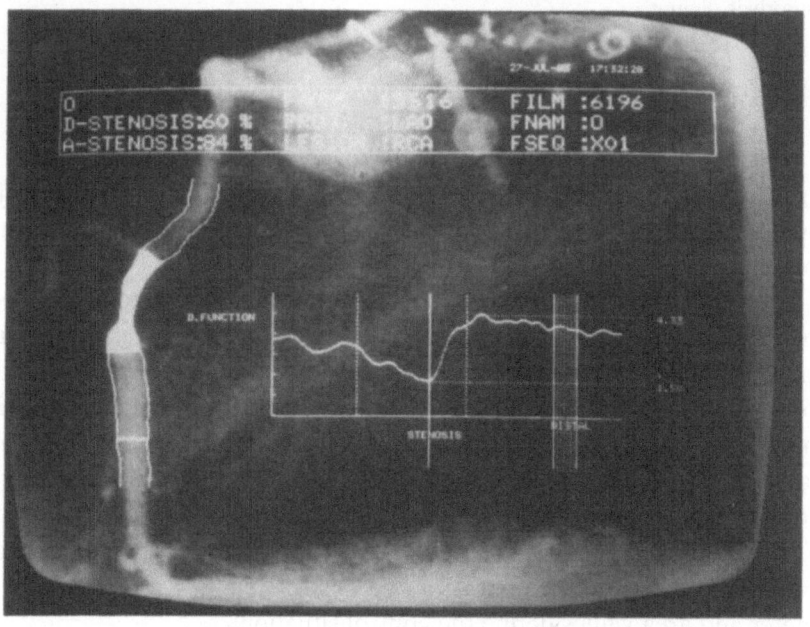

b

376

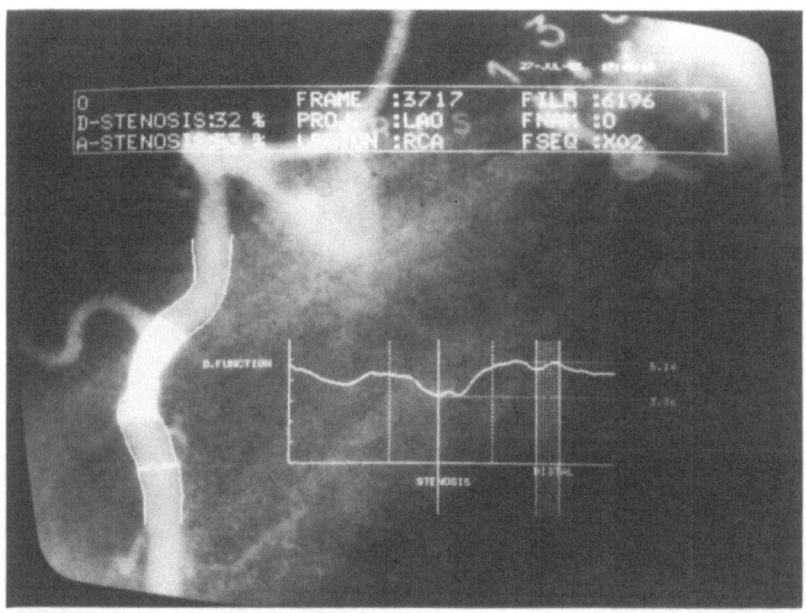

c

Fig. XIX.1. Computer measurements of an atherosclerotic lesion in the right coronary artery at different states of vasomotion. a: control state; b: after intravenous ergometrine; c: after intracoronary isosorbide dinitrate.

Geometric considerations: dynamic vascular wall thickening

The geometric principle to predict the narrowing expected at a lesion site, given the severity of the lesion and the degree of vasoconstriction of the adjacent normal segment, is shown in Fig. XIX.2 and XIX.3. From it the degree of vasomotion is estimated [11, 12, 13].

If a coronary artery is circular in cross section when it is distended by normal blood pressure, the outer diameter, denoted 2Ro and given an arbitrary value of 2.4 mm, includes the media but excludes the adventitia. In Fig. XIX.2 there is a coronary obstruction with a minimal luminal obstruction diameter of 2ri (e.g. 1.4 mm); the luminal reference diameter in the normal prestenotic segment equals 2Ri (e.g. 2.0 mm.) The cross sections at the reference position and at the site of the obstruction with the definitions of the different radii are given in figure XIX.3. The area A_R of the arterial wall at the reference cross section equals $A_R = \pi (Ro^2 - Ri^2)$ and the area A_s at the obstruction $A_s = \pi (Ro^2 - ri^2)$. These diameter and area values define the control situation.

A new situation is created when vasoconstriction occurs. (Fig. XIX.2 and XIX.3). Since the components of the arterial wall are considered to be incompressible, and since we assume that no change in the length of the artery occurs as the result of changes in its diameter, nor that intrusion of tissue from the

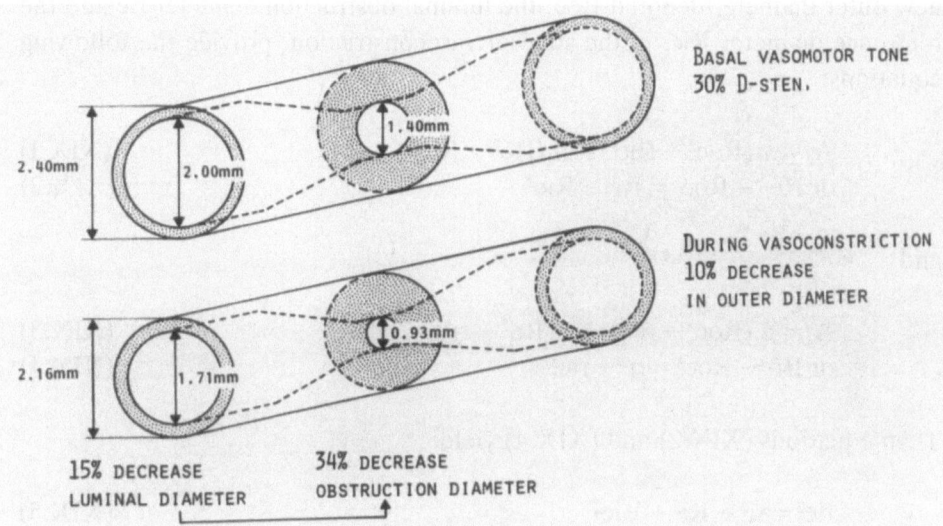

Fig. XIX.2. The geometric principle: if one assumes that the wall area of the transverse section of the coronary artery remains constant, a basal 30% diameter stenosis (upper drawing) will cause a 34% decrease of obstruction diameter (lower drawing) if the luminal diameter of the prestenotic segment decreases by 15%.

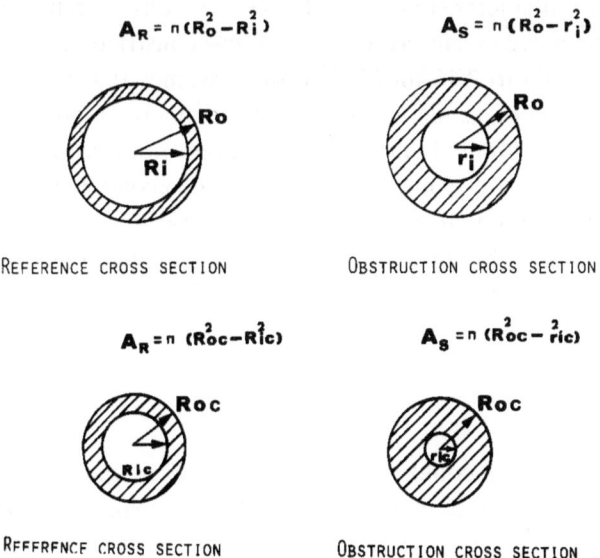

Fig. XIX.3. Circular cross sections of a hypothetical prestenotic, reference (R) segment and stenotic (S) segment of a coronary artery before (upper part) and after vasoconstriction (c, lower part). The wall area (A) of the coronary artery is calculated using outer (o) and inner (i) diameters.

constricted area into nonconstricted adjacent parts of the artery occurs, the area of the arterial wall on a transverse cross section of the vessel at any point of the artery will be constant regardless of the state of its contraction or dilation. The new outer diameter denoted Roc, the luminal obstruction diameter ric and the reference diameter Ric, in the state of vasoconstriction, provide the following equations:

$$A_r = \pi \, (\text{Roc}^2 - \text{Ric}^2) = \pi \, (\text{Ro}^2 - \text{Ri}^2) \qquad\qquad (XIX.1)$$
$$\text{or Ro}^2 - \text{Roc}^2 = \text{Ri}^2 - \text{Ric}^2 \qquad\qquad (XIX.2)$$

and

$$A_s = \pi \, (\text{Roc}^2 - \text{ric}^2) = \pi \, (\text{Ro}^2 - \text{ri}^2) \qquad\qquad (XIX.3)$$
$$\text{or Ro}^2 - \text{Roc}^2 = \text{ri}^2 - \text{ric}^2 \qquad\qquad (XIX.4)$$

Then equations (XIX.2) and (XIX.4) yield:

$$\text{ric}^2 = \text{ri}^2 - \text{Ri}^2 + \text{Ric}^2 \qquad\qquad (XIX.5)$$

Therefore, provided we know the reference diameter in the control state (Ri) and after vasoconstriction (Ric), and the obstruction diameter ri in the control state, the minimal obstruction diameter ric after vasoconstriction can be predicted from equation (XIX.5). It should be clear, that the equations (XIX.1) to (XIX.5) are equally valid during vasodilation. The coronary stenotic lesion shown in figure XIX.2 has a 30% diameter stenosis in the basal condition. When a 10% decrease in the outer diameter occurs as a result of vasoconstriction, its absolute value decreases from 2.40 to 2.16 mm. When one assumes that the wall area of the transverse cross section remains constant, the geometric model would indicate a 15% decrease in the luminal diameter of the prestenotic segment. At the site of the stenosis, there is modest intramural thickening secondary to the atherosclerotic plaque and the luminal diameter will decrease to a larger degree. In the present example a 34% decrease in obstruction diameter would be predicted from equation (XIX.5).

Results

Twenty stenotic lesions could be identified and were analyzed. (Table XIX.1) The effects of the two interventions on the mean proximal diameter and on the minimal obstruction diameter are shown in Figure XIX.4. After the admini stration of ergometrine the mean proximal diameter decreased significantly ($p<0.005$) with respect to the basal condition, from 3.7 to 3.3 mm (11%), whereas the minimal obstruction diameter was reduced by more than 50% from 2.2 to

mean proximal diameter and minimal obstruction diameter

n=20 , mean ± SD

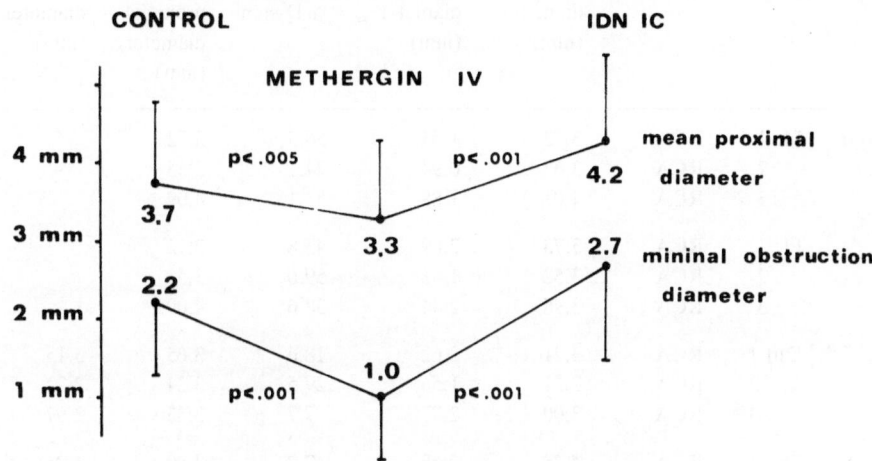

Fig. XIX.4. Effects of ergometrine (Methergin) iv and of isosorbide dinitrate (IDN) ic on the mean proximal diameter and on the minimal obstruction diameter in 20 observations.

Table XIX.1. Results from quantitative analysis of coronary arteries in different states of vasomotion.

Name		Artery	Reference diameter (mm)	Obstruction diameter (mm)	User-defined % D-sten	Mean proximal diameter (mm)	Mean distal diameter (mm)
No 1	VA 1	RCA	4.93	4.20	14.9	4.89	4.75
	2	RCA	5.39	2.79	28.3	5.24	4.33
	3	RCA	6.03	4.88	19.0	5.76	5.19
no 2	Gh 1	LAD	2.80	0.90	68.0	2.70	3.70
	2	LAD	totally occluded			2.10	
	3	LAD	3.01	1.76	41.4	2.99	3.48
no 3	Ol 1	RCA	4.48	3.34	25.4	4.1	3.8
	2	RCA	3.22	1.68	47.8	3.14	4.21
	3	RCA	4.15	3.57	14.0	4.36	4.99
	Ol 1	RCA	4.04	3.34	17.3	4.1	3.8
	2	RCA	4.14	1.68	59.4	3.14	4.21
	3	RCA	5.02	3.57	28.8	4.36	4.99
no 4	Be 1	RCA	5.96	2.79	53.2	5.82	4.46
	2	RCA	totally occluded			4.98	
	3	RCA	6.36	2.88	54.7	6.52	5.97
no 5	Cr 1	RCA	5.34	3.16	40.9	5.21	
	2	RCA	5.11	1.37	73.1	4.85	
	3	RCA	5.29	3.90	26.3	5.26	

Table XIX.1. Results from quantitative analysis of coronary arteries in different states of vasomotion.

Name		Artery	Reference diameter (mm)	Obstruction diameter (mm)	User-defined % D-sten	Mean proximal diameter (mm)	Mean distal diameter (mm)
no 6	Flc 1	RCA	3.73	1.63	56.3	3.72	
	2	RCA	3.63	0.94	74.1	3.55	
	3	RCA	4.01	1.88	53.1	4.09	
	Flc 1	RCA	3.73	2.09	43.8	3.72	
	2	RCA	3.52	1.42	59.6	3.55	
	3	RCA	3.98	2.44	38.6	4.09	
no 7	Duf 1	RCA	3.21	2.62	18.6	3.65	3.15
	2	RCA	2.21	1.56	29.5	3.24	2.22
	3	RCA	3.00	2.77	7.7	3.83	2.97
no 8	Flm 1	RCA	4.75	2.48	47.7	4.80	4.25
	2	RCA	4.02	1.36	66.2	4.00	2.54
	3	RCA	5.30	4.59	13.3	5.29	4.21
no 9	Dup 1	LCX	5.88	2.65	54.9	6.11	3.69
	2	LCX	4.94	2.14	56.7	4.73	3.62
	3	LCX	7.01	4.59	34.6	7.02	5.11
no 10	Ti 1	LAD	2.38	1.22	48.7	2.36	2.62
	2	LAD	totally occluded			2.16	
	3	LAD	3.39	1.44	57.6	3.18	2.69
no 11	No 1	RCA	3.16	1.83	42.0		3.16
	2	RCA	2.89	0.38	86.7		2.76
	3	RCA	3.31	1.79	45.9		3.16
no 12	De 1	RCA	3.11	1.49	52.0	3.04	3.54
	2	RCA	totally occluded			2.38	
	3	RCA	3.94	0.99	74.9	3.88	3.77
no 13	Dum 1	LAD	3.23	1.29	60.1	3.08	
	2	LAD	2.67	1.14	57.3	2.70	
	3	LAD	3.97	2.03	49.0	3.96	
no 14	Paz 1	LAD	2.43	1.27	47.6		2.41
	2	LAD	totally occluded			2.64	
	3	LAD	3.58	2.32	35.4	2.60	3.22
no 15	Pat 1	LAD	2.85	2.09	26.8		2.70
	2	LAD	2.31	1.23	46.6		2.05
	3	LAD	2.82	2.19	22.2		2.71
no 16	Me 1	RCA	3.75	2.96	21.0	2.83	
	2	RCA	4.24	1.50	64.6	3.94	2.70
	3	RCA	3.60	3.44	4.5	3.55	3.69

Table XIX.1. Results from quantitative analysis of coronary arteries in different states of vasomotion.

Name		Artery	Reference diameter (mm)	Obstruction diameter (mm)	User-defined % D-sten	Mean proximal diameter (mm)	Mean distal diameter (mm)
no 17	Gr 1	LAD	3.24	1.65	49.0	3.06	3.36
	2	LAD	totally occluded			2.70	
	3	LAD	3.38	1.33	60.8	3.50	3.00
no 18	Jo 1	RCA	2.94	1.41	51.9		2.98
	2	RCA	1.98	1.37	30.7		1.94
	3	RCA	2.90	1.56	46.3	2.88	3.39

1 = control
2 = ergometrine
3 = isosorbide dinitrate
Abbreviations: RCA, right coronary artery, LAD, left anterior descending artery, LCX, left circumflex artery.

1.0 mm ($p<10^{-7}$). The intracoronary injection of isosorbide dinitrate provoked a very significant vasodilation of the obstructive lesion from 1.0 mm to 2.7 mm ($p<10^{-8}$), as well as a significant increase in mean proximal diameter from 3.3 mm to 4.2 mm ($p<10^{-6}$).

The individual changes in minimal obstruction diameter are given in Fig. XIX.5. After ergometrine, six of the twenty analyzed stenotic lesions became transiently occluded (Fig. XIX.5), whereas after isosorbide dinitrate i.c. the luminal diameters of all the obstructive lesions, which had been vasoconstricted during the provocative test, increased in size.

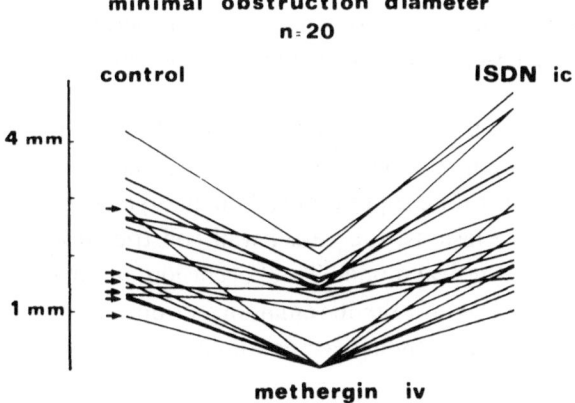

Fig. XIX.5. Individual changes in minimal obstruction diameter after ergometrine (Methergin) iv and isosorbide dinitrate (ISDN) ic. Six (marked with arrows) of the twenty analyzed stenotic lesions became transiently occluded during the provocative test.

382

changes in percentages diameter stenosis

methergin   iv

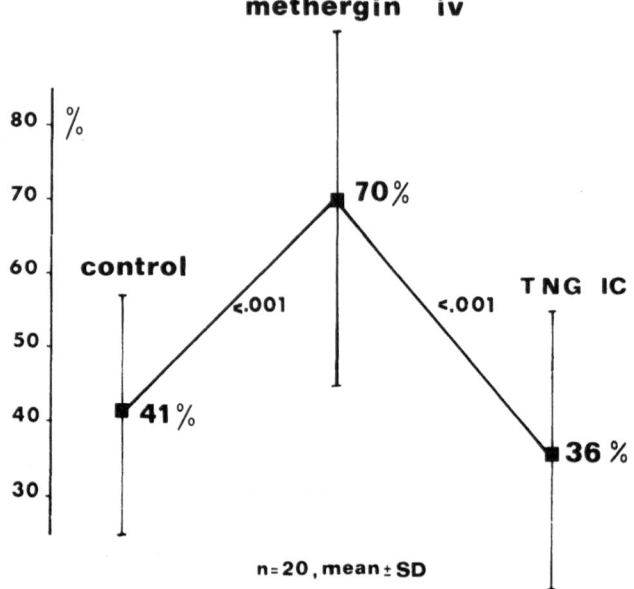

Fig. XIX.6. Changes in percentage diameter stenosis during the provocative test and after the intracoronary injection of isosorbide dinitrate (TNG).

In terms of percentage diameter stenosis, the severity of the obstructive lesions increased on the average from 41% to 70% (p<.0001) after ergometrine, but returned to an average value of 36% after the intracoronary injection of isosorbide dinitrate (Fig. XIX.6).

In Fig. XIX.7, the geometric concept has been visualized for a stenotic lesion with a 20% diameter stenosis. When this theoretical relationship was applied to the different states of vasomotion measured in all patients, the behavior of the stenotic lesions during vasoconstriction deviated considerably from the expected, since some stenotic lesions were hyperreactive and others hyporeactive (Fig. XIX.8).

As only four stenotic lesions reacted as predicted by the theory, it was concluded that the decrease in luminal diameter at the stenotic site was the result of an increase in vasomotor tone superimposed on an organically narrowed vessel. In the six hyporeactive lesions, the vessel wall constricted less than had been suggested from the theoretical model. Total occlusion, predicted to occur in five cases, was not observed. As for the 10 remaining lesions, they all showed arterial hyperreactivity, while four of them became totally occluded during vasoconstriction.

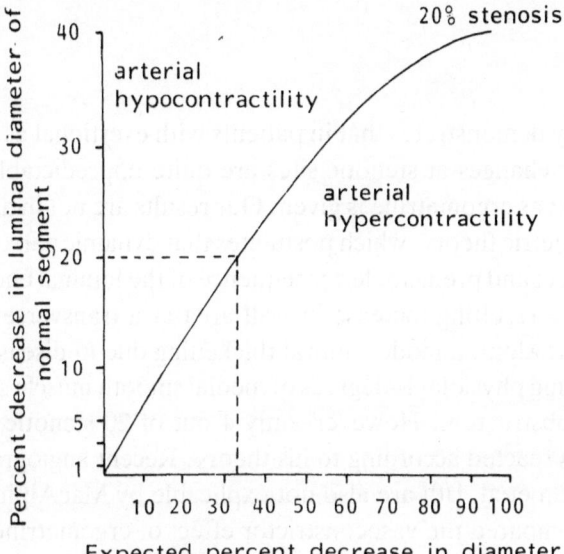

Fig. XIX.7. Relationship between expected changes in diameter of a stenotic segment as a result of a decrease in luminal diameter of the adjacent nonstenotic segment, according to geometric principles. In this example a 20% decrease in diameter of the normal segment will reduce the obstruction diameter of the stenotic segment by 33%.

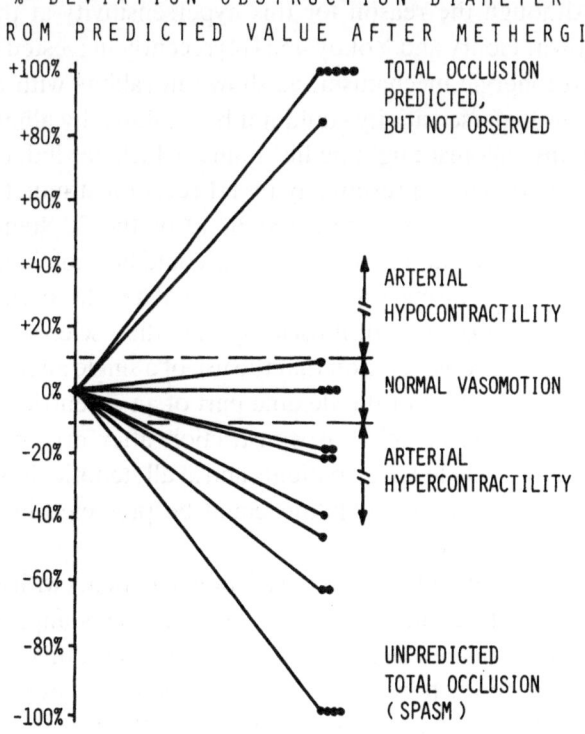

Fig. XIX.8. Percentage deviation of the obstruction diameters from predicted values after ergometrine (Methergin).

Discussion

The present study demonstrates that in patients with exertional as well as resting angina, diameter changes at stenotic sites are quite unpredictable when a vasoconstrictor agent as ergometrine is given. Our results are not in agreement with MacAlpin's geometric theory, which postulates that dynamic narrowing of stenotic lesions is a direct and predictable consequence of the luminal encroachment by atheroma and the resulting increase in wall area at a transverse cross section. According to MacAlpin, a modest mural thickening due to disease may act as a 'lever' in translating physiologic degrees of medial smooth muscle shortening into critical luminal obstruction. However, only 4 out of 20 stenotic lesions in our group of patients reacted according to his theory. Recent angiographic observations by Freedman et al. [10] are also not explicable by MacAlpin's hypothesis. These authors compared the vasoconstrictor effect of ergometrine in 11 patients with variant angina to those in 21 patients with atypical chest pain. The dynamic response of the stenotic lesions in patients with variant angina, in contrast to the reaction in the patients with atypical complaints, was always more pronounced than had been predicted by the geometric theory, even though the severity of the atheromateous lesions in both populations was similar. Their results suggest an increased sensitivity of the obstructive lesion to ergometrine in patients with variant angina. Although the reason for this hypersensitivity at the site of an atheroma is unknown, Henry and Yokoyama [14] recently suggested that this was mediated by a serotonergic mechanism, as shown in rabbits with diet induced atherosclerosis. This hypersensitivity could not be inhibited by alpha adrenergic blockers [14]. Another agonist might be histamine, which has induced coronary artery spasm in some patients, presumably by H1 receptor stimulation [15].

While a hyperreactive response occurred in 10 of the 20 stenotic lesions, hyporeactivity was observed at 6 other sites. This could be explained either by a decreased pliability of the coronary artery at the site of an atherosclerotic plaque [11] or by the destruction of smooth muscle by the atherosclerotic process.[10] Furthermore, there is the consideration that the use of a single angiographic view underestimates the contraction of the flexible part of an eccentric stenosis.

In contrast to the unpredictable vasoconstriction after ergometrine, intracoronary isosorbide dinitrate led in all patients and at all stenotic sites to vasodilation. However, the extent of vasodilation could be predicted by MacAlpin's theory in only half of the cases.

It is concluded that the extent of vasoconstriction in patients with exertional as well as resting angina after administration of ergometrine is unpredictable and cannot adequately be explained by geometric principles. Vasodilation at stenotic sites by isosorbide dinitrate, however, is a more predictable event, which to a large extent can be accounted for by MacAlpin's hypothesis.

References

1. Serruys PW, Steward R, Booman F, Michels R, Reiber JHC, Hugenholtz PG: Can unstable angina pectoris be due to increased coronary vasomotor tone? Eur Heart J 1(Suppl B): 71–85, 1980.
2. Epstein SE, Talbot TL: Dynamic coronary tone in precipitation, exacerbation and relief of angina pectoris. Am J Cardiol 48: 797–803, 1981.
3. Maseri A, Severi S, De Nes M, L'Abbate A, Chierchia S, Marzilli M, Ballestra AM, Parodi O, Biagini A, Distante A: 'Variant' angina: one aspect of a continuous spectrum of vasospastic myocardial ischaemia. Am J Cardiol 42: 1019–1035, 1978.
4. MacAlpin RN: Relation of coronary arterial spasm to sites of organic stenosis. Am J Cardiol 46: 143–153, 1980.
5. Heupler FA, Proudfit WL, Razavi M, Shirey EK, Greenstreet R, Sheldon WC: Ergonovine maleate provocative test for coronary arterial spasm. Am J Cardiol 41. 631–640, 1978.
6. Schroeder JS, Bolen JL, Quint RA, Clark DA, Hayden WG, Higgins CB, Wexler L: Provocation of coronary spasm with ergonovine maleate. Am J Cardiol 40: 487–481, 1977.
7. Waters DD, Theroux P, Szlachcic J, Dauwe F, Crittin J, Bonan R, Mizgala HF: Ergonovine testing in a coronary care unit. Am J Cardiol 46: 922–930, 1980.
8. Curry RC, Pepine CJ, Sabom MB, Feldman RL, Christie LG, Conti CR: Effects of ergonovine in patients with and without coronary artery disease. Circulation 56: 803–809, 1977.
9. Freedman SB, Dunn RF, Bernstein L, Richmond DR, O'Neill G, Kelly DT: Coronary artery spasm: use of ergonovine in diagnosis. Aust NZ J Med 10: 6–11, 1980.
10. Freedman B, Richmond DR, Kelly DT: Pathophysiology of coronary artery spasm. Circulation 66: 705–709, 1982.
11. MacAlpin RN: Contribution of dynamic vascular wall thickening to luminal narrowing during coronary arterial constriction. Circulation 61: 296–301, 1980.
12. Folkow B, Grimby G, Thulesius O: Adaptive structural changes of the vascular walls in hypertension and their relation to the control of the peripheral resistance. Acta Physiol Scand 44: 255–272, 1958.
13. Conway J: Vascular reactivity in experimental hypertension measured after hexamethonium. Circulation 17: 807–810, 1958.
14. Henry PD, Yokoyama M: Supersensitivity of atherosclerotic rabbit aorta to ergonovine: mediation by a serotonergic mechanism. J Clin Invest 66: 306–313, 1980.
15. Ginsburg R, Bristow MR, Kantrowitz N, Baim DS, Harrisson DC: Histamine provocation of clinical coronary artery spasm: Implications concerning pathogenesis of variant angina pectoris. Am Heart J 102: 819–822, 1981.

XX. Responses of normal and obstructed coronary arterial segments to cold stimulation; a quantitative angiographic study*

Summary

This study describes the quantitative coronary angiographic response to one minute hand immersion in ice water, the cold pressor test (CPT). The study population consisted of 20 patients with insignificant coronary disease (<50% diameter narrowing), 26 patients with exertional angina and 18 patients with angina at rest. A total of 49 obstructive lesions and 203 nonobstructed segments in the left coronary arterial system were analyzed with the CAAS.

Overall, CPT decreased the mean diameters of nonobstructed coronary segments from 2.76 to 2.68 mm (-3%, $p<0.001$). Relative changes in mean coronary arterial dimensions were similar among the three groups of patients. The diameter of the left main artery was not influenced by CPT. The relative magnitude of change by CPT was greatest (-6%) in the distal segments of the circumflex artery.

The overall size of stenotic arterial segments demonstrated comparable vasoconstriction (-3%) as nonobstructed coronary segments. Focal spasm was not observed after CPT. Increases in percentages luminal narrowing at stenotic lesions never exceeded 25%. At the average, the minimal obstruction diameter increased slightly, but not significantly after CPT (1.47 vs 1.52 mm, n.s.).

The results from this study thus indicate that CPT may not be a reliable provocative manoeuvre to induce focal coronary spasm.

Introduction

When exposed to a low environmental temperature, patients with coronary artery disease often experience angina pectoris at a lower threshold than at more moderate temperatures. As cold stimulation, even to a small part of the body,

* This study was supported by the Dutch Heart Foundation under grant no. 82.058.

increases heart rate and arterial pressure, this increase in cardiac workload has been held responsible for the aggravation of symptoms in cold weather by previous investigators [1–3]. Other studies, however, have demonstrated that one minute hand immersion in ice water (cold pressor test (CPT)) does not lead to a reflex increase in coronary blood flow in patients with coronary artery disease, suggesting that inappropriate coronary vasoconstriction causes the deleterious effects of cold in these patients [4, 5]. In addition, a high incidence of focal coronary vasospasm after cold stimulation has been reported in a number of studies [6–7]. As a result, CPT has been proposed as an alternative provocative test to ergonovine [7].

The purpose of the present study was to quantify angiographic changes induced by CPT in normal and obstructed coronary arteries.

Methods

Study population

Sixty-four patients who underwent routine cardiac catheterization for evaluation of chest pain were studied following informed consent. In all subjects treatment with beta-blocking agents, nitrates and calcium antagonists was withheld at least 16 hours before catheterization. No patient had symptoms or clinical signs of heart failure or valvular disease.

Excluded from this study were patients with electrocardiographic evidence of variant angina, patients with significant narrowing of the left main coronary artery, and those with spontaneous angina during catheterization.

The study population was categorized into three groups according to symptoms and angiographic findings. A luminal diameter narrowing greater than 50% in one of the major coronary arteries was considered significant. Group A included 20 patients without significant coronary artery disease. Group B consisted of 26 patients with significant coronary disease and exertional angina pectoris, defined as transient episodes of angina precipitated only by exercise. Group C included 18 patients with coronary disease and angina at rest, characterized by episodes of pain occurring not only with exercise, but also in circumstances without apparent increased myocardial oxygen demand.

Coronary angiography and cold stimulation

Catheterization was performed in a fasting state without premedication. Before cold stimulation, multiple coronary angiographic views, including at least two with a sagittal tilt, were obtained using the Sones or Judkins technique. After electrocardiographic and pressure changes induced by selective injection of the contrast material had reverted to baseline levels, a control coronary angiogram was obtained in a projection with minimal overlap of proximal coronary segments and with optimal visualization of any proximal coronary stenoses. Five minutes after the control angiogram, the patient's left hand and lower forearm were submerged in ice water for a period of one minute. Immediately thereafter, a second selective angiogram was repeated in exactly the same view as the control angiogram. Coronary spasm induced by CPT was considered to be present if a stenotic lesion in the control angiogram progressed to complete or subtotal (91–99% diameter narrowing) occlusion, or if a nonsignificant lesion became significant (>50% diameter narrowing) by an increase of at least 25% after cold stimulation.

Quantitative angiographic analysis

The quantitative analyses of selected coronary segments were carried out with the CAAS. The left epicardial coronary artery was divided into various segments as proposed by the American Heart Association [8]. In this study, each obstructive lesion was characterized by its minimal obstruction diameter and user-defined percentage diameter stenosis; for obstructed as well as nonobstructed coronary segments the overall mean arterial dimension was also computed. The percentage change in arterial dimension induced by cold stimulation was calculated as:

$$\frac{(\text{arterial diameter after CPT}) - (\text{control diameter})}{\text{control diameter}} \times 100\%.$$

Figure XX.1 is an example of the quantitative measurements of a nonobstructed coronary segment before and after cold stimulation.

Statistical analysis

Student's t-test was used to compare measurements obtained before and after cold stimulation. Results are expressed as mean ± s.d. P-values <0.05 were considered significant.

Results

Details of the study population and data obtained during catheterization are summarized in Table XX.1. Twenty patients had insignificant coronary disease or normal angiograms. Forty-four patients had coronary disease considered hemodynamically significant. In both groups, left ventricular ejection fraction was within normal limits (Table XX.1).

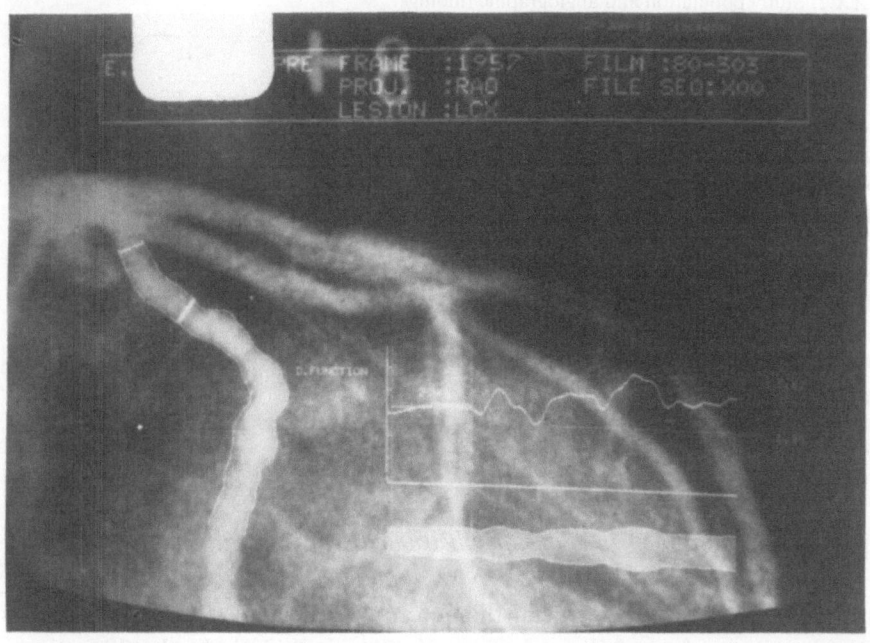

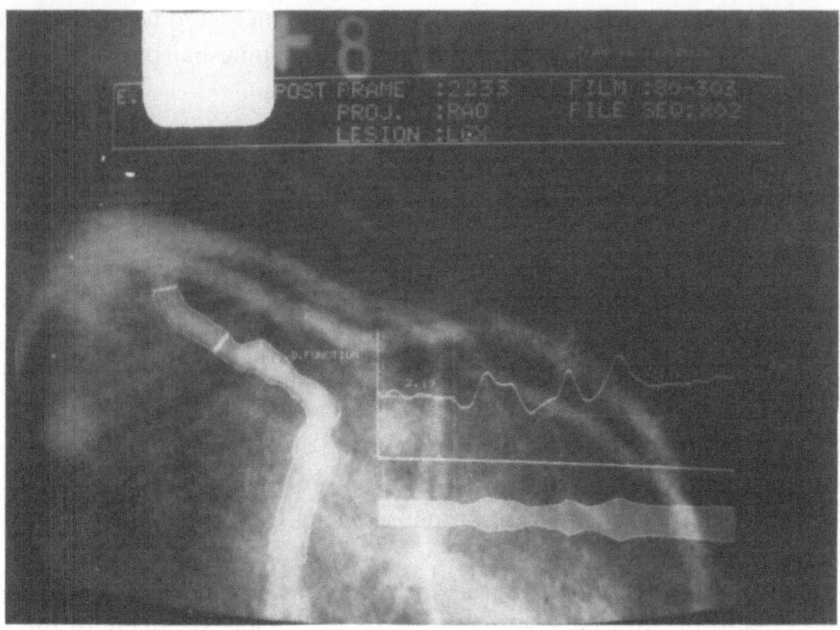

Fig. XX.1. The mean diameter of the proximal non-obstructed segment of the circumflex artery decreased from 2.40 mm before (upper photograph) to 2.19 mm after (lower photograph) cold stimulation.

Table XX.1. Study population and angiographic findings.

	No CAD	CAD	
		AP at exercise	AP at rest
Number of patients	20	26	18
Males (%)	13 (65)	24 (92)	16 (89)
Age* (years)	52 ± 11	53 ± 10	55 ± 6
Ejection fraction* (%)	63 ± 6	60 ± 10	62 ± 6
Number of patients with:			
one vessel disease		14	7
two vessel disease		7	5
three vessel disease		5	6

* = Mean ± s.d., CAD, coronary artery disease.

Changes in arterial dimensions in non-obstructed segments induced by CPT

Overall, CPT decreased the mean diameters of 203 analyzed non-obstructed coronary segments from 2.76 to 2.68 mm (-3%, $p<0.001$). In the 20 patients without coronary disease, the mean diameter of 57 coronary segments decreased from 2.93 to 2.84 mm after CPT (-3%, $p<0.002$). In patients with coronary disease, 146 non-obstructed coronary segments were measured before and after CPT. In this group, the mean coronary diameter also diminished by 3% from 2.70 to 2.62 mm ($p<0.001$) after cold stimulation.

Diameter changes by CPT in different non-obstructed segments

The magnitude of change in coronary artery diameters varied among the various segments analyzed. In the study population as a whole, the diameter of the left main coronary artery was not influenced by CPT (4.19 vs 4.19 mm, p = n.s.). In all other segments of the left coronary artery, CPT induced a decrease in mean diameter. This change reached statistical significance in all branches, except in the distal segment of the left anterior descending artery and the postero-lateral branch of the circumflex artery. Table XX.2 provides the details about the absolute and relative changes in the various segments in patients with and without coronary artery disease.

In patients without coronary disease, the relative magnitude of change in mean coronary diameter after CPT was greatest in the middle segments of the left anterior descending artery (-6%, $p<0.05$) and in the distal segments of the circumflex artery (-8%, n.s.). In patients with coronary disease, decreases in coronary dimensions after CPT varied between -2% and -6% and were also greatest ($p<0.05$) in the distal segments of the circumflex artery. Comparing

Table XX.2. Changes in average arterial dimensions in nonobstructed segments before and after cold stimulation.

Coronary segment	Patients without CAD			Patients with CAD		
	Before CPT	After CPT	% Change	Before CPT	After CPT	% change
Left main	4.33 ± 0.70	4.35 ± 0.75	+1%	4.12 ± 0.66	4.11 ± 0.69	0%
Left anterior descending artery						
Proximal	3.05 ± 0.40	2.97 ± 0.42	−3%	2.81 ± 0.52	2.68 ± 0.49	−4%
Middle	2.47 ± 0.31	2.33 ± 0.30	−6%	2.32 ± 0.40	2.28 ± 0.44	−2%
Distal	1.70 ± 0.32	1.69 ± 0.35	−1%	1.93 ± 0.34	1.85 ± 0.36	−4%
Circumflex artery						
Proximal	2.99 ± 0.77	2.92 ± 0.77	−2%	2.76 ± 0.52	2.68 ± 0.51	−3%
Distal	2.52 ± 0.34	2.31 ± 0.29	−8%	2.15 ± 0.67	2.01 ± 0.56	−6%
Marginal branch	2.79 ± 0.68	2.53 ± 0.55	−9%	1.99 ± 0.29	1.91 ± 0.33	−4%
Postero-lateral branch	1.98 ± 0.45	1.91 ± 0.45	−3%	2.04 ± 0.23	1.94 ± 0.28	−5%

All values: mean ± s.d; CAD = coronary artery disease.

segments from patients with exertional angina (Group B) to those with angina at rest (Group C) revealed that CPT decreased the coronary diameters in both groups in a similar manner. Figure XX.2 illustrates the diameter changes by CPT in different segments of the left anterior descending and circumflex arteries in these patients.

Responses of stenotic segments and lesions to CPT

In the patients with significant coronary obstructions, 49 lesions were analyzed. At the average, the overall mean diameter of the coronary segments in which these stenoses were located, decreased from 2.49 to 2.42 mm (-3%, $p<0.05$), and was thus comparable to the diameter change of nonstenotic segments. Focal coronary spasm was not observed in any patient, neither at a stenosis nor in segments with only luminal irregularities. Although six initially insignificant lesions became significant after CPT, the increase in luminal narrowing after cold stimulation never exceeded 25%. This response was seen in 2 patients with angina at rest, and in 4 patients with exertional angina.

In the 49 abnormal segments, the average percentage diameter stenosis did not change after cold stimulation (50% vs 48%, n.s), whereas the average minimal obstruction diameter of the 49 lesions increased slightly, but not significantly after CPT (1.47 vs 1.52 mm, n.s.).

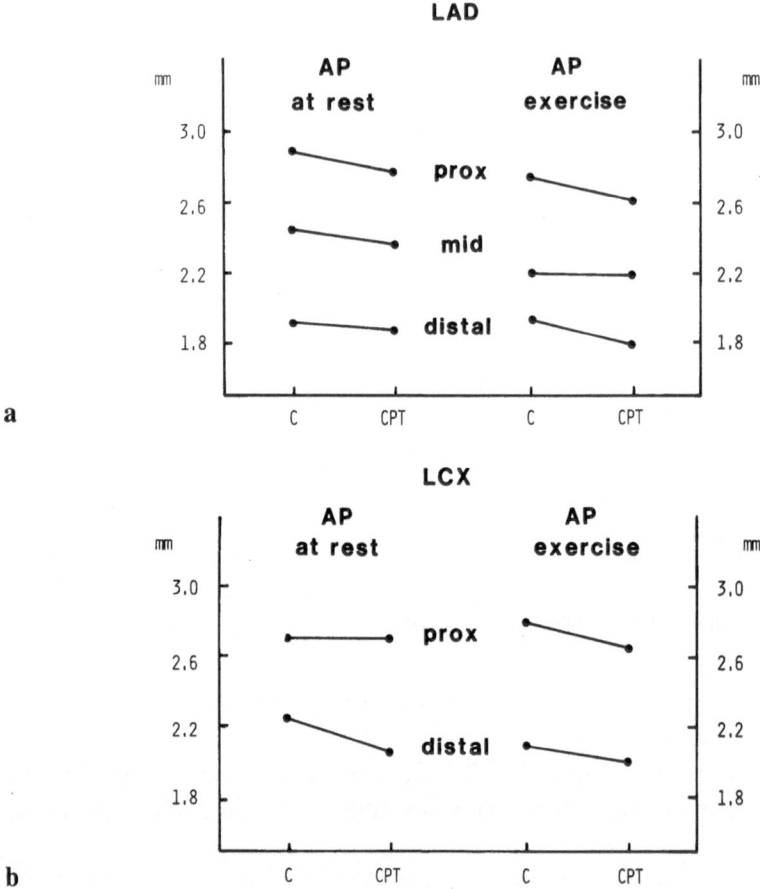

Fig. XX.2. Changes induced by one minute cold stimulation on the mean dimensions of non-obstructed segments of the left anterior descending (Fig. XX.2a) and circumflex arteries (Fig. XX.2b) in 26 patients with exertional angina and in 18 patients with angina at rest.

Discussion

Coronary arterial spasm, probably the most important feature of variant angina [9, 10], may also play a significant role in other aspects of ischemic heart disease [11]. During the past years, evidence has cumulated that not only acute myocardial infarction, but also angina at rest may be caused by coronary arterial spasm [11–13]. Demonstration of coronary spasm usually involves pharmacological provocation during coronary angiography; intravenous administration of methergine has been used most widely for this purpose [14].

Recently, the application of cold to induce a reflex sympathic effect and provoke spasm has been proposed as a test which would be easier to perform and lead to less complications than the injection of ergot alkaloides [6, 15]. Previous studies have demonstrated that in response to cold, blood pressure and peripheral vascular resistance generally increase [1]. Although cold stimulation may thus increase the oxygen requirements of the myocardium, an unexpected decrease in coronary sinus blood flow and an increase in coronary vascular resistance have been reported after CPT in some patients with coronary disease, but without variant angina [5]. Cold induced spasm of epicardial vessels have been held responsible for this response by some authors [6]. The present analysis was thus undertaken in an attempt to establish the influence of cold on the large epicardial coronary vessels in different groups of patients.

Our data demonstrate that one minute hand immersion in ice water causes a small, but significant reduction of the mean diameters of the epicardial coronary vessels. The decrease in coronary dimensions was largest in the medium sized coronary segments, but focal coronary spasm in these vessels was not observed. Changes in mean coronary diameter were similar among patients with and without coronary disease and the relative magnitude of vasoconstriction was comparable among patients with exertional angina and patients with symptoms suggestive of increased vasoactivity. No significant differences in vasoconstriction induced by CPT were found between stenotic and nonstenotic segments. Finally, as the absolute minimal obstruction diameters of the analyzed coronary lesions did not decrease after CPT, cold stimulation did not augment the severity of coronary stenoses, nor did the stimulus provoke focal coronary spasm. It seems therefore unlikely, that the observed changes in coronary diameter after CPT would cause an increase in coronary vascular resistance as the contribution of the epicardial vessels to total coronary resistance is small [16]. Percent decreases in epicardial coronary diameters as large as 15% have been shown to be too small to elicit an increase in coronary resistance [17]. Diffuse narrowing of small, intra-myocardial vessels could explain an increase in coronary vascular resistance, but such vessels can not be visualized by coronary angiography.

Measurements of global coronary sinus blood flow during CPT have indicated that coronary flow can indeed decrease during cold stimulation [5], but it is unsure whether such a response occurs frequently [17, 18]. As Feldman et al. recently demonstrated that increases in coronary resistance may be limited only to abnormally perfused left ventricular regions [17], it may be relevant that left ventricular function was within normal limits in our study population.

Few other studies have also assessed the angiographic response to cold; however, the reported results are generally in agreement with those presented here. Raizner et al. studied 35 patients, including six considered to have variant angina, and 14 patients with classical angina [6]. Focal coronary spasm after CPT developed in 4 patients with variant angina, in 2 patients with exertional angina and in 1 patient without significant coronary disease. The coronary angiographic response to CPT in patients without variant angina varied between 5% and 8% decrease in diameter. Feldman et al. performed quantitative coronary angiography before and after cold stimulation in 12 patients with exertional chest pain [19]. An average diameter reduction of 6% was observed after CPT, both in normals as well as in patients with coronary disease. The degree of vasoconstriction in their study was largest (-10%) in distal segments. Finally, Wendt et al. found no differences in coronary diameters before and after CPT in 16 patients, but reported an incidence of spasm in all 4 patients with a history of angina at rest [20].

In our analysis, CPT was unable to provoke focal coronary spasm in any patient. This may be partly explained by the selection of our patients, as we excluded subjects with evidence of variant angina. Demonstration of coronary spasm during catheterization in these patients, however, is often unnecessary, as clinical evidence suggesting the presence of spasm can usually be obtained from electrocardiography. It is probably more appropriate to test the potential of a new provocative test in a population with a lower likelihood of inappropriate vasoconstriction. Nevertheless, although our study included a considerable number of patients with angina at rest, in some of whom the administration of ergot alkaloides would have resulted in coronary vasospasm [14], cold stimulation was unable to provoke focal spasm in any of them. Our results thus indicate that CPT may not be a reliable provocative manoeuvre to induce focal coronary spasm.

References

1. Epstein SE, Stampfer M, Beiser GD, Goldstein RE, Braunwald E: Effects of a reduction in environmental temperature on the circulatory response to exercise in man. Implications concerning angina pectoris. N Engl J Med 280: 7–11, 1969.
2. Neill WA, Duncan DA, Kloster F, Mahler DJ: Response of coronary circulation to cutaneous cold. Am J Med 56: 471–476, 1974.
3. Lassvik C, Areskog N-H: Angina pectoris during inhalation of cold air. Reactions to exercise. Br Heart J 43: 661–667, 1980.
4. Hattenhauer M, Neill WA: The effect of cold air inhalation on angina pectoris and myocardial oxygen supply. Circulation 51: 1053–1058, 1975.
5. Mudge GH Jr, Grossman W, Mills RM Jr, Lesch M, Braunwald E. Reflex increase in coronary vascular resistance in patients with ischemic heart disease. N Engl J Med 295: 1333–1337, 1976.
6. Raizner AE, Chahine RA, Ishimori T, Verani MS, Zacca N, Jamal N, Miller RR, Luchi RJ: Provocation of coronary artery spasm by the cold pressor test. Hemodynamic, arteriographic and quantitative angiographic observations. Circulation 62: 925–932, 1980.
7. Rasmussen K, Bagger JP, Bøttzauw J, Henningsen P: Prevalence of vasospastic ischaemia induced by the cold pressor test or hyperventilation in patients with severe angina. Eur Heart J 5: 354–361, 1984.
8. Austen WG, Edwards JE, Frye RL, Gensini GG, Gott VL, Griffith LSC, McGoon DC, Murphy ML, Roe BB: A reporting system on patients evaluated for coronary artery disease. Report of the Ad Hoc Committee for Grading of Coronary Artery Disease, Council on Cardiovascular Surgery, American Heart Association. Circulation 51: 7–40, 1975.
9. Chahine RA: Prinzmetal's variant angina. A syndrome apart or another clinical presentation of atheromatous heart disease. Arch Intern Med 139: 26–27, 1979.
10. Maseri A, Severi S, de Nes M, l'Abbate A, Chierchia S, Marzilli M, Ballestra AM, Parodi O, Biagini A, Distante A: 'Variant' angina: one aspect of a continuous spectrum of vasospastic myocardial ischemia. Pathogenetic mechanisms, estimated incidence and clinical and coronary

arteriographic findings in 138 patients. Am J Card 42: 1019–1035, 1978.

11. Maseri A, l'Abbate A, Chierchia S, Parodi O, Severi S, Biagini A, Distante A, Marzilli M, Ballestra AM: Significance of spasm in the pathogenesis of ischemic heart disease. Am J Card 44: 788–792, 1979.

12. Oliva PB, Breckinridge JC: Arteriographic evidence of coronary arterial spasm in acute myocardial infarction. Circulation 56: 366–374, 1977.

13. Maseri A, l'Abbate A, Baroldi G, Chierchia S, Marzilli M, Ballestra AM, Severi S, Parodi O, Biagini A, Distante A, Pesola A: Coronary vasospasm as a possible cause of myocardial infarction. A conclusion derived from the study of 'preinfarction' angina. N Engl J Med 299: 1271–1277, 1978.

14. Bertrand ME, LaBlanche JM, Tilmant PY, Thieuleux FA, Delforge MR, Carre AG, Asseman P, Berzin B, Libersa C, Laurent JM: Frequency of provoked coronary arterial spasm in 1089 consecutive patients undergoing coronary arteriography. Circulation 65: 1299–1306, 1982.

15. Bauman D: Complications after provocation of coronary spasm with ergonovine maleate. Am J Cardiol 42: 694–695, 1978.

16. Kelley KO, Feigl EO: Segmental α-receptor-mediated vasoconstriction in the canine coronary circulation. Circ Res 43: 908–917, 1978.

17. Feldman RL, Curry RC Jr, Pepine CJ, Mehta J, Conti CR: Regional coronary hemodynamic effects of ergonovine in patients with and without variant angina. Circulation 62: 149–159, 1980.

18. Feldman RL, Whittle JL, Marx JD, Pepine CJ, Conti CR: Regional coronary hemodynamic responses to cold stimulation in patients without variant angina. Am J Cardiol 49: 665–673, 1982.

19. Guiomard A, Zygelman M, Evstigneff T, Bréaud N, Roland E, Pansard Y, Mérillon JP, Gourgon R: Effets hémodynamiques et métaboliques coronaires du test au froid avant et après acébutolol. Arch Mal Coeur 76: 77–85, 1983.

20. Feldman RL, Whittle JL, Pepine CJ, Conti CR: Regional coronary angiographic observations during cold stimulation in patients with exertional chest pain: Comparison of diameter responses in normal and fixed stenotic vessels. Am Heart J 102: 822–830, 1981.

21. Wendt Th, Schutz W, Kaltenbach M, Kober G: Auswirkung von Kältereizen auf Hämodynamik und Koronargefässweite. Provokation von Koronarspasmen. Z Kardiol 72: 24–31, 1983.

XXI. Quantitative angiography of the left anterior descending coronary artery: correlations with pressure gradient and exercise thallium scintigraphy

Summary

In order to evaluate during cardiac catheterization what constitutes a physiologically significant obstruction to blood flow in the human coronary system, computer based quantitative analysis of coronary angiograms was performed in 31 patients with isolated proximal left anterior descending coronary artery disease. The angiographic severity of the stenosis was compared with the transstenotic pressure gradient measured with the dilatation catheter during angioplasty and the results of exercise thallium scintigraphy. A curvilinear relation was found between the pressure gradient across the stenosis (normalized for the mean aortic pressure) and the residual minimal obstruction area (after subtracting the area of the angioplasty catheter). This relation was best fitted by the equation: normalized mean pressure gradient $= a + b \cdot \log$ [obstruction area], $r = 0.74$. The measurements of the percent area stenosis (cut-off 80%) and of the transstenotic pressure gradient (cut-off 0.30) obtained at rest, correctly predicted the occurrence of thallium perfusion defects induced by exercise in 83% of the patients.

Introduction

It is uncertain which degree of narrowing of a major epicardial coronary artery will consistently lead to myocardial ischemia during exercise [1]. Under experimental conditions, a 50% reduction in the luminal diameter can diminish the vasodilatory reserve of the coronary vascular bed, but the resting blood flow is unaffected until the diameter stenosis exceeds 80–90% [2]. Moreover, an estimation of the severity of a stenosis based on the minimal cross-sectional area of the vessel is a more accurate descriptor of its hemodynamic impact than the percent diameter narrowing, which is the traditional method for grading coronary stenoses [3, 4].

In the clinical setting, more precise assessment of the relationship between the arteriographic degree of stenosis and the actual impairment in the perfusion is hampered by several limitations, the major one being the large intra- and interobserver variability in interpretation of coronary angiograms [5, 6]. Other limitations include the inconstant vasomotor tone [7, 8], the frequently irregular luminal geometry and the extent to which collaterals are present.

In order to study the relation between the stenotic diameter of a coronary artery and the pressure gradient across its stenosis on the one hand, and the extent of myocardial ischemia induced by exercise on the other hand, we selected patients with single left anterior descending coronary artery disease. In these patients, angiograms were obtained after intracoronary injection of nifedipine. The severity of the residual stenosis was measured by a computerized quantitative analysis procedure, while exercise induced ischemia was assessed by means of stress thallium scintigraphy.

Methods

Patients selection

Thirty-one consecutive patients with stable exertional angina pectoris were studied; all were candidates for percutaneous transluminal angioplasty of an isolated proximal left anterior descending stenosis. All subjects gave informed consent and no complications resulted from the study. Details regarding the procedure used in our laboratory have been previously described [9, 10].

Quantitative coronary angiography

The quantitative analysis of selected coronary segments was carried out with the Cardiovascular Angiography Analysis System (CAAS). From the obstruction diameter and the reference diameter computed by the interpolated measurement technique, the percentage area reduction, assuming circular cross sections, is computed as: %-A stenosis = $(1 - (\text{minimal diameter/reference diameter})^2) \times 100\%$ (XXI.1).

A representative analysis with the detected contours and the diameter function superimposed on the original video image is shown in Fig. XXI.1A. The results by the interpolated percentage diameter stenosis measurement are shown in Fig. XXI.1B.

In this study, the coronary angiograms were obtained within five minutes after intracoronary injection of nifedipine (0.1 to 0.2 mg) in order to obtain a vasodilatation of the epicardial vessels and the relief of a possible spasm [11, 12]. Since the luminal cross section at the site of the coronary obstruction is frequently irregular in shape especially after angioplasty [13, 14], the average obstruction

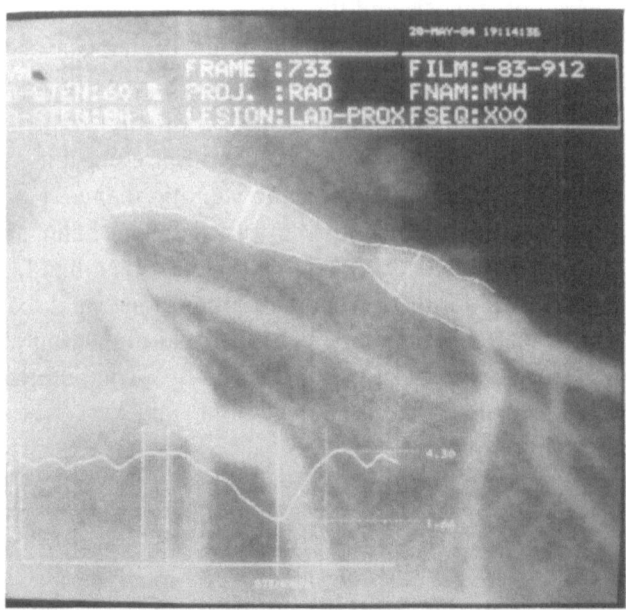

FRAME :733   FILM:-83-912
PROJ. :RAO   FNAM:MVH
LESION:LAD-PROX FSEQ:XOO

A

Fig. XXI.1. Detected contours for a representative left anterior descending coronary artery stenosis superimposed on the original video image. The diameter function is shown at the bottom. The calibrated diameter values in mm are plotted along the ordinate starting from the proximal to the distal part of the analyzed segment along the abscissa.

Fig. XXI.1A. The reference diameter (or area) was selected proximal to the stenosis. A %-area stenosis of 84% results.

area and percent area reduction obtained from multiple views were used (mean of 1.7 views per segment). Since the presence of the dilatation catheter within the stenotic lumen further reduces lumen area, the difference between the luminal area measured from the coronary angiograms and the area of the balloon catheter (0.64 mm^2) was used as an approach to the actual residual lumen and related to the pressure gradient measurements. The mean pressure gradient across the stenotic lesion was measured with the dilatation catheter (mean diameter of 0.9 mm, Schneider 20–30 or 20–37) before and after angioplasty and calculated on line after a data acquisition period of 20 seconds [15].

Noninvasive testing

Exercise thallium-201 myocardial scintigraphy was performed before angioplasty in 7 patients, after angioplasty in 13 patients and before and after in 11 patients. Sequential imaging was performed according to a standard protocol immediately after a symptom limited exercise test and again 4 hours later. Scintigraphy was

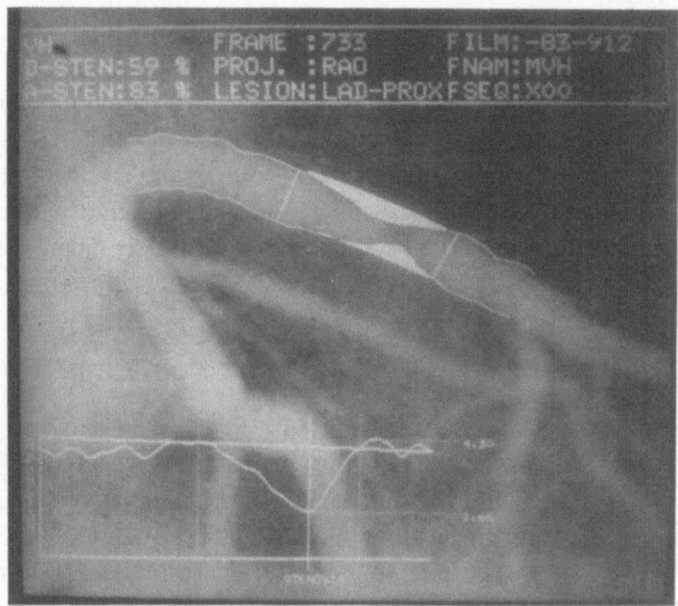

B

Fig. XXI.1B. The normal size of the artery over the obstruction has been estimated by the interpolated method. The resulting reference contours are shown and the difference in area between these boundaries and the detected contours is a measure of the atherosclerotic plaque (shaded area). A %-area stenosis of 83% results.

performed in the week before angiography (n = 18) and in the three weeks after successful angioplasty (n = 24). No patient had recurrence of angina pectoris during this time interval. During exercise, three orthogonal leads (X, Y, Z) were monitored and analyzed as previously described [16]. The scintigraphic images were processed on a DEC gamma-11 system [17]. Basically, circumferential profiles were computed in three projections (anterior, LAO 45, LAO 65) within the automatically detected contour of the left ventricle following background subtraction according to Watson [18]. The circumferential profiles, the processed images and the analog polaroid images were interpreted by three independent observers, who were unaware of the angiographic data. The myocardial uptake of thallium was scored in 13 segments both for early and late exercise scintigrams in the following manner: 0 = no thallium uptake; 1 = severely abnormal; 2 = definitely abnormal; 3 = doubtfully abnormal; 4 = normal. These scores were summed per patient and the difference between late and early postexercise sums was taken as a measure of the amount of redistribution. Using this approach, ischemia was considered to be present if at least two observers found that the redistribution score was two or more points higher than the early postexercise one. Since only patients with single vessel disease were included, the left anterior descending artery stenosis was taken responsible for the regional defects observed in the antero-septal, anterior, antero-lateral as well as apical segments [19].

Statistical analysis

Simple regressions were used to attempt the best fit relation between the pressure gradient and the obstruction area. The Student t-test for paired data and linear least squares regressions were used to compare the interpolated and user-defined percent area stenosis measurements. One-way analysis of variance followed by multiple comparisons was used to compare the angiographic measurements between three subgroups of patients. Data are expressed as mean ± standard deviation (s.d.).

Results

The absolute dimensions of the minimal obstruction area are given in Table XXI.1, ranked from the minimal obstruction area value of 0.15 mm^2 to the maximal value of 17.9 mm^2. The interpolated and user-defined percent area stenoses are shown as well. The user-defined reference was taken proximal to the stenosis in all but 10 cases where it was taken distally due to the take-off of the left circumflex artery just before the stenosis. There was no significant difference between the interpolated and user-defined percent area stenosis: the difference between paired data was 1.7 ± 10 and the correlation coefficient was 0.91 (interpolated %-Area st. = 0.95 user %-Area st. + 4.8; SEE = 10). When the mean pressure gradient across the stenosis, normalized for the mean aortic pressure ($\overline{AoP}$), is compared to the residual obstruction area after subtracting the balloon area (Fig. XXI.2), a nonlinear relation is found which can be described by the equation:

$$\Delta P/\overline{AoP} = a + b \cdot \log [\text{obstruction area}] \tag{XXI.2},$$

where a = 0.35 and b = −0.12 (r = 0.74). It is shown that there is a steep increase in pressure gradient once a critical value of 2.5 mm^2 of the stenotic segment is reached. In seven cases, the angioplasty catheter almost totally obstructed the vessel. The computed cross-sectional area reduction is also related to the pressure gradient (Fig. XXI.3). Here, the steep increase in pressure gradient is observed once the critical reduction of 80% in cross-sectional area is reached.

During the exercise test, the maximal workload averaged 85 ± 17% of the predicted value. According to the results of the thallium scintigraphy, three types of responses are observed. In group I (N = 25), the scintigram is normal, with either normal or abnormal exercise ECG. In group II (N = 7), thallium scintigraphy is abnormal while the exercise test results are normal. In group III (N = 10), both thallium scintigraphy and exercise test results (angina and/or ST-segment changes) are abnormal. The percent area stenosis is 55 ± 23 in group I, 74 ± 17 in group II and 90 ± 4 in group III. The mean pressure gradient was: 0.18 ± 0.13 in group I, 0.44 ± 0.23 in group II and 0.62 ± 0.15 in group III. The pressure

Table XXI.1. Quantitative angiography and exercise test results.

Patient			Obstr. Area	A st. inter	A st. user	$\triangle P/\overline{AoP}$	AP	ECG	TL 201
1	HD	b	0.15	98	96	0.75	−	−	+
2	FA	b	0.30	98	94	0.49	+	+	−
3	HO	b	0.36	97	97	0.87	+	+	+
4	PL	b	0.45	96	84	0.46	+	+	+
5	EN	b	0.58	96	94	0.54	−	−	+
6	KS	b	0.58	92	91	0.55	−	−	−
7	BO	b	0.65	93	90	0.74	−	+	+
8	VD	b	0.80	90	(-)	0.38	−	BB	−
9.	HN	b	0.88	89	89	0.63	−	+	+
10	EL	b	0.92	90	75	0.73	+	−	+
11	MS	b	0.98	80	85	0.67	−	−	+
12	HO	a	1.23	70	75	0.29	−	−	−
13	EM	a	1.58	72	55	0.16	−	+	−
14	KT	b	1.65	89	84	0.43	−	+	+
15	HE	b	1.74	91	89	0.65	+	+	+
16	SK	b	1.77	89	(-)	0.60	+	−	+
17	GI	b	2.06	88	90	0.39	+	BB	+
18	SR	b	2.09	88	87	0.72	−	+	+
19	DA	b	2.38	62	69	0.39	−	BB	+
20	RS	a	2.75	75	72	0.10	+	BB	−
21	MS	a	2.83	38	65	0.13	−	−	−
22	DA	a	2.95	34	50	0.18	+	−	−
23	HP	a	3.00	55	65	0.10	−	−	−
24	FN	a	3.11	54	64	0.13	−	+	−
25	HD	a	3.14	60	(-)	0.09	−	−	−
26	BE	a	3.14	44	32	0.06	−	−	−
27	WI	a	3.17	66	65	0.28	−	−	−
28	KL	b	3.33	65	65	0.15	−	−	+
29	MO	a	3.70	56	54	0.34	−	−	+
30	NS	a	3.94	61	30	0.16	−	−	−
31	BV	a	4.12	48	39	0.11	−	−	−
32	HT	a	4.16	66	48	0.16	−	+	−
33	FA	a	4.26	37	45	0.21	−	+	−
34	HN	a	4.34	65	56	0.04	−	−	−
35	KL	a	4.95	37	52	0.00	−	−	−
36	OW	a	5.68	44	43	0.16	−	−	−
37	SK	a	6.20	62	67	0.18	−	−	−
38	HE	a	7.07	64	53	0.21	−	−	+
39	SE	a	7.50	60	57	0.10	−	−	−
40	KN	a	8.29	6	14	0.21	−	+	−
41	KT	a	9.90	30	21	0.07	−	−	−
42	GI	a	17.87	6	6	0.06	−	−	−

Abbreviations: b = before PTCA; a = after PTCA; Obstr. Area = obstruction area in mm²; A st. = percent area stenosis; inter = interpolated, and user = user-defined reference; (-) = missing data; $\triangle P/\overline{AoP}$ = mean pressure gradient normalized for mean aortic pressure; AP = angina pectoris; ECG = ST depression $\geqslant 0.1\,\text{mV}$; 201 Tl = redistribution from exercise to rest scintigram; + = present; − = absent; BB = bundle branch block.

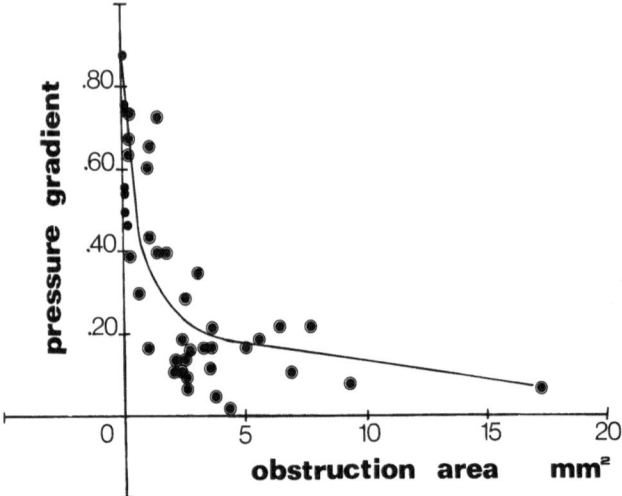

Fig. XXI.2. The relation between the mean pressure gradient normalized for the mean aortic pressure and the residual obstruction area in mm² (after subtraction of the area of the angioplasty catheter) is nonlinear; the best fit is obtained by the logarithmic function (r = 0.74). Filled symbols represent stenoses in which the angioplasty catheter totally obstructed the vessel.

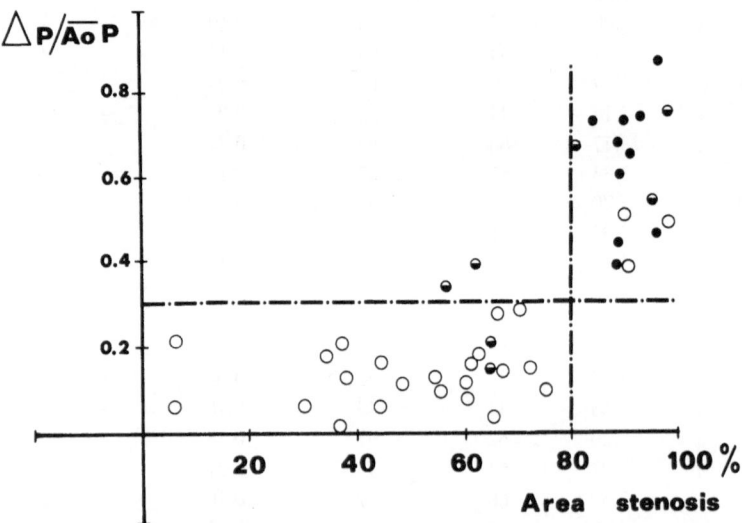

Fig. XXI.3. The relation between mean normalized pressure gradient, percentage area stenosis and the results of the thallium scintigraphy is shown. Open circles are patients with a normal scintigram (group I, N = 25), while half filled circles represent patients with an abnormal thallium but normal exercise test (group II, N = 7). Filled circles represent patients with both abnormal thallium and exercise test (group III, N = 10).

gradient measurements discriminated better between the groups than the area stenosis measurements (Table XXI.2). When combining both parameters, two groups of data points are delineated as shown in Fig. XXI.3. Using cut-off values of 0.30 for the pressure gradient and 80% for the cross-sectional area reduction, the result of the exercise thallium scintigram was correctly predicted from the angiographic data in 83% of the patients. An abnormal scintigraphy is observed in 13 of the 16 patients with a pressure gradient of at least 0.30 and a percent area stenosis equal to or greater than 80% (sensitivity of 81%). Two out of three patients with a normal thallium uptake and exercise test had important collaterals shown by angiography. Conversely, the thallium uptake is normal in 22 of the 24 patients with a pressure gradient less than 0.30 together with an area stenosis less than 80% (specificity 92%). Similar figures were found when the user-defined percent area was used instead of the interpolated method (sensitivity 85%, specificity 87%).

Discussion

In this study, we selected the simplest human model available to assess the relationship between the angiographic stenosis severity and the inducibility of regional perfusion defects during exercise thallium scintigraphy. Attempts to correlate closely the anatomy of a coronary stenosis and its physiologic signifi- cance are hampered by the large intra- and interobserver variability [5, 6] due to subjective visual scoring of coronary angiograms and to the inconstant vasomotor tone. To circumvent these limitations, the coronary angiograms were performed after intracoronary injection of nifedipine and the cinefilms were quantitatively analyzed with the help of automated edge detection techniques. Since part of the results are expressed in terms of percent area (or diameter) stenosis, a critical point is the choice by the user of an appropriate reference area (or diameter). When a large vessel gives rise to a major daughter branch, the cross-sectional area of the main vessel distal to the branch point is significantly less than its area proximal to the branch point; hence, the choice of a proximal reference would not be appropriate. Conversely, the choice of an appropriate distal reference is often

Table XXI.2. Noninvasive test results and angiographic estimates of stenosis severity.

		N	% Area stenosis	mean pressure gradient
Group I	(Tl−)	25	55 ± 23	0.18 ± 0.13 #
Group II	(Tl+/ET−)	7	* 74 ± 17 n.s.	* 0.44 ± 0.23
Group III	(Tl+/ET+)	10	90 ± 4 n.s.	0.62 ± 0.15 n.s.

Abbreviations as previously; N, number of patients; ET, exercise test result; +, abnormal; −, normal; n.s., nonsignificant; symbols refer to p-values: # $p < 0.005$; * $p < 0.001$.

hampered by the presence of poststenotic ectasia and by anatomical tapering. Therefore, an alternative method was developed, similar to that used by Crawford et al. [20], which is based on the computer estimation of the 'original contour of the pre-atherosclerotic lumen' and allows the vessel to taper. The difference in area between the original lumen and the contours of the obstruction is a measure for the atherosclerotic plaque. Crawford et al. have demonstrated that such angiographic assessment of the atherosclerotic plaque by computer densitometry correlated with the cholesterol content of the corresponding human arterial specimen. Their approach includes both density and edge measurements; among these, the computer detected lumen with taper yielded the best correlation with the pathologic data [20]. In the present as well as in earlier studies [13, 21], the user-defined and interpolated measurements are closely correlated. However, for the analysis of repeated angiograms [22, 23], the knowledge of the exact location of the reference, either proximal or distal to the stenosis, is not required when the interpolated method is used. For these theoretical and practical reasons, we favor the use of an automated definition of the reference area (or diameter) with the interpolated technique [10, 14].

From these data, obtained in a clinical setting, a curvilinear relation was found between the pressure drop across the stenosis and the minimal obstruction area as well as the percent cross-sectional area reduction. Both relations are similar to those calculated on theoretical grounds by Brown et al. [24] as well as to those experimentally derived from isolated human arteries [25] or dog experiments [3]. Such curvilinear relation is expected from the general equation of fluid dynamics showing that the pressure drop across a stenosis is influenced mainly by viscous losses in the stenotic segment and separation losses at the exit of the stenosis. For a given level of flow, the single most important determinant of stenosis resistance is its minimal cross-sectional area which appears as a second order term in both viscous and separation losses equations. In the animal laboratory, a coronary stenosis can be characterized precisely by simultaneous measurements of flow and stenosis gradient and related to the quantitative assessment of stenosis geometry. In such experimental setting, blood flow velocity and pressure drop across the stenosis are correlated in an exponential fashion [26]. Recently, coronary blood flow velocity measurements were obtained in patients during heart surgery and related to the computer-based analysis of their coronary angiograms [4, 27]. It was shown that the minimal cross-sectional area was the best predictor of the physiological significance of a coronary stenosis. During cardiac catheterization, the pressure-flow relation across a coronary stenosis cannot be determined, although the feasibility of transluminal measurements of coronary blood flow velocity has been reported recently [28]. However, the pressure distal to a coronary stenosis is measured routinely during the transluminal angioplasty procedure. This has stimulated the development of very small catheters for the in vivo investigation of the functional significance of pressure gradient measurements [29]. The physiological value of these measurements, even those obtained with the smallest catheters, must be questioned since the catheter impedes flow through the obstruction. Experimental data obtained in dog femoral arteries suggest that the 'true' lesional gradient is overestimated in a predictable manner dependent on the ratio of the catheter diameter over the stenosis diameter [30]. In addition, the mean pressure gradient is affected by phasic changes in flow velocity [26]. The distal coronary pressure may be affected by collaterals and is entirely determined by collateral flow when the angioplasty catheter totally obstructs the vessel. In spite of these limitations, Vogel et al. have shown that the mean pressure gradient measured across the stenosis during angioplasty predicted accurately the coronary flow reserve measured as the ratio of hyperemic over control myocardial contrast appearance times by digital angiography [31]. In the present study, the gradient was related in a curvilinear way with the actual luminal area obtained by subtracting the area of the deflated balloon catheter from the minimal obstruction area as assessed by quantitative angiography. The major finding of this study was that the combination of pressure drop measurements across the stenosis with quantitative assessment of the luminal narrowing predicted the occurrence of exercise thallium perfusion abnormalities better than the measurements of the stenosis alone. Using the cut-off values of 0.30 for the pressure gradient and 80 for the percent cross-sectional area reduction, the result of the exercise thallium scintigram was correctly predicted from the angiographic data in all but six patients. In four of them, thallium perfusion abnormalities occurred without signs of ischemia in the presence of a noncritical cross-sectional area stenosis of about 60%. These discrepancies are not surprising since many other factors such as blood density, viscosity, stenosis length and divergence angle were not accounted for [24, 25]. Two patients had normal scintigrams and exercise tests while ischemia was expected from the angiographic measurements. This can be due to the presence of coronary collaterals as shown by angiography since previous work suggests that they could prevent the occurrence of thallium perfusion defects during exercise [32, 33].

In summary, the functional significance of a coronary stenosis can be evaluated at rest by quantitative analysis of coronary dimensions and transstenotic pressure gradient measurements. In patients with single left anterior descending coronary artery disease this allowed identification, at rest, of those lesions responsible or not for thallium perfusion defects induced by exercise.

References

1. Gould KL: Noninvasive assessment of coronary stenoses by myocardial perfusion imaging during pharmacologic coronary vasodilatation. I. Physiologic basis and experimental validation. Am J Cardiol 41: 267–278, 1978.
2. Gould KL, Lipscomb K: Effects of coronary stenoses on coronary flow reserve and resistance. Am J Cardiol 34: 48–55, 1974.
3. Mates RE, Gupta RL, Bell AC, Klocke FJ: Fluid dynamics of coronary artery stenosis. Circ Res 42: 152–162, 1978.

4. Harrison DG, White CW, Hiratzka LF, Doty DB, Barnes DH, Eastham CL, Marcus ML: The value of lesion cross-sectional area determined by quantitative coronary angiography in assessing the physiologic significance of proximal left anterior descending coronary arterial stenoses. Circulation 69: 1111–1119, 1984.

5. Detre KM, Wright E, Murphy ML, Takaro T: Observer agreement in evaluating coronary angiograms. Circulation 52: 979–986, 1975.

6. Zir LM, Miller SW, Dinsmore RE, Gilbert JP, Harthhorne JW: Interobserver variability in coronary angiography. Circulation 53: 627–632, 1976.

7. Gould KL: Dynamic coronary stenosis. Am J Cardiol 45: 286–292, 1980.

8. Serruys PW, Steward R, Booman F, Michels R, Reiber JHC, Hugenholtz PG: Can unstable angina pectoris be due to increased coronary vasomotor tone? Eur Heart J 1(Suppl B): 71–85, 1980.

9. Serruys PW, Brand M van den, Brower RW, Hugenholtz PG: Regional cardioplegia and cardioprotection during transluminal angioplasty, which role for nifedipine? Eur Heart J 4(Suppl. C): 115–121, 1983.

10. Serruys PW, Wijns W, Brand M van den, Ribeiro V, Fioretti P, Simoons ML, Kooijman CJ, Reiber JHC, Hugenholtz PG: Is transluminal coronary angioplasty mandatory after successful thrombolysis? Br Heart J 50: 257–265, 1983.

11. Serruys PW, Hooghoudt TEH, Reiber JHC, Slager C, Brower RW, Hugenholtz PG: Influence of intracoronary nifedipine on left ventricular function, coronary vasomotility, and myocardial oxygen consumption. Br Heart J 49: 427–441, 1983.

12. Amende I, Simon R, Hood WP, Hetzer R, Lichtlen PR: Intracoronary nifedipine in human beings: magnitude and time course of changes in left ventricular contraction/relaxation and coronary sinus blood flow. J Am Coll Cardiol 6: 1141–1145, 1983.

13. Serruys PW, Booman F, Troost GJ, Reiber JHC, Gerbrands JJ, Brand M van den, Cherrier F, Hugenholtz PG: Computerized quantitative coronary angiography applied to percutaneous transluminal coronary angioplasty; advantages and limitations. In: Transluminal Coronary Angioplasty and Intracoronary Thrombolysis. M Kaltenbach, A Gruentzig, K Rentrop, WD Bussmann (Eds.) Springer-Verlag, Berlin/Heidelberg/New York: 110–124, 1982.

14. Serruys PW, Reiber JHC, Wijns W, Kooijman CJ, Brand M van den, Katen HJ ten, Hugenholtz PG: Assessment of percutaneous transluminal coronary angioplasty by quantitative coronary angiography: Diameter vs densitometric area measurements. Am J Cardiol 54: 482–488, 1984.

15. Brower RW, Meester GT, Zeelenberg C, Hugenholtz PG: Automatic data processing in the cardiac catheterization laboratory. Comp Progr in Biomed 7: 99–110, 1977.

16. Simoons ML, Hugenholtz PG: Estimation of the probability of exercise-induced ischemia by quantitative ECG analysis. Circulation 56: 552–559, 1977.

17. Reiber JHC, Lie SP, Simoons ML, Wijns W, Gerbrands JJ: Computer quantification location, extent and type of thallium-201 myocardial perfusion abnormalities. Proc. First IEEE Comp. Society Int. Symp. on Medical Imaging and Image Interpretation. IEEE Cat No. 82 CH1804-4: 123–128, 1982.

18. Watson DD, Beller GA, Berger BC, Teates CD: Notes on the quantitation of sequential T1-201 images. Softwhere 6: 4–5, 10, 1979.

19. Rigo P, Bailey IK, Griffith LSC, Pitt B, Burow RD, Wagner HN Jr, Becker LC: Value and limitations of segmental analysis of stress thallium myocardial imaging for localization of coronary artery disease. Circulation 61: 973–981, 1980.

20. Crawford DW, Brooks SH, Selzer RH, Barndt R, Beckenbach ES, Blankenhorn DH: Computer densitometry for angiographic assessment of arterial cholesterol content and gross pathology in human atherosclerosis. J Lab Clin Med 89: 378–392, 1977.

21. Cherrier F, Booman F, Serruys PW, Cuillière M, Danchin N, Reiber JHC: L'angiographie coronaire quantitative. Application à l'évaluation des angioplasties transluminales coronaires. Arch Mal Coeur 74: 1377–1387, 1981.

22. Wijns W, Serruys PW, Brand M van den, Suryapranata H, Kooijman CJ, Reiber JHC, Hugen-holtz PG: Progression to complete coronary obstruction without myocardial infarction in patients who are candidates for percutaneous transluminal angioplasty: a 90-day angiographic follow-up. In: Prognosis of Coronary Heart Disease. Progression of Coronary Arteriosclerosis, H Roskamm (Ed.) Springer-Verlag, Berlin/Heidelberg/New York/Tokyo: 190–195, 1983.

23. Serruys PW, Lablanche JM, Reiber JHC, Bertrand ME, Hugenholtz PG: Contribution of dynamic vascular wall thickening to luminal narrowing during coronary arterial vasomotion. Z Kardiol 72: 116–123, 1983.

24. Brown BG, Bolson EL, Dodge HT: Arteriographic assessment of coronary atherosclerosis. Review of current methods, their limitations, and clinical applications. Arteriosclerosis 2: 2–15, 1982.

25. Logan SE: On the fluid mechanics of human coronary artery stenosis. IEEE Trans on Biomed Eng BME-22: 327–334, 1975.

26. Gould KL: Pressure-flow characteristics of coronary stenoses in unsedated dogs at rest and during coronary vasodilation. Circ Res 43: 245–253, 1978.

27. Marcus M, Wright C, Doty D, Eastham C, Laughlin D, Krumm P, Fastenow C, Brody M: Measurements of coronary velocity and reactive hyperemia in the coronary circulation of humans. Circ Res 49: 877–891, 1981.

28. Wilson RF, Hartley CJ, Laughlin DE, Marcus ML, White CW: Transluminal subselective measurement of coronary blood flow velocity and coronary vasodilator reserve in man. J Am Coll Cardiol 3: 529 (Abstract), 1984.

29. Ganz P, Gaspar G, Barry BH: Phasic coronary stenosis pressure gradients in man; correlations with arteriography. Circulation 68: III–164 (Abstract), 1983.

30. Leiboff R, Bren G, Katz R, Korkegi R, Ross A: Determinants of transstenotic gradients observed during angioplasty: an experimental model. Am J Cardiol 52: 1311–1317, 1983.

31. Vogel RA, Colfer HT, O'Neill WW, Walton JA, Aueron FM, Bates ER, Kirlin PC, LeFree MT, Pitt B: Correlations of arteriographically measured coronary cross-sectional area and coronary flow reserve with translesional gradient. J Am Coll Cardiol 1: 672 (Abstract), 1983.

32. Eng C, Patterson RE, Horowitz SF, Halgash DA, Pichard AD, Midwall J, Herman MV, Gorlin R: Coronary collateral function during exercise. Circulation 66: 309–316, 1982.

33. Rigo P, Becker LC, Griffith LSC, Alderson PO, Bailey IK, Pitt B, Burow RD, Wagner HN Jr: Influence of coronary collateral vessels on the results of thallium-201 myocardial stress imaging. Am J Cardiol 44: 452–458, 1979.

XXII. Quantitative coronary angiography in a lipid intervention study (The Leiden Diet Intervention Trial)

Summary

Postheparin lipoprotein lipase activities, lipid fractions and atherosclerosis linked hormones were studied in 35 male patients with advanced coronary artery disease, who participated in a two year diet only, lipid lowering intervention program, The Leiden Diet Intervention Trial. Sequential angiographies, one at the beginning of the trial and one two years later, were performed to assess the degree of progression or regression of the disease; the coronary angiograms were analyzed with the CAAS. In each patient film a total of nine coronary segments in the major coronary arteries were analyzed in at least two angiographic views. From the obstruction diameters and mean diameter values in nonobstructed segments, an absolute coronary score was derived. A patient was considered to have progressive disease, if the absolute coronary score showed a decrease over the study period. No lesion growth or regression of the disease was assumed if the coronary score showed an increase. Specific response patterns to dietary therapy were measured for total cholesterol, triglycerides, HDL cholesterol and the postheparin lipases, sex-, and thyroid hormones, insulin and cortisol.

At the termination of the study fourteen men showed no lesion growth or regression of atherosclerosis, whereas twenty-one men showed further progression of their underlying disease. Lipoprotein lipase (LPL) was not significantly different in the two groups studied, while liver lipase activity (LLA) was significantly lower ($p<0.01$) in the progression group ($314 \pm 166 \, \text{mU/ml}$) as compared to the no lesion growth group ($470 \pm 169 \, \text{mU/ml}$); LLA was inversely correlated with the degree of progression ($r = -0.601$, $p<0.01$). Cholesterol and triglycerides were higher and HDL cholesterol lower in the progression group as compared to the no lesion growth group. The measured hormones, testosterone, estradiol-17β, cortisol, insulin, thyroid stimulating hormone, thyroxine and T_3 resin uptake were not different between the two groups of patients. Triiodothyronine (T_3) appeared to be significantly higher in the no lesion growth group (2.34 ± 0.41 vs 1.78 ± 0.28). Linear regression analysis showed a poor correlation between LLA and T_3 ($r = 0.306$, $p = \text{n.s.}$). When the individual responses to dietary intervention were assessed, LLA appeared to be the only indicator of an inducibility of regression of atherosclerosis by dietary means only.

We infer from this study, in which for the first time a diet only therapy in coronary atherosclerosis was prescribed, in which sequential coronary angiograms were analyzed quantitatively and in which atherogenesis linked hormones, lipid fractions and lipoprotein lipases were measured, the following:

(a) Regression due to diet therapy only appears to be feasible.
(b) Liver lipase activity is a possible marker for the success of dietary intervention to induce a deceleration of the natural course of coronary atherosclerosis.
(c) Testosterone, estradiol, thyroxine, thyroid stimulating hormone, cortisol and insulin seem to be of no great additional importance, when lipid fractions are manipulated by dietary means to induce regression of coronary atherosclerosis. The triiodothyronine level seems to reflect the usage of beta blocking agents.

Introduction

Coronary atherosclerosis resulting in angina pectoris, myocardial infarction and sudden death remains a major contributor to the epidemic of cardiovascular disease in the industrialized world [1]. One of the major factors that determine the rate of development of progression of coronary atherosclerosis is a disordered lipid metabolism [2–5].

The total cholesterol (TC) is considered to be causal to coronary artery disease (CAD) for the reasons as stated by the WHO Expert Committee on the Prevention of Coronary Heart Disease [6]: 'The manifestation of its strength, graded character, consistency and independence, the demonstration that the trait precedes the disease; the coherence with clinical and experimental data; and the fact that logical mechanisms have been deliniated for the effect'.

The major lipid fraction within TC is the low density lipoprotein (LDL) fraction. This fraction has been implicated as the atherogenetic fraction, while another lipoprotein fraction, the high density lipoprotein (HDL), has been considered as anti-atherogenetic for many reasons, among these the inverse relation to coronary atherosclerosis and its clinical manifestations [7]. Modulators of lipoprotein metabolism, that codetermine the ratio between 'good' (HDL) and 'bad' (LDL) cholesterol are therefore of great importance. Postheparin lipoprotein lipase activities are important modulators in the process of atherosclerotic development [8–12]. Another group of factors that influence directly or indirectly this process are certain hormones, e.g. the sex, thyroid and stress hormones [13–17].

Until recently only more or less specific clinical manifestations of the atherosclerotic lesion growth, such as angina pectoris, acute myocardial infarction or sudden death, could be studied. It is also well-known that a direct positive relationship exists between the number of vessels diseased and the level of the ratio of total cholesterol and HDL cholesterol [18]. However, an accurate method to study growth or possibly regression of atherosclerotic plaques itself, which is strongly related in living human subjects to the clinical manifestations mentioned above, was unavailable.

Visual interpretation of sequential coronary angiographies was one method by means of which one has tried to measure directly the natural growth of coronary atherosclerosis in humans. By this means one did not want to wait for manifestations of atherosclerosis, but attempted to observe the process of growth itself. However, the method of visual interpretation is very much limited by the relatively large inter- and intraobserver variations in the judgement of the severity of the disease; these variations in itself are usually larger than the absolute anatomical changes present in the serial angiograms [19–21].

With the CAAS, differences in the atherosclerotic plaques between two sequential angiograms can be measured with high accuracy. To demonstrate the applicability and the value of the CAAS in such studies, the coronary angiograms in the Leiden Intervention Trial were measured with this system [22].

Methods

Patients

Thirty-five male patients with chronic stable angina pectoris who had undergone coronary arteriography to assess their suitability for coronary bypass grafting surgery were selected for the study after having been rejected for surgery for technical reasons [22]. They were offered to participate in a diet intervention study. At the end of the two year study period a repeat coronary arteriography was performed.

Although both sexes could be admitted according to the original design of the study, in practice only four women entered the study. As postheparin lipoprotein lipase activities and hormone levels differ between the sexes, only the 35 men who completed the study were ultimately evaluated. The study lasted from 1978 until 1982 and each patient was on dietary intervention for a period of 2 years, with – if needed – individual therapy for angina pectoris or hypertension.

All patients were seen monthly during the first half year at the outpatient clinic and bimonthly thereafter. They were seen by a cardiologist and a dietician for a total of fifteen times during the two year period. At each visit lipid fractions were measured, and a routine physical examination and dietary re-evaluation were performed.

Diet

A diet advice was given to all patients participating in the study and active encouragement to comply with this advice was also given to the partners of the patients. The diet was vegetarian with a total fat content of 33 energy(cal) percent (e%) with a low saturated fat content of 7.0 e%. It contained 100 mg cholesterol or less and was low caloric if appropriate. Adherence to the diet was assessed by the determination of the fatty acid content of cholesterol esters.

Dietary instruction was individualized and based on a 24 hour recall which was carried out in the first weeks following study admittance. Adherence to the diet was further checked by evaluation of the food consumed during a period of one week. Further measures that were undertaken to try to mitigate coronary risk factors were the following. Smoking was strongly discouraged. An advice to exercise at least half an hour daily was given. Hypertension (RR≥160/95 mmHg) if present, was treated with hygienic methods; if this failed, a step-up medication was prescribed consisting of beta-blocking agents, diuretics, and vasodilating drugs.

Biochemical measurements

Serum total cholesterol (TC) and HDL cholesterol (HDL-C) were determined at the Gaubius TNO Research Laboratory in Leiden in accordance with Abell's method [23]. HDL-C was isolated by precipitating other lipoproteins with magnesiumphosphotungstate; cholesterol was determined in the supernatant [24].

Baseline readings were defined by the mean values of the measurements on two different days prior to entry into the study; for the interpretation of the results due to the intervention, the mean values of the total of fifteen measurements performed over the following two years were determined.

Triglycerides were measured at the end of the study following an overnight fast in a basal resting state [25]. Also at the termination of the study, postheparin lipoprotein lipase activities – liver lipase activity (LLA) and lipoprotein lipase (LPL) – were measured as follows: Thirty minutes after introduction of an intravenous catheter in the right brachial vein, heparin* (50 IU/kg bodyweight) was administered intravenously. Blood was collected from the left brachial vein in disodium EDTA (2.7 mmol/l) on ice. Twenty minutes after the administration of heparin, blood was centrifuged at 4° C for 30 minutes at 3000 r.p.m. and plasma was stored at −20° C. LPL and LLA were measured at the Department of Internal Medicine III of the Erasmus University Rotterdam [26].

At the end of the study hormone measurements were performed in blood drawn 30 minutes after introduction of an intravenous catheter prior to heparin

---

*   Thromboliquine, Organon, Oss.

administration according to the following methods: cortisol* * (C), estradiol-17β (E2) [27], testosterone (T) [28], triiodothyronine (T_3) [29], thyroxine (T_4) [30], T_3-resin-uptake [29], thyroid stimulating hormone (TSH) [30], and insulin* * * (In).

Quantitative coronary arteriography

The coronary angiographic investigation was performed at the Department of Cardiology of Leiden University via the Judkins technique. The initial and sequential coronary arteriographies were performed by the same angiographer. At the second arteriography special care was taken to obtain projections identical to those of the first angiography. At the time of the first angiography the angulations of the X-ray systems in the different projections had been registered. Angiograms were recorded on 35 mm cinefilm using the 6 inch mode of a Philips image intensifier.

All patients had constant dose maintenance therapy with vasodilatory drugs (isosorbide-dinitrate and nifidipine), thereby reducing any possible effects on diameter measurements due to a change in vasomotor tone.

Quantitative analysis of coronary arterial segments was carried out with the CAAS at the Thoraxcenter in Rotterdam. An example of the quantitative analyses of the pre- and post-intervention coronary angiograms is shown in Figure XXII.1. The severity of a coronary obstruction was expressed as a percentage diameter reduction with respect to a user-defined reference position proximal or distal to the stenosis and by means of the absolute value of the minimal obstruction diameter. For arterial segments showing no focal obstruction the mean diameter value over a user-defined length was computed.

Cineframes to be analyzed were selected as closely as possible to the end-diastolic phase. In cases of overlap of a particular segment with other vessels, a frame was selected at another instant in time.

Coronary angiographic scoring method

The large coronary arteries were divided into a total of nine coronary segments according to the recommendations by the American Heart Association (right coronary artery: proximal, mid and distal portions; left anterior descending artery: proximal, mid and distal portions; left circumflex artery: proximal and distal portions; and the main-stem) [31]. These nine coronary segments were analyzed in at least two angiographic views.

* * I.R.E., Holland.
* * * I.M.C., Holland, MRC 66/304.

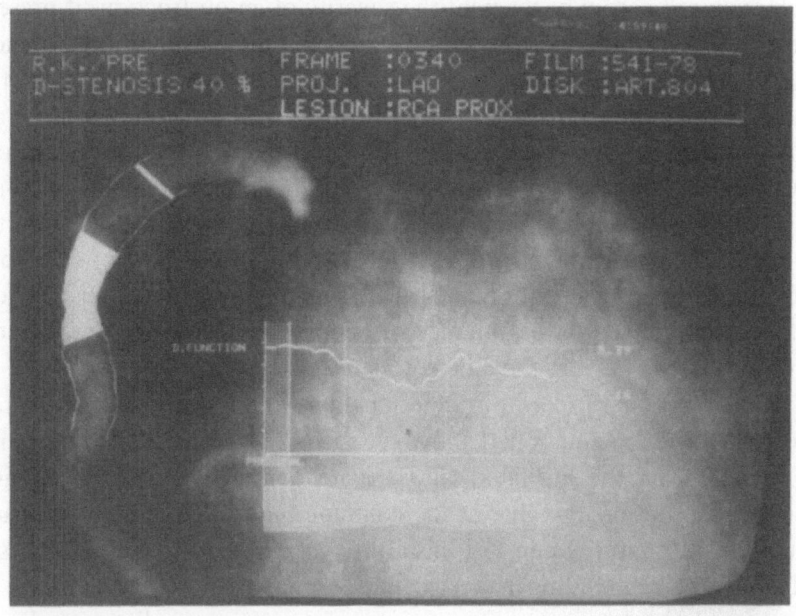

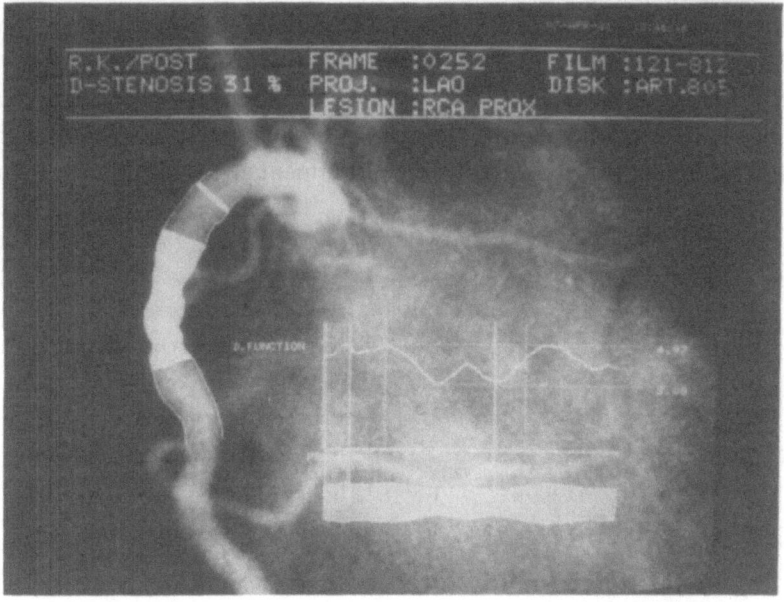

Fig. XXII.1. Example of quantitative results of one particular coronary segment (proximal part of right coronary artery) in the pre(upper photograph)- and post(lower photograph)-study situation. Note that a decrease of approximately 0.1 mm in the minimal obstruction diameter was found at the end of the study (obstruction diameter 3.08 mm) as compared to the initial situation (obstruction diameter 3.18 mm). Due to the fact that the reference diameter showed a larger decrease in size than the obstruction diameter, the percentage diameter stenosis decreased as well from 40% to 31%.

For each analyzed coronary segment the severity of an obstruction, if present, was computed in terms of relative and absolute measures; in addition, the mean diameters over the remaining normal proximal and distal parts were computed. From all data two coronary scores were derived, a percentage coronary score and an absolute coronary score; an example is given in Table XXII.1. The percentage score was determined as follows: for each obstruction the percentage area stenosis was computed from the percentages diameter stenoses assessed from two projections, assuming elliptical cross sections, and multiplied by a flow dependent weighting factor specific for that particular coronary segment [32]. The total percentage coronary score was obtained by adding these weighted area stenosis values for all obstructions in the nine coronary segments.

The absolute coronary score was determined as follows: for each of the four large coronary arteries mentioned above the mean obstruction diameter in mm was computed from the available views. If no obstruction was present in a coronary artery, the mean value of the computed average diameter measurements for the different segments of this artery was substituted. Adding these 4 mean diameter values resulted in the absolute coronary score. The changes in the percentage and absolute coronary scores over the two year diet period were simply determined as the differences in the pre- and post-diet coronary scores.

A patient was considered to have progressive disease, if the absolute coronary score showed a decrease. No lesion growth or regression of the disease was assumed if the coronary score showed an increase. Since we were particularly interested in changes of absolute dimensions of coronary obstructions and of nonobstructed segments, only absolute measurements were used for this study.

Statistical Analysis

Mean values and their standard deviations were used as descriptive statistics for the total group or subgroups of patients. Mean values were compared by the two sample t-test (two-sided) or when appropriate by paired t-tests. Relations between continuous variables were analyzed by linear regression analysis. All results are expressed as mean $\pm$ standard deviation (m $\pm$ s.d.). Multivariate analysis was performed by stepwise discriminant analysis [33].

Results

No significant difference was found in the initial coronary scores between the no lesion growth group of patients (N = 14) and the progression group (N = 21) (Table XXII.2); neither were weight, age, blood pressure or smoking habits significantly different. Persistance of anginal complaints in the progression group was much higher than in the no lesion growth group.

Table XXII.1. Example computation of percentage and absolute coronary scores.

| Analyzed lesion | | Percentage coronary score | | | | | |
| | | Pre-study | | | Post-study | | |
Branch	Section	%-A sten.	WF	Cor. score	% A-sten.	WF	Cor. score
RCA	mid 1	0.31	1.0	0.31	0.23	1.0	0.23
RCA	mid 2	0.15	1.0	0.15	0.39	1.0	0.39
RCA	mid 3	0.89	1.0	0.89	0.88	1.0	0.88
RCA	mid 4	0.87	1.0	0.87	0.78	1.0	0.78
LAD	prox	0.64	3.5	2.24	0.53	3.5	1.86
LAD	mid 1	0.93	2.5	2.33	0.91	2.5	2.28
LAD	mid 2	0.92	2.5	2.30	0.90	2.5	2.25
CX	dist 1	0.45	1.0	0.45	0.42	1.0	0.42
CX	dist 2	0.73	1.0	0.73	0.45	1.0	0.45
			Total	10.27		Total	9.54

Mean obstr. diameter	Pre	Post	Mean diameter. art.segm.	Pre	Post
RCA	2.50	2.11	RCA	3.59	3.54
MAIN	–	–	MAIN	4.66	4.27
LAD	1.65	1.75	LAD	2.77	2.80
CX	2.21	2.22	CX	3.42	3.01

Absolute coronary score (mm)	Pre	Post
RCA	2.50	2.11
MAIN	4.66	4.27
LAD	1.65	1.75
CX	2.21	2.22
Absol. score	11.02	10.35 +

Abbreviations: RCA: right coronary artery; LAD: left anterior descending artery; CX: circumflex artery; %-A sten: percentage area stenosis computed from the measured percentages diameter stenosis in two views; WF: flow dependent weighting factor.

In Table XXII.3 the pre- and post-study values of several lipid fractions and of the postheparin lipoprotein lipase activities are given for both groups of patients. At the start of the intervention trial total cholesterol (TC) was significantly higher in the progression group, while high density lipoprotein cholesterol (HDL-C) was the same in both groups. At the end of the study a significant difference was observed in the triglycerides (TG) values. TC levels showed a relatively larger drop in the progression group than in the no lesion growth group (although not

Table XXII.2. Clinical data and coronary scores in patients showing no lesion growth and those with progression of coronary atherosclerosis.

	No lesion growth group (N = 14)		Progression group (N = 21)	
Age (years; m ± s.d.)	49.8 ± 8.0		52.4 ± 7.8	
Number of patients	Pre-study	Post-study	Pre-study	Post-study
Smoking	9 (64%)	6 (42%)	10 (48%)	5 (23%)
Angina pectoris	14 (100%)	4 (28%)	21 (100%)	14 (67%)
Syst. BP (mmHg; mean)	130	124	131	128
Diast. BP (mmHg; mean)	83	80	85	85
Quetelet index (kg/m²; mean)	23.9	23.9	24.1	23.4
CS (mm; mean ± s.d.)	10.17 ± 1.72	11.14 ± 1.79	10.38 ± 2.29	9.17 ± 2.12
△CS (mm; mean ± s.d)	+1.02 ± 0.69		−1.20 ± 0.96	

Abbreviations: N, number of patients; BP, blood pressure; CS, coronary score; △CS, the difference (mm) in absolute coronary scores between the pre- and post-study angiograms.

significant). Liver lipase activity (LLA) in the progression group was significantly lower than in the no lesion growth group of patients, while lipoprotein lipase (LPL) was not different in the two groups of patients. LLA was inversely correlated with the degree of progression in the total population (Fig. XXII.2). LPL did not show any significant linear regression relation to the changes in coronary scores of the total population. Multivariate stepwise discriminant analy-

Table XXII.3. Serum lipids and lipases in patients showing no lesion growth and those with progression of coronary atherosclerosis.

	No lesion growth group (N = 14)		Progression group (N = 23)	
	Pre-study	Post-study	Pre-study	Post-study
TC	6.37 ± 1.05 – * –	5.80 ± 1.03	7.22 ± 1.57 – * –	6.43 ± 1.55
HDL-C	1.00 ± 0.15	1.01 ± 0.19	0.99 ± 0.23	0.96 ± 0.11
TG		1.59 ± 1.14		2.02 ± 1.04*
LLA		470 ± 169		314 ± 166**
LPL		86 ± 36		87 ± 34

(TC row: p<0.05 between no lesion growth pre-study and progression pre-study; p<0.05 between post-study values)

Abbreviations: TC: total cholesterol (normal values: 4.5–8.0 mmol/l); HDL-C: high density lipoprotein cholesterol (normal values: 0.80–1.20 mmol/l); TG: triglycerides (normal values: 0.50–2.50 mmol/l); LLA: liver lipase activity (mU/ml) (normal values: 472 ± 127); LPL: lipoprotein lipase (mU/ml) (normal values: 87 ± 32); 1mU: mmoles free fatty acids released/min. All values are mean ± s.d.; *p<0.05; **p<0.01.

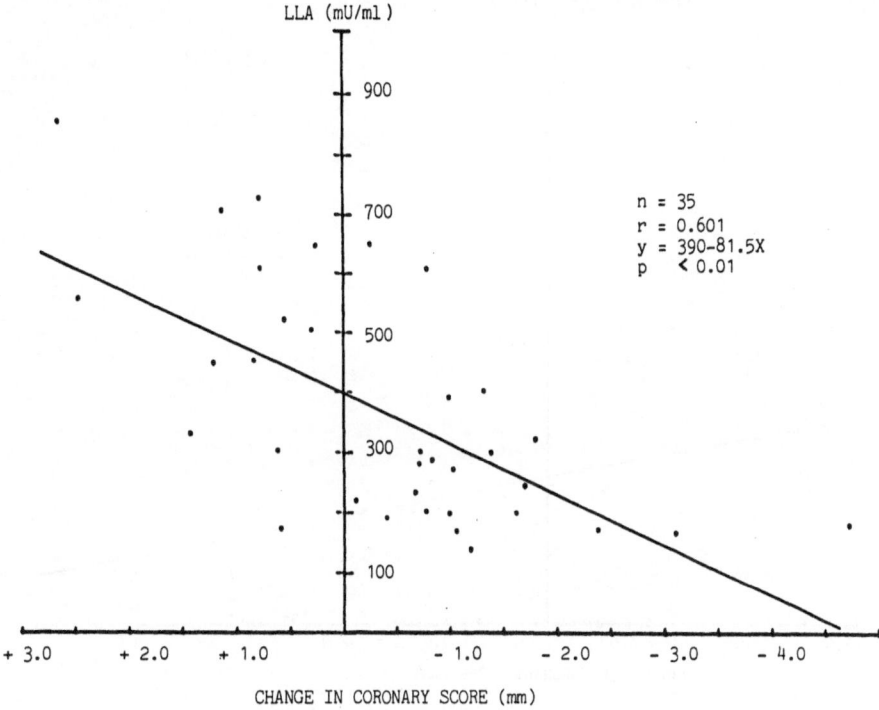

LLA (mU/ml)

n = 35
r = 0.601
y = 390–81.5X
p < 0.01

CHANGE IN CORONARY SCORE (mm)

Fig. XXII.2. This figure shows the relationship between the change in absolute coronary score (mm) and liver lipase activity at the end of the study period. LLA = liver lipase activity (mU/ml). 1 mU: mmoles free fatty acids released/min.

sis showed LLA to be the strongest parameter to progression or regression of atherosclerosis, independently from other pre- or post-study parameters (TC, HDL-C, TG). The change in the degree of coronary atherosclerosis expressed in terms of differences in absolute coronary scores, was not related to the change in TC or to the change in the TC to HDL-C ratio ($r = -0.196$) (Fig. XXII.3).

Table XXII.4 shows the absence of any significant difference in basal cortisol, estradiol-17β, testosterone and insulin values between the no lesion growth and progression groups of patients. Similarly, there were no significant differences in thyroid hormone values as indicated by thyroxine, T_3-resin-uptake and the thyroid stimulating hormone between these two groups of patients (Table XXII.5). However, triiodothyronine (T_3), another thyroid hormone, appeared to be significantly ($p<0.01$) higher in the no lesion growth group, although T_3 remained within the normal ranges for both groups. Linear regression analysis showed a poor correlation between LLA and T_3 ($r = 0.306$, $p = $ n.s.).

When the total male population was categorized according to the lipid lowering effects of the diet, three response patterns became apparent (Table XXII.6). The group (N = 15 patients) with an initial low TC to HDL-C ratio (<6.9) remained so during dietary treatment; this behavior was accompanied by a high LLA value.

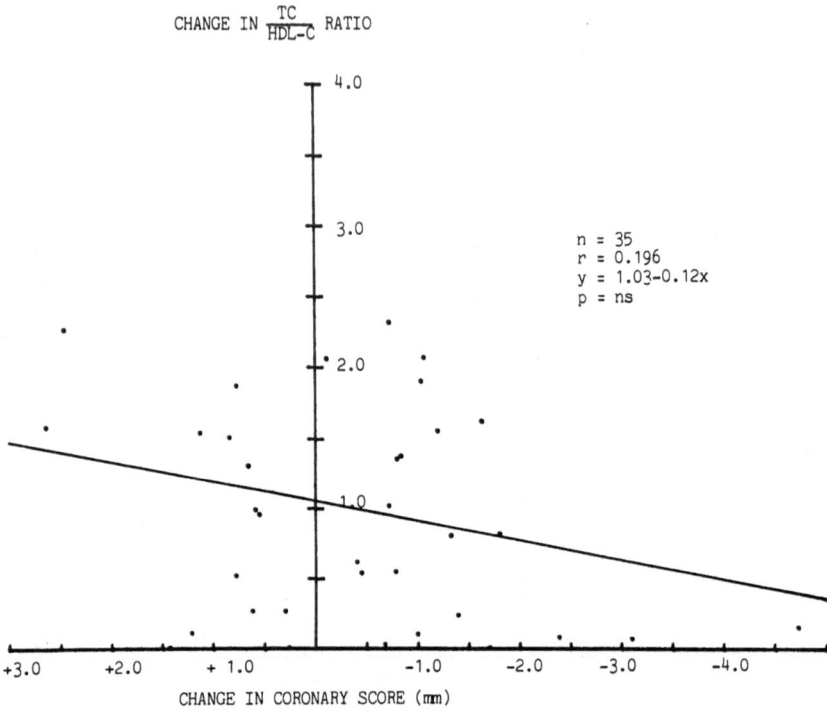

CHANGE IN $\frac{TC}{HDL-C}$ RATIO

n = 35
r = 0.196
y = 1.03-0.12x
p = ns

CHANGE IN CORONARY SCORE (mm)

Fig. XXII.3. In this figure the relationship between the change in absolute coronary scores (mm) and the change in the ratio of total cholesterol (TC) to HDL-C from baseline values is shown. HDL-C = high density lipopotein cholesterol (mmol/l).

The second group (N = 11 patients) showed an initial high value of the TC of HDL-C ratio (>6.9), which was nonresponsive to the diet, and a low LLA value. Of particular interest is the third group (N = 9 patients) in which an initial high TC to HDL-C ratio (>6.9) fell to below 6.9 in reaction to the dietary intervention, while the LLA was as high as in the first mentioned group of patients. LPL was not different in these three groups of patients showing different responses to dietary intervention.

Table XXII.4. Insulin, sex hormones and cortisol in the no lesion growth and progression groups of patients.

	No lesion growth group (N = 14)	Progression group (N = 21)
Testosterone (nmol/l)	23.6 ± 12.0	22.3 ± 10.6
Estradiol − 17 (pmol/l)	118 ± 37	129 ± 31
Cortisol (nmol/l)	455 ± 97	479 ± 138
Insulin (mU/l)	12.4 ± 1.3	13.9 ± 1.9

All values: mean ± s.d.

Table XXII.5. Thyroid hormone values in the no lesion growth and progression groups of patients.

	No lesion growth group (N = 14)	Progression group (N = 21)
T_3 (nmol/l)	2.34 ± 0.41	1.78 ± 0.28*
T_4 (nmol/l)	103 ± 16	111 ± 17
T_3-resin-uptake (%)	27.8 ± 2.5	27.1 ± 2.9
TSH (mU/ml)	1.9 ± 2.5	2.4 ± 2.8

Abbreviations: T_3, Triiodothyronine; T_4, Thyroxine; TSH, Thyroid Stimulating Hormone. All values: mean ± s.d.; *$p<0.01$.

The values of the endocrine parameters in relation to the three different response patterns are given in Table XXII.7. No specific major effect on dietary lowering of TC could be found for insulin, estradiol-17β, testosterone, cortisol, tyroxine, T_3-resin-uptake and the thyroid stimulating hormone. In the group of patients that were responsive to the dietary intervention triiodothyronine was higher than in both other groups.

Table XXII.8 shows the average initial coronary score values and the mean changes over the study period for the three different lipid lowering patterns.

Table XXII.6. Dietary lipid lowering effects on the postheparin lipoprotein lipase activities and on the lipid fractions.

TC/HDL ratio					
Initial value	>6.9		>6.9		<6.9
Value during study	<6.9		>6.9		<6.9
	(N = 9)		(N = 11)		(N = 15)
TC/HDL-C	6.20 ± 0.70	*	8.38 ± 1.09	**	5.10 ± 0.72
			$p<0.05$		
TG	1.21 ± 0.54	*	2.46 ± 1.04	*	1.13 ± 0.42
			n.s.		
LLA	380 ± 149	*	244 ± 104	**	426 ± 144
			n.s.		
LPL	85 ± 38	n.s.	78 ± 20	n.s.	89 ± 23
			n.s.		

Abbreviations: TC, total cholesterol (mmol/l); HDL-C, high density lipoprotein cholesterol (mmol/l); TG, triglycerides (mmol/l); LLA, liver lipase activity (mU/ml); LPL, lipoprotein lipase (mU/ml); 1 mU, mmoles free fatty acids released/min. All values: mean ± s.d.; n.s., not significant; *, $p<0.01$; ** $p<0.001$.

Table XXII.7. Dietary lipid lowering effects and endocrine parameters.

TC/HDL ratio			
Initial value	>6.9	>6.9	>6.9
Value during study	<6.9	>6.9	<6.9
	(N = 9)	(N = 11)	(N = 15)
In (mU/l)	11.2 ± 1.4	13.7 ± 2.9	14.3 ± 40
		⌊————— $p<0.05$ —————⌋	
E2 (pmol/l)	114 ± 37	120 ± 38	124 ± 4.3
T (nmol/l)	19.6 ± 4.2	18.0 ± 75	19.9 ± 4.3
C (nmol/l)	398 ± 89	480 ± 134	472 ± 121
T_3 (nmol/l)	2.2 ± 0.4 *	1.7 ± 0.2	1.9 ± 0.9
		⌊——————— * ———————⌋	
T_4 (nmol/l)	109 ± 1.9	109 ± 24	106 ± 16
T_3-resin uptake (%)	26.1 ± 2.6	28.8 ± 2.9	28.1 ± 2.7
TSH (mU/l)	2.2 ± 2.4	1.0 ± 2.6	1.8 ± 2.0

Abbreviations: In, Insulin; E2, Estradiol-17β; T, Testosterone; C, Cortisol; T_3, Triiodothyronine; T_4, Thyroxine; TSH, Thryoid Stimulating Hormone; All values: mean ± s.d. *, $p<0.01$; Other relations were all nonsignificant.

Discussion

Although this study is hampered by the fact that no pre-study endocrine and postheparin lipoprotein lipase activities were available, the following conclusions may be drawn taking into account comparable data from other studies [34]:

Firstly, in the presence of advanced coronary atheroclerosis, progression of the disease i.e. its natural progressive course, apparently may be halted or even reversed by dietary intervention.

Secondly, LLA and not LPL is negatively correlated to the degree of progression of coronary atherosclerosis, suggesting a key role for the former enzyme

Table XXII.8. Dietary lipid lowering effect and the initial average coronary score and the changes therein over the study period.

TC/HDL ratio			
Initial value	>6.9	>6.9	<6.9
Value during study	<6.9	>6.9	<6.9
	(N = 9)	(N = 11)	(N = 15)
Average initial coronary score	10.88 ± 1.52 n.s.	10.71 ± 1.40 $p<0.05$	9.64 ± 1.92
		⌊————— $p<0.05$ —————⌋	
Mean change in mm	+0.38	−1.09	+0.07
Range of changes	(−1.09, +2.47)	(−3.10, +0.26)	(−1.25, +2.05)

All values: mean ± s.d.

[35]. The levels of all analyzed hormones, with the exception of T_3 were not different when the no lesion growth group was compared to the progression group.

With respect to the first conclusion, it should be noticed that although the two groups studied were comparable with respect to complaints, age, weight, biochemical status and lipid profile (except for a initial slightly higher TC-value in the progression group), it cannot be excluded that the two groups of patients differed in other parameters. The interpretation of the results from this study is also limited to some extent by the lack of a control group.

However, as has been shown before, coronary atherosclerosis is an almost unequivocally progressive disease and therefore any evidence of nonprogression may be considered as an indication of a deviation from the natural course of the disease [36, 37]. Difficulties in quantitative evaluation of atherosclerosis have been described elsewhere [38, 39].

The purpose of this study was threefold:
(1) To assess the relationship between the diet induced changes in lipid values and the progression of coronary atherosclerosis.
(2) To assess the relationship between the postheparin lipoprotein lipase activities and the progression of coronary atherosclerosis on the one hand and the diet induced lipid value changes on the other hand.
(3) To assess the role of several atherosclerosis related hormones and the progression of coronary atherosclerosis.

Concerning the first question, a clear and powerful positive relationship has been established between diet (the amount of cholesterol and poly-unsaturated fatty acids) and lipid level changes and the rate of progression of coronary atherosclerosis [22]. As has been stated before, the postheparin lipoprotein lipase activities are important modulators in lipid metabolism determining to a certain degree the ratio between 'good' HDL and 'bad' LDL cholesterol.

To study the possible relationship between LLA and LPL, and the degree of change of coronary atherosclerosis in men with advanced atherosclerosis, a lowered LLA and a normal LPL level may be assumed for the reasons mentioned before [34]. This seems valid as the initial coronary atherosclerotic values, expressed in terms of coronary scores, were essentially not different (Table XXII.2). As may be derived from the results, LLA was significantly higher in the no lesion growth group of patients but still within the normal range, independently from all other lipoprotein parameters including LPL (Table XXII.3).

The results may suggest a possible threshold value for cholesterol for the induction of nonprogression of advanced coronary atherosclerosis; this is based on the fact that the decrease in TC level in the progression group was even larger than in the no lesion growth group (Table XXII.3). A lowered LLA may impair the mobilization of TC from peripheral cells by HDL by hampering with the excretion of cholesterol in the liver to be converted to bile acids. Therefore, a lowered LLA may contribute to a higher cholesterol pool and as a result contribute to the progression of atherosclerosis.

Although LLA was only measured at the end of the study, results clearly demonstrate that those patients that responded to diet with a lowering of the TC values, show no further lesion growth or possibly even regression. This may indicate those patients that may benefit from the prescribed diet and those who do not. In the future a period of only three to six months may be sufficient to discriminate those who may profit from diet alone and those who do not by measuring the LLA level, although this requires further study.

It is of interest to note that those patients with an initial and continuing low TC/HDL-C ratio, had the lowest coronary scores, hence the most extensive atherosclerotic disease (Table XXII.8). Since they did not appear to be the patients with the greatest tendency to regression of the atheroclerotic process, as measured by the average change (mm) in coronary scores, other factors besides the lipoprotein lipase, have to be assumed (Table XXII.8).

The Leiden Intervention Trial showed that LLA measured following dietary intervention is strongly correlated to changes in coronary atherosclerotic lesion size (Fig. XXII.2). However, whether a causal relationship may be assumed between LLA and the changes observed cannot be concluded from these data. A strong relationship between the changes in TC/HDL-C ratio and those in the coronary scores was not observed (Fig. XXII.3).

As far as the third question concerning endocrine parameters is concerned, a differentiation must be made between the various possibly atherosclerotic growth related hormones and the progression of coronary atherosclerosis. Diabetes mellitus or abnormal levels of insulin (relative or absolute) are correlated to accelleration of progression of coronary atherosclerosis [40]. Cortisol, the main adrenal cortical stress hormone, is also positively related to the rate of progression of coronary atherosclerosis [41]. No significant difference between the groups mentioned could be established at the end of our study, suggesting that no important role for both of these atherogenic hormones exists (Table XXII.4).

Estradiol-17β (E2) has been considered to be anti-atherogenic and was even administered in pharmacologic doses in the Coronary Drug Project [42], but was later withdrawn for reasons that in those patients receiving estradiol a significantly higher percentage suffered sudden death. Nevertheless, E2 which in men is mainly derived from testosterone (T), is known to show a positive correlation to the degree of coronary atheroclerosis [43]. Our study showed that after two years of dietary intervention no significant difference could be found in E2 and T values between the no lesion growth and the progression groups (Table XXII.4).

Of particular interest is thyroid hormone action in relation to atherosclerosis. The TC measurement used to be a marker for the metabolic state. When TC was high, a low thyroid function was presumed [44]. Although it is well-known that in hypothyroidism coronary atherosclerosis is severe, a clear benefit from thyroxine administration has not been shown to benefit a general population. The Coronary Drug Project even withdrew thyroxine administration as therapeutic drug after the establishment of severe side effects in coronary atherosclerosis [45].

Nevertheless, it is of interest to derive from the results that patients showing no lesion growth apparently have a normal although higher metabolic state than the progression group patients, as measured by T_3 levels (Table XXII.5). A possible explanation may be that at the end of the study, those patients showing progression were using beta blocking agents to a greater extent than the patients from the no lesion growth group, signaling the fact that more patients in the first group suffered angina pectoris. As all patients were suffering from angina at the beginning of the study and were taking beta blocking agents, only those patients that did not respond to dietary treatment and showed further progression of their disease were finally in need of beta blocking agents to alleviate their symptoms. As beta blocking agents inhibit the conversion of T_4 to T_3, this may explain to some degree the higher metabolic state of these patients in the no lesion growth group as compared to the progression group.

Finally, it may be concluded from this study, that the levels of insulin, cortisol, estradiol, testosterone or of the thyroid hormones, with the exception of T_3, were not essentially different in the no lesion growth and progression groups, suggesting no major atherogenetic modulating effect of these hormones.

References

1. Pyörälä K, Epstein FH, Korentzer M: Changing trends in coronary heart disease mortality; possible explanations. S Karger Berlin, 1985.
2. Lipid Research Clinics Program: The Lipid Research Clinics Coronary Primary Prevention Trial Results. I. Reduction in incidence of coronary heart disease. JAMA 251: 351–364, 1984.
   Lipid Research Clinics Program. The Lipid Research Clinics Coronary Primary Prevention Trial Results. II. The relationship of reduction in incidence of coronary heart disease to cholesterol lowering. JAMA 251: 365–374, 1984.
3. Consensus Conference. Lowering blood cholesterol to prevent heart disease. JAMA 253: 2080–2086, 1985.
4. Levy RI: Cholesterol and disease – what are the facts? JAMA 248: 2888–2890, 1982.
5. Glueck CJ: Relationship of lipid disorders to coronary heart disease. Am J Med 74 (No. 5A): 10–14, 1983.
6. Report of a WHO Expert Committee: Prevention of coronary heart disease. Technical Report Series 678, World Health Organization, Geneva: 14–24, 1982.
7. Levy RI: Cholesterol, lipoproteins, apoproteins and heart disease: present status and future prospects. Clin Chem 27: 653–662, 1981.
8. Nilsson-Ehle P, Garfinkel AS, Schotz MC: Lipolytic enzymes and plasma lipoprotein metabolism. Ann Rev Biochem 49: 667–693, 1980.
9. Jansen H, Hülsmann WC: Heparin-releasable (liver) lipase(s) may play a role in the uptake of cholesterol by steroid-secreting tissues. Trends in Biochemical Sciences: 265–268, 1980.
10. Nikkilä EA: Metabolic regulation of plasma high density lipoprotein concentrations. Eur J Clin Invest 8: 111–113, 1978.
11. Kekki M: Lipoprotein-lipase action determining plasma high density lipoprotein cholesterol level in adult normolipaemics. Atherosclerosis 37: 143–150, 1980.
12. Jansen H, Tol A van, Hülsmann WC: On the metabolic function of heparin-releasable liver lipase. Biochem Biophys Res Commun 92: 53–59, 1980.

424

13. Phillips GB: Sex hormones, risk factors and cardiovascular disease. Am J Med 65: 7–11, 1978.
14. Tunbridge WMG, Evered DC, Hall R, Appleton D, Brewis M, Clark F, Grimley Evans J, Young E, Bird T, Smith PA: The spectrum of thyroid disease in a community: The Whickham survey. Clin Endocrinol 7: 481–493, 1977.
15. Raziel A, Rosenzweig B, Botvinic V, Beigel I, Landau B, Blum I: The influence of thyroid function on serum lipid profile. Atherosclerosis 41: 321–326, 1982.
16. Schwertner HA, Troxler RG, Uhl GS, Jackson WG: Relationship between cortisol and cholesterol in men with coronary artery disease and type A behavior. Arteriosclerosis 4: 59–64, 1984.
17. Luria MH, Johnson MW, Pego R, Seuc CA, Manubens SJ, Wieland MR, Wieland RG: Relationship between sex hormones, myocardial infarction, and occlusive coronary disease. Arch Intern Med 142: 42–44, 1982.
18. Jenkins PJ, Harper RW, Nestel PJ: Severity of coronary atherosclerosis related to lipoprotein concentration. Brit Med J 2: 388–391, 1978.
19. Zir LM, Miller SW, Dinsmore RE, Gilbert JP, Harthorne JW: Interobserver variability in coronary angiography. Circulation 53: 627–632, 1976.
20. De Rouen TA, Murray JA, Owen W: Variability in the analysis of coronary arteriograms. Circulation 55: 324–328, 1977.
21. Detre KM, Wright E, Murphy ML, Takaro T: Observer agreement in evaluating coronary angiograms. Circulation 52: 979–986, 1975.
22. Arntzenius AC, Kromhout D, Barth JD, Reiber JHC, Bruschke AVG, Buis B, Gent CM van, Kempen-Voogd N, Strikwerda S, Velde EA van der: Diet, lipoproteins, and the progression of coronary atherosclerosis. The Leiden Intervention Trial. N Eng J Med 312: 805–811, 1985.
23. Abell LL, Levy BB, Brodie BB, Kendall FE: A simplified method for the estimation of total cholesterol in serum and demonstration of its specificity. J Biol Chem 195: 357–366, 1952.
24. Lopes-Virella MF, Stone P, Ellis S, Colwell JA: Cholesterol determination in high-density lipoproteins separated by three different methods. Clin Chem 23: 882–884, 1977.
25. Wahlefeld AW: Triglycerids determination after enzymatic hydrolysis. In: Methods in enzymatic analysis Vol. D. HU Bergmayer (Ed.). Academic Press New York N.Y.: 1831, 1974.
26. Huttunen JK, Ehnholm C, Kinnunen PK, Nikkilä EA: An immunochemical method for the selective measurement of two triglyceride lipases in human postheparin plasma. Clin Chim Acta 63: 335–347, 1975.
27. Murphy BEP: Some studies of the protein-binding of steroids and their applications to the routine micro and ultramicro measurement of various steroids in body fluids by competitive protein-binding radioassay. J Clin Endocr 27: 973–990, 1967.
28. Jong FH de, Hey AH, Molen HJ van der: Oestradiol-17β and testosterone in rat testis tissue: effect of gonado-trophins, localization and production in vitro. J Endocr 60: 409–419, 1974.
29. Docter R, Hennemann G, Bernard H: A radioimmunoassay for measurement of T_3 in serum. Israel J Med Sci 8: 1870 (Abstract), 1972.
30. Visser TJ, Hout-Goemaat NL van den, Docter R, Hennemann G: Radio-immunoassay of thyroxine in unextracted serum. Neth J Med 18: 111–115, 1975.
31. Austen WG, Edwards JE, Frye RL, Gensini GG, Gott VL, Griffith LSC, McGoon DC, Murphy ML, Roe BB: A reporting system on patients evaluated for coronary artery disease: Report of the Ad Hoc Committee for Grading of Coronary Artery Disease, Council on Cardiovascular Surgery. American Heart Association, 1975. Circulation 51-2: 7–40, 1975.
32. Leaman DM, Brower RW, Meester GT, Serruys P, Brand M van den: Coronary artery atherosclerosis: severity of the disease, severity of angina pectoris and compromised left ventricular function. Circulation 63: 285–292, 1981.
33. BMPD statistical software: University of California Press, Berkeley, U.S.A.
34. Barth JD, Jansen H, Hugenholtz PG, Birkenhäger JC: Post-heparin lipases, lipids and related hormones in men undergoing coronary arteriography to assess atheroclerosis. Atherosclerosis 48: 235–241, 1983.

35. Hülsmann WC, Jansen H: High myocardial and low hepatic lipoprotein lipase activities responsible for the initiation of atherosclerosis. Biochem Med 13: 293–297 (Letter to the Editor), 1975.

36. Bruschke AVG, Wijers ThS, Kolsters W, Landmann J: The anatomic evolution of coronary artery disease demonstrated by coronary arteriography in 256 nonoperated patients. Circulation 63: 527–536, 1981.

37. Proudfit WL, Bruschke AVG, Sones FM Jr: Natural history of obstructive coronary artery disease: ten-year study of 601 nonsurgical cases. Prog Cardiovasc Dis 21: 53–78, 1978.

38. Brown BG, Bolson EL, Dodge HT: Arteriographic assessment of coronary atherosclerosis. Review of current methods, their limitations and clinical applications. Arteriosclerosis 2: 2–15, 1982.

39. Chandler AB, Bond MG, Insull W Jr, Glagov S, Cornhill JF, Barnes RW, Greenleaf JF, Daoud AS, Newman III WP, Blankenhorn DH: Quantitative evaluation of atherosclerosis. Arteriosclerosis 3: 183–186, 1983.

40. Stout RW: The relationship of abnormal circulating insulin levels to atherosclerosis. Arteriosclerosis 27: 1–13, 1977.

41. Troxler RG, Sprague EA, Albanese RA, Fuchs R, Thompson AJ: The association of elevated plasma cortisol and early atherosclerosis as demonstrated by coronary angiography. Atherosclerosis 26: 151–162, 1977.

42. The Coronary Drug Project Research Group: The Coronary Drug Project. Clofibrate and Niacin in coronary heart disease. JAMA 231: 360–381, 1975.

43. Phillips GB: Evidence for hyperoestrogenaemias as a risk factor for myocardial infarction in men. Lancet 2: 14–18, 1976.

44. Blumgart HL, Freedberg AS, Kurland GS: Hypercholesterolemia, Myxedema and Atherosclerosis. Am J Med 14: 665–673, 1953.

45. The Coronary Drug Project Research Group: The Coronary Drug Project. Findings leading to further modifications of its protocol with respect to Dextrothyroxine. JAMA 220: 996–1008, 1972.

XXIII. Asynchrony in regional filling dynamics as a consequence of uncoordinated segmental contraction during coronary transluminal occlusion

Summary

The effects of brief periods of a major coronary artery occlusion on the global and regional peak filling rates were studied during angioplasty in 14 patients. None had had a previous myocardial infarction. High-fidelity left ventricular pressure and volume (by angiography) were obtained before, 20 and 50 seconds after the onset of transluminal coronary occlusion and shortly after the last balloon inflation. Segmental wall motion was analyzed frame-by-frame along 20 hemiaxes. Global peak filling rate decreased significantly both after 20 (-25%; $p<.05$) and 50 seconds (-24%; $p<.05$) from the onset of the occlusion. The term $\sum \triangle t_1$ was defined as the sum of the absolute values of the time differences from the occurrence of global peak filling rate and the segmental peak filling rate, in 20 segments. This parameter increased significantly during both periods of transluminal occlusion (by 64%; $p<.005$ and by 54%; $p<.005$, respectively) thus indicating an asynchrony in the occurrence of regional peak filling rate. Simultaneously, the sum of time intervals between the aortic valve closure (end systole) and the occurrence of peak segmental shortening, $\sum \triangle t_2$, measured in the 20 segments, increased to a similar extent, thus demonstrating an asynchrony in segmental contraction. A significant, negative correlation was found between the global peak filling rate and both $\sum \triangle t_1$ and $\sum \triangle t_2$ ($r = -.68$; $p<.0001$ and $r = -.73$; $p<.0001$, respectively). Our findings suggest that during coronary transluminal occlusion an early asynchrony in regional peak filling rate occurs which is strictly related to a delayed and asynchronous peak segmental shortening.

Introduction

It is well known, that in patients with coronary artery disease, abnormalities may occur in left ventricular filling dynamics, even in the presence of normal systolic function [1–4]. Recently, the relationship between the regional and global filling has been investigated in patients with one vessel disease using radionuclide angiography; an asynchrony in diastolic filling of the ischemic regions in the absence of regional systolic dyshomogeneity was reported [5, 6].

We previously observed that transient ischemia induced by luminal occlusion of a major coronary artery during percutaneous transluminal angioplasty (PTCA) caused a shift in timing of the peak inward wall displacement of the ischemic segments from end systole to early diastole [7]. In order to investigate the relationship, if any, between such temporal nonuniformity of contraction and abnormalities in filling dynamics during ischemia, we studied regional wall displacement in systole and diastole during transient ischemia induced by balloon inflation at PTCA.

Materials and methods

Study population

After a preliminary study to confirm the absence of effects of nonionic contrast media (metrizamide-Amipaque®) on left ventricular function, permission was obtained from the Thoraxcenter Ethics Committee to perform left ventricular angiography during balloon inflation at PTCA. All patients involved in the study gave informed consent and no complications related to the research procedure occurred. Fourteen patients with coronary artery disease undergoing PTCA, with the following selection criteria, were studied:
(1) isolated, obstructive lesion in one coronary artery (in ten patients in the left anterior descending artery, in three patients in the right coronary artery and in one patient in the left circumflex artery), without angiographically demonstrable collateral circulation.
(2) normal left ventricular wall motion at rest, as determined from prior diagnostic catheterization.
(3) no intraventricular conduction abnormalities on the resting ECG.
Four patients had mild essential hypertension and an elevated left ventricular end-diastolic pressure ($\geqslant 25$ mmHg). Standard anti-anginal therapy was allowed until the day of the study. An evaluation of the systolic function in the same series of patients had been reported previously [7].

Study protocol

Left ventricular pressure was recorded during ventriculography (30° right anterior oblique view at 50 frames/second) carried out before balloon dilatation, at a mean occlusion time of 20 seconds during the second dilatation, at a mean occlusion time of 48 seconds during the fourth dilatation and at a mean of 12 minutes after the last dilatation. Angiography during the fourth dilatation was performed in only 9 patients. A total of 3 to 10 occlusions were performed and the duration of balloon inflation ranged from 15 to 75 seconds. Each consecutive balloon inflation was made only when end-diastolic pressure and left ventricular pressure-derived isovolumic parameters of contractility and relaxation, which were available on line during the procedure [8, 9], had returned to basal values. Care was taken to maintain the patient's position relative to the X-ray equipment during sequential angiograms which were performed with the patient helding his/her breath in shallow inspiration.

Analysis of pressure and pressure-derived indices

Left ventricular pressure was measured with a tipmanometer on an 8 F pigtail catheter and digitized at 250 samples/sec, allowing a beat-to-beat analysis. End-diastolic pressure was defined as that point on the pressure trace at which the derivative of the pressure first exceeded 200 mmHg/sec; end systole or aortic valve closure was assumed to occur simultaneously with the dicrotic notch on the central aortic pressure. Details regarding the off-line analysis of pressure – derived indices of relaxation used in our laboratory have been published previously [7, and Ch. XVIII]. The isovolumic relaxation period was defined as the time interval between the aortic valve closure and the mitral valve opening. This latter was defined during left ventriculography, as occurring in the last frame preceding the entry of nonopacified blood into the left ventricle from the left atrium. The left ventricular pressure corresponding to this frame was considered to reflect left atrial pressure [10].

Analysis of regional and global left ventricular function

A complete cardiac cycle was analyzed frame-by-frame from each angiogram with the Contouromat. Over a full cardiac cycle, beginning at end diastole, segmental wall displacement was determined in the 20 segments, 10 in the anterior and 10 in the infero-posterior wall. Peak segmental inward and outward velocity was computed as the first-derivative relative to time of the segmental wall displacement after a 3-points smoothing had been applied to the data (Fig. XXIII.1). Peak ejection rate was taken as the peak negative dV/dt value after end diastole; peak global filling rate as the peak dV/dt value after mitral valve opening, and the time to peak filling rate was the time interval between the aortic valve closure and the moment of peak dV/dt. The time interval was measured between the occurrence of the global peak filling rate and the peak velocity of segmental outward displacement (Fig. XXIII.2). We defined $\sum \Delta t_i$ as the sum of the absolute values of the time differences between global peak filling rate and

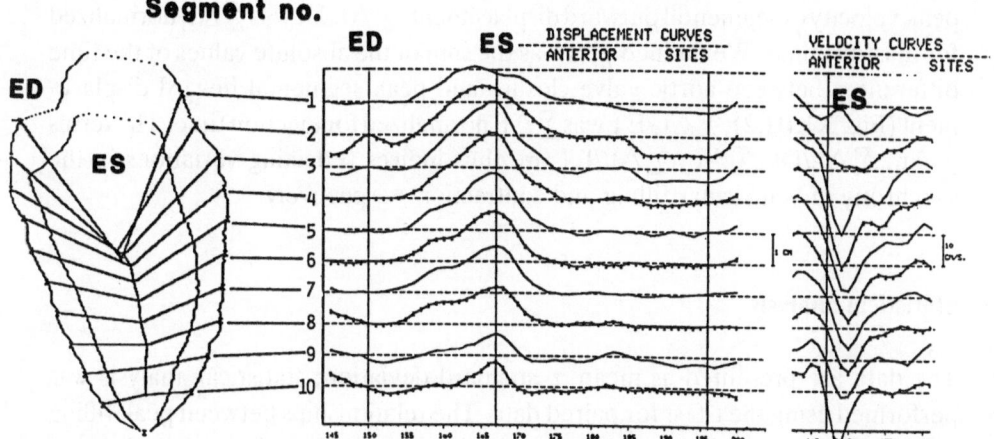

Fig. XXIII.1. Example of computer output showing the end-diastolic and end-systolic contours of the 30° RAO left ventriculography. Left ventricular segmental wall displacement is determined along a system of coordinates derived from endocardial landmark trajectories in normal individuals and is studied in 20 separate segments, 10 in the anterior and 10 in the infero-posterior wall. Left ventricular wall velocity, the first-derivative of wall displacement, is derived from these data.

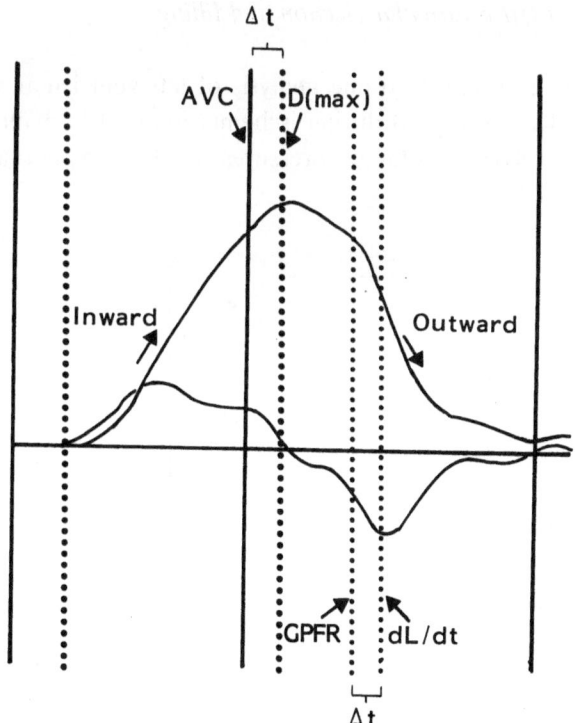

Fig. XXIII.2. Segmental wall displacement and its first-derivative are superimposed to show the temporal relationship between inward and outward phases with the moment of aortic valve closure (AVC). The time intervals (△t) between AVC and the maximal inward wall displacement (Dmax), and between the occurrence of global peak filling rate (GPFR) and the peak velocity of outward displacement (dL/dt) were measured in every segment.

peak velocity of segmental outward displacement; $\sum \triangle t_1/Dt$ was $\sum \triangle t_1$ normalized for diastolic time. We defined $\sum \triangle t_2$ as the sum of the absolute values of the time differences between aortic valve closure and peak segmental inward displacement (Fig. XXIII.2); $\sum \triangle t_2/ET$ was $\sum \triangle t_2$ normalized for ejection time. The terms $\sum \triangle t_1$, $\sum \triangle t_1/Dt$, $\sum \triangle t_2$, $\sum \triangle t_2/ET$ are thus indices reflecting variations in the synchrony of ventricular filling and contraction, respectively.

Statistical analysis

The data are presented as mean ± standard deviation; statistical analysis was performed using the t-test for paired data. The relationships between peak filling rate and the regional indices reflecting asynchrony of contraction and filling were analyzed by regression analysis.

Results

Global indices of left ventricular ejection and filling

An example of the frame-to-frame analysis of left ventricular volume and its derivative (dV/dt) before and during ischemia induced by balloon inflation is shown in Figure XXIII.3. Volumes, pressures and derived parameters measured

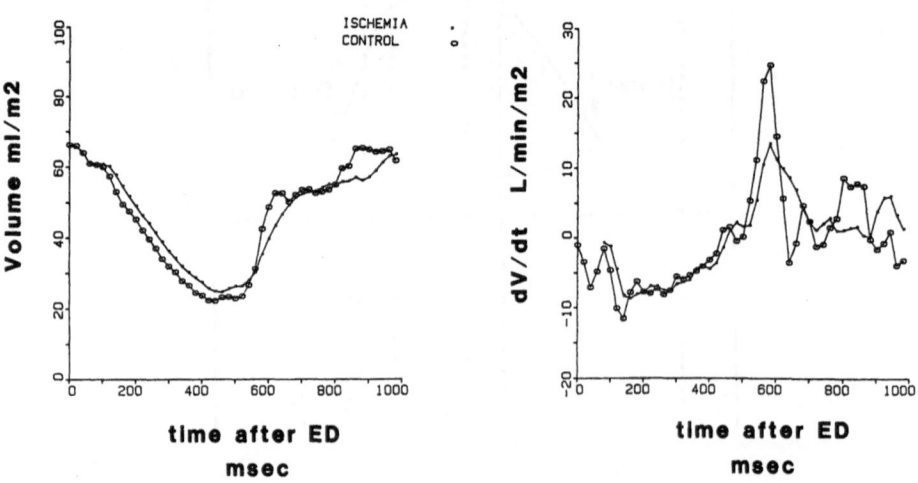

Fig. XXIII.3. Left: Left ventricular volume curves for the same patient, derived from angiographic cineframes 20 msec apart analyzed over a complete cardiac cycle, before and during transluminal occlusion. *Right:* Instantaneous left ventricular volume derivative (dV/dt) curves for the same patient, measured every 20 msec throughout a complete cardiac cycle, before and during transluminal occlusion. During ischemia a decrease in peak dV/dt was observed. ED = end diastole.

Table XXIII.1A. Global systolic function before PTCA, 20 and 50 sec after the onset of occlusion and after PTCA.

Variables	Before PTCA Total group (N=14)	Before PTCA Subgroup (N=9)	20 sec occlusion (total group; N=14)	50 sec occlusion (subgroup; N=9)	After PTCA Subgroup (N=9)	After PTCA Total group (N=14)
Ejection fraction (%)	61 ± 8	62 ± 6	54 ± 8*	48 ± 12*	66 ± 6	64 ± 7
Stroke volume (ml/m²)	50 ± 11	49 ± 11	44 ± 12°	39 ± 14°	52 ± 10	50 ± 9
Mean systolic ejection rate (ml/sec)	129 ± 24	127 ± 24	125 ± 32	116 ± 67	165 ± 48	147 ± 27
Peak ejection rate (ml/sec)	251 ± 97	255 ± 106	222 ± 69	185 ± 61°	248 ± 77	240 ± 68
Time to peak ejection rate (msec)	172 ± 44	175 ± 50	172 ± 56	153 ± 34	170 ± 88	166 ± 76
Peak ejection rate 1** (sec⁻¹)	5 ± 1	5.4 ± 1	5 ± 0.7	5 ± 0.9	5 ± 0.6	4.7 ± 0.6
Peak ejection rate 2*** (sec⁻¹)	3 ± 0.8	3.3 ± 0.9	2.7 ± 0.5	2.3 ± 0.5*	3.2 ± 0.5	3 ± 0.5
End-systolic pressure (mmHg)	95 ± 18	92 ± 22	90 ± 19	98 ± 24	91 ± 15	90 ± 14
End-systolic volume (ml/m²)	31 ± 9	29 ± 7	37 ± 9*	41 ± 9*	26 ± 15	27 ± 7

° p <.05;
* p <.005 (compared with before PTCA, paired Student t-test);
** normalized by stroke volume;
*** normalized by end-diastolic volume.

Table XXIII.1B. Global diastolic function before PTCA, 20 and 50 sec after the onset of occlusion and after PTCA.

Variables	Before PTCA		20 sec occlusion (total group; N=14)	50 sec occlusion (subgroup; N=9)	After PTCA	
	Total group (N=14)	Subgroup (N=9)			Subgroup (N=9)	Total group (N=14)
Tau_1 (msec) [7]	55 ± 8	55 ± 6	79 ± 17*	68 ± 16*	56 ± 7	54 ± 7
Tau_2 (msec) [7]	44 ± 7	43 ± 7	51 ± 8°	59 ± 8*	45 ± 8	45 ± 9
IRP (msec)	71 ± 18	77 ± 18	85 ± 16°	80 ± 17	77 ± 16	71 ± 15
MVO pressure (mmHg)	19 ± 5	18 ± 3	23 ± 8	25 ± 6°	19 ± 5	21 ± 6
MVO volume (ml/m²)	37 ± 9	35 ± 7	41 ± 9°	45 ± 10*	30 ± 6	31 ± 8
Peak filling rate (ml/sec)	311 ± 83	296 ± 84	234 ± 82°	225 ± 93°	297 ± 117	277 ± 109
Time to peak filling rate (msec)	128 ± 20	133 ± 22	145 ± 38	151 ± 26	130 ± 18	126 ± 23
Peak filling rate (SV/sec)	6.5 ± 1	6 ± 0.9	5.9 ± 1	6 ± 2	5.8 ± 0.8	5.7 ± 1
Peak filling rate (EDV/sec)	4 ± 1	3.7 ± 0.8	3 ± 8°	2.8 ± 0.7*	3.8 ± 0.9	3.6 ± 1
Pmin (mmHg)	10 ± 5	8 ± 3	11 ± 4	16 ± 6*	8 ± 5	8 ± 4
Volume at Pmin (ml/m²)	51 ± 13	48 ± 11	53 ± 10	55 ± 10	45 ± 11	45 ± 9
MRVI (ml/sec)	179 ± 82	198 ± 78	98 ± 78*	104 ± 69*	161 ± 131	138 ± 113

Tau_1 and Tau_2 = time constant of relaxation (biexponential fitting), Tau_1 fit of first 40 msec, Tau_2 fit after 40 msec; IRP = isovolumic relaxation period; MVO = mitral valve opening; Pmin = minimal left ventricular diastolic pressure; MRVI = mean rate of volume inflow during the time interval between MVO and Pmin. ° $p < .05$; * $p < .005$ (compared with before PTCA, paired Student t-test).

before, during and after transluminal occlusion are listed in Tables XXIII.1a and XXIII.1b. The global indices of the ejection phase decreased during the two periods of coronary occlusion; the ejection fraction fell from 61% to 54% over 20 seconds (p<.005) and from 62% to 48% (p<.005) over 50 seconds, this reduction being mainly due to the increase in end-systolic volume over 20 seconds (from 31 ± 9 ml/m² to 37 ± 9; p<.005) and 50 seconds (from 29 ± 7 ml/m² to 41 ± 9; p<.005). Consequently, the stroke volume was significantly decreased from 50 ± 11 ml/m² to 44 ± 12 (p<.05) during the first period of occlusion and from 49 ± 11 ml/m² to 39 ± 14 (p<.05) during the second. A slight but not significant reduction in peak ejection rate was observed over 20 seconds, but after 50 seconds it had decreased from 255 ± 106 ml/m² to 185 ± 61 (p<.05) (Fig. XXIII.4). Normalization for end-diastolic volume and stroke volume did not render the change in peak ejection rate at 20 seconds significant. The relaxation parameters Tau$_1$ and Tau$_2$ [7] significantly increased (Table XXIII.1b) during both periods of occlusion and returned to basal values at the end of the PTCA procedure. The isovolumic relaxation period increased from 71 ± 18 msec to 85 ± 16 (p<.05) over 20 seconds and from 77 ± 18 msec to 80 ± 17 (p = n.s.) over 50 seconds. The left ventricular pressure at the time of mitral valve opening increased from 19 ± 5 mmHg to 23 ± 8 (p = n.s.) over 20 seconds and from 18 ± 3 mmHg to 25 ± 6 (p<.05) over 50 seconds. Peak filling rate was reduced from 311 ± 85 ml/sec to 234 ± 82 (p<.05) after 20 seconds of ischemia (Fig. XXIII.4) and from 296 ± 84 ml/sec to 225 ± 93 (p<.05) after 50 seconds. When normalized for stroke volume, peak filling rate was unchanged after 20 and 50

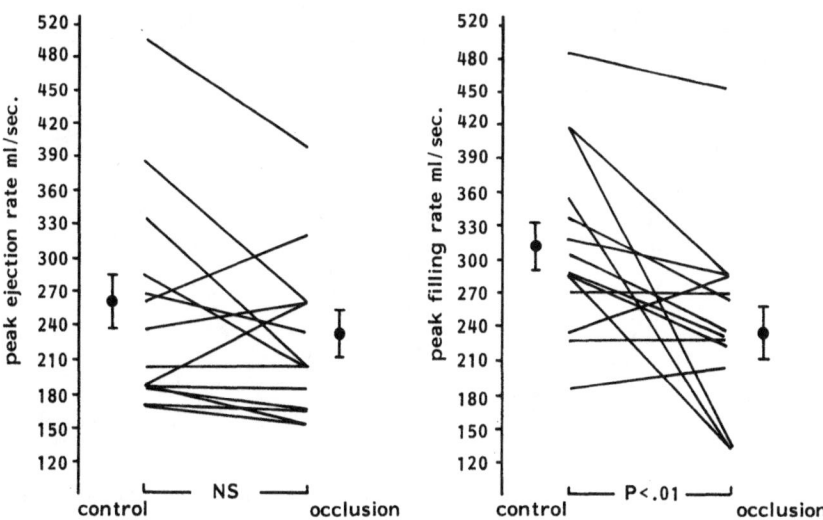

Fig. XXIII.4. Individual and mean changes ($\pm$ SEM) in peak ejection rate and peak filling rate during transluminal occlusion (20 msec). Only the peak filling rate showed a significant decrease during the early phase of coronary occlusion.

434

seconds of occlusion, whereas after normalization for end-diastolic volume it was significantly decreased after 20 (from 4 ± 1 EDV/sec to 3 ± 0.8; p<.05) and 50 seconds (from 3.7 ± 0.8 EDV/sec to 2.8 ± 0.7; p<.005). The mean rate of volume inflow, measured during the early filling period between the mitral valve opening and the occurrence of minimal diastolic pressure, declined significantly both at 20 (from 179 ± 82 ml/sec to 98 ± 78; p<.005) and 50 seconds (from 198 ± 94 ml/sec to 104 ± 69; p<.005) from the onset of occlusion.

Regional indices of left ventricular ejection and filling

As previously demonstrated [7], during occlusion of the left anterior descending artery the time of maximal inward wall displacement of the anterior wall shifts from end systole to early diastole (Fig. XXIII.5). In the present study a delay was observed in the occurrence of peak velocity of outward displacement (dL/dt) with respect to aortic valve closure after 20 seconds of ischemia, particularly in the apical region (segments 10 and 20 in Fig. XXIII.5) and the absolute value of the dL/dt was reduced in the ischemic segments (Fig. XXIII.6). In the nonischemic segments a compensatory increase in dL/dt was observed. In order to test whether this decrease in the absolute value of dL/dt was in fact intrinsically

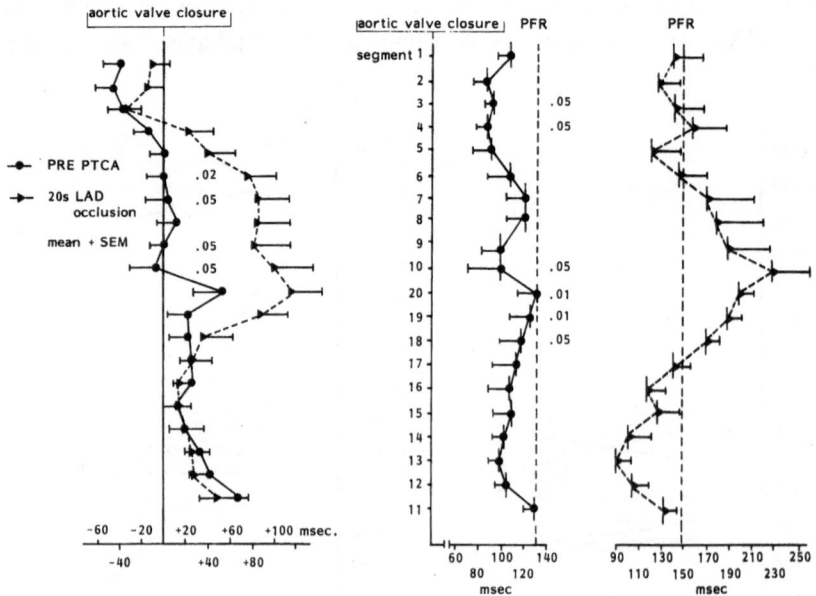

Fig. XXIII.5. Left panel: Time relationship between aortic valve closure and the occurrence of maximal inward wall displacement before and after 20 msec of occlusion of the left anterior descending artery. *Center and right panel:* Time relationship between aortic valve closure and the occurrence of peak velocity of segmental outward displacement before (center panel) and after 20 sec of occlusion (right panel) of the left anterior descending artery. PFR = global peak filling rate.

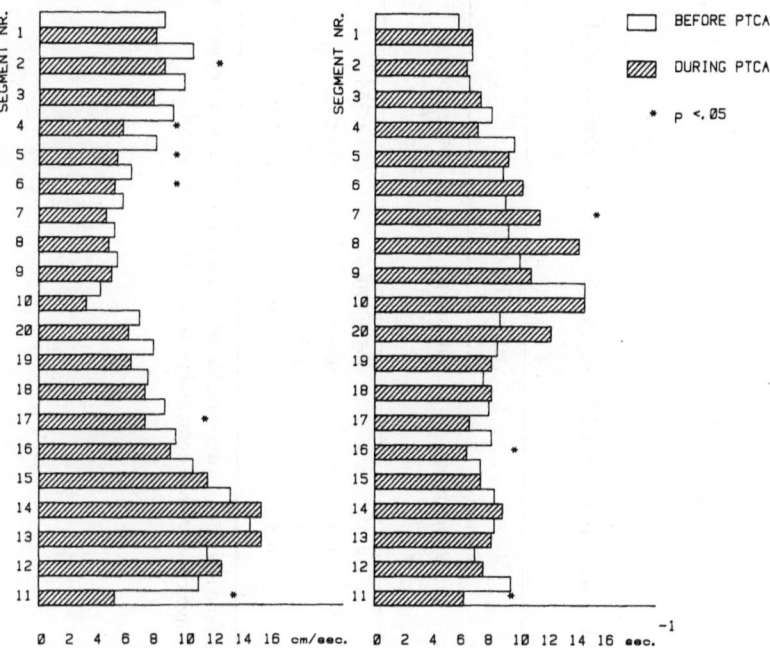

Fig. XXIII.6. *Left panel:* Mean changes in peak velocity of segmental outward displacement (dL/dt) in 10 anterior and 10 posterior segments before and during occlusion of the left anterior descending artery. *Right panel:* Mean changes in the ratio dL/dt/ maximal outward displacement in 10 anterior and 10 posterior segments before and during occlusion of the left anterior descending artery.

related to a reduction in the amplitude of the peak outward displacement, we normalized segmental dL/dt for the corresponding value of maximal outward displacement. After normalization we observed an increase in the ischemic segments, while no major changes were apparent in the nonischemic segments (Fig. XXIII.6). Therefore, a relationship between the asynchrony of segmental dL/dt and the reduction of global peak filling rate was sought by measuring the sum of the absolute values of the time differences from global peak filling rate to the occurrence of peak dL/dt in each of the 20 segments $(\sum \triangle t_1)$. This sum increased significantly during both the first (from 572 ± 194 msec to 940 ± 264 msec; p<.005) and the second occlusion (from 546 ± 198 msec to 842 ± 224 msec; p<.005); increases were also found for $\sum \triangle t_1/Dt$, thus indicating an asynchrony in filling (Table XXIII.2). To elucidate whether the decrease in global peak filling rate was related to the asynchrony in regional peak filling rate rather than to other causes, we correlated global peak filling rate with $\sum \triangle t_1$ and found a significant negative correlation ($r = -.68$; p<.001), demonstrating that a greater degree of asynchrony was associated with a reduction in peak filling rate (Fig. XXIII.7). To determine whether the asynchrony in regional filling was an isolated phenomenon or the effect of a temporal nonuniformity in inward wall displacement, we quantified this systolic nonuniformity be measuring the time

Table XXIII.2. Measurement of regional asynchrony in inward and outward wall displacement before PTCA, 20 and 50 sec after the onset of occlusion and after PTCA.

Variables	Before PTCA		20 sec occlusion (total group; N = 14)	50 sec occlusion (subgroup; N = 9)	After PTCA	
	Total group (N = 14)	Subgroup (N = 9)			Subgroup (N = 9)	Total group (N = 14)
$\sum \triangle t_1$ (msec)	572 ± 194	546 ± 198	940 ± 264*	842 ± 224*	495 ± 179	645 ± 355
$\sum \triangle t_2$ (msec)	965 ± 348	948 ± 415	1442 ± 314*	1472 ± 370°	985 ± 171	978 ± 281
$\sum \triangle t_1$/diastolic time	1.1 ± 0.7	1.3 ± 0.8	1.8 ± 0.8*	1.9 ± 1*	1.3 ± 0.7	1.2 ± 0.6
$\sum \triangle t_2$/ejection time	2.6 ± 0.9	2.8 ± 0.7	4.2 ± 0.9*	4.5 ± 0.9°	3 ± 0.9	2.8 ± 0.8

° p <.05; * p <.005 (compared with before PTCA, paired Student t-test). $\sum \triangle t_1$ = sum of the time intervals between global peak filling rate and peak velocity of segmental outward displacement (dL/dt). $\sum \triangle t_2$ = sum of the time intervals between aortic valve closure and segmental peak inward displacement.

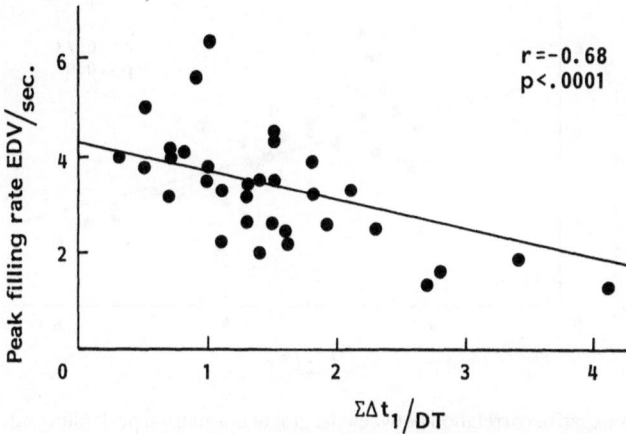

Fig. XXIII.7. The negative correlation between the global normalized peak filling rate and the $\sum \triangle t_1 /$ diastolic time as an index of segmental asynchrony in filling, in patients with left anterior descending artery disease.

relationship between end systole and the occurrence of the segmental peak inward displacement. The sum of the absolute time differences between aortic valve closure and the peak regional inward wall displacement ($\sum \triangle t_2$) was used as an index of systolic asynchrony, and during coronary occlusion both $\sum \triangle t_2$ and $\sum \triangle t_2 / ET$ increased in the same fashion as $\sum \triangle t_1$ and $\sum \triangle t_1 / Dt$ (Table XXIII.2). In addition, we found a significant correlation ($r = .66$; $p < .001$) between $\sum \triangle t_2$ and $\sum \triangle t_1$ (Fig. XXIII.8), suggesting an interdependance between the asynchrony of contraction and the abnormalities of filling dynamics. This temporal interdependance between inward and outward wall displacement is illustrated in Fig. XXIII.5. Further supportive evidence for the interrelationship between con-

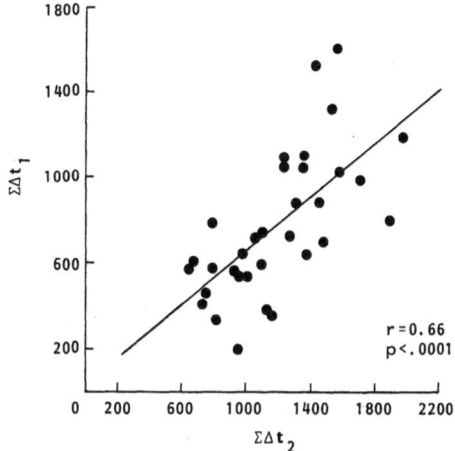

Fig. XXIII.8. The correlation between the $\sum \triangle t_1$ as an index of segmental asynchrony in filling and the $\sum \triangle t_2$ as an index of segmental asynchrony in contraction.

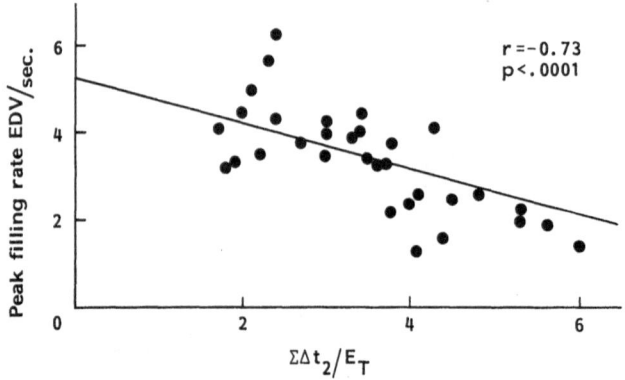

Fig. XXIII.9. The negative correlation between the global normalized peak filling rate and the $\sum \triangle t_2 /$ ejection time as an index of segmental asynchrony in contraction, in patients with left anterior descending artery disease.

traction and filling was given by the significant negative correlation between the global peak filling rate and $\sum \triangle t_2$ ($r = -.73$; p<.001) (Fig. XXIII.9). Thus the greater the asynchrony in the pattern of contraction, the greater the decrease in peak filling rate. All these data indicate that the asynchrony in the occurrence of the regional filling with subsequent decreases in peak filling rate, reflects non-uniformity of left ventricular contraction and occurs within 20 seconds of the onset of ischemia. To further elucidate the dynamic interplay between asynchrony in contraction and abnormalities in early diastolic phase we correlated $\sum \triangle t_2$ with parameters of the relaxation phase and these latter parameters with the peak filling rate. A significant correlation was observed between $\sum \triangle t_2$ and Tau_1 ($r = .75$, p<.0001) and between Tau_1 and the duration of isovolumic relaxation period ($r = .58$; p<.0001). On the other hand, no correlation or only weak correlations were observed between parameters of the relaxation phase and peak filling rate (Table XXIII.3).

Table XXIII.3. Correlation between parameters of left ventricular relaxation and filling.

Comparison	Correlation coefficient	p-value
Tau_1–PFR	−0.33	0.06
Tau_2–PFR	−0.152	0.37
IRP–PFR	−0.53	0.009
MVO*–PFR	−0.23	0.2

* = pressure. For legends see Table XXIII.1B.

Discussion

Variability in the temporal sequence of regional left ventricular contraction in normal subjects has been previously observed and attributed to variations in the sequence of electrical activation or to other factors playing an important role in determining ventricular geometry such as ventricular volume and fiber orientation [11, 12]. In patients with coronary artery disease the completion of ejection was found to be delayed, whereas the onset of ejection was not and the severity of coronary artery disease was positively correlated with the persistence of these contraction abnormalities into early diastole [13]. During spontaneous angina, a significant prolongation of left ventricular ejection time with an accompanying shortening of diastole has also been observed [14]. All these observations dictate that studies of relaxation and filling in early diastole should be correlated with the pattern of contraction. Further insight into this relationship was given by the study of Smalling in the canine model [15]. A biphasic expansion and contraction in both endocardial wall motion and myocardial wall thickening was observed during acute and graded ischemia. This combined biphasic wall motion effect was attributed to a loss of the early diastolic distending forces of coronary pressure (the 'erectile' effect) or to a persistent contraction of the ischemic zone during early diastole. On the basis of these previous studies, we investigated the relationship between the ejection phase and early diastolic filling.

Methodological considerations

Contrast angiography was used rather than radionuclide angiography, because the acquisition time required for radionuclide angiography precludes the detection of acute changes in left ventricular performance [16], although reliable information on segmental wall motion can be derived from changes in regional counts [6, 17]. Recently, the nonimaging nuclear probe has been proved useful in a study of ventricular filling phase during PTCA [18], permitting a beat-to-beat noninvasive assessment of cardiac function 10 seconds after radionuclide injection. However, this technique has two important limitations: (1) the inability to measure absolute volume changes; and (2) the inability to measure regional volume-derived parameters. On the other hand, contrast angiography does not allow a continuous beat-to-beat assessment of the changes in left ventricular function during the early phase of ischemia, but only provides a snapshot of this rapidly evolving situation.

Analysis of the left ventricular angiograms was performed by an automated, high resolution, frame-to-frame edge detection system allowing fast and reliable acquisition of single left ventricular contours over a complete cardiac cycle. Many wall motion models have been proposed to approximate actual endocardial motion, which reflects the problems investigators have had to establish a geo-

440

metric framework upon which to determine whether the motion of the endocardial contour is normal or abnormal [19, 20]. All these methods assess wall motion in terms of extent of shortening at specific points on an axis reference system and it is highly unlikely that a particular endocardial site will coincide with one of these points during an entire cardiac cycle. The wall motion analysis system we used is based on the motion pattern of small irregularities at the left ventricular endocardial border (endocardial landmarks) which can be detected in the contrast cineangiogram with the automated endocardial outlining system. Such endocardial landmark pathway has been tested previously in 23 normal human left ventricles and validated in pigs with metal endocardial markers inserted via a percutaneous, retrograde, transvascular approach [21, Ch. XI]. The major advantage of this wall motion analysis is that it is unaffected by the translation and rotation of the heart, thus permitting an accurate study of segmental wall motion and derived parameters.

Determinants of filling dynamics

It has been suggested that the peak filling rate is dependent on the rate of left ventricular relaxation and on the left atrial pressure [22]. Under normal conditions the relaxing left ventricle produces a rapid change in the atrio-ventricular pressure gradient, which is the driving force for the inflow [23]. Thus, a prolonged relaxation phase as observed during acute ischemia, causes a delay in the development of the atrio-ventricular pressure gradient, and consequently, a greater left atrial pressure is required to open the mitral valve. In fact, we observed a consistent delay in the relaxation rate occurring 20 seconds after the onset of ischemia and concomitantly both the isovolumic relaxation period and the left atrial pressure required for mitral valve opening increased. The significant relationship existing between $\sum \triangle t_2$ and Tau_1, and between this latter parameter and the duration of the isovolumic relaxation period, suggests that during acute ischemia the atrio-ventricular dynamic interplay occurring during the early diastole is affected by the asynchronous left ventricular contraction. Yellin et al. [22], demonstrated in the dog that under conditions of similar left atrial pressure at valve opening, the prolongation of the time constant of relaxation decreases the rate and amplitude of filling, whereas under conditions of similar left ventricular pressure during relaxation an increase of left atrial pressure increases the amplitude of early filling. Thus the lack of correlation between peak filling rate and any single parameter of the relaxation phase, such as time constants of relaxation, isovolumic relaxation period or mitral valve opening pressure was expected since these latter parameters are changing in opposite direction during acute ischemia.

A decrease in peak filling rate has been extensively reported in patients with coronary artery disease with or without previous myocardial infarction. Until recently no data were available in the literature regarding the relationship between global and regional left ventricular filling. Yamagishi et al. [5] investigated this relationship using radionuclide angiography in normal subjects and in patients with left anterior descending coronary artery disease without previous myocardial infarction and found differences in peak filling rate differentiating normals from those with coronary artery disease. To explain this difference they analyzed regional filling dynamics and identified that asynchrony in regional filling was a major determinant of decrease in peak filling rate. The sum of the absolute time differences between the global and regional peak filling rate was inversely correlated to the global peak filling rate and proposed as an index of asynchrony in diastolic filling. More recently Bonow et al. [6] studied with radionuclide angiography the relationship between regional left ventricular diastolic asynchrony and global diastolic filling, before and after PTCA in patients with single vessel coronary artery disease. Before PTCA, impaired global diastolic filling was found and was related to regional variations in the timing of left ventricular relaxation and filling determined by variations in phase among sectors and by regional quadrant analysis. In addition, they demonstrated a negative correlation between the magnitude of global peak filling rate and the extent of regional asynchrony. Reevaluation one day to one month after PTCA showed an improvement of the above mentioned changes in diastolic global and regional function.

Role of the asynchronous contraction

In the present study, we demonstrated that ischemia occurring early during coronary occlusion severely alters filling dynamics and that the major determinant of this change is asynchrony in regional filling. This diastolic asynchrony was secondary to a nonuniformity of inward wall displacement, but the crucial question remains whether this diastolic asynchrony was a direct, intrinsic manifestation of altered relaxation properties of the myocardium (inactivation) or a consequence of dysfunction of the contractile properties of the myocardium (activation) [24, 25].

Recently we evaluated the beat-to-beat myocardial shortening changes accompanying acute coronary occlusion in one patient undergoing PTCA of a coronary artery bypass graft, in whom pairs of epicardial wall markers had been placed at the time of his original cardiac surgery [26]. Their motion reflecting epicardial transverse shortening was characterized, in ischemic myocardium, by the early appearance of a late systolic lengthening followed by an early diastolic shortening (Fig. XXIII.10). We referred to this biphasic motion as the 'W' phenomenon due to its morphologic characteristics, transient duration, and frequency of appearance in studies of endocardial wall thickness motion during regional ischemia. This polyphasic wall motion pattern appears to be similar to

442

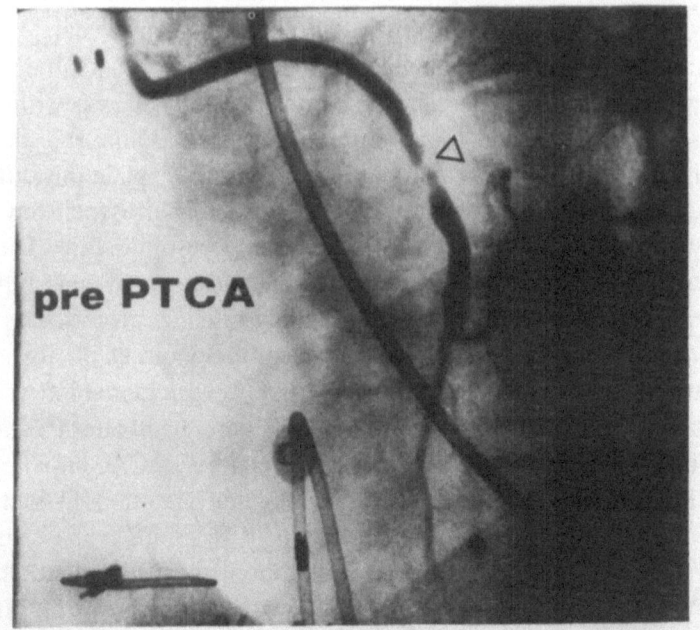

A

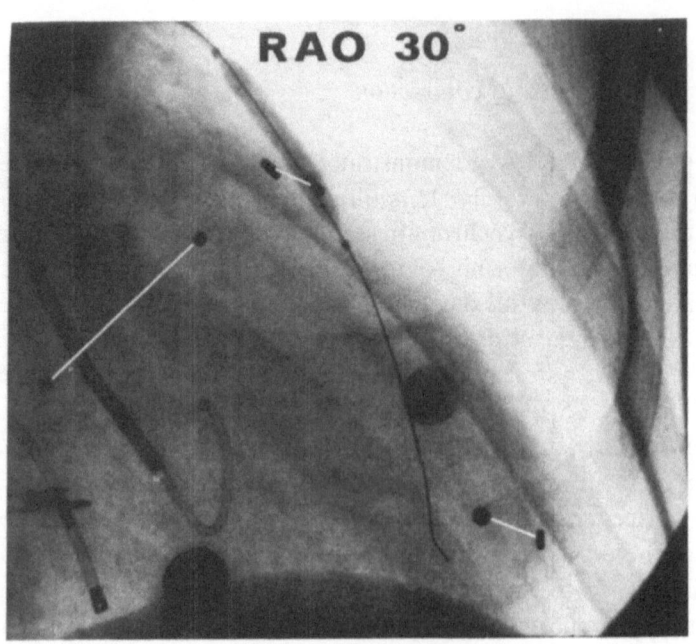

B

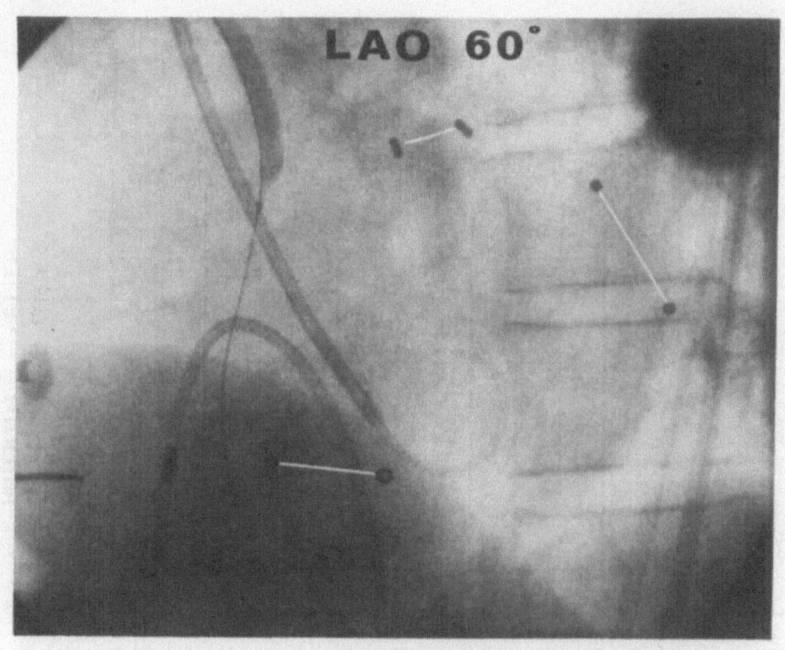

C

EPICARDIAL MARKER PAIR SHORTENING

D   LEFT VENTRICULAR PRESSURE

Fig. XXIII.10. Angiogram of left anterior descending bypass graft stenosis and markers before PTCA (Fig. XXIII.10A). Figures XXIII.10B and 10C show the inflated angioplasty catheter in place, in RAO 30° and LAO 60° respectively. In Fig. XXIII.10D changes in epicardial marker pair shortening in region of bypass graft and left ventricular pressure during graft occlusion. The W phenomenon (see text) is evident.

444

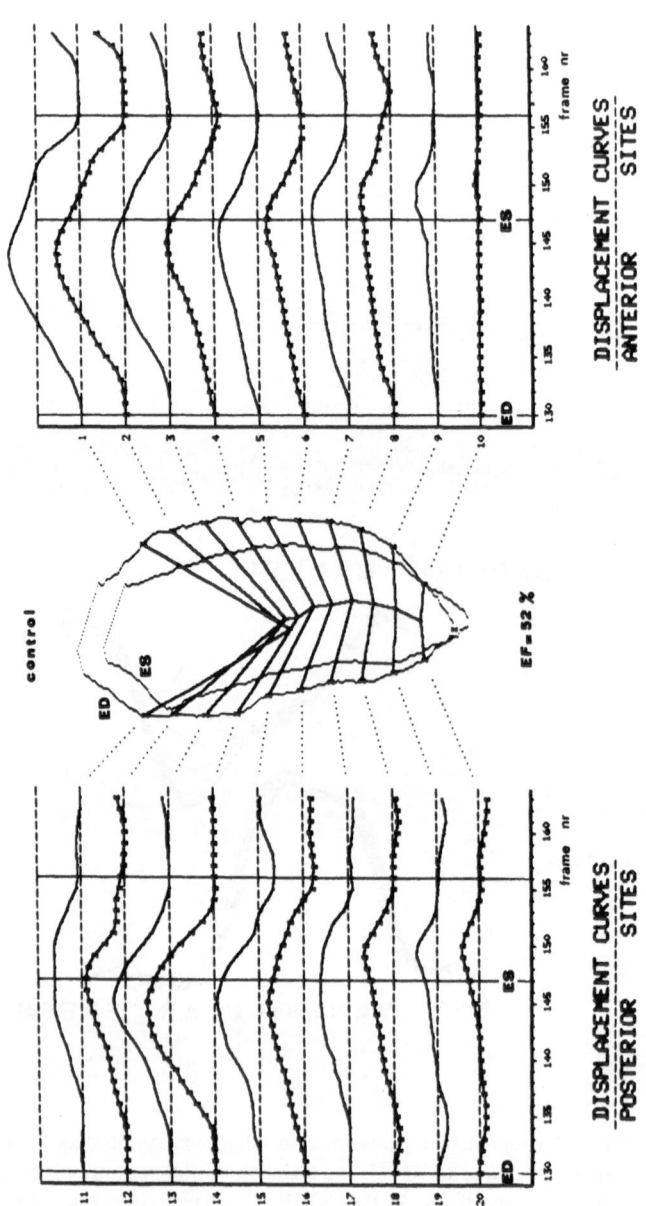

445

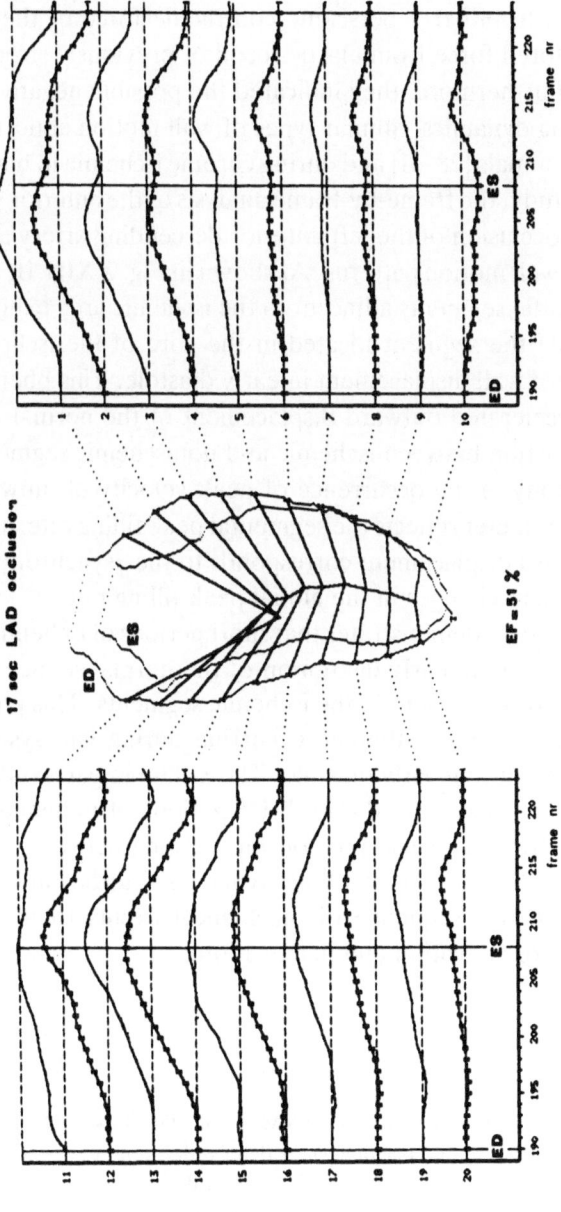

Fig. XXIII.11. Left ventricular wall displacement in 10 anterior (right) and 10 infero-posterior (left) segments in the control state (upper figures) and after 17 sec of occlusion of the left anterior descending (LAD) artery (lower figures). After 17 sec of occlusion of the LAD. A biphasic pattern of contraction is observed in the anterior segments, while the apical segments (anterior and inferoposterior) show a late inward wall displacement occurring in the early diastole. In the nonischemic segments an accelerated outward displacement is observed.

that described by Wiegner et al. [27], who studied the interaction of normal and hypoxic myocardial muscles in series. They identified a biphasic pattern of motion of the hypoxic muscle analogous to that observed in the ischemic region of the intact left ventricle. The early lengthening phase of the hypoxic muscle was attributed to a premature onset of force decline and the second late shortening phase was ascribed to either a persisting contractile force of the muscle or a manifestation of stored force from elastic recoil of previously stretched passive muscle elements. Furthermore, they indicated the possible negative role of late shortening on filling dynamics. Similar types of wall motion abnormalities have been described in animals [28–31] and during chronic ischemia in man [32, 33]. In our angiographic study, the frame-by-frame analysis of the anterior wall displacement during brief occlusion of the left anterior descending artery also showed a variety of biphasic wall motion patterns. As shown in Fig. XXIII.11, after 17 sec of occlusion, some of the segments adjacent to the ischemic area exhibited the 'W' phenomenon, while the segment located in the core of the ischemic area exhibited a late inward wall displacement in early diastole. This phenomenon was mirrored by an accelerated outward displacement of the normal segment. Ultimately, the interaction between ischemic and nonischemic segments results in segmental asynchrony in the occurrence of peak velocity of outward displacement. Since this parameter reflects the segmental peak filling rate, an asynchrony in segmental outward displacement corresponds to the asynchrony in the filling phase with consequent changes in the global peak filling rate.

In summary, our study demonstrates that short periods of ischemia, induced by balloon inflation, cause an early disruption of the normal sequence of inward-outward segmental displacement in the ischemic segments. This phenomenon is characterized by an early lengthening occurring during late systole with late shortening occurring during early diastole. These data in part confirm an 'asynchronous contraction' occurring during brief periods of ischemia [34] and, in particular, demonstrate the close relationship existing between uncoordinated contraction and the impairment of filling dynamics. Further investigations are needed to correlate this sequence of mechanical events to the intracellular biochemical events of activation and inactivation.

References

1. Bonow RO, Bacharach SL, Green MV, Kent KM, Rosing DR, Lipson LC, Leon MB, Epstein SE: Impaired left ventricular diastolic filling in patients with coronary artery disease: assessment with radionuclide angiography. Circulation 64: 315–323, 1981.
2. Bonow RO, Leon MB, Rosing DR, Kent KM, Lipson LC, Bacharach SL, Green MV, Epstein SE: Effects of Verapamil and Propranolol on left ventricular systolic function and diastolic filling in patients with coronary artery disease: radionuclide angiographic studies at rest and during exercise. Circulation 65: 1337–1350, 1981.
3. Polak JF, Kemper AJ, Bianco JA, Parisi AF, Tow DE: Resting early peak diastolic filling rate: a

sensitive index of myocardial dysfunction in patients with coronary artery disease. J Nucl Med 23: 471–478, 1982.

4. Mancini GBJ, Slutsky RA, Norris SL, Bhargava V, Ashburn WL, Higgins CB: Radionuclide analysis of peak filling rate, filling fraction, and time to peak filling rate: response to supine bycicle exercise in normal subjects and patients with coronary disease. Am J Cardiol 51: 43–51, 1983.

5. Yamagishi T, Ozaki M, Kumada T, Ikezono T, Shimizu T, Furutani Y, Yamaoka H, Ogawa H, Matsuzaki M, Matsuda Y, Arima A, Kusukawa R: Asynchronous left ventricular diastolic filling in patients with isolated disease of the left anterior descending coronary artery: assessment with radionuclide ventriculography. Circulation 69: 933–942, 1984.

6. Bonow RO, Vitale DF, Bacharach SL, Frederick TM, Kent KM, Green MV: Asynchronous left ventricular regional function and impaired global diastolic filling in patients with coronary artery disease: reversal after coronary angioplasty. Circulation 71: 297–307, 1985.

7. Serruys PW, Wijns W, Brand M van den, Meij S, Slager C, Schuurbiers JCH, Hugenholtz PG, Brower RW: Left ventricular performance, regional blood flow, wall motion, and lactate metabolism during transluminal angioplasty. Circulation 70: 25–36, 1984.

8. Meester GT, Bernard N, Zeelenberg C, Brower RW, Hugenholtz PG: A computer system for real time analysis of cardiac catheterization data. Cathet Cardiovasc Diagn 1: 113–132, 1975.

9. Brower RW, Meij S, Serruys PW: A model of asynchronous left ventricular relaxation predicting the bi-exponential pressure decay. Cardiovasc Res 17: 482–488, 1983.

10. Fioretti P, Brower RW, Meester GT, Serruys PW: Interaction of left ventricular relaxation and filling during early diastole in human subjects. Am J Cardiol 46: 197–203, 1980.

11. Clayton PD, Bulawa WF, Klausner SC, Urie PM, Marshall HW, Warner HR: The characteristic sequence for the onset of contraction in the normal human left ventricle. Circulation 59: 671–679, 1979.

12. Klausner SC, Blair TJ, Bulawa WF, Jeppson GM, Jensen RL, Clayton PD: Quantitative analysis of segmental wall motion throughout systole and diastole in the normal human left ventricle. Circulation 65: 580–590, 1982.

13. Holman BL, Wynne J, Idoine J, Neill J: Disruption in the temporal sequence of regional ventricular contraction. I. Characteristic and incidence in coronary artery disease. Circulation 61: 1075–1083, 1980.

14. Ferro G, Piscione F, Carella G, Betocchi S, Spinelli L, Chiariello M: Systolic and diastolic time intervals during spontaneous angina. Clin Cardiol 7: 588–592, 1984.

15. Smalling RW, Kelley KO, Kirkeeide RL, Gould KL: Comparison of early systolic and early diastolic regional function during regional ischemia in a chronically instrumented canine model. J Am Coll Cardiol 2: 263–269, 1983.

16. Crawford MH, Amon KW, Vance WS, Sorensen SG, Rabinowitz AC: Advantages of the two-dimensional echo over radionuclide angiography for detecting acute changes in LV performance during exercise. Circulation 64 (Supp IV): IV-13 (Abstract), 1981.

17. Green MV, Jones-Collins BA, Bacharach SL, Findley SL, Patterson RE, Larson SM: Scintigraphic quantification of asynchronous myocardial motion during the left ventricular isovolumic relaxation period: a study in the dog during acute ischemia. J Am Coll Cardiol 4: 72–79, 1984.

18. Monteferrante JC, Stein JH, Ro JH, Blake JW, McCrossan J, Bontemps RA, Herman MV, Weiss MB: Systolic and diastolic left ventricular function by nuclear probe during transluminal coronary angioplasty. Circulation 70 (Supp II): II-37 (Abstract), 1984.

19. Brower RW, Meester GT: Computer based methods for quantifying regional left ventricular wall motion from cine ventriculograms. Comp Cardiol: 55–62, 1976.

20. Brower RW, Meester GT: Quantitative analysis and subjective scoring of regional wall motion: an application for discriminant function classification theory. Comp Cardiol: 3–7, 1982.

21. Slager CJ, Hooghoudt TEH, Reiber JHC, Schuurbiers JCH, Verdouw PD, Hugenholtz PG: Left ventricular wall motion as derived from endocardially implanted radiographic markers and from

contrast angiograms. In: Ventricular wall motion. U Sigwart and PH Heintzen (Eds.). Georg Thieme Verlag, Stuttgart/New York: 150–159, 1984.

22. Yellin EL, Yoran C, Sonnenblick EH, Frater RWM: The relation between left ventricular relaxation and early diastolic filling in the intact dog heart. Eur Heart J 1 (Suppl B): 179–180, 1980.

23. Yellin EL, Peskin C, Yoran C, Koeningsberg M, Matsumoto M, Laniado S, McQueen D, Shore D, Frater RWM: Mechanisms of mitral valve motion during diastole. Am J Physiol 214: H389–H400, 1981.

24. Brutsaert DL, Housmans PR, Goethals MA: Dual control of relaxation. Its role in the ventricular function in the mammalian heart. Circ Res 47: 637–652, 1980.

25. Brutsaert DL, Rademakers FE, Sys SU: Triple control of relaxation: implications in cardiac disease. Circulation 69: 190–196, 1984.

26. Jaski BE, Serruys PW: Epicardial wall motion and left ventricular function during transluminal angioplasty in man. J Am Coll Cardiol 6: 695–700, 1985.

27. Wiegner AW, Allen GJ, Bing OHL: Weak and strong myocardium in series: implications for segmental dysfunction. Am J Physiol 235: H776–H783, 1978.

28. Pagani M, Vatner SF, Baig H, Braunwald E: Initial myocardial adjustment to brief periods of ischemia and reperfusion in the conscious dog. Circ Res 43: 83–92, 1978.

29. Kumada T, Karliner JS, Pouleur H, Gallagher KP, Shirato K, Ross J Jr: Effects of coronary occlusion on early ventricular diastolic events in conscious dogs. Am J Physiol 237: H542–H549, 1979.

30. Forrester JS, Wyatt HL, da Luz PL, Tyberg PV, Diamond GA, Swan HJC: Functional significance of regional ischemic contraction abnormalities. Circulation 54: 64–70, 1976.

31. Heyndrickx GR, Millard RW, McRitchie RJ, Maroko PR, Vatner SF: Regional myocardial functional and electrophysiological alterations after brief coronary artery occlusion in conscious dogs. J Clin Invest 56: 978–985, 1975.

32. Sasayama S, Nonogi H, Fujita M, Sakurai T, Wakabayashi A, Kawai C, Eiho S, Kuwahara M: Analysis of asynchronous wall motion by regional pressure-length loops in patients with coronary artery disease. J Am Coll Cardiol 4: 259–267, 1984.

33. Gibson DG, Prewitt TA, Brown DJ: Analysis of left ventricular wall movement during isovolumic relaxation and its relation to coronary artery disease. Br Heart J 38: 1010–1019, 1976.

34. Gaasch WH, Blaustein AS, Bing OHL: Asynchronous (segmental early) relaxation of the left ventricle. J Am Coll Cardiol 5: 891–897, 1985.

Index of subjects